Pharmacology in Rehabilitation
Edition 2

Contemporary Perspectives in Rehabilitation

Steven L. Wolf, PhD, FAPTA, Editor-in-Chief

Pharmacology in Rehabilitation
Edition 2

Charles D. Ciccone, PhD, PT
Associate Professor
Department of Physical Therapy
School of Health Sciences and Human Performance
Ithaca College
Ithaca, New York

 F.A. DAVIS COMPANY • Philadelphia

F. A. Davis Company
1915 Arch Street
Philadelphia, PA 19103

Copyright © 1996 by F. A. Davis Company

Printed in the United States of America

Last digit indicates print number: 10 9 8 7 6 5 4 3 2 1

Acquisitions Editor: Jean-François Vilain
Developmental Editor: Crystal S. McNichol
Production Editor: Nancee A. Vogel
Cover Designer: Louis J. Forgione

As new scientific information becomes available through basic and clinical research, recommended treatments and drug therapies undergo changes. The author and publisher have done everything possible to make this book accurate, up to date, and in accord with accepted standards at the time of publication. The author, editors, and publisher are not responsible for errors or omissions or for consequences from application of the book, and make no warranty, expressed or implied, in regard to the contents of the book. Any practice described in this book should be applied by the reader in accordance with professional standards of care used in regard to the unique circumstances that may apply in each situation. The reader is advised always to check product information (package inserts) for changes and new information regarding dose and contraindications before administering any drug. Caution is especially urged when using new or infrequently ordered drugs.

Library of Congress Cataloging-in-Publication Data

Ciccone, Charles D., 1953–
    Pharmacology in rehabilitation / Charles D. Ciccone. —Ed. 2.
      p. cm. —(Contemporary perspectives in rehabilitation)
    Includes bibliographical references and index.
    ISBN 0-8036-0030-5
    1. Pharmacology.   2. Medical rehabilitation.   I. Title.
  II. Series
    [DNLM: 1. Drug Therapy.   2. Rehabilitation.   3. Pharmacokinetics.
  4. Pharmacology.   WB 330 C568p 1996]
    RM301.C515   1996
    615.5'8—dc20
    DNLM/DLC
    for Library of Congress   95-22130
                                            CIP

Dedicated to Penny, Katie, and Alex for providing constant faith, support, and inspiration.

Foreword

When we first approached Chuck Ciccone in late 1986 about his exceptional knowledge regarding pharmacology and its relevance to physical therapy practice, we were overwhelmed by his desire to integrate his wealth of knowledge on this subject in teaching his students. There were grave trepidations on my part about whether rehabilitation practitioners or students would be ready for such a text. After all, seldom is a course designed to specifically address the role of drug interactions in therapeutic applications. Moreover, some question existed about the desire of clinicians to invest in a book about pharmacology if their formal training had been void of this information and if book purchases themselves were restricted predominantly to new clinical approaches. In short, would anyone besides Chuck and his students have enough interest to look at this creative effort, let alone buy the text?

As it turns out, my thoughts on how important teachers perceived the need for rehabilitation students to know about such issues as drug-response curves, over-medication, the influence of polypharmacy on treatment, drug contraindications, and the influence of pharmacological management on intervention efficacy or changes in biological system behavior was a profound and resounding underestimation. The first edition of *Pharmacology in Rehabilitation* has been a totally unprecedented success when one considers the unique content relative to traditional course content or the primary interests among clinicians. But why was this book so successful? The answer undoubtedly resides in the attentiveness of instructors, students, and practitioners to an emergent sense of urgency to be accountable for patient responsiveness to treatment and the role that multiple influences may have on that success. A primary element in that accountability equation is the influence that drugs can have on patient outcomes to therapeutic interventions. Intuitively we have come to recognize that a dynamically evolving health care system causes us to bring to consciousness all factors that can impact on our livelihood. Paramount in our quest to relate treatment to outcome is the need to understand patient reaction to medications, for without awareness of this important variable we cannot effectively comprehend for ourselves, or explain to others, the therapeutic value of our service.

So why proceed with a second edition? Why run the risk of disrupting a good thing? There are several reasons, not the least of which is Dr. Ciccone's extraordinary ability to provide an accounting of potentially difficult material in easily readable portions. More significantly, during the past 5 years not only have substantial changes occurred in the health-care field, but new drugs that can profoundly influence our treatments have been synthesized. Clearly a need exists for us to know their names, their actions, and the impact they will have on how successful our interventions may be perceived.

The clarity of expression and the need for multiple sources to assist readers in understanding typical drugs they encounter persist in this second edition. Drugs no longer in use have been discarded, and new medications have been incorporated within relevant chapters. None of the helpful aids have been eliminated. In fact, an additional appendix on common drug suffixes has been added. The text retains its eight sections, and Dr. Ciccone continues his practice of providing chapter components that address the relevance of content to rehabilitation care at each appropriate opportunity. Of course the problem solving format and case history presentations have been retained.

Two entirely new chapters have been added and one has been enlarged substantially. Chapter 17, "Patient-Controlled Analgesia," is a contemporary and welcomed addition, especially for those of us attempting to enhance functional independence for pain patients with subcutaneous, epidural, or intrathecal analgesia medications. Section VIII, "Chemotherapy of Infectious and Neoplastic Diseases," offers a new chapter on immunosuppressive agents (Chapter 37). Once again, this timely addition will provide students and clinicians insights into the interrelationship between treatment and response for patients with weakened immune systems. Chapter 16 on pharmacologic management of arthritic patients has been expanded to include detailed descriptions of osteoarthritic as well as rheumatoid arthritic individuals.

Revisions and updates are plentiful, but many would go undetected without careful comparison with the first edition. For example, the pharmacokinetics of drug administration (Chapter 2), discusses in more detail how drugs are distributed within the body and addresses new techniques for drug delivery. Chapter 4 offers greater detail from contemporary findings on surface receptor interfaces to drugs, while the discussions on use of antiepileptic drugs and treatment considerations (Chapter 9) have been abundantly expanded. Treatment of patients with Parkinson's disease (Chapter 10) now includes a section on tissue transplants. Physical and occupational therapists and students will be particularly interested in the updates for Chapter 13, "Skeletal Muscle Relaxants," which now includes discussions on the application of intrathecal baclofen and use of botulinum toxin to treat spasticity and dystonia. The presentation on opioid analgesia (Chapter 14) presents an enlightened conceptualization of opioid drug addiction and the impact that this occurrence may have for treatment. Many changes have been made in subsequent treatment-oriented chapters, such as inclusion of hyperlipidemia in the management of coagulation disorders (Chapter 25), but the reader is encouraged to self-explore these enhancements.

This second edition of *Pharmacology in Rehabilitation* is a definitive labor of love, and undoubtedly, Chuck Ciccone's obsession with perfection and clarity of expression is born out of caring for physiological pharmacology, rehabilitation, and the resoundingly positive feedback he received from the first edition. As was noted in the Foreword to the first edition, this text is the first and only compendium of pharmacology written by a rehabilitation health-care professional for his present and future colleagues. This second edition reaffirms the conviction that the material herein is superlative, relevant to rehabilitation practice, and of such remarkable quality as to allow skeptical and hard-headed editors like me to rescind our misgivings and enthusiastically endorse this monumental contribution to professional enhancement.

Steven L. Wolf, PhD, FAPTA
Series Editor

Preface to the Second Edition

Pharmacology is perhaps the most dynamic of all the basic and applied sciences. New drugs are being developed on a regular basis, and existing drugs are constantly being re-examined to help provide the most effective management of various diseases. Likewise, increased knowledge about certain diseases and the emergence of new pathogens necessitates an ongoing search for medications that are effective in preventing and treating these diseases. Hence, this edition of *Pharmacology in Rehabilitation* has been expanded to provide physical therapists and occupational therapists with a current and comprehensive treatise on pharmacotherapeutics.

The drug information described in this second edition was updated to reflect advancements in our understanding of how these drugs work and what potential adverse effects can occur. As with the first edition, emphasis was placed on describing the beneficial and adverse effects that are especially relevant in patients receiving physical therapy and occupational therapy. Important new drugs that were approved since the first edition of this text were also incorporated into the appropriate chapters. The methods for drug administration and the rationale for using specific drugs in specific situations were also updated to reflect contemporary pharmacologic practice.

Several specific additions were also made to this text to expand the scope of this information and to increase the applicability to rehabilitation specialists. Chapter 4 was expanded to include more depth and detail about cellular mechanisms of drug-receptor interactions, and Chapter 16 was expanded to include treatment of osteoarthritis as well as rheumatoid arthritis. A new chapter (Chapter 17) was created to describe the use of patient-controlled analgesia (PCA) as a method for controlling postoperative and chronic pain. Methods used to control blood coagulation (Chapter 25) were expanded to include treatment of hyperlipidemias. The information on treatment of HIV and AIDS (Chapter 34) was expanded to reflect the most current pharmacologic strategies used in this important disease. A new chapter was created to describe drugs used to suppress the immune system (Chapter 37), and a new appendix (Appendix E) was created to help readers recognize drug classes by the suffix attached to the drug's generic name.

Hence, this edition of *Pharmacology in Rehabilitation* is meant to provide students and clinicians with a comprehensive, accurate, and relevant resource on how contemporary drug therapy can affect patients receiving physical therapy and occupational therapy. It is hoped that this information will be useful in helping clinicians design and implement effective therapeutic strategies based on a better understanding of the beneficial and adverse effects that medications can have on our patients.

Charles Ciccone

Preface to the First Edition

Pharmacology is currently recognized as an area that has direct relevance to the practice of physical and occupational therapy. Therapeutic drugs may provide beneficial effects that act synergistically with the rehabilitation treatment, or they can generate adverse side effects that may directly interfere with the goals of physical rehabilitation. Physical therapists, occupational therapists, and other rehabilitation specialists must have an adequate background in pharmacology in order to understand how various drugs may influence their patients. Many educational programs have acknowledged the importance of this topic by instituting a formal course in pharmacology into their PT and OT curricula.

This book was written to provide physical and occupational therapists with a resource text in basic and clinical pharmacology. To date there has been a relative lack of texts that deal with pharmacology on a level consistent with the educational background and clinical experiences of physical and occupational therapists. Most of the pharmacology texts that are currently available are focused towards other health care professionals such as physicians and nurses. In contrast, this text is intended to provide therapists with a comprehensive yet understandable survey of contemporary pharmacology, with special emphasis on the relationship of drug therapy to rehabilitation.

- The purpose of this text is twofold: to serve as a basic text in pharmacology for physical and occupational therapy students and to serve as a reference source for practicing clinicians. As a pharmacology text, this book should draw on the student's knowledge of biology, chemistry, physiology, and pathology. In this sense, this text will help integrate and expand the student's knowledge in these basic sciences while exposing the student to the importance and relevance of pharmacology in rehabilitation. For the practicing clinician, this text will serve as a reference for virtually all pertinent aspects of drug therapy including which drugs are used to treat specific disorders, the rationale for their use, how specific drugs work, and the manner in which these drugs may impact on various rehabilitation treatments.
- This text is organized into eight parts. In Part I, a discussion of basic pharmacologic principles sets a foundation for the rest of the text. Part II consists of drugs that act primarily by influencing the central nervous system. Chapters in this part of the text deal with several diverse topics including psychological disorders (depression, psychosis), epilepsy, Parkinson's disease, and anesthesia. Part III contains a single chapter on drugs affecting skeletal muscle, and examines the treatment of spasticity and skeletal muscle spasms. In Part IV, the pharmacologic management of pain and in-

flammation is discussed. Chapters in Part IV cover narcotic and non-narcotic anal-gesics and the treatment of rheumatoid arthritis.

Part V begins by examining the autonomic nervous system and the pharmaco-logic methods used to alter autonomic function. The remainder of Part V is devoted to cardiovascular pharmacology and the treatment of specific disorders incuding hypertension, angina pectoris, cardiac arrhythmias, congestive heart failure and co-agulation disorders. Part VI consists of two chapters that discuss respiratory and gastrointestinal drugs, respectively. Part VII addresses endocrine pharmacology and the use of drugs to treat hormonal disorders as well as to manipulate endogenous endocrine function. Finally, Part VIII reviews the pharmacologic management of in-fectious disease and the use of chemotherapy in the treatment of cancer.

- The following basic format is used to describe drug therapy within each chapter. A chapter typically begins with a brief review of the pathophysiologic processes that necessitate the use of therapeutic drugs. By understanding the physiologic changes underlying a certain disease, the reader can better comprehend how pharmacologic agents may serve to prevent or resolve the disease process. This is followed by a de-tailed description of individual agents used to treat the disease, and the physiologic mechanisms by which specific drugs work. The way in which a drug exerts its ef-fects on a cellular or even subcellular level is examined according to the most cur-rent theories of drug action. This knowledge of the biochemical and molecular basis of drug action is crucial in understanding how a drug ultimately affects systemic function and the patient's overall well-being. (At the risk of exposing a personal bias of the author, it can also be stated that the molecular mechanism of drug action is one of the most fascinating aspects of pharmacology). Each chapter concludes by relating aspects of individual drugs as they may impact on physical rehabilitation. Case studies, which use a problem-solving format, are also included to illustrate practical situations that may arise because of an interaction of drug therapy and specific rehabilitation treatments.
- Finally, pharmacology is an extremely dynamic and rapidly changing area. New drugs are being developed and introduced on virtually a daily basis. Hence, the ma-jor focus of this text is to provide a general foundation in drug use and actions rather than a comprehensive listing of specific agents. Although examples of cur-rently used drugs are included in the appropriate chapters, it is inevitable that newer agents will soon be available which can be added to the types of drugs de-scribed in this text. However, it is hoped that the material in this text will provide the reader with a solid background in understanding the current as well as future status of pharmacology, especially as it relates to contemporary physical rehabilita-tion.
- The book ends with five appendices for quick reference (Drugs Administered by Iontophoresis and Phonophoresis, Potential Interactions between Physical Agents and Therapeutic Drugs, How to Use the Physician's Desk Reference, Drugs of Abuse), a glossary, and an extensive index. A Drug and Agent Index follows imme-diately after the Table of Contents.

ACKNOWLEDGMENTS TO THE SECOND EDITION

The author would like to thank the following reviewers:

Sandra B. Levine, PhD, PT, OTR, Associate Professor, University of Illinois at Chicago, Department of Physical Therapy, Chicago, Illinois; Jeffrey Rothman, EdD, PT, Professor and Director of Physical Therapy Program, The College of Staten Island of the City University of New York, Staten Island, New York; and Barbara Mac-Dermott Costa, MS, RN, Professor Emeritus, Syracuse University, Syracuse, New York.

Thanks also to Bonnie DeSombre for her help in developing the figures and tables that appear in this edition.

Additional thanks to Jean-François Vilain, Publisher, Allied Health, and his staff at F. A. Davis, for their encouragement and support.

ACKNOWLEDGMENTS TO THE FIRST EDITION

I am deeply indebted to everyone who offered assistance, encouragement, and support during the preparation and completion of this text. I would especially like to thank the following people:

Linda D. Crane, John F. Decker, Mark Greve, Sandra Levine, Donald L. Merrill, Grace Minerbo, Jeffrey Rothman, and Steven L. Wolf for their excellent suggestions and feedback during the review of this manuscript.

Bonnie DeSombre and Cheryl Tarbell for their help in compiling various tables and charts in this text.

All of my family and friends for their patience and tolerance throughout this project.

The students I have taught for the challenge and privilege of helping them assimilate this body of knowledge.

Steve Wolf, Jean-François Vilain, and everyone at F. A. Davis for giving me the opportunity to write this book and helping me maintain the conviction that this project could actually become a reality.

TABLE OF CONTENTS

DRUG AND AGENT INDEX

An "f" following a page number indicates a figure; a "t" following a page number indicates a table.

General Principles
of Pharmacology

CHAPTER 1

Basic Principles of Pharmacology

Pharmacology is the study of drugs. In its broadest definition, a drug can be described as "any chemical agent that affects processes of living."[2] In this sense, a drug includes any substance that alters physiologic function in the organism, regardless of whether the effect is beneficial or harmful. In terms of clinical pharmacology, it has traditionally been the beneficial or therapeutic effects that have been of special interest. Throughout history, certain naturally occurring chemicals have been used to relieve pain or treat disease in humans. Within the past century, the use of natural, semisynthetic, and synthetic chemical agents has expanded to the point where many diseases can be prevented or cured, and the general health and well-being of many individuals have improved dramatically through the use of therapeutic drugs.

Because of the extensive clinical use of therapeutic medications, members of the medical community must have some knowledge of the basic types of drugs and the mechanisms of their actions. Although this has always been true for individuals who prescribe and administer drugs (i.e., physicians and nurses), it is now recognized that members of other health-related professions must also have a fundamental knowledge of pharmacology.

An understanding of basic drug mechanisms can help practitioners such as physical therapists, occupational therapists, and other rehabilitation specialists better understand the patient's response to the drug. In addition, the knowledge of how certain rehabilitative procedures may interact with the medication will be helpful in getting the optimal response from the patient to both the drug and the therapy treatment. For instance, scheduling the patient for therapy when certain drugs reach their peak effect may improve the therapy session dramatically. This may be true for drugs that decrease pain (analgesics) or improve the patient's motor skills (antiparkinson drugs). Conversely, some therapy sessions that require the patient's active participation may be rendered useless if scheduled when medications such as sedatives reach their peak effect. Also, any adverse responses that may occur because of a direct interaction between the therapy treatment and certain medications may be avoided or controlled by understanding the pharmacologic aspects of specific drugs. For example, the patient taking a peripheral vasodilator may experience a profound decrease in blood pressure when he or she is placed in a hot whirlpool. By understanding the implications of such an interaction, the therapist can be especially alert for any detrimental effects on the patient, or a different therapy treatment may be instituted in some patients.

In order to help the reader have a more focused approach to the study of drugs, pharmacology is often divided into several areas of concern (Fig. 1–1). **Pharmacotherapeutics** is the area of pharmacology that refers to the use of specific drugs to prevent, treat, or diagnose disease. For the purposes of this text, the effects of drugs on humans will be of primary concern, with animal pharmacology mentioned only in reference to drug testing and research in animals.

When drugs are used therapeutically in humans, information must be known about the way in which the body interacts with the drug and what specific effect the drug has on the individual. Consequently, pharmacotherapeutics is divided into two functional areas: pharmacokinetics and pharmacodynamics (see Fig. 1–1). **Pharmacokinetics** is the study of how the body deals with the drug in terms of the way the drug is absorbed, distributed, and eliminated. **Pharmacodynamics** is the analysis of what the drug does to the body, including the mechanism by which the drug exerts its effect. In this text, the basic principles of pharmacokinetics will be outlined in Chapters 2 and 3, and the pharmacodynamics and pharmacokinetics of specific drugs will be discussed in their respective chapters.

Toxicology is the study of the harmful effects of chemicals. Although it can be viewed as a subdivision of pharmacology, toxicology has evolved into a separate area of study because of the scope of all the adverse effects of therapeutic agents as well as environmental toxins and poisons. However, because virtually every medication can produce some adverse effects, a discussion of toxicology must be included in pharmacotherapeutics. For the purposes of this text, discussions of drug toxicity are limited to the unwanted "side effects" of therapeutic drugs. The toxic side effects of individual

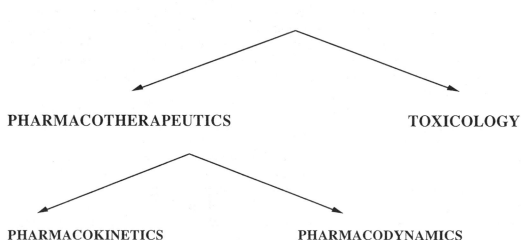

FIGURE 1–1. Areas of study within pharmacology.

drugs are covered in the respective chapter describing the therapeutic effects of that drug.

Pharmacy deals with the preparation and dispensing of medications. Although pharmacy is also frequently considered a subdivision of pharmacology, this area has evolved into a distinct professional discipline. Care must be taken not to use the terms "pharmacy" and "pharmacology" interchangeably, because these are quite different areas of study.

DRUG NOMENCLATURE

One of the most potentially confusing aspects of pharmacology is the variety of names given to different drugs or even to the same compound. Students of pharmacology as well as clinicians are often faced with myriad terms that represent the same drug.[8] Most of the problems in drug terminology arise from the fact that each drug can be identified according to its *chemical, generic,* or *trade* name[1] (Table 1–1). **Chemical names** refer to the specific structure of the compound and are usually fairly long and cumbersome. The **generic name** (also known as the "official" or "nonproprietary" name) tends to be somewhat shorter and is often derived from the chemical name. **Trade names** are assigned to the compound by the pharmaceutical company and may or may not bear any reference at all to the chemical and generic terminology. An additional problem with trade names is that several manufacturers may be marketing the same compound under different names, thus adding to the confusion. If there is no existing patent for that compound or if the patent has expired, the same drug may be marketed by separate drug companies. For practical purposes, the generic name is often the easiest and most effective way to refer to a drug, and this terminology will be used most frequently in this text.

WHAT CONSTITUTES A DRUG: DEVELOPMENT AND APPROVAL OF THERAPEUTIC AGENTS

In the United States, the **Food and Drug Administration** (FDA) is responsible for monitoring the use of existing drugs as well as the development and approval of new drugs.[3,11] The analogous body in Canada is the Drugs Directorate of Health Protection Branch, Department of Health and Welfare. The two primary concerns of these agencies are (1) whether or not the drug is effective in treating a certain condition and (2) whether the drug is reasonably safe for human use.

TABLE 1–1 Examples of Drug Nomenclature

Chemical	Generic (Nonproprietary)	Trade (Proprietary)
N-Acetyl-p-aminophenol	Acetaminophen	Tylenol, Panadol, many others
3,4-Dihydroxyphenyl-L-alanine	Levodopa	Larodopa
5,5-Phenylethylbarbituric acid	Phenobarbital	Luminal, Eskabarb
7-Chloro-1,3-dihydro-1-methyl-5-phenyl-2H-1,4-benzodiazepin-2-one	Diazepam	Valium

Drug Approval Process

The development of a new drug involves extensive preclinical (animal) and clinical (human) studies.[3,11] The basic procedure for testing a new drug is outlined here and is summarized in Table 1–2.

PRECLINICAL STUDIES

Drugs are tested initially in animals, often using several different species. Initial information on the basic pharmacokinetic and pharmacodynamic properties of the compound is obtained. Information on dosage and toxicity is also obtained from these animal trials.

HUMAN (CLINICAL) STUDIES

If the results from animal trials are favorable, the drug sponsor files an investigational new drug (IND) application with the FDA. If approved as an IND, the sponsor may begin testing the drug in humans. Human or "clinical" testing is divided into three primary phases.

Phase I: The drug is tested in a relatively small number of healthy volunteers. Initial information about the effects of the drug on humans is determined.
Phase II: The drug is tested in a small, select patient population (10 to 150 subjects) to evaluate the effect of the drug in treating a specific disease or pathologic condition.

TABLE 1–2 Drug Development and Approval

Testing Phase	Purpose	Subjects	Usual Time Period
Preclinical testing	Initial laboratory tests to determine drug effects and safety	Laboratory animals	1–2 yr
Investigational New Drug (IND) Application			
Human (clinical) testing:			
Phase I	Determine effects, safe dosage, pharmacokinetics	Small number of healthy volunteers	<1 yr
Phase II	Assess drug's effectiveness in treating a specific disease/disorder	Limited number (200–300) patients with target disorder	2 yr
Phase III	Assess safety and effectiveness in a larger patient population	Large number (1000–3000) of targeted patients	3 yr
New Drug Application (NDA) Approval			
Phase IV (postmarketing surveillance)	Monitor any problems that occur after NDA approval	General patient population	Indefinite

Phase III: Clinical evaluation is expanded to include more patients (several hundred to several thousand) as well as more evaluators. Additional information is obtained regarding the drug's safety and effectiveness in a large patient population.

At the end of phase III, the drug sponsor applies for a new drug application (NDA). Results from clinical testing are reviewed extensively by the FDA, and if found favorable, the NDA is approved. At this point, the drug can be marketed and prescribed for use in the general population.

A fourth phase known as "postmarketing surveillance" should be instituted after the NDA is approved. Here the marketing company continues to monitor use of the drug and collect information from physicians about drug safety and effectiveness. Results from postmarketing surveillance are then reported periodically to the FDA with a description of any problems encountered when the drug is used in the general population. This phase may be very helpful in detecting problems that were not apparent when the drug was tested on a relatively limited number of patients during clinical testing. For instance, many drugs will cause a specific adverse effect in only 1 in 10,000 patients taking the drug.[3] It is very likely that such an adverse effect could be missed during phase I through phase III of the clinical trials because the drug is typically tested only in a few thousand subjects (e.g., 1000 to 3000 people). Hence, postmarketing surveillance has been advocated as being critical in ensuring that the safety and efficacy of the drug continues to be monitored when the drug is actually being used by the general patient population.[3,13,14]

The development of a new drug in the United States is an extremely expensive and time-consuming process. The time course for the entire testing process from the beginning of animal trials to the end of phase III human testing may be as long as 7 to 9 years. The FDA has made provisions, however, to shorten the review process in cases where the drug shows exceptional promise or there is a critical need for the immediate clinical use of the drug.[9] For example, certain drugs that have shown promise in treating conditions such as cancer or acquired immunodeficiency syndrome (AIDS) may be made available for patient use even before clinical testing is completed.[3,18] Likewise, the approval process can be expedited if a drug has already received approval for treating one condition, but the drug is now being considered for use in other "supplemental" conditions.[5,16]

The process of drug testing and approval does seem to be fairly rigorous in its ability to screen out ineffective or potentially harmful drugs. Out of every 10,000 compounds, only 10 make it to the stage of human clinical trials. Of the 10 tested clinically, only 1 will ever be released as a prescription drug.[6]

Prescription Versus Over-the-Counter Medications

In the United States, pharmacotherapeutic agents are divided into those requiring a prescription for use and those available as nonprescription, **over-the-counter** (OTC) drugs.[7] Nonprescription drugs can be purchased directly by the consumer, whereas prescription medications may be ordered or dispensed only by an authorized practitioner (i.e., physician or dentist). The classification as a prescription or a nonprescription drug falls under the jurisdiction of the FDA.[10,11] In general, OTC medications are used to treat relatively minor problems and to make the consumer more comfortable until the condition is resolved. These medications have been judged to be safe for use by the consumer without direct medical supervision, and the chances of toxic effects are usually small when the medications are taken in the recommended amounts.[10] Of course, the patient may ingest more than the recommended amount, and in the case of an overdose, the danger always exists for potentially harmful effects, even if the drug is nonprescription in nature.

Frequently, the concern with OTC products is not with their safety but with whether the drugs really do what their manufacturers claim. The OTC medication may be said to exert effects that cannot be achieved either because appropriate ingredients are lacking or because the ingredients are below therapeutic dosage levels. In many cases, there is a relative lack of **placebo**-controlled clinical studies that document the effectiveness of specific OTC products. There is also a lack of well-designed clinical research that documents the efficacy of OTC products in a variety of age groups. For example, OTC products such as certain cold medications have been shown to be effective in alleviating symptoms in adolescents and adults, but the efficacy of these drugs in younger children remains unknown.[15] Hence, the effectiveness of OTC medications is an issue that must be examined continually in order to protect the consumer from purchasing products that are essentially worthless.

Most OTC medications have a much lower pharmacologic impact than their prescription counterparts. Some OTC compounds do, however, require significant attention either because they are able to exert an important effect at the recommended dosage or because they may interact with prescription drugs in an adverse manner.[12] Such OTC compounds are discussed in this text in the appropriate chapters.

Controlled Substances

In 1970, federal legislation was enacted to help control the abuse of legal and illegal drugs. The Comprehensive Drug Abuse Prevention and Control Act (or Controlled Substances Act, as it is also known) placed drugs into specific categories, or "schedules," according to their potential for abuse.[11,17] Descriptions of these schedules for controlled drugs follow.

Schedule I: These drugs are regarded as having the highest potential for abuse, and the legal use of agents in this category is restricted to approved research studies or therapeutic use in a very limited number of patients (e.g., use of marijuana as an antiemetic). Examples of schedule I drugs include heroin, lysergic acid diethylamide (LSD), psilocybin, mescaline, peyote, marijuana, tetrahydrocannabinols, and several other hallucinogens.

Schedule II: Drugs in this category are approved for specific therapeutic purposes but still have a high potential for abuse and possible addiction. Examples include opioids such as morphine and meperidine, barbiturates such as pentobarbital and secobarbital, and drugs containing amphetamines.

Schedule III: Although these drugs have a lower abuse potential than those in schedules I and II, there is still the possibility of developing mild to moderate physical dependence or strong psychologic dependence, or both. Drugs in schedule III include opioids (e.g., codeine, hydrocodone) that are combined in a limited dosage with other nonopioid drugs. Other drugs in this category are certain barbiturates and amphetamines that are not included in schedule II.

Schedule IV: These drugs supposedly have a lower potential for abuse than schedule III drugs, with only a limited possibility of physical dependence, psychologic dependence, or both. Examples include the benzodiazepines (diazepam, chlordiazepoxide), certain opioids (pentazocine, propoxyphene), barbiturates not included in other schedules, and a variety of other depressants and stimulants.

Schedule V: These drugs have the lowest relative abuse potential. Drugs in this category consist primarily of low doses of opioids that are used in cough medications and antidiarrheal preparations.

Several other criteria relate to the different controlled substance schedules, such as restrictions on prescription renewal and penalties for illegal possession of drugs in different schedules. For a further discussion of controlled substances, the reader is referred to another source.[1]

BASIC CONCEPTS IN DRUG THERAPY

All drugs exert their beneficial effects by reaching some specific target cell or tissue. On the cellular level, the drug in some way changes the function of the cell either to help restore normal physiologic function or to prevent a disease process from occurring. In general, the **dose** of the drug must be large enough to allow an adequate concentration to reach the target site, thus producing a beneficial response. However, the administered **dosage** must not be so excessive that toxicologic effects are produced. Some aspects of the relationship between dosage and response are discussed here.

Dose-Response Curves and Maximal Efficacy

The relationship between the dosage of a drug and a specific response to the drug is illustrated in Figure 1–2. Typically, very low doses do not produce any observable effect. At some threshold dose, the response begins to occur and continues to increase in magnitude before reaching a plateau. The plateau in the response indicates that

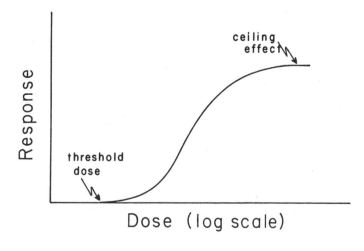

FIGURE 1–2. Dose-response curve.

there will be no further increment in the response even if the dosage continues to be increased. The point at which there is no further increase in the response is known as **ceiling effect,** or **maximal efficacy**, of the drug.[4]

Dose-response curves are used to provide information about the dosage range over which the drug is effective, as well as the peak response that can be expected from the drug. In addition, the characteristic shape of the dose-response curve and the presence of the plateau associated with maximal efficacy can be used to indicate specific information about the binding of the drug to cellular receptors. The relevance of dose-response curves to drug-receptor interactions is discussed further in Chapter 4.

Potency

One criterion used frequently when comparing drugs is the concept of **potency**. Potency is related to the dosage that produces a given response in a specific amplitude.[4] When two drugs are compared, the more potent drug requires a lower dosage to produce the same effect as a higher dose of the second drug. For instance, in Figure 1–3, a dosage of 10 mg of drug A would lower blood pressure by 25 percent,

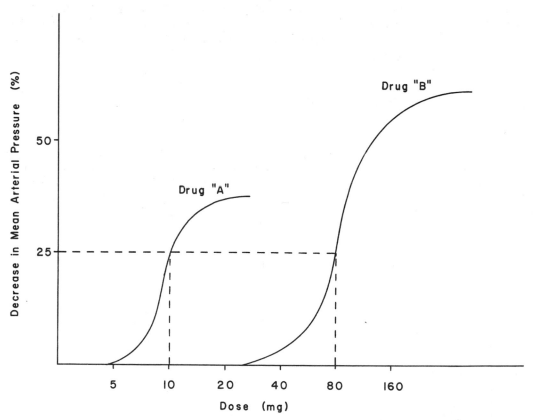

FIGURE 1–3. Relative potency and maximal efficacy of two drugs. Drug A is more potent, and drug B has a greater maximal efficacy.

whereas 80 mg of drug B would be required to produce the same response. Consequently, drug A would be described as being the more potent drug. It should be noted that potency is not synonymous with maximal efficacy. Drug B is clearly able to exert a greater maximal effect than drug A. Consequently, the term "potency" is often taken to be much more significant than it really is. The potency of a drug is often misinterpreted by the layperson as an indication of the drug's overall therapeutic benefits, whereas potency really just refers to the fact that less of the compound is required to produce a given response. In fact, neither potency nor maximal efficacy fully indicates a drug's therapeutic potential. Other factors such as the therapeutic index (described further on) and drug selectivity (see Chapter 4) are also important in comparing and ultimately choosing the best medication for a given problem.

ELEMENTS OF DRUG SAFETY

Quantal Dose-Response Curves and the Median Effective Dose

The dose-response curves shown in Figures 1–2 and 1–3 represent the graded response to a drug as it would occur in a single individual or in a homogeneous population. In reality, variations in the response to a drug that are caused by individual differences in the clinical population need to be considered when trying to assess whether a drug is safe as well as effective. Consequently, the relationship between the dose of the drug and the occurrence of a certain response is measured in a large group of people (or animals if the drug is being tested preclinically). When plotted, this relationship yields a cumulative, or *quantal*, dose-response curve (Fig. 1–4).[4] This curve differs from the dose-response curve discussed previously in that it is not the magnitude of the response that increases with increasing dosage, but the percentage of the population who exhibit a specific response as the dose is increased. The response is not graded; it is either present or it is absent in each member of the population. For example, a headache medication is administered in an increasing dosage to 1000 people. At some dose, some of the individuals will begin to respond to the drug by reporting the absence of their headache. As the dosage is increased, more and more individuals will experience pain relief because of the medication, until finally 100 percent of the population report that their headaches are gone. Again, it is the percentage of the population who respond in a specific way (e.g., reporting loss of their headaches) that is measured relative to the dose of the drug. An important reference point in this type of cumulative dose-response curve is the **median effective dose** (ED_{50}). This is the dose at which 50 percent of the population respond to the drug in a specified manner.

Median Toxic Dose

In the aforementioned example, relief from pain was the desired response, which is often termed the "beneficial" effect. As doses of the drug continue to be increased, however, adverse or toxic effects may become apparent. To continue the earlier example, higher doses of the same medication may be associated with the appearance of a specific toxic effect such as acute gastric hemorrhage. As the dosage is increased, more and more individuals will then begin to exhibit that particular adverse effect. The

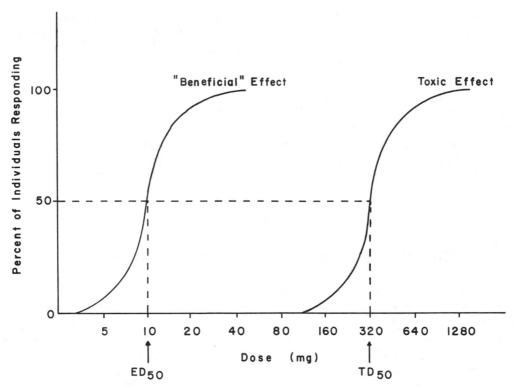

FIGURE 1–4. Cumulative dose-response curve. The median effective dose (ED_{50}) is 10 mg, and the median toxic dose (TD_{50}) is 320 mg. The therapeutic index (TI) for this drug is 32.

dosage at which 50 percent of the group exhibits the adverse effect is termed the **median toxic dose** (TD_{50}). In animal studies, the toxic effect studied is often the death of the animal. In these cases, high doses of the drug are used to determine the **median lethal dose** (LD_{50}), the dose that causes death in 50 percent of the animals studied. Of course, the LD_{50} is not a relevant term in clinical use of the drug in humans, but it does serve to provide some indication of the drug's safety in preclinical animal trials.

Therapeutic Index

The median effective and toxic doses are used to determine the **therapeutic index** (TI). The TI is calculated as the ratio of the TD_{50} to the ED_{50}:

$$TI = \frac{TD_{50}}{ED_{50}}$$

In animal studies in which the median lethal dose is known, the TI is often calculated using the LD_{50} in place of the TD_{50}. In either human or animal studies, the TI is used as an indicator of the drug's safety.[4] The greater the value of the TI, the safer the drug is considered to be. In essence, a large TI indicates that it takes a much larger dose to evoke a toxic response than it does to cause a beneficial effect.

It should be noted, however, that the TI is a relative term. Acetaminophen, a nonprescription analgesic, has a TI of approximately 27 (i.e., the ratio of the median toxic dose to the median effective dose equals 27). Prescription agents tend to have lower TIs. For instance, the narcotic analgesic meperidine (Demerol) has a TI of 8, and the sedative-hypnotic diazepam (Valium) has a TI equal to 3. Other prescription agents such as the cancer chemotherapeutic agents (methotrexate, azathioprine, and so on) may have a very low TI, some being close to 1. However, a low TI is often acceptable in these agents, considering the critical nature of cancer and similar serious conditions. The consequences of not using the drug outweigh the risks of some of the toxic effects.

To help keep the risk of toxicity to a minimum with low-TI drugs, it is generally advisable to periodically monitor blood levels of the drug. This helps prevent concentrations from quickly reaching toxic levels. This precaution is usually not necessary with high-TI drugs, because there is a greater margin of error (i.e., blood levels can rise quite a lot above the therapeutic concentration before becoming dangerous).

SUMMARY

In its broadest sense, pharmacology is the study of the effects of chemicals on living organisms. Most discussions of clinical pharmacology deal primarily with the beneficial effects of specific drugs on humans, and the manner in which these drugs exert their therapeutic effects. Since all drugs have the potential to produce unwanted or toxic responses, some discussion of the adverse effects of drugs is also essential in pharmacology. Drugs used therapeutically are subjected to extensive testing prior to approval for use in humans and are classified as either prescription or over-the-counter depending on their dosage, effectiveness, and safety profile. Finally, certain characteristic relationships exist between the dosage of a drug and the response or effect it produces. Such relationships can provide useful information about drug efficacy and potency and about the relative safety of different compounds.

REFERENCES

1. Benet, LZ: Appendix I. Principles of prescription order writing and patient compliance instructions. In Gilman, AG, et al (eds): The Pharmacological Basis of Therapeutics, ed 8. Pergamon Press, New York, 1990.
2. Benet, LZ, Mitchell, JR, and Sheiner, LB: Introduction. In Gilman, AG, et al (eds): The Pharmacological Basis of Therapeutics, ed 8. Pergamon Press, New York, 1990.
3. Berkowitz, BA and Katzung, BG: Basic and clinical evaluation of new drugs. In Katzung, BG (ed): Basic and Clinical Pharmacology, ed 5. Appleton & Lange, Norwalk, CT, 1992.
4. Bourne, HR and Roberts, JM: Drug receptors and pharmacodynamics. In Katzung, BG (ed): Basic and Clinical Pharmacology, ed 5. Appleton & Lange, Norwalk, CT, 1992.
5. DiMasi, JA, et al: New indications for already approved drugs: An analysis of regulatory review times. J Clin Pharmacol 31:205, 1991.
6. Grabowski, HG and Vernon, JM: The regulation of pharmaceuticals: Balancing the benefits and risks. American Enterprise Institute for Public Policy Research, Washington, DC, 1983.
7. Handbook of Nonprescription Drugs, ed 9. American Pharmaceutical Association, Washington, DC, 1990.
8. Hemminki, E, et al: Trade names and generic names: Problems for prescribing physicians. Scand J Prim Health Care 2:84, 1984.
9. Kaitlin, KI, et al: Therapeutic ratings and end-of-phase II conferences: Initiatives to accelerate the availability of important new drugs. J Clin Pharmacol 31:17, 1991.
10. Koda-Kimble, MA: Therapeutic and toxic potential of over-the-counter agents. In Katzung, BG (ed): Basic and Clinical Pharmacology, ed 5. Appleton & Lange, Norwalk, CT, 1992.

11. Kuhn, MA and Moraca-Sawicki, AM: Pharmacology and the nurse's role. In Kuhn, MA (ed): Pharmacotherapeutics: A Nursing Process Approach, ed 3. FA Davis, Philadelphia, 1994.
12. Lake, KD, et al: Over-the-counter medications in cardiac transplant recipients: Guidelines for use. Ann Pharmacother 26:1566, 1992.
13. Mellinger, GD, et al: Survey method for post-marketing drug surveillance: A demonstration. J Clin Psychopharmacol 8:168, 1988.
14. Smart, AJ and Walters, L: The importance of postmarketing drug surveillance. S Afr Med J 82:383, 1992.
15. Smith, MBH and Feldman, W: Over-the-counter cold medications: A critical review of clinical trials between 1950 and 1991. JAMA 269:2258, 1993.
16. Spivey, RN, Lasagna, L, and Trimble, AG: New applications for already approved drugs: Time trends for the new drug application review phase. Clin Pharmacol Ther 41:368, 1987.
17. United States Pharmacopeia XXII National Formulary XVII. United States Pharmacopeia Convention, Inc., Rockville, MD, 1990, pp 1629–1665.
18. Vanchieri, C: Speedier drug approval modeled after FDA's cancer drug review system. J Nat Cancer Instit 84:666, 1992.

CHAPTER 2

Pharmacokinetics I: Drug Administration, Absorption, and Distribution

Pharmacokinetics is the study of the way in which the body deals with pharmacologic compounds. In other words, what does the body do to the drug? This includes the manner in which the drug is administered, absorbed, distributed, and eventually eliminated from the body. These topics are discussed in this chapter and the next.

ROUTES OF ADMINISTRATION

In general, drugs can be administered via two primary routes: through the alimentary canal (**enteral administration**) or through nonalimentary routes (**parenteral administration**). Each major route has several variations, and each offers distinct advantages and disadvantages (Table 2–1). The primary features of some of the major routes are discussed here. For a more detailed description of the specific methodology involved in drug administration, the reader is referred to several excellent discussions of this topic.[7,30,48]

Enteral

ORAL

The primary way drugs are given enterally is through the oral route. This is the most common method of administering most medications and offers several distinct advantages. Oral administration is by far the easiest method of taking medications, especially when self-administration is necessary or desired. The oral route is also relatively safe because drugs enter the system in a fairly controlled manner. This avoids the large, sudden increase in plasma drug levels that can occur when the drug is ad-

15

TABLE 2–1 Routes of Drug Administration

Route	Advantages	Disadvantages	Examples
Enteral			
Oral	Easy, safe, convenient	Limited or erratic absorption of some drugs; chance of first-pass inactivation in liver	Analgesics, sedative-hypnotics, many others
Sublingual	Rapid onset; not subject to first-pass inactivation	Drug must be easily absorbed from oral mucosa	Nitroglycerin
Rectal	Alternative to oral route; local effect on rectal tissues	Poor or incomplete absorption; chance of rectal irritation	Laxatives, suppository forms of other drugs
Parenteral			
Inhalation	Rapid onset; direct application for respiratory disorders; large surface area for systemic absorption	Chance of tissue irritation; patient compliance sometimes a problem	General anesthetics; antiasthmatic agents
Injection	Provides more direct administration to target tissues; rapid onset	Chance of infection if sterility is not maintained	Insulin, antibiotics, anticancer drugs, narcotic analgesics
Topical	Local effects on surface of skin	Only effective in treating outer layers of skin	Antibiotic ointments, creams used to treat minor skin irritation and injury
Transdermal	Introduces drug into body without breaking the skin	Drug must be able to pass through dermal layers intact	Nitroglycerin, motion sickness medications, drugs used with phonophoresis and iontophoresis

ministered by other methods such as intravenous injection. Most medications administered orally are absorbed from the small intestine, thus utilizing the large surface area of the intestinal microvilli to enhance entry into the body.

Several disadvantages may preclude drugs from being given orally. Drugs that are administered by mouth must have a relatively high degree of lipid solubility in order to pass through the gastrointestinal mucosa into the bloodstream. Large, non–lipid-soluble compounds are absorbed very poorly from the alimentary canal and will eventually be lost from the body in the feces. Certain medications may irritate the stomach to the extent that discomfort, vomiting, or even damage to the gastric mucosa may occur. The acidic environment and presence of digestive proteases in the stomach may also cause various compounds to be degraded and destroyed prior to absorption from the gastrointestinal tract.

Drugs that are given orally are subject to a phenomenon known as the **first-pass effect**.[6,27] After absorption from the alimentary canal, the drug is transported directly to the liver via the portal vein, where a significant amount of the drug may be metabolized and destroyed prior to reaching its site of action. The dosage of the orally administered drug must be sufficient to allow an adequate amount of the compound to survive hepatic degradation and eventually to reach the target tissue.[9] Some drugs such as nitroglycerin undergo such extensive inactivation from the first-pass effect that it is usually preferable to administer them by nonoral routes.

A final limitation of the oral route is that the amount and rate at which the drug eventually reaches the bloodstream tends to be somewhat less predictable with oral administration compared with more direct routes such as injection. Factors that affect intestinal absorption (intestinal infection, presence of food, rate of gastric emptying, amount of visceral blood flow, and so on) can alter the usual manner in which a drug is absorbed into the body from the gastrointestinal tract.[4,7,39,54]

SUBLINGUAL

Drugs are administered sublingually by placing the drug under the tongue. The drug is absorbed through the oral mucosa into the venous system draining the mouth region. These veins eventually carry blood to the superior vena cava, which in turn carries blood to the heart. Consequently, a drug administered sublingually can reach the systemic circulation without being subjected to first-pass inactivation in the liver. This provides an obvious advantage for drugs, such as nitroglycerin, that would be destroyed in the liver when absorbed from the stomach or intestines. The sublingual route also offers a means of enteral administration to people who have difficulty swallowing or to patients who cannot be given drugs rectally.[20] The restrictions of the sublingual route are that the amount of drug that can be administered is somewhat limited, and the drug must be able to pass easily through the oral mucosa in order to reach the venous drainage of the mouth.

RECTAL

A final method of enteral administration is via the rectum. Many drugs are available as rectal suppositories to allow administration through this route. This method is less favorable because many drugs are absorbed poorly or incompletely, and irritation of the rectal mucosa may occur.[7] Rectal administration does offer the advantage of allowing drugs to be given to a patient who is unconscious, or when vomiting prevents drugs from being taken orally. However, the rectal route is used most often for treating local conditions such as hemorrhoids.

Parenteral

All methods of drug administration that do not use the gastrointestinal tract are termed *parenteral*. Parenteral administration generally allows the drug to be delivered to the target site more directly, and the quantity of the drug that actually reaches the target site is often more predictable.[7,53] Also, drugs given parenterally are not usually subject to first-pass inactivation in the liver. Other advantages and disadvantages of various parenteral routes are discussed further on.

INHALATION

Drugs that exist in a gaseous or volatile state or that can be suspended as tiny droplets in an aerosol form may be given via inhalation. Pulmonary administration offers the advantage of a large (alveolar) surface area for diffusion of the drug into the pulmonary circulation and is generally associated with rapid entry of the drug into the bloodstream.[19] This method is used extensively in administering the volatile general anesthetics (e.g., halothane) and is also advantageous when applying medications directly to the bronchial and alveolar tissues for the treatment of specific pulmonary pathologies. One limitation of the inhalation route is that the drug must not irritate the alveoli or other areas of the respiratory tract. Also, some patients have trouble administering drugs by this route, and drug particles tend to be trapped by cilia and mucus in the respiratory tract. Both of these factors tend to limit the ability to predict exactly how much drug eventually reaches the lungs.

INJECTION

Various types of injection can be used to introduce the drug either systemically or locally. If sterility is not maintained, all types of injection have the disadvantage of possible infection, and certain types of injection are more difficult, if not impossible, for the patient to self-administer. Specific types of injection include the following routes:

Intravenous. The bolus injection of a medication into a peripheral vein allows an accurate, known quantity of the drug to be introduced into the bloodstream over a short period of time, frequently resulting in peak levels of the drug appearing almost instantaneously in the peripheral circulation and thus reaching the target site rapidly. This occurrence is advantageous in emergency situations when it is necessary for the medication to exert an immediate effect. Of course, adverse reactions may also occur because of the sudden appearance of large titers of the drug in the plasma. Any unexpected side effects or miscalculation in the amount of the administered drug are often difficult to deal with after the full dosage has been injected. In certain situations, an indwelling intravenous cannula (IV "line") can be used to allow the prolonged, steady infusion of a drug into the venous system. This method prevents large fluctuations in the plasma concentration of the drug and allows the dose of the drug to be maintained at a specific level for as long as desired.

Intra-arterial. The injection of a drug directly into an artery is understandably a difficult and dangerous procedure. This method permits a large dose of the medication to reach a given site, such as a specific organ, and may be used to focus the administration of drugs into certain tissues. Intra-arterial injections are used occasionally in cancer chemotherapy to administer the anticancer drug directly to the tumor site with minimal exposure of the drug to other healthy tissues. This route may also be used to focus the administration of other substances such as radiopaque dyes for various diagnostic procedures.

Subcutaneous. Injecting medications directly beneath the skin is used when a local response is desired, such as in certain situations requiring local anesthesia. Also, a slower, more prolonged release of the medication into the systemic circulation can be achieved in situations where this is the desired effect. A primary example is insulin injection in the patient with diabetes mellitus. Subcutaneous administration provides a relatively easy route of parenteral injection that can be performed by patients themselves, providing they are properly trained. Some limitations are that the amount of drug that can be injected in this fashion is fairly small and that the injected drug must not irritate or inflame the subcutaneous tissues. The subcutaneous route can also be used when certain types of drug preparations are implanted surgically beneath the skin so that the drug is slowly dispersed from the implanted preparation and absorbed into the bloodstream for prolonged periods. An example of this form of subcutaneous administration is the use of implanted hormonal contraceptive products (Norplant). The use of this drug is discussed in more detail in Chapter 30.

Intramuscular. The large quantity of skeletal muscle in the body allows this route to be an easily accessible site for parenteral administration. Intramuscular injections can be used to treat a problem located directly in the injected muscle, or as a method for a relatively steady, prolonged release of the drug into the systemic circulation.

Intramuscular injection offers the advantage of providing a relatively rapid effect (i.e., within a few minutes), while avoiding the sudden, large increase in plasma levels seen with intravenous injection. The major problem with intramuscular administration is that many drugs injected directly into a muscle cause a significant amount of local pain and prolonged soreness, tending to limit the use of this route for repeated injections.

Intrathecal. Intrathecal injections are given by injecting the medication within a sheath, and frequently refer to injections within the spinal subarachnoid space. This particular type of intrathecal route allows drugs such as narcotic analgesics, local anesthetics, and antispasticity drugs to be applied directly to the spinal cord. Also, intrathecal injections allow certain drugs such as antibiotics and anticancer drugs to bypass the blood-brain barrier and reach the central nervous system (see Chapter 5). Other intrathecal injections include administration of the drug within a tendon sheath or bursa, which may be used to treat a local condition such as an inflammation within those structures.[43]

TOPICAL

Drugs given topically are applied to the surface of the skin or mucous membranes. Most medications applied directly to the skin are absorbed fairly poorly through the epidermis and into the systemic circulation and are used primarily to treat problems that exist on the skin itself. Topical application to mucous membranes is also usually done to treat the membrane itself, although significant amounts of the drug can be readily absorbed through the membrane and into the bloodstream. This point must be considered if adverse effects will result when the topical drug is absorbed into the body.[49,52]

TRANSDERMAL

Unlike topical administration, transdermal application consists of applying drugs directly to the surface of the skin with the intent that they *will* be absorbed through the dermal layers and into either the subcutaneous tissues or the peripheral circulation. A transdermally administered drug must possess two basic properties: (1) it must be able to penetrate the skin, and (2) it must not be degraded to any major extent by drug-metabolizing enzymes located in the dermis.[17,28] Absorption may be enhanced by mixing the drug in an oily base, thus increasing solubility and permeability through the dermis.

Transdermal administration provides a slow, controlled release of the drug into the body that is effective in maintaining plasma levels of the drug at a relatively constant level for prolonged periods of time.[10,22] Drugs that can be administered transdermally are often delivered through medicated "patches" that can be adhered to the skin much like a small bandage. This method has been used for some time to allow the prolonged administration of drugs such as nitroglycerin and some anti–motion sickness medications such as scopolamine. The use of transdermal patches has been expanded recently to include other medications such as hormonal agents (estrogen)[5,12] and opioid analgesics (fentanyl).[3,55] Likewise, transdermal nicotine patches have received a great deal of attention for their use in helping people quit smoking cigarettes.[21,22] Researchers continue to explore the use of the transdermal route, and the use of transdermal patches continues to gain acceptance as a safe and effective method of administering many medications.

The transdermal route also includes the use of iontophoresis and phonophoresis to administer the drug. In iontophoresis, electric current is used to "drive" the ionized form of the medication through the skin.[11] Phonophoresis uses ultrasound waves as the driving force to propel the medication through the dermis.[56] Both phonophoresis and iontophoresis are often used to treat pain and inflammation by transmitting specific medications to a subcutaneous tissue such as a muscle, tendon, or bursa. These forms of transdermal administration are important in a rehabilitation setting since they are often administered by a physical therapist following prescription by a physician. Specific medications that can be administered via iontophoresis or phonophoresis are listed in Appendix A. For a more detailed description of how these transdermal routes are employed, the reader is referred to several additional sources.[11,24,56]

DRUG ABSORPTION AND DISTRIBUTION: BIOAVAILABILITY

Although several routes exist for the administration of drugs, merely introducing the drug into the body does not ensure that the compound will reach all tissues uniformly or even that the drug will reach the appropriate target site. For instance, oral administration of a drug that affects the myocardium will not have any pharmacologic effect unless the drug is absorbed from the gastrointestinal tract into the bloodstream. The extent to which the drug reaches the systemic circulation is referred to as **bioavailability**, which is a parameter that is expressed as the percentage of the drug administered that reaches the bloodstream.[6] For instance, if 100 g of a drug is given orally, and 50 g eventually makes it to the systemic circulation, the drug is said to be 50 percent bioavailable. If 100 g of the same compound were injected intravenously, the drug would be 100 percent bioavailable by that route.

Consequently, bioavailability depends on the route of administration as well as the drug's ability to cross membrane barriers. Once in the systemic circulation, further distribution into peripheral tissues may also be important in allowing the drug to reach the target site. Many drugs must eventually leave the systemic capillaries and enter other cells. Thus, drugs have to move across cell membranes and tissue barriers to get into the body and be distributed within the body. In this section, the ability of these membranes to affect absorption and distribution of drugs is discussed.

Membrane Structure and Function

Throughout the body, biologic membranes act as barriers that permit some substances to pass freely, while others pass through with difficulty or not at all. This dif-

FIGURE 2–1. Schematic diagram of the cell membrane. (Adapted from Singer and Nicolson,[50] p 723. Copyright 1972 by the AAAS.)

ferential separation serves an obvious protective effect by not allowing certain substances to enter the body or by limiting the distribution of the substance within the body. In effect, the body is separated into various "compartments" by these membranes. In the case of pharmacotherapeutics, there is often the need for the drug to cross one or more of these membrane barriers to reach the target site.

The ability of the membrane to act as a selective barrier is related to the membrane's normal structure and physiologic function. The cell membrane is composed primarily of lipids and proteins. Membrane lipids are actually *phospholipids*, which are composed of a polar, hydrophilic "head" (which contains a phosphate group) and a lipid, hydrophobic "tail" (Fig. 2–1). The phospholipids appear to be arranged in a bilayer, with the hydrophobic tails of the molecule oriented toward the membrane's center, and the hydrophilic heads facing away from the center of the membrane.[50] Interspersed throughout the lipid bilayer are membrane proteins, which can exist primarily in the outer or inner portion of the membrane or can span the entire width of the cell membrane (see Fig. 2–1).

The lipid bilayer that composes the basic structure of the cell membrane acts as a water barrier. The lipid portion of the membrane is essentially impermeable to water and other non–lipid-soluble substances (electrolytes, glucose). Lipid-soluble compounds (including most drugs) are able to pass directly through the membrane by becoming dissolved in the lipid bilayer. Non–lipid-soluble substances including water may be able to pass through the membrane because of the presence of membrane pores. Small holes or channels appear to exist in the membrane, thereby allowing certain substances to pass from one side of the membrane to the other. These channels are believed to be formed by some of the membrane proteins that span the width of the membrane.[37] The ability of a substance to pass through a specific pore depends primarily on the size, shape, and electrical charge of the molecule. Also, in excitable membranes (nerve, muscle) some of these pores are dynamic in nature and appear to have the ability to "open" and "close," thus regulating the flow of certain ions in and out of the cell.[1,32,44]

Movement Across Membrane Barriers

Drugs and other substances that pass through biologic membranes usually do so via passive diffusion, active transport, facilitated diffusion, or some "special" process such as endocytosis (Fig. 2–2). Each of these mechanisms is discussed here.

FIGURE 2–2. Schematic diagram summarizing the ways in which substances may cross the cell membrane. Energy is expended during active transport by hydrolyzing adenosine triphosphate (ATP) into adenosine diphosphate (ADP) and inorganic phosphate (Pi). The three other mechanisms do not require any net energy expenditure. See text for further discussion of how and when each mechanism is utilized.

PASSIVE DIFFUSION

Drugs and other substances will pass through a membrane by way of diffusion, providing two essential criteria are met. First, there must be a difference between the concentration of substance on one side of the membrane and that on the other side. When this occurs, the diffusing substance will move "downhill" from the area of high concentration to that of low concentration. In addition to a concentration difference, diffusion can also occur because of the presence of a pressure gradient or, in the case of charged particles, an electrical potential gradient. The rate of the diffusion is dependent on several factors, including the magnitude of the concentration difference, the size of the diffusing substance, the distance over which diffusion occurs, and the temperature at which diffusion occurs.[23] The term *passive diffusion* is often used to emphasize the fact that this movement occurs without any energy being expended. The driving force in passive diffusion is the electrochemical or pressure difference on the two sides of the membrane.

For passive diffusion through a membrane to occur, the second essential factor is that the membrane must be permeable to the diffusing substance. As mentioned earlier, non–lipid-soluble compounds can diffuse through the membrane via specific pores. Some non–lipid-soluble drugs such as lithium are small enough to diffuse through these pores. Many drugs, however, are able to diffuse directly through the lipid bilayer; hence, they must be fairly lipid soluble. Passive lipid diffusion is nonselective, and a drug with a high degree of lipid solubility can gain access to many tissues because of its ability to pass directly through the lipid portion of the cell membrane.

Effect of Ionization on Lipid Diffusion. Passive lipid diffusion of certain drugs is also dependent on whether or not the drug is ionized. Drugs will diffuse more readily through the lipid layer if they are in their neutral, nonionized form. Most drugs are weak acids or weak bases,[15,29] meaning that they have the potential to become positively charged or negatively charged depending on the pH of certain body fluids. In the plasma and in most other fluids, most drugs remain in their neutral, nonionized form because of the relatively neutral pH of these fluids. In specific fluids, however, a drug may exist in an ionized state, and the absorption of the drug will be affected because of the decreased lipid solubility associated with ionization. For instance, when a weak acid is in an acidic environment (e.g., gastric secretions of the stomach), it tends to be in its neutral, nonionized form. The same drug will become positively charged if the pH of the solution increases and becomes more basic (e.g., the digestive fluids in the duodenum). For example, a weak acid like aspirin will be nonionized and therefore absorbed fairly easily from the stomach because of its lipid solubility (Fig. 2–3). This same drug will be poorly absorbed if it reaches the basic pH of the duodenum and becomes ionized. Conversely, a drug that is a weak base will be ionized and poorly absorbed from the acidic environment of the stomach. The same drug will be nonionized and therefore lipid soluble when it reaches the duodenum, allowing it to be absorbed from the proximal small intestine.

Diffusion Trapping. Changes in lipid solubility caused by ionization can also be important when the body attempts to excrete a drug in the urine. Here the situation becomes slightly more complex because the urine can sometimes be acidic and other times basic in nature. In either situation, it is often desirable for the drug to *remain* ionized while in the urine so that the drug will be excreted from the body. If the drug becomes nonionized while in the nephron, it may be reabsorbed back into the body because of its increased lipid solubility. An ionized form of the drug will remain "trapped" in the nephron and will eventually be excreted in the urine.[29] Thus, if the urine is basic, weak acids will become trapped in the nephron and will be excreted more readily. Weak bases will be excreted better if the urine is acidic. The importance of the kidneys in excreting drugs from the body is discussed further in Chapter 3.

Diffusion Between Cell Junctions. So far, the diffusion of drugs and other substances through individual cell membranes has been discussed. Often groups of cells will join together to form a barrier that separates one body compartment from another. In some locations, cells form "tight junctions" with each other and do not allow any appreciable space to exist between adjacent cells. In these cases, the primary way a

FIGURE 2–3. Effect of pH and ionization on absorption of drugs from the gastrointestinal tract. Weak acids and bases are absorbed from the stomach and duodenum, respectively, when they are in their neutral, nonionized form. (From Clark, JB, Queener, SF, and Karb, VB: Pharmacological Basis of Nursing Practice, ed 4. CV Mosby, St. Louis, 1993, p 8, with permission.)

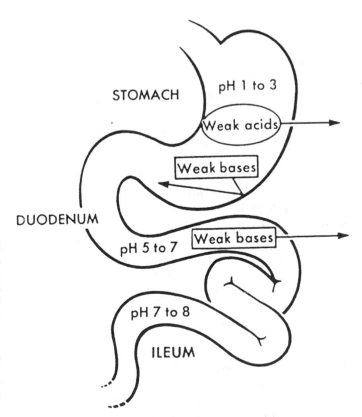

drug may diffuse across the barrier is by diffusing first into and then out of the other side of the cells comprising the barrier. Such locations include the epithelial lining of the gastrointestinal tract and the capillary endothelium of the brain (one of the reasons for the **blood-brain barrier**). In other tissues, such as peripheral capillaries, there may be relatively large gaps between adjacent cells. Here, relatively large substances with molecular weights as high as 30,000 may be able to diffuse across the barrier by diffusing between adjacent cells.

Osmosis. Osmosis refers to the special case of diffusion where the diffusing substance is water. In this situation, water moves from an area where it is highly concentrated to an area of low concentration. Of course, permeability is still a factor when osmosis occurs across a membrane or tissue barrier. During osmosis, certain drugs may simply travel with the diffusing water, thus crossing the membrane by the process of "bulk flow." This is usually limited to osmosis through the gaps between adjacent cells because membrane pores are often too small to allow the passage of the drug molecule along with the diffusing water.

ACTIVE TRANSPORT

Active or carrier-mediated transport involves using membrane proteins to transport substances across the cell membrane (see Fig. 2–2). Membrane proteins that span the entire membrane may serve as some sort of carrier that shuttles substances from one side of the membrane to the other.[2,25] Characteristics of active transport include the following:

Carrier specificity: The protein carrier exhibits some degree of specificity for certain substances, usually discriminating among different compounds according to their shape and electrical charge. This specificity is not absolute, and some compounds that resemble one another will be transported by the same group of carriers.

Expenditure of energy: The term *active* transport implies that some energy must be used to fuel the carrier system. This energy is usually in the form of ATP hydrolysis.

Ability to transport substances against a concentration gradient: Carrier-mediated active transport may be able to carry substances "uphill," that is, from areas of low concentration to areas of high concentration.

The role of active transport in moving drugs across cell membranes is somewhat limited. Essentially, the drug has to bear a good deal of resemblance to the endogenous substance that the transport system routinely carries. However, some drugs, such as theophylline, are apparently absorbed from the intestine via active transport,[26] and active transport systems in the kidney may be important in the excretion of certain drugs into the urine.[7] Also, some drugs may exert their effect by either facilitating or inhibiting endogenous transport systems that affect cellular homeostasis.

FACILITATED DIFFUSION

Facilitated diffusion, as the name implies, bears some features of both active transport and passive diffusion. A protein carrier is present in facilitated diffusion, but no net energy is expended in transporting the substance across the cell membrane. As a result, in most cases of facilitated diffusion there is an inability to transport substances "uphill" against a concentration gradient. The entry of glucose into skeletal muscle cells via facilitated diffusion is probably the primary example of this type of transport in the body. As in active transport, the movement of drugs across membranes through facilitated diffusion is fairly infrequent, but certain medications may affect the rate at which endogenous facilitated diffusion occurs.

SPECIAL PROCESSES

Certain cells have the ability to transport substances across their membranes through processes such as endocytosis. Here the drug is engulfed by the cell via an invagination of the cell membrane. Although limited in scope, this method does allow certain large non–lipid-soluble drugs to enter the cell.

DISTRIBUTION OF DRUGS WITHIN THE BODY

Factors Affecting Distribution

Following administration, the extent to which a drug is uniformly distributed throughout the body or sequestered in a specific body compartment depends on several factors:

1. *Tissue permeability:*   As discussed earlier, the ability to pass through membranes radically affects the extent to which a drug moves around within the body. A highly lipid-soluble drug can potentially reach all the different body compartments and enter virtually every cell it reaches.[38,51] A large non–lipid-soluble compound will remain primarily in the compartment or tissue to which it is administered. Also, certain tissues such as the brain capillary endothelium have special characteristics that limit the passage of drugs. This so-called blood-brain barrier limits the movement of drugs out of the bloodstream and into the central nervous system tissue.
2. *Blood flow:*   If a drug is circulating in the bloodstream, it will gain greater access to tissues that are highly perfused. More of the drug will reach organs that receive a great deal of blood flow, such as the brain, kidneys, and exercising skeletal muscle, than other, less active tissues such as adipose stores.[7]
3. *Binding to plasma proteins:*   Certain drugs will form reversible bonds to circulating proteins in the bloodstream such as albumin.[7,15,45] This fact is significant because only the unbound or "free" drug is able to reach the target tissue and exert a pharmacologic effect. Basically, the fraction of the drug that remains bound to the circulating proteins is sequestered within the vascular system and not available for therapeutic purposes in other tissues and organs.
4. *Binding to subcellular components:*   In a situation similar to plasma protein binding, drugs that are bound within specific cells are unable to leave the cell and be distributed throughout other fluid compartments. An example of this is the antimalarial drug quinacrine, which binds to nucleoproteins located within liver and muscle cells.[6]

Volume of Distribution

The distribution of a given drug within the body is often described by calculating the **volume of distribution** (V_d) for that drug.[6,33] V_d is the ratio of the amount of drug administered to the concentration of drug in the plasma:

V_d = amount of drug administered ÷ concentration of drug in plasma

V_d is used to estimate a drug's distribution by comparing the calculated V_d with the total amount of body water in a normal person. A normal 70-kg man has a total body fluid content of approximately 42 L (5.5 L blood, 12.0 L extracellular fluid, 24.5 L intracellular fluid). If the calculated V_d of a drug is approximately equal to the total amount of body water, then the drug is distributed uniformly throughout all of the body fluids. If the V_d of the drug is far less than 42 L, then the drug is being retained in the bloodstream because of factors such as plasma protein binding. A V_d much greater than 42 L indicates that the drug is being concentrated in the tissues. It should be noted that V_d is not a "real" value; that is, it does not indicate the actual amount of fluid in the body, but is merely an arbitrary figure that reflects the apparent distribution of a drug using total body water as a reference point. Table 2–2 gives some examples of the calculation of the V_d for three different types of drugs.

DRUG STORAGE

Storage Sites

Following administration and absorption, many drugs are "stored" to some extent at certain locations in the body[7]; that is, prior to drug elimination, the drug may be sequestered in its active form in a relatively inert tissue that may be different from the target site of the drug. Some storage sites include the following:

1. *Adipose:*   The primary site for drug storage in the body is adipose tissue. Because many drugs are lipid soluble, fat deposits throughout the body can serve as a considerable reservoir for these compounds. In some individuals, the amount of fat in the body can reach as high as 40 to 50 percent of body weight, thus creating an extensive storage compartment. Once drugs have been stored in adipose tissue, they tend to remain there for long periods because of the low metabolic rate and poor blood perfusion of these tissues. Examples of drugs that tend to be stored in fat include the highly lipid-soluble anesthetics such as the barbiturates (thiopental) and inhalation anesthetics (halothane).
2. *Bone:*   Bone acts as a storage site for several toxic agents, especially the heavy metals like lead. Also, drugs such as the tetracyclines, which bind to and form molecular complexes with heavy metals, are stored within bone.
3. *Muscle:*   Binding of drugs to components within the muscle may create the long-term storage of these compounds. Various agents may be actively transported into the muscle cell and may form reversible bonds to intracellular structures such as proteins, nucleoproteins, or phospholipids. An example is the antimalarial drug quinacrine.
4. *Organs:*   Drugs are often stored within certain organs such as the liver and kidneys. As in muscle cells, the drug may enter the cell passively or by active transport and then form bonds to subcellular components. Examples include the antimicrobial aminoglycoside agents (such as gentamicin and streptomycin), which accumulate in renal proximal tubular cells.

TABLE 2–2 Examples of Volume of Distribution

Drug	Amount Administered	Plasma Concentration	Volume of Distribution	Indication	Examples
A	420 mg	0.01 mg/mL	$\dfrac{420 \text{ mg}}{0.01 \text{ mg/mL}} = 42,000 \text{ mL} = 42 \text{ L}$	Uniform distribution	Erythromycin, lithium
B	420 mg	0.05 mg/mL	$\dfrac{420 \text{ mg}}{0.05 \text{ mg/mL}} = 8400 \text{ mL} = 8.4 \text{ L}$	Retained in plasma	Aspirin, valproic acid
C	420 mg	0.001 mg/mL	$\dfrac{420 \text{ mg}}{0.001 \text{ mg/mL}} = 420,000 \text{ mL} = 420 \text{ L}$	Sequestered in tissues	Morphine, quinidine

Adverse Consequences of Drug Storage

High concentrations of drugs and toxic compounds within tissues can cause local damage to the tissues in which they are stored. This event is particularly true for toxic compounds that are incorporated and stored in the matrix of bone or that are highly concentrated within specific organs. For instance, aluminum may be stored in organs such as the liver and kidney, as well as in certain central neurons.[34] Since aluminum is neurotoxic, some neurologic disorders such as Alzheimer's disease, Parkinson's disease, and amyotrophic lateral sclerosis have been associated with the accumulation of this metal in certain nerve cells.[14,40,41] Continued research will be necessary to determine the exact relationship between specific neurologic disorders and aluminum and other neurotoxins.

Another problem of drug storage occurs when the storage site acts as a reservoir that "soaks up" the drug and prevents it from reaching the target site. For instance, a highly lipid-soluble drug such as a general anesthetic must be administered in a sufficient dose to ensure that there will be enough drug available to reach the CNS, despite the tendency for much of the drug to be sequestered in the body's fat stores. Storage sites may also be responsible for the redistribution of drugs. This occurrence is seen when the drug begins to leak out of the storage reservoir after plasma levels of the drug have begun to diminish. In this way, the drug may be reintroduced to the target site long after the original dose should have been eliminated. This redistribution may explain why certain individuals experience prolonged effects of the drug or extended adverse side effects.

NEWER TECHNIQUES FOR DRUG DELIVERY

Controlled-Release Preparations

Controlled-release preparations, also known as *timed-release* or *extended-release preparations*, are generally designed to permit a slower and more prolonged absorption of the drug from the gastrointestinal tract. This may offer several advantages such as decreasing the number of doses needed each day, preventing large fluctuations in the amount of drug appearing in the plasma, and sustaining plasma levels throughout the night.[7] This type of preparation has been used successfully with several types of drugs, including cardiovascular medications (beta blockers, calcium channel blockers)[16,18] and narcotic analgesics such as morphine.[13] Controlled-release preparations will probably continue to gain popularity as a means for administering these and other medications in the future.

Implanted Drug Delivery Systems

Several techniques have been developed whereby some type of drug "reservoir" is implanted surgically within the body and the drug is then released in a controlled fashion from the implanted reservoir.[36,42,47] These drug reservoirs typically consist of a small container placed under the skin in the abdomen. These containers are often programmed to allow a small, measured dose of the drug to be released periodically from the reservoir. Alternatively, the reservoir can be controlled electronically from outside the body through the use of small, remote-control devices, thus allowing the patient to regulate release of the drug as needed. In some cases, the drug reservoir may be connected by a small cannula to a specific body compartment, such as the subarachnoid space or epidural space, and the drug can be delivered directly into that space. This type of system appears to be very helpful in applying certain drugs such as analgesics, anesthetics, and muscle relaxants to the spinal cord.[36,42,47]

Another type of implantable system has been developed recently that incorporates the drug into some type of biodegradable substance such as a polymer matrix or gel.[31,35] The drug-polymer complex is then implanted in the body and the drug is slowly released into the surrounding tissues as the matrix gradually dissolves. This type of system is still fairly experimental, but it has shown promise in being able to deliver hormones such as insulin and local anesthetics such as bupivacaine.[31,35]

Hence, implantable drug delivery systems are being considered as a potential means of administering several drugs including analgesics, muscle relaxants, and insulin. Improvements in the technology of this type of drug delivery will hopefully permit increased clinical applications of these systems in the near future. The use of implantable drug delivery systems with specific types of medications will be discussed in more detail when these medications are addressed in subsequent chapters in this book.

Targeting Drug Delivery to Specific Cells and Tissues

Some very innovative approaches have been attempted on a molecular level to try to target the drug specifically to the cells that require treatment. For instance, specific types of antibodies (monoclonal antibodies) can be synthesized and attached to certain drugs such as the cytotoxic agents often used in cancer chemotherapy.[8] The antibodies are then attracted to antigens located on the surface of the tumor cells. This offers the distinct advantage of focusing the drug more directly on the cancerous cells rather than on healthy human tissues. Other cellular techniques have been investigated that could also help direct the drug to the affected tissues. One such technique involves the possibility that white blood cells can be used to transport antibacterial drugs to the site of infection.[46] The white blood cells engulf the medication by phagocytosis. Then, by normal chemotactic mechanisms, these cells are drawn to the infection site, where the cells will ultimately be degraded, thus releasing the drug.

The idea of targeting drugs to specific tissues through various cellular and molecular mechanisms is still fairly experimental at this point. These techniques have shown considerable promise, however, and may ultimately be extremely useful in increasing the effectiveness of certain drugs while decreasing their side effects.

SUMMARY

In order for any drug to be effective, it must be able to reach specific target tissues. The goal of drug administration is to deliver the drug in the least complicated manner that will still allow sufficient concentrations of the active form of the drug to arrive at the desired site. Each route of administration has certain advantages and disadvantages that will determine how much and how fast the drug is delivered to specific tissues. In addition to the route of administration, the distribution of the drug within the body must be taken into account. Simply introducing the drug into certain body fluids such as the bloodstream does not ensure its entry into the desired tissues. Factors such as tissue permeability and protein binding may influence how the drug is dispersed within the various fluid compartments within the body. Finally, some drugs have a tendency to be stored in certain tissues for prolonged periods of time. This may produce serious toxic effects because of high concentrations of the compound damaging the cells in which it is stored.

REFERENCES

1. Agnew, WS: Voltage-regulated sodium channel molecules. Annu Rev Physiol 46:517, 1984.
2. Almers, W and Stirling, C: Distribution of transport proteins over animal cell membranes. J Membr Biol 77:169, 1984.
3. Ashburn, MA and Stanley, TH: Non-invasive drug delivery systems for the management of postoperative pain. Prog Anesth 5:146, 1991.
4. Bailey, DG, et al: Interaction of citrus juices with felodipine and nifedipine. Lancet 337:268, 1991.
5. Balfour, JA and McTavish, D: Transdermal estradiol: A review of its pharmacological profile, and therapeutic potential in the prevention of postmenopausal osteoporosis. Drugs and Aging 2:487, 1992.
6. Benet, LZ: Pharmacokinetics: Absorption, distribution and excretion. In Katzung, BL (ed): Basic and Clinical Pharmacology, ed 5. Appleton & Lange, Norwalk, CT, 1992.
7. Benet, LZ, Mitchell, JR, and Sheiner, LB: Pharmacokinetics: The dynamics of drug absorption, distribution and elimination. In Gilman, AG, et al (eds): The Pharmacological Basis of Therapeutics, ed 8. Pergamon Press, New York, 1990.
8. Blakely, DC: Drug targeting with monoclonal antibodies: A review. Acta Oncologica 31:91, 1992.
9. Brockmeier, D and Ostrowski, J: Mean time and first pass metabolism. Eur J Clin Pharmacol 29:45, 1985.
10. Brown, L and Langer, R: Transdermal delivery of drugs. Annu Rev Med 39:221, 1988.
11. Ciccone, CD: Iontophoresis. In Robinson, AJ and Snyder-Mackler, L: Clinical Electrophysiology, ed 2. Williams & Wilkins, Baltimore, 1994.
12. Corson, SL: A decade of experience with transdermal estrogen replacement therapy: Overview of key pharmacologic and clinical findings. Int J Fertil 38:79, 1993.
13. Deschamps, M, et al: The evaluation of analgesic effects in cancer patients as exemplified by a double-blind, cross-over study of immediate-release versus controlled-release morphine. J Pain Symptom Management 7:384, 1992.
14. Doll, R: Review: Alzheimer's disease and environmental aluminum. Age Ageing 22:138, 1993.
15. Ebadi, M: Pharmacology: A Review with Questions and Answers, ed 2. Little, Brown, & Co, Boston, 1993.
16. Feliciano, NR, et al: Pharmacokinetic and pharmacodynamic comparison of an osmotic release oral metoprolol tablet and the metoprolol conventional tablet. Am Heart J 120(2, suppl):483, 1990.
17. Finnen, MJ, Herdman, ML, and Shuster, S: Distribution and sub-cellular localization of drug metabolizing enzymes in the skin. Br J Dermatol 113:713, 1985.
18. Frishman, WH: A new extended-release formulation of diltiazem HCl for the treatment of mild-to-moderate hypertension. J Clin Pharmacol 33:612, 1993.
19. Gillis, CN: Pharmacologic aspects of metabolic processes in the pulmonary microcirculation. Ann Rev Toxicol 26:183, 1986.
20. Gong, L and Middleton, RK: Sublingual administration of opioids. Ann Pharmacotherapy 26:1525, 1992.
21. Gora, ML: Nicotine transdermal systems. Ann Pharmacotherapy 27:742, 1993.
22. Gorsline, J, et al: Steady-state pharmacokinetics and dose relationship of nicotine delivered from Nicoderm. J Clin Pharmacol 33:161, 1993.
23. Guyton, AG: Textbook of Medical Physiology, ed 8. WB Saunders, Philadelphia, 1990.
24. Henley, EJ: Transcutaneous drug delivery: Iontophoresis, phonophoresis. CRC Crit Rev Phys Rehabil Med 2:139, 1991.
25. Hobbs, AS and Albers, RW: The structure of proteins involved in active membrane transport. Annu Rev Biophys Bioeng 9:259, 1980.
26. Johansson, O, Lindberg, T, and Melander, A: In-vivo absorption of theophylline and salicylic acid from rat small intestine. Acta Pharmacol Toxicol 55:335, 1984.
27. Kaneniwa, N, Hiura, M, and Funaki, T: The absorption kinetics of barbiturates in rabbits. Int J Pharmacol 26:157, 1985.
28. Kao, J, Patterson, FK, and Hall, J: Skin penetration and metabolism of topically applied chemicals in six mammalian species, including man: An in-vitro study with benzo(a)pyrene and testosterone. Toxicol Appl Pharmacol 81:502, 1985.
29. Katzung, BG: Introduction. In Katzung, BG (ed): Basic and Clinical Pharmacology, ed 5. Appleton & Lange, Norwalk, CT, 1992.

30. Kuhn, MA (ed): Pharmacotherapeutics: A Nursing Process Approach, ed 3. FA Davis, Philadelphia, 1994.
31. Kwon, IC, Bae, YH, and Kim, SW: Electrically erodible polymer gel for controlled release of drugs. Nature 354:291, 1992.
32. Latore, R and Alvarez, O: Voltage-dependent channels in lipid bilayer membranes. Physiol Rev 61:77, 1981.
33. Levy, RH and Bauer, LA: Basic pharmacokinetics. Therapeutic Drug Monitoring 8:47, 1986.
34. Lione, A: Aluminum toxicity and the aluminum containing medications. Pharmacol Ther 29:255, 1985.
35. Masters, DB, et al: Prolonged regional nerve blockade by controlled release of local anesthetic from a biodegradable polymer matrix. Anesthesiology 79:340, 1993.
36. Meythaler, JM, et al: Continuous intrathecal baclofen in spinal cord spasticity: A prospective study. Am J Phys Med Rehabil 71:321, 1992.
37. Miller, C: Intergral membrane channels: Studies in model membranes. Physiol Rev 63:1209, 1983.
38. Ochs, HR, et al: Cerebrospinal fluid uptake and peripheral distribution of centrally acting drugs: Relation to lipid solubility. J Pharm Pharmacol 37:428, 1985.
39. Oguey, D, et al: Effect of food on the bioavailability of low-dose methotrexate in patients with rheumatoid arthritis. Arthritis Rheum 35:611, 1992.
40. Perl, DP and Brody, AR: Alzheimer's disease: X-ray spectrometric evidence of aluminum accumulation in neurofibrillary tangle-bearing neurons. Science 208:299, 1980.
41. Perl, DP, et al: Intraneuronal accumulation in amyotrophic lateral sclerosis and parkinsonism dementia of Guam. Science 217:1053, 1982.
42. Penn, SD, et al: Intrathecal baclofen for severe spinal spasticity. N Engl J Med 320:1517, 1989.
43. Rizk, TE, Pinals, RS, and Talaiver, AS: Corticosteroid injections in adhesive capsulitis: Investigation of their value and site. Arch Phys Med Rehabil 72:20, 1991.
44. Rogart, R: Sodium channels in nerve and muscle membranes. Annu Rev Physiol 43:711, 1981.
45. Routledge, PA: Factors contributing to variability in drug pharmacokinetics: II. Drug distribution. J Clin Hosp Pharm 10:15, 1983.
46. Schentag, JJ and Ballow, CH: Tissue-directed pharmacokinetics. Am J Med 91(suppl 3A):5S, 1991.
47. Shaw, HL: Treatment of the patient with cancer using parenteral electrical drug administration. Cancer 70(4, suppl):993, 1992.
48. Sheridan, E, Patterson, HR, and Gustafson, EA: Falconer's: The Drug, the Nurse, the Patient, ed 7. WB Saunders, Philadelphia, 1985.
49. Shohat, M, et al: Adrenocortical suppression by topical application of glucocorticoids in infants with seborrheic dermatitis. Clin Pediatr 25:209, 1986.
50. Singer, SJ and Nicolson, GL: The fluid-mosaic model of the structure of membranes. Science 175:720, 1972.
51. Theodorsen, L and Brors, O: The importance of lipid solubility and receptor selectivity of beta-adrenoceptor blocking drugs for the occurrence of symptoms and side effects in out-patients. J Intern Med 226:17, 1989.
52. Urtti, A and Salminen, L: Minimizing systemic absorption of topically administered ophthalmic drugs. Surv Ophthalmol 37:435, 1993.
53. Weiss, M: On pharmacokinetics in target tissues. Biopharm Drug Dispos 6:57, 1985.
54. Yammamoto, A, et al: Immunological control of drug absorption from the gastrointestinal tract: Effect of local anaphylaxis on the intestinal absorption of low molecular weight drugs in the rat. J Pharmacobiodyn 8:830, 1985.
55. Yee, LY and Lopez, JR: Transdermal fentanyl. Ann Pharmacother 26:1393, 1992.
56. Ziskin, MC, McDiarmid, T, and Michlovitz, SL: Therapeutic ultrasound. In Michlovitz, SL (ed): Thermal Agents in Rehabilitation, ed 2. FA Davis, Philadelphia, 1990.

CHAPTER 3

Pharmacokinetics II: Drug Elimination

All drugs must eventually be eliminated from the body to terminate their effect and to prevent excessive accumulation of the drug. Drugs are usually eliminated by chemically altering the original compound while it is still in the body so that it is no longer active (*biotransformation*), by excreting the active form of the drug from the body (*excretion*), or by a combination of biotransformation and excretion. These methods of drug elimination will be discussed here.

BIOTRANSFORMATION

Drug metabolism, or **biotransformation**, refers to chemical changes that take place in the drug following administration. Enzymes located within specific tissues are responsible for catalyzing changes in the drug's structure and subsequently altering the pharmacologic properties of the drug. The location of these enzymes and the reactions involved in biotransformation are discussed later in this chapter.

Biotransformation usually results in an altered version of the original compound known as a **metabolite,** which is usually inactive or has a greatly reduced level of pharmacologic activity. Occasionally, the metabolite has a higher level of activity than the original compound. In cases where the metabolite has a higher level of activity, the drug may be given in an inactive, or "prodrug," form that will be activated via biotransformation following administration. However, termination of the drug after it has exerted its pharmacologic effect is the primary function of drug biotransformation.

Inactivation of a drug and termination of its effect once the drug is no longer needed are often essential. For instance, the effects of general and local anesthetics must eventually wear off and allow the patient to resume normal function. Although termination of drug activity can occur when the active form of the drug is excreted from the body via organs such as the kidneys, excretory mechanisms are often too slow to effectively terminate the activity of most drugs within a reasonable time period. If excretion were the only way to terminate drug activity, some compounds would continue to exert their effects for several days or even weeks. Biotransformation of the drug into an inactive form usually occurs within a matter of minutes or hours, thus reducing the chance for toxic effects caused by drug accumulation or prolonged drug activity.

Cellular Mechanisms of Drug Biotransformation

The chemical changes that occur during drug metabolism usually are caused by oxidation, reduction, hydrolysis, or conjugation of the original compound.[5] Examples of each type of reaction are listed in Table 3–1. Each type of reaction and the location of the enzymes catalyzing the reaction are also discussed here.

TABLE 3–1 Examples of Drug Biotransformation Reactions

	Examples
I. Oxidation	
A. Side chain (aliphatic) hydroxylation	
$RCH_2CH_3 \xrightarrow{[O]} RCHCH_3$ (OH)	Ibuprofen
B. N-oxidation	
$(R)_2N \xrightarrow{[O]} R_2N = 0$	Acetaminophen
C. Deamination	
$RCH_2NH_2 \xrightarrow{[O]} RCHO + NH_3$	Diazepam
II. Reduction	
A. Nitro reductions	
$RNO_2 \rightarrow RNH_2$	Dantrolene
B. Carbonyl reductions	
$RCR' \rightarrow RCHR'$ (O → OH)	Methadone
III. Hydrolysis	
A. Esters	
$RCOR' \rightarrow RCOOH + R'OH$ (O)	Aspirin
B. Amides	
$RCNR' \rightarrow RCOOH + R'NH_2$ (O)	Lidocaine
IV. Conjugation	
A. Acetylation	
$RNH_2 + AcetylCoA \rightarrow RNHCCH_3 + CoA\text{-}SH$ (O)	Clonazepam
B. Glycine conjugation	
$RCOOH \rightarrow RCSCoA + NH_2CH_2COOH \rightarrow$ (O)	
$RCNHCH_2COOH + CoA\text{-}SH$ (O)	Benzoic acid

Parent drug compounds are represented by the letter "R." Examples are types of drugs that undergo biotransformation via the respective type of chemical reaction.

FIGURE 3–1. Drug oxidation catalyzed by drug microsomal metabolizing system (DMMS) enzymes.

1. *Oxidation:* Oxidation occurs because of the addition of oxygen or the removal of hydrogen from the original compound. Oxidation reactions comprise the predominant method of drug biotransformation in the body. The enzymes responsible for this type of drug metabolism are located on the smooth endoplasmic reticulum of specific cells and are referred to as the **drug microsomal metabolizing system** (DMMS). The general scheme of drug oxidation as catalyzed by the DMMS is shown in Figure 3–1.
2. *Reduction:* Reduction reactions consist of removing oxygen or adding hydrogen to the original compound. Enzymes that are located in the cell cytoplasm are usually responsible for reducing the drug.
3. *Hydrolysis:* The original compound is broken into separate parts. The enzymes responsible for hydrolysis of the drug are located at several sites within the cell (i.e., the endoplasmic reticulum and cytoplasm) as well as extracellularly (e.g., circulating in the plasma).
4. *Conjugation:* In conjugation reactions, the intact drug, or the metabolite of one of the reactions described earlier, is coupled to an endogenous substance such as acetyl coenzyme A (acetyl CoA), glucuronic acid, or an amino acid. Enzymes catalyzing drug conjugations are found in the cytoplasm and on the endoplasmic reticulum.

The chemical reactions involved in drug biotransformation are also classified as either phase I or phase II reactions.[12] Phase I reactions consist of those using oxidation, reduction, or hydrolysis. Phase II reactions involve conjugation of the parent drug or the metabolite of a drug that was already metabolized using a phase I reaction.

Regardless of the type of chemical reaction used, biotransformation also helps in the excretion of the metabolite from the body by creating a more polar compound.[5] After one or more of the reactions just described, the remaining drug metabolite usually has a greater tendency to be ionized in the body fluids. The ionized metabolite is more water soluble, thus becoming more easily transported in the bloodstream to the kidneys. Upon reaching the kidneys, the polar metabolite can be excreted from the body in the urine. The contribution of biotransformation toward renal excretion is discussed in a later section.

Organs Responsible for Drug Biotransformation

The primary location for drug metabolism is the liver.[5,34] DMMS enzymes are abundant on hepatic smooth endoplasmic reticulum, and liver cells also contain other cytoplasmic enzymes responsible for drug reduction and hydrolysis. Other organs that contain metabolizing enzymes and exhibit considerable ability for drug transformation include the lungs, kidneys, gastrointestinal epithelium, and skin. Drug metabolism can be radically altered in conditions where these tissues are damaged. For instance, inactivation of certain drugs may be significantly delayed in the patient with hepatitis or cirrhosis of the liver.[17,42,45] As would be expected, dosages in these patients must be adjusted accordingly to prevent drug accumulation and toxicity.

Enzyme Induction

A frequent problem in drug metabolism is the phenomenon of **enzyme induction**.[12] Prolonged use of certain drugs "induces" the body to be able to enzymatically destroy the drug more rapidly, usually because of either more of the metabolizing enzymes being manufactured or less being degraded. Enzyme induction may cause drugs to be metabolized more rapidly than expected, thus decreasing their therapeutic effect. This may be one reason why **tolerance** to some drugs occurs when the drug is used for extended periods (tolerance is the need for increased dosages of the drug to produce the same effect). Long-term ingestion or inhalation of other exogenous compounds such as alcohol, cigarette smoke, or environmental toxins may also cause enzyme induction.[15,28,33] When this occurs, medicinal drugs may be more rapidly metabolized even when they are first administered because of the preexisting enzyme induction.

DRUG EXCRETION

The kidneys are the primary site for drug excretion.[5] The functional unit of the kidney is the nephron (Fig. 3–2), and each kidney is composed of approximately 1 million nephrons. Usually the metabolized or conjugated version of the original drug reaches the nephron and is then filtered at the glomerulus. Following filtration at the glomerulus, the compound traverses the proximal convoluted tubule, loop of Henle, and distal convoluted tubule before reaching the collecting ducts. If the drug is not reabsorbed while moving through the nephron, it will ultimately leave the body in the urine. As discussed earlier, biotransformation plays a significant role in creating a polar, water-soluble metabolite that is able to reach the kidneys through the bloodstream. Only drugs or their metabolites that are relatively polar will be excreted in significant amounts by the kidney because the ionized metabolite has a greater tendency to remain in the nephron and not be reabsorbed into the body.[39] Nonpolar compounds that are filtered by the kidneys are relatively lipophilic and can easily be passively reabsorbed back into the body by diffusing through the wall of the nephron. However, the polar metabolite is relatively impermeable to the epithelium lining the nephron and tends to remain "trapped" in the nephron following filtration, where it will eventually be excreted in the urine (see Fig. 3–2).

In addition to filtration, some drugs may be secreted into the nephron by active transport mechanisms located in the proximal convoluted tubule. Two basic transport systems exist, one for the secretion of organic acids (e.g., uric acid) and one for the secretion of organic bases (e.g., choline, histamine).[5] (A third transport system that ac-

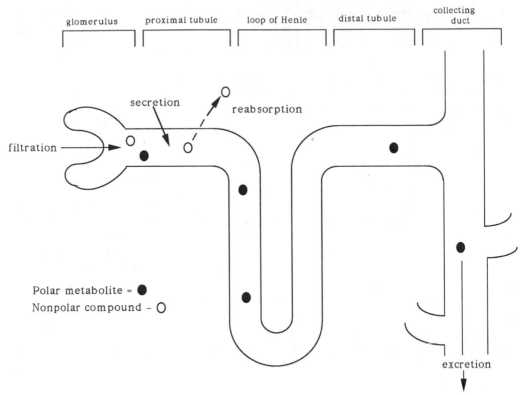

FIGURE 3–2. Drug excretion at the nephron. Compounds reach the nephron by filtration and/or secretion. Polar metabolites remain trapped in the nephron and are eventually excreted. Nonpolar compounds are able to diffuse back into the body (reabsorption).

tively secretes the chelating agent EDTA* has also been identified, but its significance is unclear). Certain drugs may be transported by one of these carrier systems so that they are actively secreted into the nephron. For example, penicillin is actively secreted via the transport system for organic acids, and hexamethonium† is secreted by the organic base transport system. In these specific cases, elimination of the drug is enhanced by the combined effects of tubular secretion and filtration in delivering the drug to the urine.

Other routes for drug excretion include the lungs and gastrointestinal tract. The lungs play a significant role in excreting volatile drugs, that is, drugs that are usually administered by inhalation. Consequently the lungs serve as the route of both administration and excretion for drugs such as the gaseous anesthetics. The gastrointestinal tract usually plays only a minor role in drug excretion. Certain drugs can be excreted by the liver into the bile and subsequently reach the duodenum via the bile duct. If the drug remains in the gastrointestinal tract, it will eventually be excreted in the feces.

---

*EDTA (ethylenediaminetetraacetate): An agent that binds to (chelates) heavy metals and is sometimes used to treat metallic poisoning (e.g., lead poisoning).

†Hexamethonium: A drug used to block transmission in autonomic ganglia; it is sometimes used to treat a hypertensive crisis (see Chapter 21).

However, most of the secreted bile is reabsorbed, and drugs contained in the bile are often reabsorbed simultaneously. Other minor routes for drug excretion include the sweat, saliva, and breast milk of lactating mothers. Although drugs excreted via lactation are considered a relatively minor route with regard to loss from the mother, the possibility that the infant may imbibe substantial concentrations of the drug does exist. Careful consideration for the welfare of the nursing infant must always be a factor when administering medications to the lactating mother.[7,44]

DRUG ELIMINATION RATES

The rate at which a drug is eliminated is significant in determining the amount and frequency of the dosage of the drug. If a drug is administered much faster than it is eliminated, the drug will accumulate excessively in the body and reach toxic levels. Conversely, if elimination greatly exceeds the rate of delivery, the concentration in the body may never reach therapeutic levels. Several parameters are used to indicate the rate at which a drug is usually eliminated so that dosages may be adjusted accordingly. Two of the primary measurements are *clearance* and *half-life*.

Clearance

Clearance of a drug (CL) can be described in terms of the ability of all organs and tissues to eliminate the drug (systemic clearance) or in terms of the ability of a single organ or tissue to eliminate the drug.[5,30] To calculate clearance from a specific organ, two primary factors must be considered. First, the blood flow to the organ (Q) determines how much drug will be delivered to the organ for elimination. Second, the fraction of drug removed from the plasma as it passes through the organ must be known. This fraction, termed the *extraction ratio*, is equal to the difference in the concentration of drug entering (Ci) and exiting (Co) the organ, divided by the entering concentration (Ci). Clearance by an individual organ is summarized by the following equation:

$$CL = Q \times \frac{Ci - Co}{Ci}$$

The calculation of clearance using this equation is illustrated by the following example. Aspirin is metabolized primarily in the liver. Normal hepatic blood flow (Q) equals 1500 mL/min. If the blood entering the liver contains 200 μg/mL of aspirin (Ci) and the blood leaving the liver contains 134 μg/mL (Co), hepatic clearance of aspirin is calculated as follows:

$$CL_{hepatic} = Q \times \frac{Ci - Co}{Ci}$$

$$= 1500 \text{ mL/min} \times \frac{200 \ \mu g/mL - 134 \ \mu g/mL}{200 \ \mu g/mL}$$

$$= 495 \text{ mL/min}$$

This example illustrates that clearance is actually the amount of plasma from which the drug can be totally removed per unit time. As calculated here, the liver would be able to completely remove aspirin from 495 mL of blood each minute. Tetracycline, a common antibacterial drug, has a clearance equal to 130 mL/min, indicating that this drug would be completely removed from approximately 130 mL of plasma each minute.

Clearance is dependent on the ability of the organ or tissue to extract the drug from the plasma as well as the perfusion of the organ. Some tissues may have an excellent ability to remove the drug from the bloodstream, but clearance is limited because of the amount of blood flow to the organ. Conversely, highly perfused organs may be ineffective in removing the drug, thus prolonging its activity.

In terms of the elimination of the drug from the entire body, systemic clearance is calculated as the sum of all the individual clearances from all organs and tissues (i.e., systemic CL = hepatic CL + renal CL + lung CL, and so on). Note that the elimination of the drug includes the combined processes of loss of the drug from the body (excretion) as well as inactivation of the drug through biotransformation.[30]

Half-Life

In addition to clearance, the **half-life** of the drug is important in describing the length of activity of the compound. Half-life is defined as the amount of time required for 50 percent of the drug remaining in the body to be eliminated.[5,27,30] Most drugs are eliminated in a manner such that a fixed portion of the drug is eliminated in a given time period. For example, a drug such as acetaminophen with a half-life of 2 hours indicates that in each 2-hour period, 50 percent of the acetaminophen still in the body will be eliminated (Fig. 3–3).

Half-life is a function of both clearance and volume of distribution (V_d)[30]; that is, the time it takes to eliminate 50 percent of the drug depends not only on the ability of the organ(s) to remove the drug from the plasma, but also on the distribution or presence of the drug in the plasma. A drug that undergoes extensive inactivation in the liver may have a long half-life if it is sequestered intracellularly in skeletal muscle. Also, disease states that affect either clearance or V_d will affect the half-life of the drug, so dosages must be altered accordingly.

DOSING SCHEDULES AND PLASMA CONCENTRATION

With some medications, it is desirable to bring plasma concentrations of the drug up to a certain level and maintain them at that level. If the drug is administered by continuous intravenous administration, this can be done fairly easily by matching the rate of administration with the rate of drug elimination (clearance), once the desired plasma concentration is achieved (Fig. 3–4). In situations where the drug is given at specific intervals, the dosage must be adjusted to provide an average plasma concentration over the dosing period. Figure 3–4 illustrates that if the dosing interval is relatively long (e.g., 12 hours), the dose must be considerably larger to provide the same relative plasma concentration that would exist in a shorter dosing interval (e.g., 8 hours). Note also that larger doses given further apart result in greater plasma fluctuations, that is, greater maximum and minimum plasma levels over the dosing period.

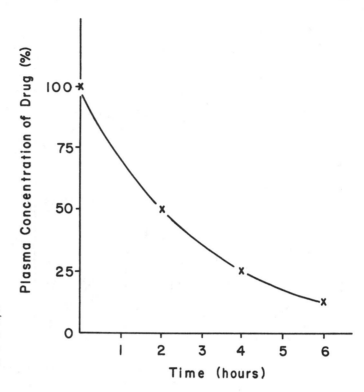

FIGURE 3–3. Elimination of a drug with a half-life of 2 hours. Fifty percent of the drug remaining in the bloodstream is eliminated in each 2-hour period.

Giving smaller doses more frequently provides an equivalent average concentration without the extreme peaks and valleys associated with longer intervals (see Fig. 3–4).

VARIATIONS IN DRUG RESPONSE AND METABOLISM

The fact that different people may react differently to the same relative dosage of a drug is an important and often critical aspect of pharmacology.[34] Two individuals who are given the same drug may exhibit different magnitudes of a beneficial response as well as different adverse effects. Several of the primary factors responsible for variations in the response to drugs are discussed here.

1. *Genetic factors:* Genetic differences are often a major factor in the way in which individuals metabolize specific compounds.[43,47] Genetic variations may result in abnormal or absent drug-metabolizing enzymes.[29,32] This can be harmful or even fatal if the drug is not metabolized and begins to exert toxic effects because of accumulation or prolonged pharmacologic activity. For example, some individuals lack the appropriate plasma cholinesterase that breaks down circulating acetylcholine and acetylcholine-like compounds. Succinylcholine is a neuromuscular blocking agent that is usually administered during general anesthesia to ensure muscular relaxation during surgery. Normally, the succinylcholine is quickly degraded by plasma cholinesterase. However, individuals lacking the appropriate form of the cholinesterase may suffer respiratory paralysis because the succinylcholine exerts its effect much longer than the expected period of time.

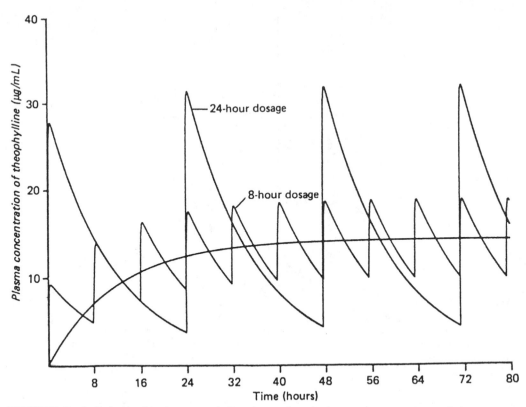

FIGURE 3–4. Relationship between dosing interval and plasma concentrations of the antiasthmatic drug theophylline. A constant intravenous infusion (shown by the smoothly rising line) yields a desired plasma level of 15 μg/ml. The same *average* plasma concentration is achieved when a dose of 340 mg is taken every 8 hours, or a dose of 1020 mg every 24 hours. However, note the fluctuations in plasma concentration seen when doses are taken at specific hourly intervals. (From Katzung, BG: Basic and Clinical Pharmacology, ed 4. Appleton & Lange, East Norwalk, CT, 1989, with permission.)

2. *Disease:* Structural or functional damage to an organ or tissue responsible for drug metabolism or excretion presents an obvious problem in pharmacology. Diseases that initiate changes in tissue function or blood flow to specific organs can dramatically affect the elimination of various drugs.[5,16,30,35,38] Certain diseases may also impair the absorption and distribution of the drug, further complicating the problem of individualized response.[40,45,46] The significance of disease in affecting the patient's response is crucial since the response to the medication may be affected by the very same pathology that the drug is being used to treat. For instance, renal excretion of antibiotics such as the aminoglycosides is altered radically in many types of bacterial infection, but these drugs are typically administered to treat the same infections that alter their own excretion.[2] Consequently, great care must be taken to adjust the dosage accordingly when administering medications in conditions where drug elimination may be altered.[6,24,35]

3. *Drug interactions:* When two or more drugs are present in the body at the same time, the chance exists that they may interact and alter each other's effects and metabolism.[21] Two similar compounds may act synergistically to produce a cumulative effect that is greater than each drug would produce alone. In some situations, this

cumulative effect may be desirable if the augmented response is anticipated and well controlled.[9,41] However, two or more drugs with similar actions may lead to an adverse response even if each individual drug is given in a nontoxic dose. For instance, taking two CNS depressants simultaneously (e.g., barbiturates and alcohol) may cause such severe CNS inhibition that the additive effects are lethal. In contrast to an additive effect, drugs with opposite actions may essentially cancel each other out, thus negating or reducing the beneficial effects of one or both medications. A drug that causes bronchodilation (i.e., for the treatment of asthma) will be negated by an agent that constricts the bronchioles.

Some of the most serious problems occurring in drug interactions have to do with one drug delaying the biotransformation of the other. If the enzymes that normally metabolize a drug are inhibited by a second compound, the original drug will exert its effect for prolonged periods, possibly leading to toxic effects.[8,23] For instance, the antiulcer drug cimetidine (Tagamet) inhibits the hepatic metabolism of oral anticoagulants such as warfarin (Coumadin). Taking these two drugs together tends to cause elevated plasma levels of the anticoagulant, which may lead to prolonged blood clotting and possible hemorrhage. Another type of interaction occurs when two or more drugs alter each other's absorption and distribution and can occur when they compete for the same active transport carrier or bind to the same plasma proteins. An example is the interaction between aspirin and methotrexate, a drug used to treat cancer and rheumatoid arthritis. Aspirin can displace methotrexate from its binding site on plasma proteins, thus allowing relatively higher amounts of unbound or "free" methotrexate to exist in the bloodstream. The increased levels of "free" methotrexate may lead to toxic effects.

The potential for drug interactions must be carefully evaluated by the prescribing physician and pharmacist. All individuals dealing with the patient must be alert for the early signs of toxic effects due to such interactions.

4. *Age.* In general, older patients are more sensitive to most drugs.[11,25] Many drugs are not metabolized as quickly in the elderly, resulting in higher plasma levels than those that would occur in younger adults given equivalent doses.[3,18,19] This fact may simply be because changes in organ structure and function are part of the aging process. Children are also subject to problems and variability in drug metabolism.[36] Adjusting the dosage appropriately for the smaller body mass of a child is often difficult. Newborns may totally lack specific drug-metabolizing enzymes, thus prolonging the effects of certain drugs in the very young patient.[31] In the elderly and the young person, the combined effects of age *and* disease dramatically increase the complexity of pharmacokinetic variability, so special care must be taken in prescribing appropriate dosages in these situations.

5. *Diet:* Diet has been shown to affect the metabolism and response to many drugs. Animal and human studies have indicated that total caloric input as well as the percentage of calories obtained from different sources (carbohydrates, proteins, and fats) will influence drug pharmacokinetics.[13,22,26] Specific dietary constituents such as cruciferous vegetables and charcoal-broiled beef can also alter drug metabolism.[1] Fortunately, most food-drug interactions are not serious and will not alter the clinical effects of the drug. However, there are a few well-known food-drug combinations that should be avoided because of their potentially serious interaction. For instance, certain foods such as fermented cheese and wine should not be ingested with drugs that inhibit the monoamine oxidase enzyme (MAO inhibitors). These foods contain high amounts of tyramine, which stimulates the release of catecholamines (norepinephrine, epinephrine) within the body. MAO-inhibiting drugs

work by suppressing the destruction of catecholamines, thus allowing higher levels of norepinephrine and epinephrine to occur. (MAO inhibitors are frequently used in the treatment of depression; see Chapter 7.) Consequently, when MAO inhibitors are taken with tyramine-containing foods, excessive levels of catecholamines may develop, leading to a dangerous increase in blood pressure (hypertensive crisis). Clinicians should be aware of this well-known interaction and be on the alert for other such interactions as new drugs arrive on the market.[10]

6. *Other factors:* A number of additional factors may alter the predicted response of the patient to a drug. Environmental and occupational hazards may induce certain toxins that alter drug absorption and metabolism.[15] Factors such as cigarette smoking and alcohol consumption have been shown to influence the metabolism of specific compounds.[28,33] Drug distribution and metabolism may be altered in the obese patient, or in response to chronic and acute exercise.[4,14,18,37] Individuals with spinal cord injuries seem to have a decreased ability to absorb certain drugs from their gastrointestinal tract, although the reasons for this are not known.[20] Clearly, the way each individual responds to a medication is affected by any number of factors, and these must be taken into account whenever possible.

SUMMARY

Drug elimination occurs because of the combined effects of drug metabolism and excretion. Elimination is essential in terminating drug activity within a reasonable and predictable time frame. Various tissues and organs (especially the liver and kidneys) are involved in drug elimination, and injury to or disease of these tissues can markedly alter the response to certain drugs. In cases of disease or injury, dosages must frequently be adjusted to prevent adverse side effects due to altered elimination rates. Many other environmental, behavioral, and genetic factors may also alter drug metabolism and disposition, and possible variability in the patient's response should always be a matter of concern when selecting the type and amount of the drug.

REFERENCES

1. Anderson, KE, et al: Nutrient regulation of chemical metabolism in humans. Fed Proc 44:130, 1985.
2. Aronson, JK and Reynolds, DJM: ABC of monitoring drug therapy: Aminoglycoside antibiotics. Br Med J 305:1421, 1992.
3. Baillie, SP, et al: Age and the pharmacokinetics of morphine. Age Ageing 18:258, 1989.
4. Benedek, IH, Blouin, RA, and McNamara PJ: Serum protein binding and the role of increased alpha-acid glycoprotein in moderately obese male subjects. Br J Clin Pharmacol 18:941, 1984.
5. Benet, LZ, Mitchell, JR, and Sheiner, LB: Pharmacokinetics: The dynamics of drug absorption, distribution, and elimination. In Gilman, AG, et al (eds): The Pharmacological Basis of Therapeutics, ed 8. Pergamon Press, New York, 1990.
6. Bennet, WM, et al: Drug prescribing in renal failure: Dosing guidelines for adults. Am J Kidney Dis 3:155, 1983.
7. Berglund, F, et al: Drug use during pregnancy and breast feeding: A classification system. Acta Obstet Gynecol Scand 126(suppl):1, 1984.
8. Bergstrom, RF, Peyton, AL, and Lemberger, L: Quantification and mechanism of the fluoxetine and tricyclic antidepressant interaction. Clin Pharmacol Ther 51:239, 1992.
9. Caranasos, GJ, Stewart, RB, and Cluff, LE: Clinically desirable drug interactions. Annu Rev Pharmacol Toxicol 25:67, 1985.
10. Carr, CJ: Food and drug interactions. Annu Rev Pharmacol Toxicol 22:19, 1982.
11. Ciccone, CD: Geriatric pharmacology. In Guccione, AA (ed): Geriatric Physical Therapy. CV Mosby, St. Louis, 1993.

12. Correia, MA: Drug biotransformation. In Katzung, B (ed): Basic and Clinical Pharmacology, ed 5. Appleton & Lange, Norwalk, CT, 1992.

13. Cuddy, PG, et al: Theophylline disposition following parenteral feeding of malnourished patients. Ann Pharmacother 27:846, 1993.

14. Dossing, M: Effect of acute and chronic exercise on hepatic drug metabolism. Clin Pharmacokin 10:426, 1985.

15. Dossing, M: Changes in hepatic microsomal function in workers exposed to mixtures of chemicals. Clin Pharmacol Ther 32:340, 1982.

16. Elston, AC, Bayliss, MK, and Park, GR: Effect of renal failure on drug metabolism by the liver. Br J Anaesth 71:282, 1993.

17. Fenyves, D, Gariepy, L, and Villeneuve, JP: Clearance by the liver in cirrhosis. Relationship between propranolol metabolism in vitro and its extraction by the perfused liver in the rat. Hepatology 17:301, 1993.

18. Greenblat, DJ, et al: Effect of age, gender and obesity on midazolam kinetics. Anesthesiology 61:27, 1984.

19. Groen, K, et al: The relationship between phenazone (antipyrine) metabolite formation and theophylline metabolism in healthy and frail elderly women. Clin Pharmacokin 25:136, 1993.

20. Halstead, LS, et al: Drug absorption in spinal cord injuries. Arch Phys Med Rehabil 66:298, 1985.

21. Hansten, PD: Appendix I. Important drug interactions. In Katzung, B (ed): Basic and Clinical Pharmacology, ed 5. Appleton & Lange, Norwalk, CT, 1992.

22. Hathcock, JN: Metabolic mechanisms of drug-nutrient interactions. Fed Proc 44:124, 1985.

23. Honig, PK, et al: Terfenadine-ketoconazole interaction: Pharmacokinetic and electrocardiographic consequences. JAMA 269:1513, 1993.

24. Hoyer, J, Schulte, KL, and Lenz, T: Clinical pharmacokinetics of angiotensin converting enzyme (ACE) inhibitors in renal failure. Clin Pharmacokin 24:230, 1993.

25. Iwamoto, K, et al: Effect of age on the hepatic clearance of propranolol. J Pharm Pharmacol 37:466, 1985.

26. Jung, D: Pharmacokinetics of theophylline in protein-calorie malnutrition. Biopharm Drug Dispos 6:291, 1985.

27. Keller, F and Scholle, J: Criticism of pharmacokinetic clearance concepts. J Clin Pharmacol Ther Toxicol 21:563, 1983.

28. Lane, EA, Guthrie, S, and Linnoila, M: Effects of ethanol on drug metabolite pharmacokinetics. Clin Pharmacokin 10:228, 1985.

29. Lennard, MS: Oxidative phenotype and the metabolism and action of beta-blockers. Klin Wochenschr 63:285, 1985.

30. Levy, RH and Bauer, LA: Basic pharmacokinetics. Ther Drug Monit 8:47, 1986.

31. Mannering, GJ: Drug metabolism in the newborn. Fed Proc 44:2302, 1985.

32. Meier, UT, et al.: Mephenytoin hydroxylation polymorphism: Characterization of the enzymatic deficiency in liver microsomes of poor metabolizers phenotyped in-vivo. Clin Pharmacol Ther 38:488, 1985.

33. Miners, JO, et al: Influence of cimetidine, sulfinpyrazone, and cigarette smoking on theobromine metabolism in man. Drug Metab Dispos 13:598, 1985.

34. Pang, KS, Xu, X, and St Pierre, MV: Determinants of metabolite disposition. Annu Rev Pharmacol Toxicol 32:623, 1992.

35. Perucca, E, Grimaldi, R, and Crema, A: Interpretation of drug levels in acute and chronic disease states. Clin Pharmacokin 10:498, 1985.

36. Prandota, J-J: Clinical pharmacokinetics of changes in drug elimination in children. Dev Pharmacol Ther 8:311, 1985.

37. Prather, RD, et al: Nicotine pharmacokinetics of Nicoderm (nicotine transdermal system) in women and obese men compared with normal-sized men. J Clin Pharmacol 33:644, 1993.

38. Putensen, C, et al: Plasma lignocaine concentrations associated with extradural analgesia in patients with and without multiple organ failure. Br J Anaesth 69:513, 1992.

39. Regardh, CG: Factors contributing to variability in drug pharmacokinetics: IV. Renal Excretion. J Clin Hosp Pharmacol 10:337, 1985.

40. Routledge, PA: Factors contributing to variability in drug pharmacokinetics: II. Drug distribution. J Clin Hosp Pharmacol 10:15, 1983.

41. Tallarida, RJ: Statistical analysis of drug combinations for synergism: A review. Pain 49:93, 1992.

42. Teunissen, MWE, et al: Antipyrine clearance and metabolite formation in patients with alcohol cirrhosis. Br J Clin Pharmacol 18:707, 1984.

43. Vesell, ES: Pharmacogenetic perspectives: Genes, drugs and disease. Hepatology 4:959, 1984.

44. Wardell, SC and Bousard, LB: Nursing Pharmacology: A Comprehensive Approach to Drug Therapy. Wadsworth Health Sciences, Monterey, CA, 1985.

45. Williams, RL: Drug administration in hepatic disease. N Engl J Med 309:1616, 1983.

46. Yamamoto, A, et al: Immunological control of drug absorption from the gastrointestinal tract: Effects of local anaphylaxis on the intestinal absorption of low molecular weight drugs in the rat. J Pharmacobiodyn 8:830, 1985.

47. Zhou, H-H, et al: Racial differences in drug response: Altered sensitivity to and clearance of propranolol in men of Chinese descent as compared with American whites. N Engl J Med 320:565, 1989.

CHAPTER 4

Drug Receptors

A **receptor** is the component of the cell to which the drug binds and through which a chain of biochemical events is initiated.[4] Most drugs exert their effect by binding to and activating such a receptor, which subsequently brings about some change in the physiologic function of the cell. These receptors can be any cellular macromolecule, but many receptors have been identified as proteins that are located on or within the cell.[1,4,21] The general mechanisms of receptor function in conjunction with their cellular location are discussed here.

RECEPTORS LOCATED ON THE CELL'S SURFACE

Proteins that are located on the outer surface of the cell may act as receptors for endogenous and exogenous compounds.[35] These receptors are responsive primarily to specific amino acid, peptide, or amine compounds.[1] Surface receptors can affect cell function (1) by acting as an ion channel and directly altering membrane permeability, (2) by acting enzymatically to directly influence function within the cell, or (3) by being linked to regulatory proteins that influence the synthesis of intracellular chemicals known as "second messengers." Each of the three basic ways that surface receptors can affect cell function is addressed here.

Surface Receptors Linked Directly to Ion Channels

Membrane receptors may be directly involved in the cellular response to the drug by acting as an ion pore and thus changing the membrane permeability. An example is the acetylcholine receptor located on the postsynaptic membrane of the neuromuscular junction (Fig. 4–1). When bound by acetylcholine molecules, the receptor increases the permeability of the muscle cell to sodium, which results in depolarization of the cell because of sodium influx. Another important example of a receptor–ion channel system is the **gamma-aminobutyric acid (GABA)**–benzodiazepine–chloride ion channel complex found on neuronal membranes in the central nervous system.[22] In this situation, the membrane's permeability to chloride is increased by the binding of both

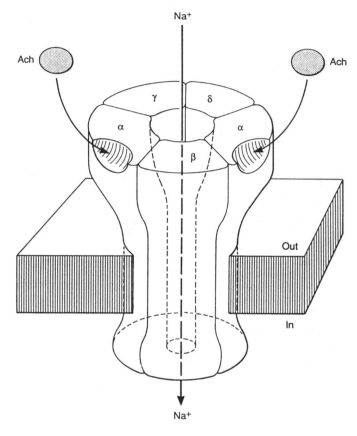

FIGURE 4-1. Schematic model of the acetylcholine receptor, an example of a surface receptor that is linked directly to an ion channel. Binding of two acetylcholine (ACh) molecules to the outer surface of the receptor protein induces opening of a central ion channel, thus allowing sodium to enter the cell. (From Bourne, HR and Roberts, JM: Drug receptors and pharmacodynamics. In Katzung, BG (ed): Basic and Clinical Pharmacology, ed 5. Appleton & Lange, Norwalk, CT, 1992, p 21, with permission.)

the neurotransmitter GABA and the benzodiazepine drugs such as diazepam (Valium) and chlordiazepoxide (Librium). The function of this chloride ion channel complex is discussed in more detail in Chapter 6.

Surface Receptors Linked Directly to Enzymes

Some proteins that span the entire width of the cell membrane may have an extracellular receptor site (binding domain) as well as an intracellular enzymatic component (catalytic domain) (Fig. 4-2). Drugs and endogenous chemicals that bind to the receptor site can change the enzyme activity of the intracellular catalytic component, thus altering the biochemical function within the cell. Receptor-enzyme systems in this category are often referred to as *protein tyrosine kinases* because binding of an appropriate substance to the outer (receptor) component initiates the phosphorylation of certain tyrosine amino acids on the inner (catalytic) component of the protein, which in turn increases the enzyme activity of the intracellular component (see Fig. 4-2). The activated enzymatic component of the receptor then catalyzes the activation of other substrates within the cell.

It appears that insulin and certain growth factors may exert their effects by acting through this type of tyrosine kinase receptor-enzyme system.[4,13] Insulin, for example, binds to the extracellular component of a protein located on skeletal muscle cells,

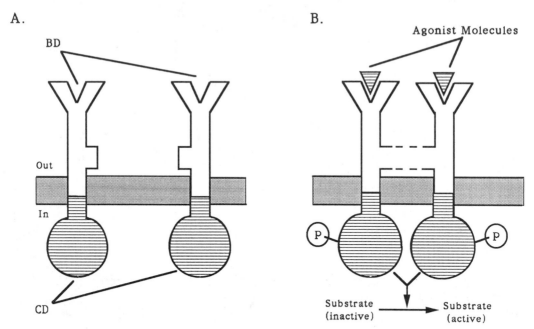

FIGURE 4–2. Example of a surface receptor that is linked directly to intracellular enzyme activity. (*A*) The receptor exists in an inactive state as two subunits: each subunit has a binding domain (BD) on the outer surface and a catalytic domain (CD) on the inner surface. (*B*) Binding of agonist molecules to the BDs causes the subunits to join together and induces phosphorylation (P) of tyrosine receptors on the CD. Tyrosine phosphorylation initiates enzymatic activity of the catalytic units, which then causes substrate activation within the cell.

thereby initiating activation of this protein's enzymatic activity on the inner surface of the cell membrane. This change in enzyme function causes further changes in cell activity, which ultimately result in increased glucose uptake in the muscle cell. The function of insulin receptors and their role in the cause and treatment of diabetes mellitus are discussed in more detail in Chapter 32.

Surface Receptors Linked to Regulatory (G) Proteins: Role of the Second Messenger

Rather than directly affecting membrane permeability or directly influencing enzyme activity, other membrane receptors affect cell function by being linked to an intermediate regulatory protein that is located on the inner surface of the cell's membrane.[12,14,41] These regulatory proteins are activated by binding guanine nucleotides, hence they are often termed **G proteins**.[3,24] When an appropriate substance binds to the surface receptor, the receptor in turn activates the regulatory G protein. The activated G protein then alters the activity of some type of intracellular effector (such as an enzyme), which then leads to a change in cell function.

There appear to be two types of regulatory G proteins: a stimulatory protein (G_s), which increases enzymatic activity in the cell, and an inhibitory protein (G_i), which decreases enzyme activity (Fig. 4–3). The two types of G proteins (stimulatory and inhibitory) are linked to different receptors, and the two receptors are responsive to dif-

FIGURE 4-3. Schematic diagram of a surface receptor–second messenger system. In this example, the second messenger is cAMP, which is synthesized from ATP by the adenylate cyclase enzyme. The enzyme is linked to surface receptors (R_1 and R_2) by regulatory G proteins. G_s stimulates the enzyme and G_i inhibits enzyme activity. Thus, a drug binding to R_1 will increase production of cAMP, while a different drug binding to R_2 will inhibit cAMP production.

ferent drugs. Certain drugs affect the cell by binding to a receptor that is linked to a G_s protein. The activated receptor activates the G_s protein, which in turn activates enzyme activity. Conversely, a drug that binds to a receptor that is linked to a G_i protein inhibits intracellular enzyme activity.

Hence, these regulatory G proteins help account for how drugs can bind to one type of receptor and stimulate cell function, whereas drugs that bind to a different receptor on the same cell can inhibit cell activity. G proteins also seem to be important in mediating other responses of the cell to stimulation or inhibition. For instance, cell function may continue to be affected through the action of G proteins even after the drug has left the binding site on the cell's surface[4]; that is, the drug may bind to the cell for only a short period of time, but this binding is sufficient to initiate the interaction of the G protein with the intracellular effector system. The sustained influence of the G protein on the effector system can help explain why the cell may continue to exhibit a response even after the drug has dissociated from the cell or even after the drug has been eliminated from the body.

Drugs and other substances that exert their effects through this type of receptor–G protein–effector system usually lead to the formation (or inhibition of the formation) of an intracellular compound known as a **second messenger**. In effect, the drug acts as the first messenger, which triggers a biochemical change in the cell, but the drug itself does not enter the cell. The second messenger, which is the substance produced inside the cell, actually mediates the change in function.

The primary example of this type of second messenger strategy is the **adenylate cyclase–cyclic adenosine monophosphate (cAMP)** system present in many cells[9,29] (see Fig. 4–3). Adenylate cyclase, which is an enzyme that is located on the inner surface of the cell membrane, is responsible for hydrolyzing adenosine triphosphate (ATP) into cAMP. Cyclic AMP acts as the second messenger in this system by activating other enzymes (i.e., protein kinases) throughout the cell. Thus, drugs that bind to a surface receptor that is linked to a G_s protein will increase adenylate cyclase activity, resulting in increased production of cAMP within the cell. Other drugs that bind to a different receptor that is linked to a G_i protein will inhibit adenylate cyclase activity, resulting in decreased production of cAMP.

The adenylate cyclase–cAMP system is associated with specific membrane receptors such as the beta-adrenergic receptors.[8,9,29] Other surface receptors may also be linked to this particular effector–second messenger system, or they may be linked to other intracellular processes that use different second messengers. Additional second messengers that have been identified in various cells include cyclic guanine monophosphate (cGMP), diacylglycerol, phosphoinositides, calcium ions, and intracellular peptides.[2,4–6,32]

Finally, alterations in the synthesis and function of G proteins have been identified in certain pathologic conditions, including alcoholism, diabetes mellitus, heart failure, and certain tumors.[20] This illustrates the fact that G proteins seem to play an integral role in mediating the cell's response to various substances in both normal and disease states. The importance of these regulatory proteins will almost certainly continue to emerge as additional information about their structure and function becomes available.

INTRACELLULAR RECEPTORS

Receptors have been identified at intracellular locations such as the cytoplasm and the nucleus. Certain drugs exert their effect by entering the cell directly and then binding with one of these receptors. For instance, steroid and steroidlike compounds usually interact with a receptor that is located in the cytoplasm.[12] Certain hormones such as thyroxin appear to act by binding primarily with a receptor that is located on the chromatin in the cell's nucleus.[21] In either case, cell function is altered because the drug-receptor complex initiates changes in nuclear messenger RNA transcription with subsequent changes in cellular protein synthesis. The role of intracellular receptors is discussed further in this text in the chapters that deal with specific drugs that bind to these intracellular components.

DRUG-RECEPTOR INTERACTIONS

The ability of a drug to bind to any receptor is dictated by factors such as the size and shape of the drug relative to the configuration of the binding site on the receptor. The electrostatic attraction between the drug and the receptor may also be important in determining the extent to which the drug binds to the receptor. This drug-receptor interaction is somewhat analogous to a key fitting into a lock. The drug acts as a "key" that will only fit into certain receptors. Once inserted into a suitable receptor, the drug activates the receptor much in the same way that a key would be able to turn and "activate" the appropriate lock. To carry this analogy one step further, unlocking a door to a room would increase the "permeability" of the room in a manner similar to the direct effect of certain activated membrane receptors (e.g., the acetylcholine receptor on the neuromuscular junction). Other types of key-lock interactions would be "linked" to some other event, such as using a key to start an automobile engine. This situation is analogous to linking a surface receptor to some intracellular process that would affect the internal "machinery" of the cell.

Although the key-lock analogy serves as a crude example of drug-receptor interactions, the attraction between a drug and any receptor is much more complex. Binding a drug to a receptor is not an all-or-none phenomenon, but is graded depending on the drug in question. Some drugs will bind readily to the receptor, some moderately, and others very little or not at all. The term **affinity** is used to describe the amount of attraction between a drug and a receptor.[38] Affinity is actually related to the amount of drug that is required to bind to the unoccupied receptors.[25] A drug with high affinity binds readily to the open receptors, even if the concentration of drug is relatively low. Drugs with moderate or low affinity require a higher concentration in the body before the receptors become occupied.

In addition to the relative degree of affinity of different drugs for a receptor, apparently the status of the receptor may also vary under specific conditions. Receptors may exist in variable affinity states (super-high, high, low) depending on the influence of local regulators such as guanine nucleotides, ammonium ions, and divalent cations.[10,36,41,42] Membrane receptors may also be influenced by the local environment of the lipid bilayer. The amount of flexibility or "fluidity" of the cell membrane is recognized as being critical in providing a suitable environment in which membrane constituents such as receptors can optimally function. Physical and chemical factors (including other drugs) may change the fluidity and organization of the membrane, thereby disrupting the normal orientation of the receptor and subsequently altering its affinity state and ability to interact with a drug.[7,15,33]

The exact way in which a drug activates a receptor has been the subject of considerable debate. Binding of a drug to the receptor is hypothesized to cause the receptor to undergo some sort of temporary change in its shape or conformation. The change in structure of the activated receptor then mediates a change in cell function, either directly or by being linked to some effector–second messenger system. Some studies have suggested that certain receptor proteins do undergo a change in structure after binding with specific chemicals.[8] This event certainly seems plausible since most receptors have been identified as protein molecules, and proteins are known to be able to reversibly change their shape and conformation as part of normal physiologic function.[23] This fact should not, however, rule out other possible ways in which an activated receptor may mediate changes in cell function. Future research will continue to clarify the role of conformational changes as well as other possible mechanisms of receptor activation.

FUNCTIONAL ASPECTS OF DRUG-RECEPTOR INTERACTIONS

The interaction between the drug and the receptor dictates several important aspects of pharmacology, including those discussed here.

Drug Selectivity

A drug is said to be *selective* if it affects only one type of cell or tissue and produces a specific physiologic response. For instance, a drug that is cardioselective will affect heart function without affecting other tissues such as the gastrointestinal tract or respiratory system. The selectivity of a particular drug is a function of the ability of that drug to interact with specific receptors on the target tissue, and not with other receptors on the target tissue or receptors on other tissues (Fig. 4–4). In reality, drug selectivity is a relative term since no drug produces only one effect. Drugs can be compared with one another, however, with the more selective drug being able to affect one type of tissue or organ with only a minimum of other responses.

Dose-Response

The shape of the typical dose-response curve discussed in Chapter 1 is related to the number of receptors that are bound by the drug (see Fig. 1–2), because within certain limits of the drug concentration, the response is proportional to the number of receptors occupied by the drug. At low dosages, only a few receptors are bound by the

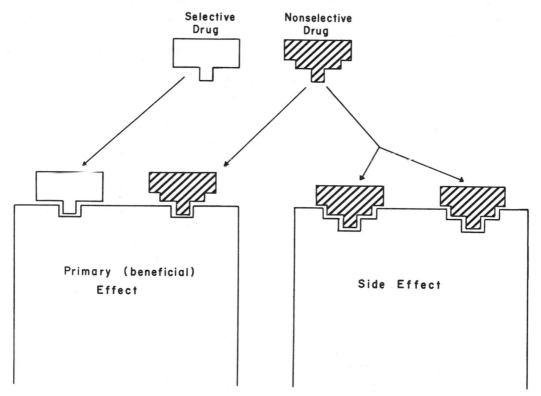

FIGURE 4–4. Drug selectivity. The diagram represents an ideal situation where the selective drug produces only beneficial effects and the nonselective drug exerts both beneficial and side effects. Drug selectivity is actually a relative term, because all drugs produce some side effects; however, a selective drug produces fewer side effects than a nonselective agent.

drug; hence, the effect is relatively small. As dosage (and drug concentration) increases, more receptors become occupied and the response increases. Finally, at some dosage, all available receptors are occupied, and the response is maximal. Increasing the dosage beyond the point at which the maximal effect is reached will not produce any further increase in response because all the receptors are bound by the drug.

Classification of Drugs: Agonist Versus Antagonist

So far, drug-receptor interactions have been used to describe the process by which a drug occupies a receptor and in some way activates the receptor. The activated receptor then brings about a change in cell function. Such a drug that binds to a receptor and initiates a change in the function of the cell is referred to as an **agonist**. An agonist is identified as having affinity and efficacy.[4] As discussed earlier, *affinity* refers to the fact that there is an attraction, or desire, for the drug to bind to a given receptor. The second characteristic, *efficacy*, indicates that the drug will activate the receptor and subsequently lead to a change in the function of the cell. Whereas an agonist has both affinity and efficacy, an **antagonist** has only affinity. This means that the drug will bind to the receptor, but it will not cause any change in the function of the receptor or cell (Fig. 4–5). Antagonists are significant because by occupying the receptor, they prevent the agonistic compound from having any effect on the cell. Antagonists are often referred to as *blockers* because of this ability to block the effect of another chemical. The primary pharmacologic significance of these antagonists has been their use in blocking the effects of certain endogenous compounds. The primary example of this is the use of the so-called beta blockers, which occupy specific receptors on the myocardium,

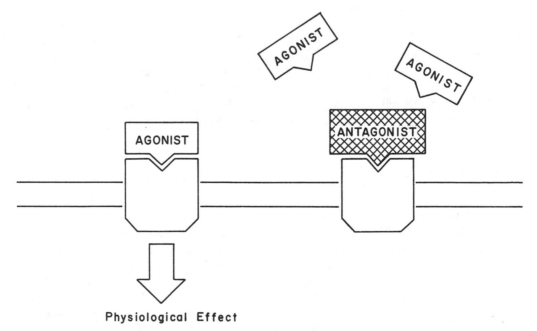

Physiological Effect

FIGURE 4–5. Drug classification: agonist versus antagonist. The antagonist (blocker) prevents the agonist from binding to the receptor and exerting a physiologic effect.

thus preventing circulating catecholamines from increasing heart rate and contractility. Other examples of antagonistic drugs are discussed in their appropriate chapters.

Competitive Versus Noncompetitive Antagonists

Pharmacologic antagonists are generally divided into two categories depending on whether they are competing with the agonist for the receptor.[4] *Competitive antagonists* are so classified because they seem to be vying for the same receptor as the agonist. In other words, both the agonist and antagonist have a more or less equal opportunity to occupy the receptor. For practical purposes, whichever drug is present in the greater concentration tends to have the predominant effect. If the number of competitive antagonist molecules far exceeds the number of agonist molecules, the antagonists will occupy most of the receptors and the overall effect will be inhibition of the particular response. Conversely, a high concentration of agonist relative to antagonist will produce a pharmacologic effect, since the agonist will occupy most of the receptors. In fact, raising the concentration of agonist in the presence of a competitive antagonist can actually overcome the inhibition that was originally present, because the competitive antagonists form rather weak bonds with the receptor and can be displaced from the receptor by a sufficient concentration of agonist molecules.[4] This is an important advantage of competitive antagonists since, if necessary, the inhibition caused by the antagonist can be overcome simply by administering high concentrations of the agonist.

In contrast to competitive antagonists, *noncompetitive antagonists* form strong, essentially permanent, bonds to the receptor. Noncompetitive antagonists have either an extremely high affinity for the receptor or actually form irreversible covalent bonds to the receptor.[4,17] Once bound to the receptor, the noncompetitive antagonist cannot be displaced by the agonist, regardless of how much agonist is present. Thus the term *noncompetitive* refers to the inability of the agonist to compete with the antagonist for the receptor site. The obvious disadvantage to this type of receptor blocker is that the inhibition cannot be overcome in cases of an overdose of the antagonist. Also, noncompetitive antagonists often remain bound for the life of the receptor, and their effect is terminated only after the receptor has been replaced as part of the normal protein turnover within the cell. Consequently, the inhibition produced by a noncompetitive blocker tends to remain in effect for long periods (i.e., several days).

Partial Agonists

Drugs are classified as *partial agonists* when they do not evoke a maximal response compared to a strong agonist. This classification is used even though the partial agonist occupies all available receptors.[4] In fact, partial agonists can be thought of as having an efficacy that lies somewhere between that of a full agonist and a full noncompetitive antagonist. The lack of a maximal response is not caused by decreased drug-receptor affinity. On the contrary, partial agonists often have a high affinity for the receptor. The decreased efficacy may be caused by the fact that the partial agonist does not completely activate the receptor after it binds, and that binding results in a lower level of any postreceptor events (e.g., less activation of G proteins, smaller changes in enzyme function).

Hence, the realization that certain drugs act as partial agonists has led to the idea that a range of efficacy can exist, depending on how specific drugs interact with their respective receptors.[38] At one end of this range are drugs that bind strongly and produce a high degree of efficacy (strong agonists), while the other end of the spectrum contains drugs that bind strongly and produce no effect (strong antagonists). Agents that fall between these two extremes (partial agonists) can have varying degrees of agonistic activity. These partial agonists can also have certain clinical advantages. For instance, certain antianxiety drugs that function as partial agonists may provide adequate anxiolytic effects without excessive side effects.[16] Other examples of how partial agonists can be used clinically are discussed elsewhere in this text.

RECEPTOR REGULATION

Receptor responses are not static but are regulated by endogenous and exogenous factors. In general, a prolonged increase in the stimulation of various receptors will lead to a *decrease* in receptor function, and decreased stimulation will lead to an *increase* in receptor numbers or sensitivity (Fig. 4–6). The mechanisms and significance of these receptor changes are described here.

Receptor Desensitization and Down-Regulation

As presented in Figure 4–6, overstimulation of postsynaptic receptors by endogenous substances (neurotransmitters, hormones) or by exogenous agonists (drugs) may lead to a functional decrease in the appropriate receptor population.[27,28,37,39] In effect,

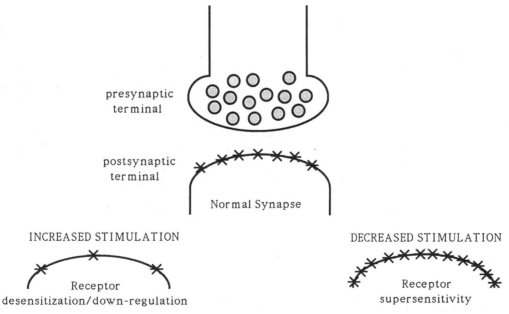

FIGURE 4–6. Receptor regulation. Functionally active receptor sites are represented by an "X." Increased stimulation results in a decrease in receptor numbers (desensitization/down-regulation), while decreased stimulation causes increased receptor numbers (supersensitivity).

the cell becomes less responsive to the prolonged stimulation by decreasing the number of active receptors. The term **desensitization** is used to describe a fairly brief and transient decrease in responsiveness. Desensitization is believed to occur because of the addition of phosphate residues (phosphorylation) or some other chemical modification to the receptor protein.[4] Adding a phosphate molecule seems to cause some membrane receptors to be uncoupled from their intermediate regulatory proteins and consequently from the rest of the cell's biochemical machinery.[26,27] Receptor desensitization helps account for the decrease in response that may be seen even though the agonist remains present in high concentration in the body. The decrease in responsiveness caused by desensitization is fairly brief, however, and a return to normal response may occur within a few minutes after the agonist is removed.

Receptor **down-regulation** describes a slower process in which the actual number of available receptors is diminished.[31,37] This results in a decrease in responsiveness that remains in effect long after the agonist is removed (i.e., several days). In some cases, this decrease in receptor numbers may be caused by receptors being sequestered within the cell's interior and hidden from further stimulation.[18,27,30] This process of receptor internalization effectively limits the ability of the agonist to stimulate the cell by decreasing the number of receptors that are available for drug binding.

Receptor desensitization and down-regulation appear to be examples of a negative feedback system used by the cell to prevent overstimulation by an agonist. The cell appears to selectively decrease its responsiveness to a particular stimulus in order to protect itself from excessive perturbation. Receptor down-regulation is important pharmacologically because it may be one of the primary reasons that a decrease in drug responsiveness occurs when certain drugs are used for prolonged periods of time.[34,40] Conversely, some drugs, such as the antidepressants, may exert their beneficial effects by intentionally causing receptor down-regulation and desensitization in certain neural pathways that cause clinical depression. These drugs are discussed in detail in Chapter 7.

Receptor Supersensitivity

A prolonged decrease in the stimulation of the postsynaptic receptors can result in a functional increase in receptor sensitivity. The best example of this is the denervation **supersensitivity** seen when a peripheral nerve is severed.[43] In this situation, the lack of presynaptic neurotransmitter release results in a compensatory increase in postsynaptic receptor numbers. A somewhat different type of denervation supersensitivity may occur when receptor antagonist drugs are used for prolonged periods. Here the postsynaptic receptors are blocked by the antagonistic drug, and they are unavailable for stimulation by the appropriate agonist. The postsynaptic neuron interprets this as if the synapse were denervated and responds by manufacturing more receptors, resulting in a compensatory *increase* in function at the synapse that was supposed to be blocked by the antagonist. Several problems may result from this pharmacologically induced supersensitivity.

NONRECEPTOR DRUG MECHANISMS

Certain drugs do not appear to exert their effects by binding to a specific cellular component. Drugs such as the general anesthetics may directly affect membrane fluidity and organization, possibly by becoming directly embedded in the lipid portion of the membrane.[15] A change in membrane structure and function would subsequently affect receptor function as well as other membrane processes such as enzymatic function and transport systems. Other drugs, such as some of the cancer chemotherapeutic agents, act as "antimetabolites" by becoming incorporated into the manufacture of specific cellular components. The drug acts as an improper ingredient in the biosynthesis of the component, so that the cell does not manufacture certain harmful or unwanted materials.[19] Other drugs may affect cell function without first binding to a receptor by directly altering enzyme function or by acting as "chelating agents," which bind to harmful compounds such as the heavy metals and prevent them from exerting toxic effects.[38] Additional nonreceptor-mediated mechanisms of specific compounds are discussed when those drugs are examined in their respective chapters.

SUMMARY

A great number of drugs and endogenous chemicals have been shown to exert their effects by first binding to and activating a cellular receptor. Cellular receptors seem to be proteins located on the cell surface or at specific locations within the cell. The primary role of the receptor is to recognize specific chemicals from the vast number of compounds that are introduced to the cell and to initiate a change in cell function by interacting with a specific agent. Activated receptors mediate a change in function by altering cell permeability or modifying the biochemical function within the cell, or both. The exact mechanism by which a receptor affects cell function depends on the type and location of the receptor.

Drug-receptor interactions are significant pharmacologically because they account for some of the basic pharmacodynamic principles such as drug selectivity and the relationship between drug dose and response. Also, the development of chemical agents that block specific receptors (antagonists) has been useful in moderating the effects of endogenous compounds on specific physiologic processes. Finally, changes in receptor number and sensitivity have been implicated as being important in the altered response seen in certain drugs with prolonged use. Information about the relationship between drugs and cellular receptors has been, and will continue to be, critical to our understanding of how drugs work, as well as to helping researchers develop new compounds.

REFERENCES

1. Baxter, JD and Funder, JW: Hormone receptors. N Engl J Med 301:1149, 1979.
2. Berridge, MJ: Inositol triphosphate and diacylglycerol as second messengers. Biochem J 220:345, 1984.
3. Birnbaumer, L: G proteins in signal transduction. Annu Rev Pharmacol Toxicol 30:675, 1990.
4. Bourne, HR and Roberts, JM: Drug receptors and pharmacodynamics. In Katzung, BG (ed): Basic and Clinical Pharmacology, ed 5. Appleton & Lange, Norwalk, CT, 1992.
5. Brostrom, CO, et al: Regulation of protein synthesis in isolated hepatocytes by calcium-mobilizing hormones. Mol Pharmacol 29:104, 1986.
6. Cheng, K and Larner, J: Intracellular mediators of insulin action. Annu Rev Physiol 47:405, 1985.
7. Cohen, RM, et al: Glutaraldehyde pretreatment blocks phospholipase A_2 modulation of adrenergic receptors. Life Sci 36:25, 1985.
8. Contreras, ML, Wolfe, BB, and Molinoff, PB: Thermodynamic properties of agonist interactions with the beta adrenergic receptor-coupled adenylate cyclase system: II. Agonist binding to soluble beta adrenergic receptors. J Pharm Exp Ther 237:165, 1986.

9. Cooper, DMF: Receptor-mediated stimulation and inhibition of adenylate cyclase. In Kleinzeller, A (ed): Current Topics in Membranes and Transport, Vol 18: Membrane Receptors. Academic Press, New York, 1983.
10. Eterovic, VA, et al: Positive modulators of muscle acetylcholine receptor. J Receptor Res 9:107, 1989.
11. Evans, RM: The steroid and thyroid hormone receptor superfamily. Science 240:889, 1988.
12. Evans, T, et al: Guanine nucleotide regulation of agonist binding to muscarinic receptors: Relation to efficacy of agonists for stimulation of phosphoinositide breakdown and calcium mobilization. Biochem J 232:751, 1985.
13. Fantl, WJ, Johnson, DE, and Williams, LT: Signalling by receptor tyrosine kinases. Annu Rev Biochem 62:453, 1993.
14. Gilman, AG: Guanine nucleotide-binding regulatory proteins and dual control of adenylate cyclase. J Clin Invest 73:1, 1984.
15. Goldstein, DB: The effects of drugs on membrane fluidity. Annu Rev Pharmacol Toxicol 24:43, 1984.
16. Haefely, W, Martin, JR, and Schoch, P: Novel anxiolytics that act as partial agonists at benzodiazepine receptors. Trends Pharmacol Sci 11:452, 1990.
17. Hahn, EF, et al: Irreversible opiate agonists and antagonists: III. Phenylhydrazone derivatives of naloxone and oxymorphone. J Pharmacol Exp Ther 235:846, 1985.
18. Harden, TK, et al: Agonist-induced alteration in the membrane form of muscarinic cholinergic receptors. J Biol Chem 260:13060, 1985.
19. Heidelberger, C: Pyrimidine and pyrimidine nucleoside antimetabolites. In Holland, JF and Frei, E (eds): Cancer Medicine, ed 2. Lea & Febiger, Philadelphia, 1982.
20. Houslay, MD: Review: G-protein linked receptors—a family probed by molecular cloning and mutagenesis. Clin Endocrinol 36:525, 1992.
21. Jaffe, RC: Thyroid receptor hormones. In Conn, PM (ed): The Receptors, Vol 1. Academic Press, New York, 1984.
22. Kandel, ER: Disorders of mood: Depression, mania, and anxiety disorders. In Kandel, ER, Schwartz, JH, and Jessell, TM (eds): Principles of Neural Science, ed 3. Appleton & Lange, Norwalk, CT, 1991.
23. Karplus, M and McGammon, JA: Dynamics of proteins: Elements of function. Annu Rev Biochem 52:263, 1983.
24. Kaziro, Y, et al: Structure and function of signal-transducing GTP-binding proteins. Annu Rev Biochem 60:349, 1991.
25. Kenakin, TP: The classification of drugs and drug receptors in isolated tissues. Pharmacol Rev 36:165, 1984.
26. Leeb-Lundberg, LM, et al: Phorbol esters promote alpha 1-adrenergic receptor phosphorylation and receptor uncoupling from inositol phospholipid metabolism. Proc Natl Acad Sci 82:5651, 1985.
27. Lefkowitz, RJ and Caron, MG: Adrenergic receptors: Molecular mechanisms of clinically relevant regulation. Clin Res 33:395, 1985.
28. Lefkowitz, RJ, Caron MG, and Stiles, GL: Mechanisms of membrane receptor regulation. Biochemical, physiological and clinical insights derived from studies of the adrenergic receptors. N Engl J Med 310:1570, 1984.
29. Lefkowitz, RJ, Stadel, JM, and Caron, MG: Adenylate cyclase-coupled beta-adrenergic receptors. Structure and mechanisms of activation and desensitization. Annu Rev Biochem 52:159, 1983.
30. Mahan, LC, Motulsky, HJ, and Insel, PA: Do agonists promote rapid internalization of beta-adrenergic receptors? Proc Natl Acad Sci 82:6566, 1985.
31. Maisel, AS, and Motulsky, HJ: Receptor redistribution does not accompany terbutaline-induced down-regulation of beta-adrenergic receptors on human mononuclear leukocytes. Clin Pharmacol Ther 42:100, 1987.
32. McKinney, M and Richelson, E: The coupling of the neuronal muscarinic receptor to responses. Annu Rev Pharmacol Toxicol 24:121, 1984.
33. Muccioli, G, Ghe, D, and DiCarlo, R: Drug-induced membrane modifications differentially affect prolactin and insulin binding in the mouse liver. Pharmacol Res Commun 17:883, 1985.
34. Overstreet, DH and Yamamura, HI: Receptor alterations and drug tolerance. Life Sci 25:1865, 1979.
35. Raffa, RB and Tallarida, RJ: The concept of a changing receptor concentration: Implications for the theory of drug action. J Theor Biol 115:625, 1985.
36. Ransnas, L, Hjalmarson, A, and Jacobsson, B: Adenylate cyclase modulation by ammonium ion: GTP-like effect on muscarinic and alpha 2-adrenergic receptors. Acta Pharmacol Toxicol 56:382, 1985.
37. Robinson, D and McGee, R: Agonist-induced regulation of the neuronal nicotinic acetylcholine receptor of PC12 cells. Mol Pharmacol 27:409, 1985.
38. Ross, EM: Pharmacodynamics: Mechanisms of drug action and the relationship between drug concentration and effect. In Gilman, AG, et al (eds): The Pharmacological Basis of Therapeutics, ed 8. Pergamon Press, New York, 1990.
39. Snavely, MD, Ziegler, MG, and Insel, PA: Subtype-selective down-regulation of rat renal cortical alpha and beta-adrenergic receptors by catecholamines. Endocrinology 117:2182, 1985.
40. Snyder, SH: Receptors, neurotransmitters and drug responses. N Engl J Med 300:465, 1979.
41. Stadel, JM and Lefkowitz, RJ: The beta-adrenergic receptor: Ligand binding studies. In Kleinzeller, A

(ed): Current Topics in Membranes and Transport, Vol 18: Membrane Receptors. Academic Press, New York, 1983.

42. Ukena, D, Poeschla, E, and Schwabe, U: Guanine nucleotide and cation regulation of radioligand binding to R(i) adenosine receptors of rat fat cells. Naunyn-Schmied Arch Pharmacol 326:241, 1984.

43. Woodcock, EA, et al: Specific increase in renal alpha 1-adrenergic receptors following unilateral renal denervation. J Recept Res 5:133, 1985.

Pharmacology of the Central Nervous System

CHAPTER 5

Central Nervous System Pharmacology: General Principles

The CNS is responsible for controlling bodily functions as well as being the center for behavioral and intellectual abilities. Neurons within the CNS are organized into highly complex patterns that mediate information through synaptic interactions. CNS drugs often attempt to modify the activity of these neurons in order to treat specific disorders or to alter the general level of arousal of the CNS. This chapter presents a simplified introduction to the organization of the CNS and the general strategies that can be used with drugs to alter activity within the brain and spinal cord.

CNS ORGANIZATION

The CNS can be grossly divided into the brain and spinal cord (Fig. 5–1). The brain is subdivided according to anatomic or functional criteria. The following is a brief overview of the general organization of the brain and spinal cord, with some indication of where particular CNS drugs tend to exert their effects, and is by no means intended to be an extensive review of neuroanatomy. A more elaborate discussion of CNS structure and function can be found in several excellent sources.[5,9,10,14]

Cerebrum

The largest and most rostral aspect of the brain is the *cerebrum* (see Fig. 5–1). The cerebrum consists of bilateral hemispheres, with each hemisphere anatomically divided into several lobes (frontal, temporal, parietal, and occipital). The outer cerebrum, or cerebral cortex, is associated with the highest order of conscious function and integration in the CNS. Specific cortical areas are responsible for sensory and motor functions, as well as intellectual and cognitive abilities. Other cortical areas are involved in

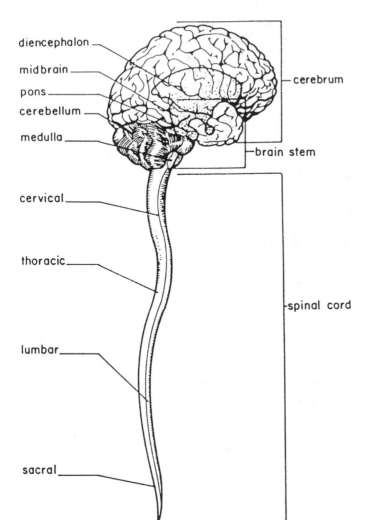

diencephalon

midbrain

pons

cerebellum

medulla

cervical

thoracic

lumbar

sacral

cerebrum

brain stem

spinal cord

FIGURE 5–1. General organization of the CNS. (From Crouch, JE: Essential Human Anatomy. Lea & Febiger, Philadelphia, 1982, with permission.)

short-term memory and speech. The cortex also seems to function in somewhat of a supervisory capacity regarding lower brain function and may influence the control of other activities such as the autonomic nervous system. With regard to CNS drugs, most therapeutic medications tend to affect cortical function indirectly by first altering the function of lower brain and spinal cord structures. An exception is the group of drugs used to treat epilepsy; these drugs are often targeted directly for hyperexcitable neurons in the cerebral cortex.

Basal Ganglia

A group of specific areas located deep within the cerebral hemispheres is collectively termed the *basal ganglia*. Components of the basal ganglia include the caudate nucleus, putamen, globus pallidus, lentiform nucleus, substantia nigra, and others. The basal ganglia are involved primarily in the control of motor activity, and deficits in this area are significant in movement disorders such as Parkinson's disease and Huntington's chorea. Certain medications used to treat these movement disorders exert their effects by interacting with basal ganglia structures.

Diencephalon

The area of brain enclosing the third ventricle is the *diencephalon*. This area consists of several important structures including the thalamus and hypothalamus. The thalamus contains distinct nuclei that are crucial in the integration of certain types of sensation and the relay of these sensations to other areas of the brain such as the somatosensory cortex. The hypothalamus is involved in the control of diverse body functions including temperature control, appetite, water balance, and certain emotional reactions. The hypothalamus is also significant in its control over the function of hormonal release from the pituitary gland. Several CNS drugs affecting sensation and control of the body functions listed here manifest their effects by interacting with the thalamus and hypothalamus.

Mesencephalon and Brainstem

The *mesencephalon,* or *midbrain,* serves as a bridge between the higher areas (cerebrum and diencephalon) and the *brainstem*. The brainstem consists of the pons and the medulla oblongata. In addition to serving as a pathway between the higher brain and the spinal cord, the midbrain and brainstem are the location of centers responsible for controlling respiration and cardiovascular function (vasomotor center). The reticular formation is also located in the midbrain and brainstem. The reticular formation is comprised of a collection of neurons that extend from the reticular substance of the upper spinal cord through the midbrain and the thalamus. The reticular formation monitors and controls consciousness and is important in regulating the amount of arousal or alertness of the cerebral cortex. Consequently, CNS drugs that affect the state of arousal of the individual tend to exert their effects on the reticular formation. Sedative-hypnotics and general anesthetics tend to decrease activity in the reticular formation, whereas certain CNS stimulants (caffeine, amphetamines) may increase arousal through a stimulatory effect on reticular formation neurons.

Cerebellum

The *cerebellum* lies posterior to the brainstem and is separated from the brainstem by the fourth ventricle. Anatomically it is divided into two hemispheres, with each hemisphere consisting of three lobes (anterior, posterior, and flocculonodular). The function of the cerebellum is to help plan and coordinate motor activity and assume responsibility for comparing the actual movement with the intended motor pattern. The cerebellum interprets various sensory input and helps modulate motor output so that the actual movement closely resembles the intended motor program. The cerebellum is also concerned with the vestibular mechanisms responsible for maintaining balance and posture. Therapeutic medications are not usually targeted directly for the cerebellum, but incoordination and other movement disorders may result if a drug exerts a toxic side effect on the cerebellum.

Limbic System

So far all of the structures described have been grouped primarily by anatomic relationships with the brain. The *limbic system* is comprised of several structures that are dispersed throughout the brain but are often considered as a functional unit or system within the CNS. Major components of the limbic system include cortical structures (such as the amygdala, hippocampus, and cingulate gyrus), the hypothalamus, certain thalamic nuclei, mamillary bodies, septum pellucidum, and several other structures and tracts. These structures share the common function of being involved in the control of emotional and behavioral activity. Certain aspects of motivation, aggression, sexual activity, and instinctive responses may be influenced by activity within the limbic system. CNS drugs affecting these aspects of behavior, including some antianxiety and antipsychotic medications, are believed to exert their beneficial effects primarily by altering activity in the limbic structures.

Spinal Cord

At the caudal end of the brainstem, the CNS continues distally as the *spinal cord.* The spinal cord is cylindrically shaped and consists of centrally located gray matter that is surrounded by white matter. The gray matter serves as an area for synaptic connections between various neurons. The white matter consists of the myelinated axons of neurons, which are grouped into tracts that ascend or descend between the brain and specific levels of the cord. Certain CNS drugs exert some or all of their effects by modifying synaptic transmission in specific areas of the gray matter, while other CNS drugs, such as the narcotic analgesics, may exert an effect on synaptic transmission in the gray matter of the cord as well as on synapses in other areas of the brain. Some drugs may be specifically directed toward the white matter of the cord. Drugs such as the local anesthetics can be used to block action potential propagation in the white matter so that ascending or descending information is interrupted (i.e., a spinal block).

THE BLOOD-BRAIN BARRIER

The *blood-brain barrier* refers to the unique structure and function of CNS capillaries.[1,11] Certain substances are not able to pass from the bloodstream into the CNS, despite the fact that these same substances are able to pass from the systemic circulation into other peripheral tissues. This fact suggests the existence of some sort of unique structure and function of the CNS capillaries that prevents many substances from entering the brain and spinal cord—hence, the term **blood-brain barrier**. This barrier effect is caused primarily by the tight junctions that occur between capillary endothelial cells; in fact, CNS capillaries lack the gaps and fenestrations that are seen in peripheral capillaries. Also, nonneuronal cells in the CNS (e.g., astrocytes) and the capillary basement membrane seem to contribute to the relative impermeability of this barrier. Functionally, the blood-brain barrier acts as a selective filter and seems to protect the CNS by limiting the entry of harmful substances into the brain and spinal cord.

The blood-brain barrier obviously plays an important role in clinical pharma-cotherapeutics. To exert their effects, drugs that are targeted for the CNS must be able to pass from the bloodstream into the brain and spinal cord. In general, nonpolar, lipid-soluble drugs are able to cross the blood-brain barrier by passive diffusion. Polar and lipophobic compounds are usually unable to enter the brain. Some exceptions occur because of the presence of carrier-mediated transport systems in the blood-brain barrier. Some substances such as glucose are transported via facilitated diffusion, while other compounds, including some drugs, may be able to enter the brain by active transport. However, these transport processes are limited to certain specific compounds, and the typical manner by which most drugs enter the brain is by passive lipid diffusion.

CNS NEUROTRANSMITTERS

The majority of neural connections in the human brain and spinal cord are characterized as chemical synapses. The term *chemical synapse* indicates that some chemical neurotransmitter is used to propagate the nervous impulse across the gap that exists between two neurons. Several distinct chemicals have been identified as neurotransmitters within the brain and spinal cord (Table 5–1). Groups of neurons within the CNS tend to use one of these neurotransmitters to produce either excitation or inhibition of other neurons. Although each neurotransmitter can be generally described as either excitatory or inhibitory within the CNS, some transmitters may have different effects, depending on the nature of the postsynaptic receptor involved. As discussed in Chapter 4, the interaction of the transmitter and the receptor dictates the effect on the postsynaptic neuron.

The facts that several distinct neurotransmitters exist and that neurons using specific transmitters are organized functionally within the CNS have important pharma-

TABLE 5–1 Central Neurotransmitters

Transmitter	Primary CNS Locations	General Effect
Acetylcholine	Cerebral cortex (many areas), basal ganglia, limbic and thalamic regions, spinal interneurons	Excitation
Norepinephrine	Neurons originating in brainstem and hypothalamus that project throughout other areas of brain	Inhibition
Dopamine	Basal ganglia, limbic system	Inhibition
Serotonin	Neurons originating in brainstem that project upward (to hypothalamus) and downward (to spinal cord)	Inhibition
GABA (gamma-aminobutyric acid)	Interneurons throughout spinal cord, cerebellum, basal ganglia, cerebral cortex	Inhibition
Glycine	Interneurons in spinal cord and brainstem	Inhibition
Glutamate, aspartate	Interneurons throughout brain and spinal cord	Excitation
Substance P	Pathways in spinal cord and brain that mediate painful stimuli	Excitation
Enkephalins	Pain suppression pathways in spinal cord and brain	Excitation

cologic implications. Certain drugs may alter the transmission in pathways using a specific neurotransmitter, while having little or no effect on other transmitter pathways. This allows the drug to exert a rather specific effect on the CNS, so many disorders may be rectified without radically altering other CNS functions. Other drugs may have a much more general effect and may alter transmission in many CNS regions. To provide an indication of neurotransmitter function, the major categories of CNS neurotransmitters and their general locations and effects are discussed subsequently.

Acetylcholine

Acetylcholine is the neurotransmitter found in many areas of the brain as well as in the periphery (skeletal neuromuscular junction, some autonomic synapses). In the brain, neurons originating in the large pyramidal cells of the motor cortex and many neurons originating in the basal ganglia secrete acetylcholine from their terminal axons. In general, acetylcholine synapses in the CNS are excitatory in nature.

Monoamines

Monoamines such as the **catecholamines** (dopamine, norepinephrine) and 5-hydroxytryptamine (serotonin) have been recognized as transmitters in several brain locations.[3] Within the basal ganglia, **dopamine** is the transmitter secreted by neurons that originate in the substantia nigra and project to the corpus striatum. Dopamine may also be an important transmitter in areas within the limbic system such as the hypothalamus. In general, dopamine inhibits neurons onto which it is released.

Norepinephrine is secreted by neurons that originate in the locus caeruleus of the pons and project throughout the reticular formation. Norepinephrine is generally regarded as an inhibitory transmitter within the CNS, but the overall effect following activity of norepinephrine synapses is often general excitation of the brain, probably because norepinephrine directly inhibits other neurons that produce inhibition. This phenomenon of *disinhibition* causes excitation by removing the influence of inhibitory neurons.

Serotonin is released by cells originating in the midline of the pons and brainstem and is projected to many different areas including the dorsal horns of the spinal cord and the hypothalamus. Serotonin is considered a strong inhibitor in most areas of the CNS and is believed to be important in mediating the inhibition of painful stimuli.

Amino Acids

Several amino acids such as glycine and gamma-aminobutyric acid (GABA) are important transmitters in the brain and spinal cord. Glycine seems to be the inhibitory transmitter used by certain interneurons located throughout the spinal cord. Likewise, GABA is released by spinal cord inhibitory interneurons and seems to be the predominant transmitter used to mediate presynaptic inhibition in the cord. GABA also has been identified as an inhibitory transmitter in areas of the brain such as the cortex and basal ganglia. Other amino acids such as aspartate and glutamate have been found in high concentrations throughout the brain and spinal cord; these substances generally cause excitation of CNS neurons. After some debate, these excitatory amino acids are believed to be true neurotransmitters, and not just precursors to protein synthesis.[4,6]

Peptides

Many peptides have already been established as CNS neurotransmitters.[12] One peptide that is important from a pharmacologic standpoint is substance P, which is an excitatory transmitter that is involved in spinal cord pathways that transmit pain impulses. Increased activity at substance P synapses in the cord serves to mediate the transmission of painful sensations, and certain drugs such as the opioid analgesics may decrease activity at these synapses. A second group of peptides that have important pharmacologic implications include three families of compounds, the endorphins, enkephalins, and dynorphins.[8] These peptides, also known as the endogenous opioids, are excitatory transmitters in certain brain synapses that inhibit painful sensations. Hence, endogenous opioids in the brain are able to decrease the central perception of pain. The interaction of these compounds with exogenous opioid drugs is discussed in Chapter 14.

Other Transmitters

In addition to the well-known substances, other chemicals are continually being identified as potential CNS neurotransmitters. Recent evidence has implicated substances such as adenosine and ATP as transmitters or modulators of neural transmission in specific areas of the brain and in the autonomic nervous system.[2,13] Peptides that are structurally and functionally similar to substance P are gaining attention as important transmitters. As the function of these chemicals and other new transmitters becomes clearer, the pharmacologic significance of drugs that affect these synapses will undoubtedly be considered.

CNS DRUGS: GENERAL MECHANISMS

The majority of CNS drugs work by modifying synaptic transmission in some way. Figure 5–2 shows a typical chemical synapse that would be found in the CNS. Most drugs that attempt to rectify CNS-related disorders do so by either increasing or decreasing transmission at specific synapses. For instance, psychotic behavior has been associated with overactivity in central synapses that use dopamine as a neurotransmitter (see Chapter 8). Drug therapy in this situation consists of agents that decrease activity at central dopamine synapses. Conversely, Parkinson's disease results from a decrease in activity at specific dopamine synapses (see Chapter 10). Antiparkinsonian drugs attempt to increase dopaminergic transmission at these synapses and to bring synaptic activity back to normal levels.

A drug that modifies synaptic transmission must somehow alter the quantity of the neurotransmitter released from the presynaptic terminal or affect the stimulation of postsynaptic receptors, or both. When considering a typical synapse, such as the one shown in Figure 5–2, there are several distinct sites at which a drug may alter activity

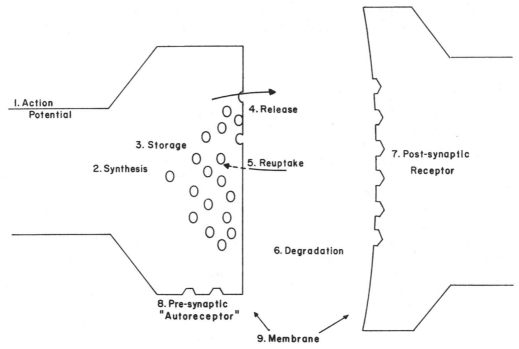

FIGURE 5-2. Sites at which drugs can alter transmission at a CNS chemical synapse.

in the synapse. Specific ways in which a drug may modify synaptic transmission are presented here.

1. *Presynaptic action potential:* The arrival of an action potential at the presynaptic terminal initiates neurotransmitter release. Certain drugs such as the local anesthetics block propagation along neural axons so that the action potential fails to reach the presynaptic terminal, which effectively eliminates activity at that particular synapse. Also, the amount of depolarization or height of the action potential arriving at the presynaptic terminal is directly related to the amount of transmitter released. Any drug or endogenous chemical that limits the amount of depolarization occurring in the presynaptic terminal will inhibit the synapse because less neurotransmitter is released. In certain situations, this is referred to as presynaptic inhibition, because the site of this effect is at the presynaptic terminal. The endogenous neurotransmitter GABA is believed to exert its inhibitory effects via this mechanism.

2. *Synthesis of neurotransmitter:* Drugs that block the synthesis of neurotransmitter will eventually deplete the presynaptic terminal and impair transmission. For example, metyrosine inhibits an enzyme essential for catecholamine biosynthesis in the presynaptic terminal. Treatment with metyrosine results in decreased synthesis of transmitters such as dopamine and norepinephrine.

3. *Storage of neurotransmitter:* A certain amount of chemical transmitter is stored in presynaptic vesicles. Drugs that impair this storage will decrease the ability of the synapse to continue to transmit information for extended periods. An example of this is the antihypertensive drug reserpine, which impairs the ability of adrenergic terminals to sequester and store norepinephrine in presynaptic vesicles.

4. *Release:* Certain drugs will increase synaptic activity by directly increasing the release of neurotransmitter from the presynaptic terminal. Amphetamines appear to exert their effects on the CNS primarily by increasing the presynaptic release of catecholamine neurotransmitters (e.g., norepinephrine). Conversely, other compounds may inhibit the synapse by directly decreasing the amount of transmitter released during each action potential. An example is botulinum toxin, which can be used as a skeletal muscle relaxant because of its ability to impair the release of acetylcholine from the skeletal neuromuscular junction (see Chapter 13).

5. *Reuptake:* After the neurotransmitter is released, some chemical synapses terminate activity primarily by transmitter reuptake. Reuptake involves movement of the transmitter molecule back into the presynaptic terminal. A drug that impairs the reuptake of transmitter allows more of the transmitter to remain in the synaptic cleft and continue to exert an effect. Consequently, blocking reuptake actually increases activity at the synapse. For instance, the tricyclic antidepressants (see Chapter 7) impair the reuptake mechanism that pumps amine neurotransmitters back into the presynaptic terminal, which allows the transmitter to continue to exert its effect, thus prolonging activity at the synapse.

6. *Degradation:* Some synapses rely primarily on enzymatic breakdown of the released transmitter to terminate synaptic activity. Inhibition of the enzyme responsible for terminating the transmitter allows more of the active transmitter to remain in the synaptic cleft, thereby increasing activity at the synapse. An example is the use of a drug that inhibits the **cholinesterase** enzyme as a method of treating myasthenia gravis. In myasthenia gravis, there is a functional decrease in activity at the skeletal neuromuscular junction. Anticholinesterase drugs such as neostigmine (Prostigmin) and pyridostigmine (Mestinon) inhibit acetylcholine breakdown, allowing more of the released neurotransmitter to continue to exert an effect at the neuromuscular synapse.

7. *Postsynaptic receptor:* As discussed in Chapter 4, chemical antagonists can be used to block the postsynaptic receptor, thus decreasing synaptic transmission. The best-known example of this is the use of the so-called beta blockers. These agents are antagonists that are specific for the beta-adrenergic receptors on the myocardium, and they are used frequently to treat hypertension and cardiac arrhythmias. Other drugs may improve synaptic transmission by directly affecting the receptor so that there is a tendency for increased neurotransmitter binding or improved receptor-effector coupling, or both. For instance, the benzodiazepines (e.g., diazepam, chlordiazepoxide) appear to enhance the postsynaptic effects of the inhibitory neurotransmitter GABA.

8. *Presynaptic autoreceptors:* In addition to postsynaptic receptors, there are also receptors on the presynaptic terminal of some types of chemical synapses. These presynaptic receptors seem to serve as a method of negative feedback in controlling neurotransmitter release.[7] During high levels of synaptic activity, the accumulation of neurotransmitter in the synaptic cleft may allow binding to these presynaptic receptors and limit further release of chemical transmitter. Certain drugs may also be able to attenuate synaptic activity through these presynaptic autoreceptors. Clonidine, for instance, may exert some of its antihypertensive effects by binding to presynaptic receptors on sympathetic postganglionic neurons and impairing the release of norepinephrine onto the peripheral vasculature. The use of drugs that alter synaptic activity by binding to these autoreceptors is still somewhat new, however, and the full potential for this area of pharmacology remains to be determined.

9. *Membrane effects:* Drugs may alter synaptic transmission by affecting membrane

organization and fluidity. Membrane fluidity is basically the amount of flexibility or mobility of the lipid bilayer. Drugs that alter the fluidity of the presynaptic membrane could affect the way that presynaptic vesicles fuse with and release their neurotransmitter. Drug-induced changes in the postsynaptic membrane would affect the receptor environment and thereby alter receptor function. Membrane modification will result in either increased or decreased synaptic transmission, depending on the drug in question and the type and magnitude of membrane change. A primary example of a drug that appears to affect membrane fluidity is alcohol (ethanol). Many, if not all, of the effects of alcohol on the CNS are probably caused by reversible changes in the fluidity and organization of the cell membranes of central neurons.

A CNS drug does not have to adhere specifically to only one of these methods of synaptic modification. Some drugs may affect the synapse in two or more ways. For example, the antihypertensive agent guanethidine impairs both the presynaptic storage and the release of norepinephrine. Other drugs such as the barbiturates may affect both the presynaptic terminal and the postsynaptic receptor in CNS synapses.

SUMMARY

Drugs affecting the brain and spinal cord usually exert their effects by somehow modifying synaptic transmission. In some instances, drugs may be targeted for specific synapses in an attempt to rectify some problem with transmission at that particular synapse. Other drugs may increase or decrease the excitability of CNS neurons in an attempt to have a more general effect on the overall level of consciousness of the individual. Specific categories of CNS drugs and their pharmacodynamic mechanisms are discussed in succeeding chapters.

REFERENCES

1. Bradbury, M: The Concept of a Blood-Brain Barrier. John Wiley & Sons, New York, 1979.
2. Burnstock, G: Purinergic mechanisms broaden their sphere of influence. Trends Neurosci 8:5, 1985.
3. Carlsson, A: Perspectives on the discovery of central monoaminergic transmission. Annu Rev Neurosci 10:19, 1987.
4. Crunelli, V, Forda, S, and Kelly, JS: Excitatory amino acids in the hippocampus: Synaptic physiology and pharmacology. Trends Neurosci 8:26, 1985.
5. DeGroot, J and Chusid, LG: Correlative Neuroanatomy and Functional Neurology, ed 20. Appleton & Lange, Norwalk, CT, 1988.
6. Fagy, GE: L-Glutamate, excitatory amino acid receptors and brain function. Trends Neurosci 8:207, 1985.
7. Gothert, M: Role of autoreceptors in the function of the peripheral and central nervous system. Arzneim-Forsch/Drug Rese 35:1909, 1985.
8. Jaffe, JH and Martin, WR: Opioid analgesics and antagonists. In Gilman, AG, et al (eds): The Pharmacological Basis of Therapeutics, ed 8. Pergamon Press, New York, 1990.
9. Kandel, ER, Schwartz, JH, and Jessell, TM: Principles of Neural Science, ed 3. Appleton & Lange, Norwalk, CT, 1991.
10. Nolte, J: The Human Brain, ed 3. CV Mosby, St Louis, 1993.
11. Rowland, LP, Fink, ME, and Rubin, L: Appendix C: Cerebrospinal fluid: Blood-brain barrier, brain edema, and hydrocephalus. In Kandel, ER, Schwartz, JH, and Jessell, TM (eds): Principles of Neural Science, ed 3. Appleton & Lange, Norwalk, CT, 1991.
12. Schwartz, JH: Chemical messengers: Small molecules and peptides. In Kandel, ER, Schwartz, JH, and Jessell, TM (eds): Principles of Neural Science, ed 3. Appleton & Lange, Norwalk, CT, 1991.
13. Stiles, GL and Olah, ME: Adenosine receptors: Annu Rev Physiol 54:211, 1992.
14. Williams, PL, et al: Gray's Anatomy, ed 37. Churchill Livingstone, New York, 1989.

CHAPTER 6

Sedative-Hypnotic and Antianxiety Agents

Drugs that are classified as sedative-hypnotics are used to relax the patient and promote sleep.[32] As the name implies, **sedative** drugs exert a calming effect and serve to pacify the patient. At a higher dose, the same drug tends to produce drowsiness and to initiate a relatively normal state of sleep (hypnosis). At still higher doses, some sedative-hypnotics (especially the barbiturates) will eventually bring on a state of general anesthesia. Because of their general CNS-depressant effects, some sedative-hypnotic drugs are also used for other functions such as treating epilepsy or producing muscle relaxation. However, the sleep-enhancing effects are of concern in this chapter.

By producing sedation, many drugs will also decrease the level of anxiety in the patient. Of course, these anxiolytic properties often occur at the expense of a decrease in the level of alertness in the individual. However, certain agents are available that can reduce anxiety without an overt sedative effect. Those medications that selectively produce antianxiety effects are discussed later in this chapter.

Even though sedative-hypnotic and antianxiety drugs are not used to directly treat any somatic disorders, many patients receiving physical and occupational therapy take these agents to help decrease anxiety and enhance relaxation. A person who becomes ill or sustains an injury requiring rehabilitation certainly has some apprehension concerning his or her welfare. If necessary, this apprehension can be controlled to some extent by using sedative-hypnotic and antianxiety drugs during the course of rehabilitation. Consequently, an understanding of the basic pharmacology of these agents will be helpful to rehabilitation specialists such as the physical therapist and occupational therapist.

SEDATIVE-HYPNOTIC AGENTS

Sedative-hypnotics fall into two general categories: barbiturates and benzodiazepines (Table 6–1). Several other nonbarbiturate, nonbenzodiazepine drugs are available (see Table 6–1), but they are typically used on only a limited basis in selected patients.

TABLE 6–1 Common Sedative-Hypnotic Drugs

Generic Name	Trade Name	Oral Adult Dose (mg)	
		Sedative	Hypnotic
Barbiturates			
Amobarbital	Amytal	30–50 BID or TID	65–200
Aprobarbital	Alurate	40 TID	40–160
Butabarbital	Butalan, Butisol, others	15–30 TID or QID	50–100
Pentobarbital	Nembutal	20 TID or QID	100
Phenobarbital	Solfoton	30–120 BID or TID	100–320
Secobarbital	Seconal	30–50 TID or QID	100
Benzodiazepines			
Estazolam	ProSom	———	1–2
Flurazepam	Dalmane, Durapam	———	15–30
Quazepam	Doral	———	7.5–15
Temazepam	Restoril	———	15–30
Triazolam	Halcion	———	0.125–0.25
Others			
Chloral hydrate	Noctec	250 TID	500–1000
Ethchlorvynol	Placidyl	———	500–1000
Glutethimide	(generic)	———	250–500
Promethazine	Phenergan (rectal)	———	25–50

The barbiturates are a group of CNS depressants that share a common chemical origin from barbituric acid. The potent sedative-hypnotic properties of these drugs have been recognized for some time, and their status as the premier medication used to promote sleep was unchallenged for many years. However, barbiturates are associated with a relatively small therapeutic index, with approximately 10 times the therapeutic dose often being fatal. These drugs are also addictive, and their prolonged use is often a problem in terms of drug abuse. Consequently, the lack of safety of the barbiturates and their strong potential for addiction and abuse necessitated the development of alternative nonbarbiturate drugs such as the benzodiazepines. Still, some barbiturates are occasionally used for their **hypnotic** properties; these drugs are listed in Table 6–1.

At present the use of barbiturates as hypnotics has essentially been replaced by other drugs, with the benzodiazepines being the current drugs of choice.[23] Several benzodiazepines are currently approved for use as hypnotics (Table 6–2). These agents exert hypnotic effects similar to those of the barbiturates, but they are generally regarded as safer because there is less chance of a lethal overdose. However, benzodiazepines are not without their drawbacks, since tolerance and physical dependence can also occur with their prolonged use (see "Benzodiazepines").[23]

Several other nonbarbiturate compounds may also be prescribed for their sedative-hypnotic properties (see Table 6–1). These compounds are chemically dissimilar but share the common ability to promote relaxation and sleep via their general ability to depress the CNS. Cyclic ethers and alcohols (including ethanol) can be included in this category, but their use specifically as sedative-hypnotics is fairly limited at present. The recreational use of ethanol in alcoholic beverages is an important topic in

TABLE 6–2 Pharmacokinetic Properties of Benzodiazepine Sedative-Hypnotics

Drug	Time to Peak Plasma Concentration (hr)*	Relative Half-Life	Comments
Estazolam (ProSom)	0.5 – 1.6	Intermediate	Rapid oral absorption
Flurazepam (Dalmane)	0.5 – 1.0	Long	Long elimination half-life because of active metabolites
Quazepam (Doral)	2.0	Long	Daytime drowsiness more likely than with other benzodiazepines
Temazepam (Restoril)	2 – 3	Short – intermediate	Slow oral absorption
Triazolam (Halcion)	Within 2	Short	Rapid oral absorption

*Adult oral hypnotic dose.

terms of abuse and long-term effects. However, this area is much too extensive to be addressed here, so this presentation will focus on the clinical use of sedative-hypnotics.

PHARMACOKINETICS

Sedative-hypnotics are usually highly lipid soluble. They are usually administered orally and are absorbed easily and completely from the gastrointestinal tract. Distribution is fairly uniform throughout the body, and these drugs reach the CNS readily because of their high degree of lipid solubility. Sedative-hypnotics are metabolized primarily by the oxidative enzymes of the drug microsomal metabolizing system (DMMS) in liver cells. Termination of their activity is accomplished either by DMMS enzymes or by storage of these drugs in non-CNS tissues; that is, by sequestering these drugs in adipose and other peripheral tissues, their CNS-depressant effects are not exhibited. However, when these drugs slowly leak out of their peripheral storage sites, they can be redistributed to the brain and can cause low levels of sedation. This occurrence may help explain the hangover-like feelings that are frequently reported the day after taking sedative-hypnotic drugs. Finally, excretion of these drugs takes place through the kidney after their metabolism in the liver. As with most types of drug biotransformation, metabolism of sedative-hypnotics is essential in creating a polar metabolite that is readily excreted by the kidney.

MECHANISM OF ACTION

Benzodiazepines

The benzodiazepines seem to exert their effects by increasing the inhibition present at CNS gamma-aminobutyric acid (GABA)–ergic synapses.[23,24,31] These inhibitory synapses are associated with a membrane protein complex containing three primary components: (1) a binding site for GABA, (2) a binding site for benzodiazepines, and (3) a chloride ion channel (Fig. 6–1).[10,11,19,30] GABA exerts its inhibitory effects by binding to its receptor site on this complex and by initiating an increase in chloride conductance through the channel. Increased chloride conductance results in hyperpolarization or a decreased ability to raise the neuron to its firing threshold. By binding to their own respective site on the complex, benzodiazepines potentiate the effects of GABA and increase the inhibition at these synapses.

Consequently, the presence of the GABA–benzodiazepine–chloride ion channel complex accounts for the specific mechanism of action of this class of sedative-hypnotics. By increasing the inhibitory effects at GABA-ergic synapses located in the reticular formation, benzodiazepines can decrease the level of arousal of the individual. In other words, the general excitation level in the reticular activating system decreases, and relaxation and sleep are enhanced.

The discovery of a CNS receptor that is specific for benzodiazepines has led to some interesting speculation as to the possible existence of some type of endogenous sedative-like agent. The presence of a certain type of receptor to indicate that the body produces an appropriate agonist for that receptor makes sense. For instance, the discovery of opiate receptors initiated the search for endogenous opiate-like substances,

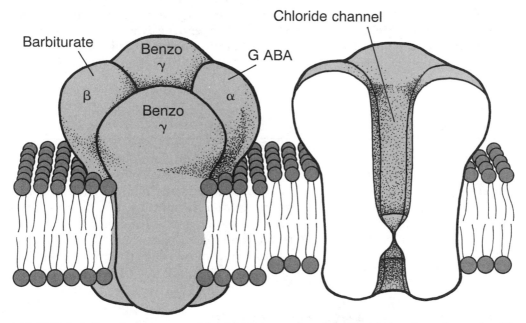

FIGURE 6-1. Putative structure of the GABA-benzodiazepine-chloride ion channel complex. The centrally located chloride ion channel is modulated by the binding of GABA to the alpha subunit of the receptor. The binding and effects of GABA are enhanced by the binding of benzodiazepines to the gamma subunits or barbiturates to the beta subunit. (From Kandel, ER: Disorders of mood: Depression, mania, and anxiety disorders. In Kandel, Schwartz, and Jessell,[10] p 882, with permission.)

which culminated in the discovery of the enkephalins. However, no endogenous substances that bind specifically to the benzodiazepine receptor have yet been identified. Continued research in this area may someday reveal such a substance, and the focus of pharmacologic treatment can then be directed toward stimulating the release of endogenous sedative-hypnotic agents.

Barbiturates

Despite their extensive use in the past, the exact mechanism of the barbiturates remains somewhat unclear. When used in sedative-hypnotic doses, barbiturates may function in a somewhat similar fashion to the benzodiazepines in that they also potentiate the inhibitory effects of GABA.[8,19] This suggests that the barbiturates may affect the benzodiazepine–GABA–chloride ion channel complex described previously. Indeed, some evidence exists that barbiturates bind directly to this complex at a site that is different from the binding site for GABA or the benzodiazepines (see Fig. 6-1).[10,23] Barbiturates may, however, also exert effects that are not mediated through an effect on the GABA–benzodiazepine–chloride ion channel. For instance, barbiturates may also directly inhibit transmitter release from presynaptic terminals (i.e., independent of their GABA-enhancing effect), and barbiturates have been shown to have an antagonist-like effect on postsynaptic receptors.[17]

Regardless of their exact mechanism, barbiturates are effective sedative-hypnotics because of their specificity for neurons in the midbrain portion of the reticular formation as well as some limbic system structures. At higher doses, the barbiturates also depress neuronal excitability in other areas of the brain and spinal cord. Their role in producing general anesthesia by this more extensive CNS depression is discussed in Chapter 11.

Other Mechanisms

The other sedative-hypnotics, which are neither benzodiazepine nor barbiturate in nature, work via poorly understood mechanisms. Alcohols seem to exert their depressant effects directly on neuronal membrane composition and fluidity. These and other highly lipid soluble substances may simply disorder the membrane in the presynaptic and postsynaptic regions of CNS neurons by becoming dissolved directly in the lipid bilayer.[4] Decreased neuronal transmission resulting from such membrane changes would account for the general CNS depression and subsequent sedative effects of such compounds.

PROBLEMS AND ADVERSE EFFECTS

Tolerance and Physical Dependence

The primary problem with many sedative-hypnotics is that prolonged use may cause tolerance and physical dependence. *Drug tolerance* is the need for more drug to be taken to exert the same effect. *Dependence* is described as the onset of withdrawal symptoms if the drug ceases to be taken. Although these problems were originally thought to be limited to the barbiturates, benzodiazepine sedative-hypnotics are now recognized as also causing tolerance and dependence when these drugs are taken continually for several weeks.

The manner and severity of withdrawal symptoms vary according to the type of drug and extent of the physical dependence.[25] Withdrawal after short-term benzodiazepine use may be associated with problems such as sleep disturbances (i.e., so-called rebound insomnia).[9,15,33] Long-term use and abuse may result in more severe problems such as psychosis and seizures if the drug is abruptly stopped.[7] When severe enough, seizures have been fatal in some cases of benzodiazepine withdrawal. Consequently, the long-term use of these drugs should be avoided, and other nonpharmacologic methods of reducing stress and promoting relaxation (e.g., mental imagery, biofeedback) should be instituted before tolerance and physical dependence become problems.[13] If the sedative-hypnotic has been used for an extended period, tapering off the dosage rather than abruptly stopping the drug has been recommended as a safer way to terminate administration.[8,25]

Residual Effects

Another problem associated with sedative-hypnotic use is the residual effects the day after administration. Individuals who take a sedative-hypnotic to get to sleep at night sometimes complain of drowsiness and decreased motor performance the next day.[5,34] These hangover-like effects may be caused by the drug being redistributed to the CNS from peripheral storage sites or may occur simply because the drug has not been fully metabolized. This problem may be resolved somewhat by taking a smaller dose or by using a drug with a shorter half-life (see Table 6–2).[33,34] Retrograde amnesia is another problem sometimes associated with sedative-hypnotic use.[27,28] The patient may have trouble recalling details of events that occurred for a certain period of time before the drug was taken. Although usually a minor problem, this can become serious if the drug-induced amnesia exacerbates an already existing memory problem, as might occur in some elderly patients.

Other Side Effects

Other **side effects** such as gastrointestinal discomfort (nausea and vomiting), dry mouth, sore throat, and muscular incoordination have been reported, but these occur fairly infrequently. Cardiovascular and respiratory depression may also occur, but these problems are dose-related and are usually not significant except in cases of overdose.

ANTIANXIETY DRUGS

Anxiety can be described as a fear or apprehension over some situation or event that the individual feels is threatening. Such events can range from a change in employment or family life to somewhat irrational phobias concerning everyday occurrences. Anxiety disorders can also be classified in several clinical categories including generalized anxiety disorder, panic disorder, obsessive-compulsive disorder, and post-traumatic stress syndrome.[1,16] Antianxiety drugs can help decrease the tension and nervousness associated with many of these syndromes until the situation is resolved or the individual is counseled effectively in other methods of dealing with his or her anxiety.

Many drugs including the sedative-hypnotics have the ability to decrease anxiety levels, but this is usually at the expense of an increase in sedation. Frequently, alleviating anxiety without producing excessive sedation is desirable so that the individual can function in his or her home, on the job, and so on. Consequently, certain drugs are available that have significant anxiolytic properties at doses that produce minimal sedation. Currently, certain benzodiazepine drugs are used most frequently in dealing with anxiety, and these are discussed here.[26,29]

Benzodiazepines

As discussed previously, because of their relative safety, the benzodiazepines have replaced the barbiturates in the treatment of nervousness and anxiety. In terms of anxiolytic properties, diazepam (Valium) is the prototypical antianxiety benzodiazepine (Fig. 6–2). The extensive use of this drug in treating nervousness and apprehension has made the trade name of this compound virtually synonymous with a decrease in tension and anxiety. When prescribed in anxiolytic dosages, diazepam and certain other benzodiazepines (Table 6–3) are associated with a decrease in anxiety without

Diazepam   FIGURE 6-2. Diazepam (Valium).

major sedative effects. The mechanism of action of the benzodiazepines has been discussed previously in this chapter. The antianxiety properties of these drugs probably involve a mechanism similar or identical to their sedative-hypnotic effects (i.e., potentiating GABA-ergic transmission). However, the relative lack of sedation suggests that appropriate doses of these particular benzodiazepines may preferentially influence limbic structures with a lesser influence on the reticular activating system. Benzodiazepines also seem to increase presynaptic inhibition in the spinal cord, which produces some degree of skeletal muscle relaxation, which may contribute to their antianxiety effects by making the individual feel more relaxed. The use of these drugs as skeletal muscle relaxants is further discussed in Chapter 13.

Nonbenzodiazepine Antianxiety Drugs

The ideal antianxiety agent is nonaddictive, safe (i.e., relatively free from harmful side effects and potential for lethal overdose), and not associated with any sedative properties. Drugs such as meprobamate (Miltown) and the barbiturates are not currently used to any great extent because they do not meet any of these criteria and are no more effective in reducing anxiety than the benzodiazepines. Newer antianxiety drugs such as the spirodecanediones (e.g., buspirone [BuSpar]) are now being evalu-

TABLE 6-3 Benzodiazepine Antianxiety Drugs

Generic Name	Trade Name	Antianxiety Dose (mg)*	Relative Half-Life
Alprazolam	Xanax	0.25–0.5 TID	Short–intermediate
Chlordiazepoxide	Librium, others	5–25 TID or QID	Long
Clorazepate	Tranxene, others	7.5–15 BID to QID	Long
Diazepam	Valium, others	15–30 OD	Long
Halazepam	Paxipam	20–40 TID or QID	Long
Ketazolam	Loftran	15 OD or BID	Long
Lorazepam	Alzapam, Ativan	1–3 BID or TID	Short–intermediate
Oxazepam	Serax	10–30 TID or QID	Short–intermediate
Prazepam	Centrax	10 TID	Long

*Doses refer to usual adult oral doses. Doses are often lower in elderly or debilitated patients.

ated as anxiolytic agents.[20] This group of drugs is believed to exert its effects by stimulating CNS serotonergic activity.[3,14] Preliminary reports indicate that buspirone may be as effective as diazepam in treating generalized anxiety disorder, but that buspirone may produce less sedation and have a lower risk of causing physical dependence. Hence, newer agents such as buspirone offer an alternative to the traditional antianxiety drugs such as the benzodiazepines.

Finally, beta-adrenergic antagonists (beta blockers, see Chapter 20) can decrease situational anxiety without producing sedation.[6,12] In particular, beta blockers such as propranolol have been used by musicians and other performing artists to decrease cardiac palpitations, muscle tremors, hyperventilation, and other manifestations of anxiety that tend to occur before an important performance.[2,18] Beta blockers probably exert their antianxiety effects through their ability to decrease activity in the sympathetic nervous system, that is, through their sympatholytic effects. These drugs may exert both peripheral sympatholytic effects (e.g., blockade of myocardial beta-1 receptors) as well as by decreasing central sympathetic tone. In any event, beta blockers may offer a suitable alternative to decrease the effects of nervousness without a concomitant decrease in levels of alertness or motivation.[2] Hence, these drugs have gained a certain popularity with performing artists as a way to blunt the symptoms of performance anxiety without actually diminishing the anticipation and excitement that is requisite for a strong performance.

Problems and Adverse Effects

Most of the problems that occur with anxiolytic drugs are similar to those mentioned regarding the use of these agents as sedative-hypnotics. Sedation is still the most common side effect of the anxiolytic benzodiazepines, even though this effect is not as pronounced as with their sedative-hypnotic counterparts.[29] Addiction and abuse are problems with chronic benzodiazepine use, and withdrawal from these drugs can be a serious problem. Also, rebound anxiety has been described when drugs like diazepam are stopped.[9] Increased anxiety levels and other symptoms were noticed in one group of patients after diazepam was discontinued following a relatively short therapeutic trial of 6 weeks.[22] This observation again reinforces the idea that these drugs are not curative but should be used only for limited periods of time and as an adjunct to other nonpharmacologic procedures such as psychologic counseling.

SPECIAL CONSIDERATION OF SEDATIVE-HYPNOTIC AND ANTIANXIETY AGENTS IN REHABILITATION

Although these drugs are not used to directly influence the rehabilitation of musculoskeletal or other somatic disorders, the prevalence of their use in patient populations is high. Any time a patient is hospitalized for treatment of a disorder, a substantial amount of apprehension and concern exists. The foreign environment of the institution as well as a change in the individual's daily routine can understandably result in sleep disturbances. Predictably, surveys reveal more than 50 percent of patients hospitalized for medical procedures receive some type of sedative-hypnotic drug.[21] Individuals who are involved in rehabilitation programs, both as inpatients and as outpatients, may also have a fairly high anxiety level because of concern about their health and their ability to resume normal function. Acute and chronic injuries can create uncertainty about a patient's future family and job obligations as well as doubts about his or her self-image. The tension and anxiety produced may necessitate pharmacologic management.

The administration of sedative-hypnotic and antianxiety drugs has several direct implications for the rehabilitation session. Obviously the patient will be much calmer and more relaxed after taking an antianxiety drug, thus offering the potential benefit of gaining the patient's full cooperation during a physical therapy treatment. Anxiolytic benzodiazepines reach peak blood levels 2 to 4 hours after oral administration, so scheduling the rehabilitation session during that time may improve the patient's participation in the treatment. Of course, this rationale will backfire completely if the drug produces significant sedative-hypnotic effects. Therapy sessions that require the patient to actively participate in activities such as gait training or therapeutic exercise will be essentially useless and even hazardous if the patient is extremely drowsy. Consequently, scheduling patients for certain types of rehabilitation within several hours after administration of sedative-hypnotics or sedative-like anxiolytics is counterproductive and should be avoided.

CASE STUDY

SEDATIVE-HYPNOTIC DRUGS

Brief History. R.S. is a 34-year-old construction worker who sustained a fracture-dislocation of the vertebral column in an automobile accident. He was admitted to an acute care facility where a diagnosis was made of complete paraplegia at the T-12 spinal level. Surgery was performed to stabilize the vertebral column. During the next 3 weeks, his medical condition improved. At the end of 1 month, he was transferred to a rehabilitation facility to begin an intensive program of physical and occupational therapy. Rehabilitation included strengthening and range-of-motion (ROM) exercises, as well as training in wheelchair mobility, transfers, and activities of daily living (ADLs). However, upon arriving at the new institution, R.S. complained of difficulty sleeping. Butabarbital (Butisol) was prescribed at a dosage of 75 mg administered each night at bedtime.

Problem/Influence of Medication. During his daily rehabilitation regimen, the therapists noted that R.S.'s performance and level of attentiveness were markedly poor during the morning sessions. He was excessively lethargic and drowsy, and his speech was slurred. These symptoms were present to a much greater extent than the normal slow starting that occurs in some patients on wakening in the morning. The therapists also found that when ADL or mobility training was taught during the morning sessions, there was poor carryover from day to day regarding these activities.

Decision/Solution. The barbiturate-hypnotic drug appeared to be producing a hangover effect, which limited the patient's cognitive skills during the early daily activities. Initially this problem was dealt with by reserving the early part of the morning session for stretching and ROM activities, and then gradually moving into upper-body strengthening. Activities that required more patient learning and comprehension were done later in the morning or in the afternoon. Also, this hangover problem was brought to the attention of the physician, and ultimately the hypnotic drug was switched to a shorter-acting barbiturate such as secobarbital (Seconal).

SUMMARY

Sedative-hypnotic and antianxiety drugs play a prominent role in today's society. The normal pressures of daily life often result in tension and stress, which affect an individual's ability to relax or cope with stress. These problems are compounded when there is some type of illness or injury present. As would be expected, a number of patients seen in a rehabilitation setting are taking these drugs. The benzodiazepines (flurazepam, diazepam) are currently the drugs of choice in reducing tension and promoting sleep. Although these drugs are generally safer than their forerunners, they are not without their problems. Because of the potential for physical and psychologic dependence, sedative-hypnotic and antianxiety drugs should not be used indefinitely. These drugs should be prescribed judiciously as an adjunct to helping patients deal with the source of their problems.

REFERENCES

1. American Psychiatric Association: Diagnostic and Statistical Manual of Mental Disorders, ed 4. American Psychiatric Association, Washington, DC, 1994.
2. Brandfonbrenner, AG: Beta-blockers in the treatment of peformance anxiety. Medical Problems Performing Artists 5:23, 1990.
3. Eison, AS, et al: Serotonergic mechanisms in the behavioral effects of buspirone and gepirone. Pharmacol Biochem Behav 24:701, 1986.
4. Goldstein, DB: The effects of drugs on membrane fluidity. Annu Rev Pharmacol Toxicol 24:43, 1984.
5. Gorenstein, C and Gentil, V: Residual and acute effects of flurazepam and triazolam in normal subjects. Psychopharmacology 80:376, 1983.
6. Gossard, D, Dennis, C, and DeBusk, RF: Use of beta-blocking agents to reduce the stress of presentation at an international cardiology meeting: Results of a survey. Am J Cardiol 54:240, 1984.
7. Harrison, M, et al: Diazepam tapering in detoxification for high-dose benzodiazepine abuse. Clin Pharmacol Ther 36:527, 1984.
8. Ho, IK and Harris, RA: Mechanism of action of barbiturates. Annu Rev Pharmacol Toxicol 21:83, 1981.
9. Kales, A, et al: Rebound insomnia and rebound anxiety: A review. Pharmacology 26:121, 1983.
10. Kandel, ER: Disorders of mood: Depression, mania, and anxiety disorders. In Kandel, ER, Schwartz, JH, and Jessell, TM (eds): Principles of Neural Science, ed 3. Appleton & Lange, Norwalk, CT, 1991.
11. Karobath, M and Supavilai, P: Interaction of benzodiazepine receptor agonists and inverse agonists with the GABA receptor complex. Pharmacol Biochem Behav 23:671, 1985.
12. Landauer, AA and Pocock, DA: Stress reduction by oxoprenolol and placebo: Controlled investigation of the pharmacological and nonspecific effects. Br Med J 289:529, 1984.
13. McClusky, HY, et al: Efficacy of behavioral versus triazolam treatment in persistent sleep-onset insomnia. Am J Psychiatry 148:121, 1991.
14. Mennini, T, et al: Neurochemical effects of buspirone in rat hippocampus: Evidence for selective activation of 5-hydroxytryptamine neurons. Arch Int Pharmacodyn Ther 279:40, 1986.
15. Merlotti, L, et al: Rebound insomnia: Duration of use and individual differences. J Clin Psychopharmacol 11:368, 1991.
16. Michels, R and Marzuk, PM: Medical progress: Progress in psychiatry. N Engl J Med 329:552 (Part I), 628 (Part 2), 1993.
17. Nicoll, R: Selective actions of barbiturates on synaptic transmission. In Lipton, MA, DiMascio, A, and Killam, KF (eds): Psychopharmacology: A Generation of Progress. Raven Press, New York, 1978.
18. Nies, AS: Clinical pharmacology of the beta-adrenergic blockers. Medical Problems Performing Artists 1:25, 1986.

19. Olsen, RW: Drug interactions at the GABA receptor-ionophore complex. Annu Rev Pharmacol Toxicol 22:245, 1982.
20. Pecknold, JC, et al: Evaluation of buspirone as an antianxiety agent: Buspirone and diazepam versus placebo. Can J Psychiatry 34:766, 1989.
21. Perry, SW and Wu, A: Rationale for the use of hypnotic agents in a general hospital. Ann Intern Med 100:441, 1984.
22. Power, KG, et al: Controlled study of withdrawal symptoms and rebound anxiety after 6 week course of diazepam for generalized anxiety. Br Med J 290:1246, 1985.
23. Rall, TW: Hypnotics and sedatives. In Gilman, AG, et al: The Pharmacological Basis of Therapeutics, ed 8. Pergamon Press, New York, 1990.
24. Richards, JG, et al: Benzodiazepine receptors resolved. Experientia 42:121, 1986.
25. Rickels, K, et al: Long-term therapeutic use of benzodiazepines: I. Effects of abrupt discontinuation. Arch Gen Psychiatry 47:899, 1990.
26. Rosenbaum, JF: The drug treatment of anxiety. N Engl J Med 306:401, 1982.
27. Roth, T, Roehrs, TA, and Zorick, FJ: Pharmacology and hypnotic efficacy of triazolam. Pharmacotherapy 3:137, 1983.
28. Shader, RI, et al: Sedative effects and impaired learning and recall after single doses of lorazepam. Clin Pharmacol 39:562, 1986.
29. Shader, RI and Greenblatt, DJ. Drug therapy: Use of benzodiazepines in anxiety disorders. N Engl J Med 328:1398, 1993.
30. Study, RE and Barker, JL: Cellular mechanisms of benzodiazepine action. JAMA 247:2147, 1982.
31. Tallman, JF and Gallager, DW: The GABA-ergic system: A locus of benzodiazepine action. Annu Rev Neurosci 8:21, 1985.
32. Trevor, AJ and Way, WL: Sedative-hypnotics. In Katzung, BG (ed): Basic and Clinical Pharmacology, ed 5. Appleton & Lange, Norwalk, CT, 1992.
33. Walsh, JK, Schweitzer, PK, and Parwatikar, S: Effects of lorazepam and its withdrawal on sleep, performance and subjective state. Clin Pharmacol Ther 34:496, 1983.
34. Woo, E, Proulx, SM, and Greenblatt, DJ: Differential side effect profile of triazolam versus flurazepam in elderly patients undergoing rehabilitation therapy. J Clin Pharmacol 31:168, 1991.

CHAPTER 7

Drugs Used to Treat Affective Disorders: Depression and Manic-Depression

Affective disorders comprise the group of mental conditions that includes depression and manic-depression.[2,20] These disorders are characterized by a marked disturbance in a patient's mood. Patients with an affective disorder typically display an inappropriate disposition, which is either excessively excited and energetic (mania) or unreasonably sad and discouraged (depression).

Because these forms of mental illness are relatively common, many rehabilitation specialists will work with patients who are receiving drug therapy for an affective disorder. Also, serious injury or illness may precipitate an episode of depression in the patient undergoing physical rehabilitation. Consequently, this chapter will discuss the pharmacologic management of affective disorders, as well as how antidepressant and antimanic drugs may influence the patient involved in physical and occupational therapy.

DEPRESSION

Clinical Picture

Depression is considered to be the most prevalent form of mental illness in the United States. Although exact calculations of the incidence of this problem are difficult, approximately 5 percent of Americans will experience major depression over a 1-year period.[6] In this sense depression is a form of mental illness characterized by intense feelings of sadness and despair. Of course, a certain amount of disappointment and sadness is part of everyday life. However, a diagnosis of clinical depression indicates that these feelings are increased in both intensity and duration to the extent that they begin to be incapacitating.[20]

Depression is characterized by a general dysphoric mood (sadness, irritability, "down in the dumps"), as well as by a general lack of interest in previously pleasurable activities. Other symptoms including anorexia, sleep disorders (either too much or too little), fatigue, lack of self-esteem, somatic complaints, irrational guilt, and recurrent thoughts of death and suicide may help lead to a diagnosis of depression. To initiate effective treatment, a proper diagnosis must be made; depression must not be confused with other mental disorders that also may influence mood and behavior (e.g., schizophrenia). To standardize the terminology and aid in recognizing depression, specific criteria for the diagnosis of a major depressive episode have been outlined by the American Psychiatric Association.[2]

The causes of depression seem to be complex and somewhat unclear. Although a recent stressful incident or misfortune can certainly exacerbate an episode of depression, some patients may become depressed for no apparent reason. The role of genetic factors in depression has been explored but remains uncertain. A great deal of evidence that a CNS neurochemical imbalance may be the underlying feature in depression, as well as in other forms of mental illness, has been developed over the past 2 decades. The importance of these findings as related to pharmacologic treatment will be discussed. However, factors responsible for initiating these changes in CNS function are unclear. Depression is undoubtedly caused by the complex interaction of a number of genetic, environmental, and biochemical factors.[18,19]

Treatment of depression is essential in minimizing the disruptive influence that this disease has on the patient's overall well-being and on his or her relationship to family and job. Depending on the severity and type of depression, procedures ranging from psychotherapy to electroconvulsive treatment have been prescribed. Drug treatment plays a major role in alleviating and preventing the occurrence of major depression, and this form of therapy is presented here.

Pathophysiology of Depression

Over the past several years, a great deal of attention has been focused on the idea that a neuronal or neurotransmitter defect may be responsible for causing depression. The emergence of such ideas was exciting in light of the fact that depression could be treated much more effectively if it were caused by a specific problem in CNS synaptic transmission.

Originally, depression was believed to be caused by a decrease in neural transmission in CNS synapses that use amine neurotransmitters[5,26]; that is, synapses containing norepinephrine, serotonin, and possibly dopamine were thought to be underactive in areas associated with mood and behavior such as the limbic system. This so-called amine hypothesis was based on the fact that most of the drugs used to treat depression increased synaptic transmission in amine synapses. However, additional research on the effects of these drugs has caused the original amine hypothesis to be modified. Depression may be caused by an increased sensitivity of the postsynaptic receptor for norepinephrine—that is, the beta-adrenoreceptor.[14,29] This modification of the original theory was based primarily on the finding that effective antidepressant drugs all seem to work by decreasing the sensitivity of the CNS postsynaptic beta-adrenoreceptors.

The current rationale for the mechanism and treatment of depression is summarized in Figure 7–1. For reasons that are still unclear, depression appears to be initiated by an increase in postsynaptic receptor sensitivity to amine neurotransmitters, particularly norepinephrine (see Fig. 7–1). Antidepressant drugs increase amine trans-

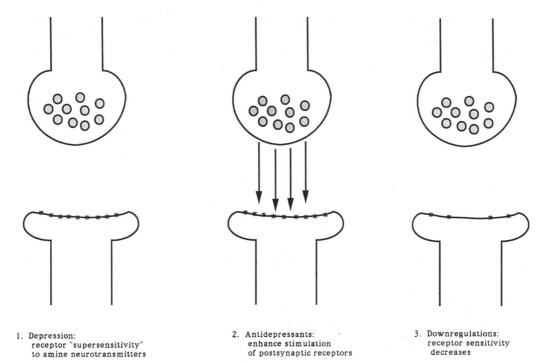

1. Depression:
   receptor "supersensitivity"
   to amine neurotransmitters

2. Antidepressants:
   enhance stimulation
   of postsynaptic receptors

3. Downregulations:
   receptor sensitivity
   decreases

FIGURE 7–1. Theoretic basis for the mechanism and treatment of depression. Functionally active receptor sites are indicated by an "∗." Depression is believed to be initiated by increased postsynaptic receptor sensitivity. Drugs that enhance stimulation of the receptors ultimately lead to receptor down-regulation, thus resolving the depression.

mission by a variety of methods, thus overstimulating the postsynaptic receptor. (The exact method by which these drugs increase amine stimulation is discussed later in this chapter.) Overstimulation of the postsynaptic receptor leads to a compensatory down-regulation and decreased sensitivity of the receptor. As discussed in Chapter 4, this down-regulation is a normal response to overstimulation by either endogenous or exogenous agonists. As receptor sensitivity decreases, the clinical symptoms of depression are resolved.

It must be emphasized that it is difficult to prove the neurochemical changes that underlie depression, and the way that antidepressant drugs help resolve depression remains theoretical at present. Still, certain aspects of drug therapy tend to support the amine hypothesis and the putative changes in receptor sensitivity induced by drug therapy. For instance, there is usually a time lag of approximately 2 to 4 weeks before antidepressant drugs begin to work.[1,23] This latency period would be necessary for a compensatory change in postsynaptic receptor sensitivity to take place after drug therapy is initiated.

Consequently, most antidepressants are believed to exert their effects by bringing about a decrease in sensitivity of the beta-adrenoreceptor at central norepinephrine synapses. The function of other amine neurotransmitters in this response requires some clarification as well. Serotonin (5-hydroxytryptamine) seems to play a permissive role in beta-receptor down-regulation, meaning that serotonergic activity must also be present for the decrease in beta-receptor sensitivity to occur.[14] In fact, certain antidepressants may exert a selective effect on serotonin. (The action of these serotonin-selective drugs is discussed later in this chapter.) The role of dopamine in the cause and treatment of depression is less obvious. Dopamine is probably not directly involved in either the pathogenesis or the drug treatment of depression, but some antidepressants may also affect dopamine synapses and produce other behavioral or motor side effects.

Antidepressant Drugs

The drugs that are currently used to treat depression are grouped into several categories according to chemical or functional criteria. These categories consist of the tricyclics, monoamine oxidase (MAO) inhibitors, and second-generation drugs (Table 7–1). All three groups attempt to increase aminergic transmission, but by different mechanisms (Fig. 7–2). Sympathomimetic stimulants such as the amphetamine drugs were also used on a limited basis to treat depression, but the powerful CNS excitation produced by amphetamine-like drugs and the potential for addiction and overdose have essentially eliminated their use as antidepressants. The pharmacologic effects of the primary antidepressant drug categories are discussed here.

Tricyclics. Drugs in this category share a common three-ring chemical structure (hence the name "tricyclic"). These drugs work by blocking the reuptake of amine neu-

TABLE 7–1 Common Antidepressant Drugs

Generic Name	Trade Name	Initial Adult Dose (mg/day)	Usual Adult Prescribing Limits* (mg/day)
Tricyclics			
Amitriptyline	Elavil, Emitrip, others	50–100	300
Desipramine	Pertofrane, Norpramin	100–200	300
Doxepin	Adapin, Sinequan	75	300
Imipramine	Janimine, Tofranil, others	75–200	300
Nortriptyline	Aventyl, Pamelor	75–100	150
Protriptyline	Vivactil	15–40	60
Trimipramine	Surmontil	75	300
MAO inhibitors			
Isocarboxazid	Marplan	10–20	30
Phenelzine	Nardil	45	90
Tranylcypromine	Parnate	10–20	60
Second-generation agents			
Amoxapine	Asendin	100–150	600
Bupropion	Wellbutrin	200	450
Fluoxetine	Prozac	20	80
Maprotiline	Ludiomil	25–75	225
Sertraline	Zoloft	50	200
Trazodone	Desyrel	150	600

*Upper limits reflect dosages administered to patients with severe depression who are being treated as inpatients.

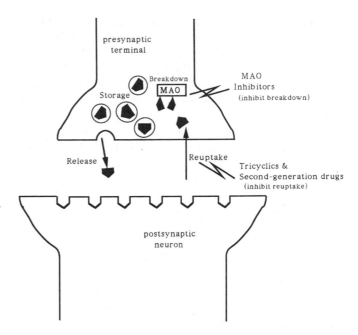

FIGURE 7–2. Effects of antidepressant drugs on amine synapses. All three types of drugs tend to increase the presence of amine transmitters (norepinephrine, dopamine, serotonin) in the synaptic cleft. Increased transmitter stimulation leads to postsynaptic receptor down-regulation/desensitization.

rotransmitters into the presynaptic terminal.[14,23] The active transport of amine neurotransmitters back into the presynaptic terminal is the method by which most (50 to 80 percent) of the released transmitter is removed from the synaptic cleft. By blocking reuptake, tricyclics allow the released amines to remain in the cleft and continue to exert their effects. The prolonged stimulation of these neurotransmitters (especially norepinephrine) leads to the compensatory decrease in receptor sensitivity, which ultimately leads to a decrease in depression.

Although other agents have been developed to treat depression, the tricyclic drugs remain the standard against which newer drugs are measured.[1] Tricyclics still seem to be the best available agents for treating several of the most common forms of depression, including melancholy depression.[23] As with all the antidepressants, the tricyclics are associated with several adverse side effects (see "Problems and Adverse Effects").

Monoamine Oxidase Inhibitors. Monoamine oxidase (MAO) is an enzyme that is located at amine synapses and helps remove the released transmitters through enzymatic destruction. Drugs that inhibit this enzyme allow more of the transmitter to remain in the synaptic cleft and continue to exert an effect. As with the tricyclics, MAO inhibitors directly increase activity at norepinephrine synapses, which brings about a subsequent receptor down-regulation. MAO inhibitors are not usually the drugs of choice in depression, but these drugs may be helpful if patients do not respond to other agents (tricyclics, second-generation drugs) or if other antidepressants produce intolerable side effects.

Second-Generation Antidepressants. Because of the limitations of first-generation drugs such as the tricyclics and MAO inhibitors, a number of diverse compounds have been developed and continue to be evaluated for their antidepressant effects. When compared with first-generation drugs, the goal of these newer drugs is threefold: (1) to have a more rapid onset in decreasing depression, (2) to have more tolerable side effects, and (3) to be safer—that is, to involve less chance of the occurrence of lethal overdose.[14] In general, the second-generation drugs have been only partially successful in meeting these goals. None of the newer antidepressants appears to have a more rapid onset than their predecessors.[29] Likewise, the newer agents have generally not proved to be more effective than standard treatment using the tricyclics.[23] The type of side effects associated with second-generation drugs may differ somewhat from the other two groups. Some of the newer agents may have a lower incidence of certain side effects (e.g., cardiovascular problems), but others do not offer any advantages in terms of decreased side effects.[8,14] Thus, when compared to other drugs such as the tricyclics, these newer drugs have not really demonstrated their superiority in the treatment of depression.

The newer antidepressants are chemically diverse, but most work by mechanisms similar to tricyclic drugs; that is, they block reuptake of norepinephrine and other monoamines. Hence, these drugs appear to exert their beneficial effects by bringing about the decrease in beta-adrenoreceptor sensitivity that seems to be the common denominator of antidepressant drugs' action. The second-generation drugs and their proposed mechanisms of action are summarized in Table 7–2.

Certain second-generation drugs (fluoxetine, sertraline, paroxetine) have received attention because of their ability to selectively block the reuptake of 5-hydroxytryptamine (serotonin). These drugs are often grouped together functionally as serotonin-selective reuptake inhibitors (SSRIs).[24] This distinguishes them from other second-gen-

TABLE 7–2 Second-Generation Antidepressants

Drug	Mechanism (Amine Selectivity)	Advantages	Disadvantages
Bupropion	Appears to inhibit dopamine reuptake	Low sedative, anticholinergic, and cardiovascular side effects	May cause overstimulation (insomnia, tremor) and induce psychotic symptoms
Fluoxetine	Strong, selective inhibition of serotonin reuptake	Low sedative, anticholinergic, and cardiovascular side effects; helpful in obsessive-compulsive disorders	May cause anxiety, nausea, insomnia; long half-life can lead to accumulation
Maprotiline	Moderate inhibition of norepinephrine reuptake	Sedating: useful in agitation	Possibility of seizures; overdoses lethal; long half-life
Sertraline	Strong selective inhibition of serotonin reuptake	Similar to fluoxetine	Similar to fluoxetine
Trazodone	Slight inhibition of serotonin reuptake	Sedating: useful in agitation; lower relative risk of overdose	May induce or exacerbate arrhythmias
Amoxapine	Moderate inhibition of norepinephrine reuptake	Low sedative and anticholinergic activity; may have more rapid onset of action	Possibility of extrapyramidal side effects (tardive dyskinesia); overdoses lethal

eration drugs and the tricyclics because these other drugs tend to be nonselective in their effect on amine neurotransmitters and block the reuptake of norepinephrine as well as serotonin. Despite this difference in amine selectivity, there does not appear to be any evidence that these SSRIs are clinically superior to the nonselective agents in resolving depression. There is, in fact, some indication that SSRIs such as fluoxetine (Prozac) may be less useful because of an increased risk of side effects including a worsening of depression in some patients.[23] Thus, the significance of the SSRIs as a subgroup of the second-generation antidepressants remains questionable at present.

Pharmacokinetics

Antidepressants are usually administered orally. Dosages vary depending not only on each drug but also on the individual patient. Initial doses generally start out relatively low and are increased slowly within the therapeutic range until beneficial effects are observed. Distribution within the body also varies with each type of antidepressant, but all eventually reach the brain to exert their effects. Metabolism takes place primarily in the liver, and metabolites of several drugs continue to show significant antidepressant activity. This fact may be responsible for prolonging the effects of the drug even after it has undergone hepatic biotransformation. Elimination takes place by biotransformation and renal excretion.

Problems and Adverse Effects

Tricyclics. A major problem with the tricyclic antidepressants is sedation (Table 7–3). Although a certain degree of sedation may be desirable in some agitated depressed patients, feelings of lethargy and sluggishness may impair patient adherence to drug therapy and result in a failure to take medication. A second major problem is that these drugs tend to have significant anticholinergic properties; that is, they act as if they are blocking certain central and peripheral acetylcholine receptors (see Table 7–3). Impairment of central acetylcholine transmission may cause confusion and delirium. The peripheral anticholinergic properties produce a variety of symptoms including dry mouth, constipation, urinary retention, and tachycardia. Other cardiovascular problems include arrhythmias and orthostatic hypotension, with the latter being particularly common in elderly patients. Finally, tricyclics have the highest potential for fatal overdose from an antidepressant. This fact leads to a serious problem when one considers the risk of suicide among depressed patients. These drugs should be dispensed in small quantities (i.e., only giving the patient a few days' worth of the drug) to diminish the risk of a fatal overdose.

MAO Inhibitors. In contrast to the tricyclics, MAO inhibitors tend to produce CNS excitation, which can result in restlessness, irritability, agitation, and sleep loss (see Table 7–3). These drugs also produce some central and peripheral anticholinergic effects (e.g., tremor, confusion, dry mouth, urinary retention), but these tend to occur to a lesser extent than with the tricyclics. Because of the systemic MAO inhibition, excess activity at peripheral sympathetic adrenergic terminals may cause a profound increase in blood pressure, leading to a hypertensive crisis. This situation is exacerbated if other drugs that increase sympathetic nervous activity are being taken concurrently. Also, there is a distinct interaction between the MAO inhibitors and certain foods such

TABLE 7–3 Side Effects of Antidepressant Drugs*

Drug	Sedation	Insomnia	Anticholinergic Effects	Orthostatic Hypotension
Tricyclic drugs				
Amitriptyline	+++	0	+++	+++
Trimipramine	+++	0	+++	++
Desipramine	+	+	+	+
Doxepin	+++	0	++	+++
Imipramine	++	0	++	++
Nortriptyline	++	0	+	+
Protriptyline	+	++	++	+
Monoamine oxidase inhibitors				
Phenelzine	+	+	0	+++
Tranylcypromine	0	++	0	+++
Isocarboxazid	0	++	0	++
Second-generation drugs				
Amoxapine	++	0	+	++
Fluoxetine	0	++	0	0
Maprotiline	++	0	+	++
Trazodone	+++	0	0	++
Bupropion	0	++	0	0

*Zero denotes no side effect, + a minor side effect, ++ a moderate side effect, and +++ a major side effect.

Source: Adapted from Potter et al,[23] p 637, by permission of *The New England Journal of Medicine.* Copyright 1991 Massachusetts Medical Society.

as fermented cheese and wines. These fermented foods contain tyramine, which stimulates the release of endogenous epinephrine and norepinephrine. The additive effect of increased catecholamine release (because of the ingested tyramine) and decreased catecholamine breakdown (because of MAO inhibition) can lead to excessive catecholamine levels and a hypertensive crisis.

Second-Generation Drugs. The type and severity of side effects associated with the newer antidepressants vary according to the specific drug in use. In general, many of the second-generation drugs have side effects similar to the earlier drugs, and many have different side effects that also make their use less than ideal. Advantages and disadvantages of these drugs as compared with the tricyclics and MAO inhibitors are summarized in Tables 7–2 and 7–3. These second-generation drugs have not been found to be more effective in treating depression than their earlier counterparts. Consequently, selection of an appropriate drug must be made on a patient-by-patient basis, with certain individuals responding best to certain antidepressants.

Use of Antidepressants in Chronic Pain

Many chronic pain syndromes (low back pain, neck pain) can be treated more effectively if antidepressants are included in the treatment regimen.[15] Some studies attribute this effect to the fact that clinical depression is present in many patients with chronic pain; administering antidepressants will help provide optimal care by resolving the depressive symptoms.[28] There is considerable evidence, however, that antidepressants will help patients with chronic pain even if no symptoms of depression are present. That is, improvements in pain have been noted even when there has been no observed effect on the patient's mood.[22] Many practitioners also feel that antidepressants may help resolve chronic pain by improving the patient's sleep patterns, but improvements in pain have been noted in patients even when no effect on sleep was seen.[22]

Hence, there is little doubt that antidepressants may be useful as an adjunct in the treatment of patients with chronic pain. However, the exact way that these drugs help diminish pain in these patients remains speculative.

TREATMENT OF MANIC-DEPRESSION: ANTIMANIC DRUGS

Bipolar Syndrome

The form of depression discussed previously is often referred to as *unipolar depression*, in contrast to bipolar or "manic-depressive" syndrome. As these terms imply, **bipolar syndrome** is associated with mood swings from one extreme (mania) to the other (depression). Manic episodes are characterized by euphoria, hyperactivity, and talkativeness, and depressive episodes are similar to those described previously. Approximately 10 percent of all depressed patients are considered to exhibit bipolar syndrome.[20]

As in unipolar depression, the exact causes of manic-depression are unknown. Certain factors initiate changes in CNS function, which eventually result in a functional increase in aminergic transmission.[4] Overactive norepinephrine and possibly serotonin pathways appear to be responsible for the manic episodes of this disorder. The subsequent depression may simply be a rebound from the general excitement of the manic episode. In any event, the treatment of bipolar syndrome focuses on preventing the start of these pendulum-like mood swings by preventing the manic episodes. Hence, drugs used to treat manic-depression are really "antimanic drugs." The primary form of drug treatment consists of lithium salts (i.e., lithium carbonate, lithium citrate). Lithium is effective in treating approximately 60 to 80 percent of manic-depressive cases.[13] In addition, lithium is a useful adjunct to other antidepressant drugs in treating resistant cases of unipolar depression.[10,25]

Lithium

Lithium (Li^+) is a monovalent cation included in the alkali metal group. Because of its small size (molecular weight 7) and single positive charge, lithium is able to pass through open neuronal sodium channels quite easily, suggesting that it may influence neural excitability by directly entering the neuron.[4,17] One theory is that lithium is able to enter the neuron through activated sodium channels during an action potential. However, the neuron is unable to remove lithium from its interior, resulting in altered ionic distribution and membrane conductance. This change may, in effect, stabilize the neuronal membrane, thereby decreasing excitability and diminishing transmission in the overactive aminergic pathways. Lithium has also been shown to directly decrease the release of amine neurotransmitters and to increase the reuptake of transmitter into the presynaptic terminal.[27] Studies have shown that lithium can diminish the function of cyclic adenosine monophosphate and other second-messenger systems that are normally stimulated by norepinephrine.[7,11,13] Obviously, lithium has the potential to influence synaptic function and neural excitability in several ways. However, exactly why this drug is able to specifically resolve overactive CNS aminergic transmission is unclear. The precise mechanism by which lithium exerts its antimanic properties remains to be determined.[4]

Absorption and Distribution

Lithium is absorbed readily from the gastrointestinal tract and distributed completely throughout all the tissues in the body. During an acute manic episode, achieving blood serum concentrations between 1.0 and 1.4 mEq/L is desirable. Maintenance doses that are somewhat lower and serum concentrations that range from 0.5 to 1.3 mEq/L are optimal.

Problems and Adverse Effects of Lithium

A major problem with lithium use is the danger of accumulation within the body.[3,16] Lithium is not metabolized, and drug elimination takes place almost exclusively through excretion in the urine. Consequently, lithium has a tendency to accumulate in the body, and toxic levels can frequently be reached during administration of this drug.

Side effects occur frequently with lithium, and the degree and type of side effects depend on the amount of lithium in the bloodstream. As Table 7–4 indicates, some side effects are present even when serum levels are within the therapeutic range. However, toxic side effects become apparent when serum concentrations approach or exceed 2.5 mEq/L, and progressive accumulation of lithium can be fatal. Consequently, individuals dealing with a patient receiving lithium therapy should be aware of any changes in behavior that might indicate that this drug is reaching toxic levels. Also, serum titers of lithium should be monitored periodically to ensure that blood levels remain within the therapeutic range.[3]

SPECIAL CONCERNS IN REHABILITATION PATIENTS

Some amount of depression is certain to be present as a result of a catastrophic injury or illness. Patients receiving physical therapy for any number of acute or chronic illnesses may be taking antidepressant medications in order to improve their mood and general well-being. Of course, therapists working in a psychiatric facility will deal with many patients taking antidepressant drugs, and severe depression may be the primary reason the patient is institutionalized in the first place. However, these drugs are also frequently prescribed to the patient suffering from a spinal cord injury, stroke, severe burn, multiple sclerosis, amputation, and so on. Different drugs have been suggested to be optimal in specific types of physical disability. For instance, the tricyclic antidepressant nortriptyline has been suggested to help patients suffering from post-

TABLE 7–4 Side Effects and Toxicity of Lithium

Mild (Below 1.5 mEq/L)	Moderate (1.5–2.5 mEq/L)	Toxicity (2.5–7.0 mEq/L)
Metallic taste in mouth	Severe diarrhea	Nystagmus
Fine hand tremor (resting)	Nausea and vomiting	Coarse tremor
Nausea	Mild to moderate ataxia	Dysarthria
Polyuria	Incoordination	Fasciculations
Polydipsia	Dizziness, sluggishness, giddiness, vertigo	Visual or tactile hallucinations
Diarrhea or loose stools	Slurred speech	Oliguria, anuria
Muscular weakness or fatigue	Tinnitus	Confusion
	Blurred vision	Impaired consciousness
	Increasing tremor	Dyskinesia-chorea, athetoid movements
	Muscle irritability or twitching	Tonic-clonic convulsions
	Asymmetric deep tendon reflexes	Coma
	Increased muscle tone	Death

Source: Adapted from Harris, E: Lithium. AJN 81(7):1312, 1981.

stroke depression.[21] Also, certain drugs may offer advantages over others in treating elderly depressed patients.[12,30] Given the variety of agents currently available, patients with various physical problems will respond differently. The physician working with the patient, family, and other health-care professionals must attempt to find the drug that produces optimal results in alleviating depression in each patient.

With regard to the impact of antidepressant and antimanic agents on the rehabilitation process, these drugs can be extremely beneficial in helping to improve the patient's outlook. The patient may become more optimistic regarding his or her future and may assume a more active role and interest in the rehabilitation process. This behavior can be invaluable in increasing patient cooperation and improving compliance with rehabilitation goals. However, certain side effects can be somewhat troublesome during physical therapy treatments. Sedation, lethargy, and muscle weakness can occur with the tricyclics and lithium, which can present a problem if the patient's active cooperation is required. Other unpleasant side effects such as nausea and vomiting can also be disturbing during treatments. A more common and potentially more serious problem is the orthostatic hypotension that occurs predominantly with the tricyclics. This hypotension can cause syncope and subsequent injury if patients fall during gait training. Blood pressure should also be monitored regularly, especially in patients taking MAO inhibitors. Care should be taken to avoid a hypertensive crisis, especially during therapy sessions that tend to increase blood pressure (e.g., certain forms of exercise).

Finally, rehabilitation specialists should remember that antidepressant treatment must often be administered for 1 month or more before an improvement in symptoms occurs.[1,23] During this period, drug therapy may actually precipitate an increase in depression, including increased thoughts of suicide in some patients.[9] Rehabilitation specialists should be alert for any signs that a patient is becoming more depressed and possibly suicidal, especially during the first few weeks after antidepressant drug therapy is initiated.

CASE STUDY

ANTIDEPRESSANT DRUGS

Brief History. J.G., a 71-year-old retired pharmacist, was admitted to the hospital with a chief complaint of an inability to move his right arm and leg. He was also unable to speak at the time of admission. The clinical impression was right hemiplegia caused by left middle cerebral artery thrombosis. The patient also had a history of hypertension and had been taking cardiac beta blockers for several years. J.G.'s medical condition stabilized, and the third day after admission he was seen for the first time by a physical therapist. Speech and occupational therapy were also soon initiated. The patient's condition improved rapidly, and motor function began to return in the right side. Balance and gross motor skills increased until he could transfer from his wheelchair to his bed with minimal assistance, and gait training activities were being initiated. J.G. was able to comprehend verbal commands, but his speech remained markedly slurred and difficult to understand. During his first 2 weeks in the hospital, J.G. had shown signs of severe depression. Symptoms increased until cooperation with the rehabilitation and nursing staffs was being compromised. Imipramine (Tofranil) was prescribed at a dosage of 150 mg/day.

Problem/Influence of Medication. Imipramine is a tricyclic antidepressant, and these drugs are known to produce orthostatic hypotension during the initial stages of drug therapy. Since the patient is expressively aphasic, he will have trouble telling the therapist that he feels dizzy or faint. Also, the cardiac beta blockers will blunt any compensatory increase in cardiac output if blood pressure drops during postural changes.

Decision/Solution. The therapist decided to place the patient on the tilt table for the first day after imipramine was started and to monitor blood pressure regularly. While the patient was on the tilt table, weight shifting and upper extremity facilitation activities were performed. The patient tolerated this well, so the therapist had him resume ambulation activities using the parallel bars on the following day. With the patient standing inside the bars, the therapist carefully watched for any subjective signs of dizziness or syncope in the patient (i.e., facial pallor, inability to follow instructions). Standing bouts were also limited in duration. By the third day, ambulation training continued with the patient outside the parallel bars, but the therapist made a point of having the patient's wheelchair close at hand in case the patient began to appear faint. These precautions of careful observation and short, controlled bouts of ambulation were continued throughout the remainder of the patient's hospital stay, and no incident of orthostatic hypotension was observed during physical therapy.

SUMMARY

Affective disorders such as depression and manic-depression are found frequently in the general population as well as in rehabilitation patients. Drugs commonly prescribed in the treatment of (unipolar) depression include the tricyclics and MAO inhibitors as well as the newer second-generation antidepressants. Lithium is the drug of choice for treating bipolar syndrome, or manic-depression. All of these drugs seem to exert their effects by modifying CNS synaptic transmission and receptor sensitivity in amine pathways. The exact manner in which these drugs affect synaptic activity has shed some light on the possible neuronal changes that may underlie these forms of mental illness. Antidepressant and antimanic drugs can improve the patient's attitude and compliance during rehabilitation, but therapists should be aware that certain side effects may alter the patient's physical and mental behavior.

REFERENCES

1. Adams, J: Drug treatment of depression. N Z Med J 106:208, 1993.
2. American Psychiatric Association: Diagnostic and Statistical Manual of Mental Disorders, ed 4. American Psychiatric Association, Washington, DC, 1994.
3. Aronson, JK and Reynolds, DJM: ABC of monitoring drug therapy—lithium. Br Med J 305:1273, 1992.
4. Baldessarini, RJ: Drugs and the treatment of psychiatric disorders. In Gilman, AG, et al (eds): The Pharmacological Basis of Therapeutics, ed 8. Pergamon Press, New York, 1990.
5. Baldessarini, RJ: The basis for amine hypothesis in affective disorders. Arch Gen Psychiatry 32:1087, 1975.
6. Bell, IR and Gelenberg, AJ: Mood disorders. In Rakel, RE (ed): Conn's Current Therapy. WB Saunders, Philadelphia, 1993.
7. Belmaker, RH: Receptors, adenylate cyclase, depression and lithium. Biol Psychiatry 16:333, 1981.
8. Coccaro, EJ and Seiver, LJ: Second generation antidepressants: A comparative review. J Clin Psychopharmacol 25:241, 1985.
9. Damluji, NF and Ferguson, JM: Paradoxical worsening of depressive symptomatology caused by antidepressants. J Clin Psychopharmacol 8:347, 1988.
10. De Montigny, C, et al: Lithium carbonate addition in tricyclic antidepressant-resistant unipolar depression: Correlations with the neurobiologic actions of tricyclic antidepressant drugs and lithium ions on the serotonin system. Arch Gen Psychiatry 40:1327, 1983.
11. Ebstein, RP, Hermoni, M, and Belmaker, RH: The effect of lithium on noradrenaline-induced cyclic AMP accumulation in the rat: Inhibition after chronic treatment and absence of supersensitivity. J Pharm Exp Ther 213:161, 1980.
12. Gwirtsman, HE, et al: Therapeutic superiority of maprotiline versus doxepin in geriatric depression. J Clin Psychiatry 44:449, 1983.
13. Hollister, LE: Antipsychotic agents and lithium. In Katzung, BG (ed): Basic and Clinical Pharmacology, ed 5. Appleton & Lange, Norwalk, CT, 1992.
14. Hollister, LE: Current antidepressants. Annu Rev Pharmacol Toxicol 26:23, 1986.
15. Jenkins, DG and Ebbutt, AF: Tofranil in the treatment of low back pain. J Int Med Res 4(suppl 2):28, 1976.
16. Johnson, FN (ed): Handbook of Lithium Therapy. University Park Press, Baltimore, 1980.
17. Johnson, FN (ed): Lithium Research and Therapy. Academic Press, New York, 1975.
18. Kandel, ER: Disorders of mood: Depression, mania, and anxiety disorders. In Kandel, ER, et al (eds): Principles of Neural Science, ed 3. Appleton & Lange, Norwalk, CT, 1991.
19. Klerman, GL: The nosology and diagnosis of depressive disorders. In Grinspoon, L (ed): Psychiatry Update, Vol II. American Psychiatric Association Press, Washington, DC, 1983.
20. Lickey, ME and Gordon, B: Drugs for Mental Illness. WH Freeman, New York, 1983.
21. Lipsey, JR, et al: Nortryptiline treatment of poststroke depression: A double blind study. Lancet 1:297, 1984.
22. McQuay, HJ, Carroll, D, and Glynn, CJ: Low dose amitriptyline in the treatment of chronic pain. Anaesthesia 47:646, 1992.
23. Potter, WZ, Rudorfer, MV, and Manji, H: Drug therapy: The pharmacologic treatment of depression. N Engl J Med 325:633, 1991.
24. Preskorn, SH: Recent pharmacologic advances in antidepressant therapy for the elderly. Am J Med 94(suppl 5A):S2–S12, 1993.
25. Price, LH, Charney, DS, and Heninger, GR: Efficacy of lithium-tranylcypromine treatment in refractory depression. Am J Psychiatry 142:619, 1985.
26. Schildkraut, JJ: Current status of the catecholamine hypothesis of affective disorders. In Lipton, MA, DiMascio, A, and Killam, KF (eds): Psychopharmacology: A Generation of Progress. Raven Press, New York, 1978.
27. Sheard, MH: The biological effects of lithium. Trends Neurosci 3:85, 1986.
28. Sullivan, MJL, et al: The treatment of depression in chronic low back pain: Review and recommendations. Pain 50:5, 1992.
29. Tyrer, P and Marsden, C: New antidepressant drugs: Is there anything new they tell us about depression? Trends Neurosci 8:427, 1985.
30. Weissman, MM, et al: A double-blind clinical trial of aprazolam, imipramine, or placebo in the depressed elderly. J Clin Psychopharmacol 12:175, 1992.

CHAPTER 8

Antipsychotic Drugs

Psychosis is the term used to describe the more severe forms of mental illness. Psychoses are actually a group of mental disorders characterized by a marked thought disturbance and an impaired perception of reality. By far the most common form of psychosis is schizophrenia, with an estimated 1.0 percent of the world population being afflicted.[15,17,18] Other psychotic disorders include psychotic depression and severe paranoid disorders. In the past, strong, sedative-like drugs were the primary method of treating patients with psychosis. The goal was to pacify these patients so that they were no longer combative and abusive to themselves and others. Such drugs were commonly referred to as "major tranquilizers" and had the obvious disadvantage of producing so much sedation that the patient's cognitive and motor skills were compromised.

As more was learned about the neurologic changes involved in psychosis, drugs were developed to specifically treat psychosis rather than simply sedate the patient. These antipsychotic drugs, or **neuroleptics** as some clinicians refer to them, represent a major breakthrough in the treatment of schizophrenia and other psychotic disorders.

Physical and occupational therapists frequently encounter patients taking antipsychotic drugs. Therapists employed in a psychiatric facility will routinely treat patients taking these medications. Therapists who practice in nonpsychiatric settings may still encounter these patients for various reasons. For instance, the patient on antipsychotic medication who sustains a fractured hip may be seen at an orthopedic facility. Consequently, knowledge of antipsychotic pharmacology will be useful to all rehabilitation specialists.

Because of the prevalence of schizophrenia, this chapter concentrates on the treatment of this psychotic disorder. Also, the pathogenesis and subsequent treatment of other forms of psychosis are similar to those of schizophrenia, and this specific condition will be used as an example of the broader range of psychotic conditions.

SCHIZOPHRENIA

The *Diagnostic and Statistical Manual of Mental Disorders* lists several distinct criteria necessary for a diagnosis of schizophrenia.[2] These include a marked disturbance in the thought process, which may include bizarre delusions and auditory hallucinations (i.e., "hearing voices"). Also, a decreased level of function in work, social relations, and self-care may be present. The duration of these and other symptoms (at least 6 months) and a differential diagnosis from other forms of mental illness (such as affective disorders and organic brain syndrome) help round out these criteria.

The exact cause of schizophrenia is unknown. Extensive research has suggested that both genetic and environmental factors are important in bringing about neurotransmitter changes in CNS dopamine pathways, but the precise role of these factors remains to be determined.[6]

The advent of antipsychotic drugs represents one of the most significant developments in the treatment of schizophrenia and similar disorders. These drugs are believed to be the single most important reason for the abrupt decrease in the number of mental patients admitted to public hospitals during the 1950s and 1960s.[13] This observation does not imply that these drugs cure schizophrenia. Schizophrenia and other psychoses are believed to be incurable, and psychotic episodes can recur throughout the lifetime of the patient. However, these drugs can normalize the patient's behavior and thinking during an acute psychotic episode, and maintenance doses are believed to help prevent the recurrence of psychosis. Consequently, the ability of these patients to take care of themselves and cooperate with others is greatly improved.

NEUROTRANSMITTER CHANGES IN SCHIZOPHRENIA

Most of the current evidence indicates that schizophrenia may be caused by overactive dopaminergic pathways in certain parts of the brain.[12,16,17,20,22] Increased dopamine transmission in areas such as the limbic system may be responsible for the behavioral changes associated with this disorder. Increased dopamine influence could be caused by excessive dopamine synthesis and release by the presynaptic neuron, decreased dopamine breakdown at the synapse, increased postsynaptic dopamine receptor sensitivity, or a combination of these and other factors.

Consequently, the currently accepted theory is that schizophrenia is caused by overactivity in dopamine synapses.[12,16,20] However, given the complexity of central neurotransmitter interaction, this belief may ultimately prove to be an oversimplification. Future research in schizophrenia and other forms of psychosis will be needed to examine the contribution of additional factors such as changes in postsynaptic dopamine receptor sensitivity and imbalances in other transmitter pathways.[6]

ANTIPSYCHOTIC CLASSES AND MECHANISMS OF ACTION

The antipsychotic drugs that are used to successfully treat schizophrenia all work by blocking central dopamine receptors (Fig. 8–1).[15–17,22] These drugs share some structural similarity to dopamine, which allows them to bind to the postsynaptic receptor, but they do not activate it. This effectively blocks the receptor from the effects of the released endogenous neurotransmitter (see Fig. 8–1). Any increased activity at central dopamine synapses is therefore negated by postsynaptic receptor blockade.

There are five major classes of antipsychotics (Table 8–1). Despite their chemical

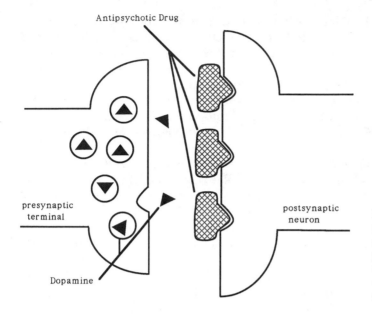

FIGURE 8-1. Effects of antipsychotic drugs on dopamine synapses. Antipsychotics act as postsynaptic receptor antagonists to block the effects of overactive dopamine transmission.

TABLE 8-1 Classes of Antipsychotic Drugs

I. Phenothiazines

Acetophenazine (Tindal)
Chlorpromazine (Thorazine)
Fluphenazine (Permitil, Prolixin)
Mesoridazine (Serentil)
Perphenazine (Trilafon, Triavil)
Prochlorperazine (Comazol, Compazine)
Promazine (Primazine, Sparine, others)
Thioridazine (Mellaril)
Trifluoperazine (Stelazine, Suprazine)
Triflupromazine (Vesprin)

II. Thioxanthenes

Chlorprothixene (Taractan)
Thiothixene (Navane)

III. Butyrophenones

Haloperidol (Haldol)

IV. Dihydroindolones

Molindone (Moban)

V. Dibenzoxazepines

Loxapine (Loxitane)
Clozapine (Clozaril)

diversity, there is no evidence indicating that one class is more effective in treating schizophrenia than another.[6] The major differences are in the potency and side effects associated with individual drugs in each class.[7,15] Antipsychotics such as haloperidol (Haldol) and fluphenazine (Prolixin) are described as having high potency, indicating that they have a fairly high affinity for CNS dopamine receptors and can exert beneficial effects when used in fairly low doses. These high-potency drugs, however, tend to be associated with a higher risk of extrapyramidal (motor) side effects, possibly because they bind effectively to several types of CNS dopamine receptors, including the receptors that influence motor function. Other agents such as chlorpromazine (Thorazine) and thioridazine (Mellaril) have lower potency and must be used in higher doses to exert an antipsychotic effect. These low-potency agents tend to cause more sedative and anticholinergic side effects (dry mouth, constipation, urinary retention, etc.).

Hence, there is generally a trade-off between sedative-anticholinergic properties and motor side effects (Table 8–2). Drugs that have fewer sedative and anticholinergic effects tend to be associated with a greater risk of motor symptoms, and vice versa. These side effects and their possible long-term implications are discussed further in this chapter.

TABLE 8–2 Antipsychotic Drugs Categorized by Side Effects*

Drug	Extrapyramidal	Sedative	Anticholinergic
Group A			
Fluphenazine	S	W	W
Perphenazine	S	W–M	W–M
Prochlorperazine	S	M	W
Trifluoperazine	S	W	W
Chlorprothixene	S	W	W
Thiothixene	S	W	W
Haloperidol	S	W	W
Molindone	S	W	W
Loxapine	S	W	W
Group B			
Triflupromazine	M–S	M–S	S
Acetophenazine	M	M	W
Group C			
Chlorpromazine	W–M	S	M–S
Promazine	W	S	S
Mesoridazine	W	M–S	M
Thioridazine	W	S	S

*Chances of side effects are classified as follows: S = Strong, M = Moderate, W = Weak. Drugs in group A tend to produce strong extrapyramidal effects but weak sedative and anticholinergic effects. Drugs in group C tend to produce moderate to strong sedative and anticholinergic side effects, but weak extrapyramidal effects. Drugs in group B tend to produce moderate to strong side effects in all three categories.

PHARMACOKINETICS

Antipsychotics are usually administered orally. During the acute stage of a psychotic episode, the daily dosage is often divided into three or four equal amounts. Maintenance doses are usually lower and can often be administered once each day. Under certain conditions, antipsychotics can be given intramuscularly. During acute episodes, intramuscular injections tend to reach the bloodstream faster than an orally administered drug and may be used if the patient is especially agitated. Conversely, certain forms of intramuscular antipsychotics that enter the bloodstream slowly have also been developed. Preparations such as fluphenazine decanoate and haloperidol decanoate can be injected every 2 to 4 weeks, respectively, and serve as a method of slow, continual release during the maintenance phase of psychosis. This method of administration may prove helpful if the patient has poor self-adherence to drug therapy and neglects to take his or her medication regularly.

Metabolism of antipsychotics is through two mechanisms: conjugation with glucuronic acid and oxidation by hepatic microsomal enzymes. Both mechanisms of metabolism and subsequent inactivation take place in the liver. Some degree of enzyme induction may occur because of prolonged use of antipsychotics and may be responsible for increasing the rate of metabolism of these drugs.

OTHER USES OF ANTIPSYCHOTICS

Occasionally these drugs are prescribed for conditions other than classic psychosis. During the acute manic stage of manic-depression, an antipsychotic combined with lithium is often more effective than lithium alone.[16] Low doses of antipsychotics may also be used in certain cases of organic brain syndrome to help control the patient's behavior.[14] These drugs are effective in decreasing the nausea and vomiting that often occur when dopamine agonists and precursors are administered to treat Parkinson's disease. The antiemetic effect of the antipsychotics is probably caused by their ability to block dopamine receptors located on the brainstem that cause vomiting when stimulated by the exogenous dopamine.

PROBLEMS AND ADVERSE EFFECTS

Extrapyramidal Symptoms

Some of the more serious problems that occur in the use of antipsychotic drugs result in the production of abnormal movement patterns.[3,4,7] Many of these aberrant movements are similar to those seen in patients with lesions of the extrapyramidal system and are often referred to as extrapyramidal side effects. The basic reason that these motor problems occur is because dopamine is an important neurotransmitter in motor pathways, especially in the integration of motor function that takes place in the basal ganglia. Since antipsychotic drugs block CNS dopamine receptors, it makes sense that motor side effects are a potential complication of these drugs. The unintentional antagonism of dopamine receptors in areas of motor integration (as opposed to the beneficial blockade of behaviorally related receptors) results in a neurotransmitter imbalance that creates several distinct types of movement problems.

Thus, most antipsychotic drugs are associated with some type of motor side effect, because these drugs are relatively nonselective in their ability to block CNS dopamine receptors. An exception may be the drug clozapine (Clozaril), which seems to be more selective for dopamine receptors in the limbic system.[4,6] Preliminary evidence has indicated that this drug may produce relatively fewer extrapyramidal side effects because of an apparent ability to bind more selectively to CNS receptors that affect behavior rather than receptors that influence motor function. In addition, research has revealed that several different subtypes of dopamine receptors may exist in the body (e.g., D_1, D_2, and D_3 receptors), and that certain subtypes such as the D_3 receptor may be located in parts of the brain that control behavior. This could help lead to the development of antipsychotic drugs that are more selective for the behavior-mediating receptors, thus decreasing the risk of extrapyramidal side effects.[23]

At present, however, extrapyramidal side effects continue to be one of the major drawbacks of antipsychotic medications. The primary types of extrapyramidal side effects, the manifestations of each type, and the relative time of their onset are shown in Figure 8–2. Some factors involved in patient susceptibility and possible treatment of these side effects are discussed here.

Tardive Dyskinesia. The disorder of **tardive dyskinesia** is characterized by a number of involuntary and fragmented movements. In particular, rhythmic movements of the mouth, tongue, and jaw are present, and the patient often produces involuntary sucking and smacking noises. Other symptoms include choreoathetoid movements of the extremities and dystonias of the neck and trunk. Tardive dyskinesia can

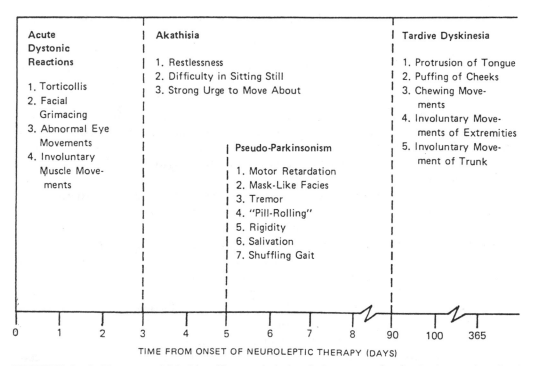

FIGURE 8–2. Extrapyramidal side effects and their relative onset after beginning antipsychotic drug therapy. (From Feigenbaum, JC and Schneider, F: Antipsychotic medications. In Mathewson, MK: Pharmacotherapeutics: A Nursing Approach. FA Davis, Philadelphia, 1986, p 404, with permission.)

begin to occur within several weeks after initiating antipsychotic therapy but is seen more frequently if the drug has been taken continually for 12 months or longer.[13] Estimates of the incidence of this problem range between 15 and 25 percent of individuals on antipsychotic medication, with elderly patients and women being especially susceptible.[3,15,25]

Tardive dyskinesia induced by antipsychotic drugs is believed to be caused by "disuse supersensitivity" of the dopamine receptor.[3,11] Although the presynaptic neurons are still intact, drug blockade of the postsynaptic receptor induces the postsynaptic neuron to respond by "up-regulating" the number or sensitivity of the receptors. This increase in receptor sensitivity causes a functional increase in dopaminergic influence, leading to a neurotransmitter imbalance between dopamine and other central neurotransmitters such as acetylcholine and gamma-aminobutyric acid (GABA). This imbalance results in the symptoms of tardive dyskinesia.

Tardive dyskinesia is the most feared side effect of antipsychotic drugs.[6] In some patients, the symptoms will disappear if the drug is stopped or the dosage is decreased, but this can take from several weeks to several years to occur. In other individuals, drug-induced tardive dyskinesia appears irreversible.[3,10] To prevent the occurrence of tardive dyskinesia, a low dose of the antipsychotic should be used, especially during the maintenance phase of drug therapy.[5,19] Also, recognition of the motor symptoms of tardive dyskinesia can be dealt with by lowering drug dosage or by substituting an antipsychotic drug that tends to produce fewer extrapyramidal side effects (see Table 8–2). Early intervention is generally believed to be the most effective way of preventing the permanent changes associated with antipsychotic-induced tardive dyskinesia.[3]

Other drugs have been used to try to alleviate the symptoms of drug-induced tardive dyskinesia.[9] Agents such as anticholinergic drugs (e.g., atropine-like drugs) and GABA-enhancing drugs (e.g., benzodiazepines) have been used to attempt to rectify the transmitter imbalance created by the increased dopamine sensitivity. Reserpine has also been used in some patients because of its ability to deplete presynaptic stores of dopamine, thus limiting the influence of this neurotransmitter.[10] However, these additional agents tend to be only marginally successful in reducing the dyskinesia symptoms, and their use tends to add complexity to the drug management of patients with psychoses. Thus, the best course of action continues to be judicious administration of these drugs, using the lowest effective dose, and early recognition and intervention if extrapyramidal symptoms appear.[3,9]

Pseudoparkinsonism. The motor symptoms seen in Parkinson's disease (see Chapter 10) are caused by a deficiency in dopamine transmission in the basal ganglia. Since antipsychotic drugs block dopamine receptors, some patients may understandably experience symptoms similar to those seen in Parkinson's disease. These symptoms include resting tremor, bradykinesia, and rigidity. Elderly patients are more susceptible to these drug-induced parkinsonian-like symptoms, probably because dopamine content (and therefore dopaminergic influence) tends to be lower in older individuals.[24] The outcome of antipsychotic-induced parkinsonism is usually favorable, and these symptoms normally disappear when the dosage is adjusted or the drug is withdrawn. Drugs used as adjuncts in treating Parkinson's disease (e.g., amantadine, benztropine mesylate) may also be administered to deal with the parkinsonian-like side effects. The primary antiparkinsonian drugs such as levodopa and dopamine agonists are not used to treat these parkinsonian-like side effects because they tend to exacerbate the psychotic symptoms.

Akathisia. Patients taking antipsychotics may experience sensations of motor restlessness and may complain of an inability to sit or lie still. This condition is known as **akathisia**. Patients may also appear agitated, may "pace the floor," and may have problems with insomnia. Akathisia can usually be dealt with by altering the dosage or type of medication. If this is unsuccessful, beta-2 adrenergic receptor blockers (propranolol) may help decrease the restlessness associated with akathisia by a mechanism involving central adrenergic receptors.[1,8]

Dyskinesia and Dystonias. Patients may exhibit a broad range of bizarre movements of the arms, legs, neck, and face including torticollis, oculogyric crisis, and opisthotonos.[3] These movements are involuntary and uncoordinated, and may begin fairly soon after initiating antipsychotic therapy (i.e., even after a single dose).[21] If they persist during antipsychotic therapy, other drugs such as antiparkinsonian adjuncts or benzodiazepines (e.g., diazepam) may be used to try to combat the aberrant motor symptoms.

Neuroleptic Malignant Syndrome. Patients taking relatively high doses of the more potent antipsychotics may experience a serious disorder known as neuroleptic malignant syndrome (NMS).[7,15] Symptoms of NMS include catatonia, stupor, rigidity, tremors, and fever. These symptoms are rather severe, and the mortality rate associated with NMS is quite high (up to 25 percent).[6] The exact causes of NMS are unclear, but men younger than 40 years of age and older patients with organic brain disease appear to be especially susceptible. Treatment typically consists of withdrawing the medication and providing supportive care.

NONMOTOR EFFECTS

Sedation

Antipsychotics have varying degrees of sedative properties. Contrary to previous beliefs, sedative properties do not enhance the antipsychotic efficacy of these drugs. Consequently, sedative side effects offer no benefit and can be detrimental in withdrawn psychotic patients.

Anticholinergic Effects

Some antipsychotics also produce significant anticholinergic effects, manifested by a variety of symptoms such as blurred vision, dry mouth, constipation, and urinary retention. Fortunately, these problems are usually self-limiting as many patients become tolerant to the anticholinergic side effects while remaining responsive to the antipsychotic properties.

Other Side Effects

Orthostatic hypotension is a frequent problem during the initial stages of antipsychotic therapy. This problem usually disappears after a few days. Certain antipsychotic drugs such as chlorpromazine are associated with photosensitivity, and care should be taken when exposing these patients to ultraviolet irradiation. Finally, abrupt withdrawal of antipsychotic drugs after prolonged use often results in nausea and vomiting, so it is advisable to decrease dosage gradually rather than to stop administration suddenly.

SPECIAL CONCERNS IN REHABILITATION PATIENTS

Antipsychotic drugs have been a great benefit to patients seen in various rehabilitation facilities. Regardless of the reason these individuals are referred to physical and occupational therapy, the improved behavior and reality perception usually provided by drug therapy will surely enhance the patient's cooperation during rehabilitation. Because these drugs tend to normalize patient behavior, the withdrawn patient often becomes more active and amiable, while the agitated patient becomes calmer and more relaxed. Also, remission of some of the confusion and impaired thinking will enable the patient to follow instructions more easily. Patients with paranoid symptoms may have fewer delusions of persecution and will feel less threatened by the entire therapy environment.

The benefits of antipsychotic drugs must be weighed against the risk of their side effects. The less serious side effects such as sedation and some of the anticholinergic effects (blurred vision, dry mouth, constipation) can be bothersome during the treatment session. Orthostatic hypotension should be guarded against, especially during the first few days after drug therapy is initiated. However, the major problems have to do with the extrapyramidal motor effects of these drugs. Therapists treating patients on antipsychotic medications should be continually on the alert for early signs of motor involvement. Chances are good that the therapist may be the first person to notice a change in posture, balance, or involuntary movements. Even subtle problems in motor function should be brought to the attention of the medical staff immediately. This early intervention may diminish the risk of long-term or even permanent motor dysfunction.

CASE STUDY

ANTIPSYCHOTIC DRUGS

Brief History. R.F., a 63-year-old woman, has been receiving treatment for schizophrenia intermittently for many years. She was last hospitalized for an acute episode 7 months ago and since then has been on a maintenance dose of haloperidol (Haldol), 25 mg/day. She is also being seen as an outpatient for treatment of rheumatoid arthritis in both hands. Her current treatment consists of gentle heat and active range-of-motion exercises, three times each week. She is being considered for possible metacarpophalangeal joint replacement.

Problem/Influence of Medication. During the course of physical therapy, the therapist noticed the onset and slow, progressive increase in writhing gestures of both upper extremities. Extraneous movements of her mouth and face were also observed, including chewinglike jaw movements and tongue protrusion.

Decision/Solution. These initial extrapyramidal symptoms suggested the onset of tardive dyskinesia. The therapist notified the patient's physician, and drug therapy was progressively shifted from haloperidol to thioridazine (Mellaril), 400 mg/day. The extrapyramidal symptoms gradually diminished over the next 8 weeks and ultimately disappeared.

SUMMARY

Antipsychotic drugs represent one of the major advances in the management of mental illness. Drugs are currently available that diminish the symptoms of psychosis and improve the patient's ability to cooperate with others and to administer self-care. Despite their chemical diversity, antipsychotics all seem to exert their beneficial effects by blocking central dopamine receptors. Therefore, psychoses such as schizophrenia may be caused by an overactivity of CNS dopaminergic pathways. Because of the rather nonspecific blockade of dopaminergic receptors, antipsychotics are associated with several adverse side effects. The most serious of these are abnormal movement patterns that resemble tardive dyskinesia, Parkinson's disease, and other lesions associated with the extrapyramidal system. In some cases, these aberrant motor activities may become irreversible and may persist even after drug therapy is terminated. Rehabilitation specialists may play a critical role in recognizing the early onset of these motor abnormalities. When identified early, potentially serious motor problems can be dealt with by altering the dosage or type of antipsychotic agent.

REFERENCES

1. Adler, L, et al: Efficacy in propranolol in neuroleptic induced akathesia. J Clin Psychopharmacol 5:164, 1985.
2. American Psychiatric Association: Diagnostic and Statistical Manual of Mental Disorders, ed 4. American Psychiatric Association, Washington, DC, 1994.
3. Baldessarini, RJ: Drugs and the treatment of psychiatric disorders. In Gilman, AG, et al (eds): The Pharmacological Basis of Therapeutics, ed 8. Pergamon Press, New York, 1990.
4. Baldessarini, RJ and Frankenburg, FR: Drug therapy: Clozapine—a novel antipsychotic agent. N Engl J Med 324:746, 1991.
5. Bollini, P, et al: High-dose neuroleptics: Uncontrolled clinical practice confirms controlled clinical trials. Br J Psychiatry 144:25, 1984.
6. Carpenter, WT and Buchanan, RW: Medical progress: Schizophrenia. N Engl J Med 330:681, 1994.
7. Dilsalver, SC: Clinical pharmacology: Antipsychotic agents—a review. Am Fam Physician 47:199, 1993.
8. Dorevitch, A, Durst, R, and Ginath, Y: Propranolol in the treatment of akathisia caused by antipsychotic drugs. South Med J 84:1505, 1991.
9. Ebadi, M: Pharmacology: A Review with Questions and Answers. Little, Brown, Boston, 1993, pp 103–112.
10. Fahn, S: A therapeutic approach to tardive dyskinesia. J Clin Psychiatry 46:19, 1985.
11. Fann, WE, et al (eds): Tardive Dyskinesia: Research and Treatment. Spectrum Publications, New York, 1980.
12. Freidhoff, AJ: A strategy for developing novel drugs for the treatment of schizophrenia. Schizophr Bull 9:555, 1983.
13. Gerner, RH: Neuroleptic drugs. In Bevan, JA, and Thompson, JH (eds): Essentials of Pharmacology, ed 3. Harper & Row, Philadelphia, 1983.
14. Gottlieb, GL and Kumar, A: Conventional pharmacological treatment for patients with Alzheimer's disease. Neurology 43(suppl 4):S56, 1993.
15. Herz, MI and Lamberti, JS: Schizophrenic disorders. In Rakel, RE (ed): Conn's Current Therapy. WB Saunders, Philadelphia, 1993.
16. Hollister, LE: Antipsychotic agents and lithium. In Katzung, BG (ed): Basic and Clinical Pharmacology, ed 5. Appleton & Lange, Norwalk, CT, 1992.
17. Kandel, ER: Disorders of thought: Schizophrenia. In Kandel, ER, Schwartz, JH, and Jessell, TM (eds): Principles of Neural Science, ed 3. Appleton & Lange, Norwalk, CT, 1991.

18. Lickey, ME and Gordon, B: Drugs for Mental Illness. WH Freeman, New York, 1983.
19. Mavroidis, ML, et al: Fluphenazine levels and clinical response. J Clin Psychiatry 45:370, 1984.
20. Meltzer, HY and Stahl, SM: The dopamine hypothesis of schizophrenia: A review. Schizophr Bull 2:19, 1976.
21. Rupniak, NMJ, Jenner, P, and Marsden, CD: Acute dystonia induced by neuroleptic drugs. Psychopharmacology 88:403, 1986.
22. Seeman, P: Dopamine receptors and the dopamine hypothesis of schizophrenia. Synapse 1:133, 1987.
23. Sokoloff, P, et al: Molecular cloning and characterization of a novel dopamine receptor (D_3) as a target for neuroleptics. Nature 347:146, 1990.
24. Stephen, PJ and Williamson, J: Drug induced parkinsonism in the elderly. Lancet 2:1082, 1984.
25. Yassa, R, et al: Tardive dyskinesia in an outpatient population: Prevalence and predisposing factors. Can J Psychiatry 28:391, 1983.

CHAPTER 9

Antiepileptic Drugs

Epilepsy is a chronic neurologic disorder characterized by recurrent seizures.[17] **Seizures** are episodes of sudden, transient disturbances in cerebral excitation that occur when a sufficient number of cerebral neurons begin to fire rapidly and in synchronized bursts.[12] Depending on the type of seizure, the neuronal activity may remain localized in a specific area of the brain, or it may spread to other areas of the brain. In some seizures, neurons in the motor cortex are activated, leading to skeletal muscle contraction via descending neuronal pathways. These involuntary, paroxysmal skeletal muscle contractions seen during certain seizures are referred to as *convulsions*. However, convulsions are not associated with all types of epilepsy, and other types of seizures are characterized by a wide variety of sensory or behavioral symptoms.

Epilepsy is associated with the presence of a group or focus of cerebral neurons that are hyperexcitable, or "irritable." The spontaneous discharge of these irritable neurons initiates the epileptic seizure. The reason for the altered excitability of these focal neurons, and thus the cause of epilepsy, varies depending on the patient.[16,22] In some patients, a specific incident such as a stroke, tumor, encephalopathy, head trauma, or other CNS injury probably caused damage to certain neurons, resulting in their altered threshold. In other patients, the reason for seizures may be less distinct or unknown, perhaps relating to a congenital abnormality, birth trauma, or genetic factor. Lastly, a systemic metabolic disorder such as infection, hypoglycemia, hypoxia, or uremia may precipitate seizure activity. In this last group of individuals, once the cause of the seizures is identified, the epilepsy is relatively easy to treat by resolving the metabolic disorder. Epilepsy resulting from these combined causes affects 1 to 2 million people in the United States and from 20 to 40 million worldwide, making this one of the most common neurologic disorders.[5,12,22]

Drug therapy is the primary form of treating epilepsy. Antiepileptic medications are successful in controlling seizures in 75 to 80 percent of the patient population.[7,15,16] Several types of drugs are currently available, and certain compounds work best in certain types of epilepsy. Consequently, the specific type of epilepsy must be determined by observing the patient and using diagnostic tests such as electroencephalography (EEG).[1,12,20] The classification system most commonly used in characterizing epilepsy is discussed here.

CLASSIFICATION OF EPILEPTIC SEIZURES

In an attempt to standardize the terminology used in describing various forms of epilepsy, the International League Against Epilepsy[3] proposed the classification scheme outlined in Table 9–1. Seizures are divided into two major categories: partial and generalized. A third category of "unclassified" seizures is sometimes included to encompass additional seizure types that do not fit into the two major groupings.

In partial seizures only part of the brain (i.e., one cerebral hemisphere) is involved, whereas in generalized seizures the whole cerebral brain is involved. Partial seizures that spread throughout the entire brain are referred to as "partial becoming generalized" or "secondarily generalized" seizures.

Partial and generalized seizures are subdivided depending on the specific symptoms that occur during the epileptic seizure (see Table 9–1). As a rule, the outward manifestations of the seizure depend on the specific area of the brain involved. Simple partial seizures that remain localized within the motor cortex for the right hand may cause involuntary, spasmlike movements of only the right hand. Other partial seizures produce motor and sensory symptoms, as well as affect consciousness and memory.

TABLE 9–1 Classification of Seizures

Seizure Type	Classification
I. Partial seizures	
A. Simple partial seizures	Limited (focal) motor or sensory signs (e.g., convulsions confined to one limb, specific sensory hallucinations); consciousness remains intact
B. Complex partial seizures	Consciousness impaired; bizarre behavior; wide variety of other manifestations; specific EEG abnormality (needed to differentiate this from absence seizures)
C. Partial becoming generalized	Symptoms progressively increase until seizure resembles a generalized (tonic-clonic) seizure
II. Generalized seizures	
A. Absence (petit mal) seizures	Sudden, brief loss of consciousness; motor signs may be absent or may range from rapid eye-blinking to symmetrical jerking movements of entire body
B. Myoclonic seizures	Sudden, brief, "shocklike" contractions of muscles in the face and trunk, or in one or more extremities; contractions may be single or multiple; consciousness may be impaired
C. Clonic seizures	Rhythmic, synchronized contractions throughout the body; loss of consciousness
D. Tonic seizures	Generalized sustained muscle contractions throughout body; loss of consciousness
E. Tonic-clonic (grand mal) seizures	Major convulsions of entire body; sustained contraction of all muscles (tonic phase) followed by powerful rhythmic contractions (clonic phase); loss of consciousness
F. Atonic seizures	Sudden loss of muscle tone in the head and neck, one limb, or thoughout the entire body; consciousness may be maintained or lost briefly
III. Unclassified seizures	
All other seizures that do not fit into one of the aforementioned categories.	

Source: Modified from Commission on Classification and Terminology of the International League Against Epilepsy,[3] 493–495, with permission.

These usually fall into the category of complex partial seizures. Generalized seizures are subclassified depending on the type and degree of motor involvement, as well as other factors such as the EEG recordings. The most well-known and dramatic of the generalized group is the tonic-clonic, or "grand mal," seizure. Absence, or "petit mal," seizures also fall into the category of generalized seizures. The drug therapy for generalized and partial seizures is discussed in "Drugs Used to Treat Epilepsy."

RATIONALE FOR DRUG TREATMENT

Even in the absence of drug therapy, individual seizures are usually self-limiting. Brain neurons are unable to sustain the high level of synaptic activity for more than a few minutes, and the seizure ends spontaneously. However, the uncontrolled recurrence of seizures is believed to cause further damage to the already injured neurons, as well as being potentially harmful to healthy cells. Certain types of seizures may be harmful if the patient loses consciousness or goes into convulsions and injures himself or herself during a fall. Certain types of convulsions are potentially fatal if cardiac irregularities result and the individual goes into cardiac arrest. Even relatively minor seizures may be embarrassing to a person, and social interaction may be compromised if the individual is afraid of having a seizure in public. Consequently, a strong effort is made to find an effective way to control or eliminate the incidence of seizures.

DRUGS USED TO TREAT EPILEPSY

Table 9–2 lists the drugs currently used to treat epilepsy according to their chemical classes and mechanisms of action. These drugs generally try to inhibit firing of certain cerebral neurons, usually by increasing the inhibitory effects of endogenous compounds such as gamma-aminobutyric acid (GABA), or by altering the movement of ions (sodium, calcium) across the neuronal membrane. However, in some cases the exact way in which antiepileptic drugs exert their beneficial effects is obscure or unknown.[11] Specific details of each chemical class of drugs are discussed here. Because these drugs tend to have many adverse side effects, however, only the frequently occurring or more serious problems are listed for each category.

Barbiturates

Phenobarbital (Solfoton) and other barbiturates such as mephobarbital (Mebaral) are prescribed in virtually all types of adult seizures but seem to be especially effective in generalized tonic-clonic and simple and complex partial seizures. These agents are considered to be very safe and effective in the treatment of seizures, but their use is often limited because of their strong tendency to produce sedation. Primidone (Mysoline) is another barbiturate-like drug that is recommended in several types of epilepsy but is particularly useful in generalized tonic-clonic seizures that have not responded to other drugs.

Mechanism of Action. The antiepileptic effects of the barbiturates are not fully understood. Barbiturates are known to increase the inhibitory effects of GABA (see Chapter 6), but whether this is the primary way in which these drugs decrease seizure

TABLE 9-2 Chemical Classification and Actions of Antiepileptic Agents

Chemical Class	Possible Mechanism of Action
Barbiturates Mephobarbital (Mebaral) Phenobarbital (Solfoton) Primidone (Mysoline)	Potentiate inhibitory effects of GABA; may also block excitatory effects of glutamate
Benzodiazepines Clonazepam (Klonopin) Clorazepate (Tranxene; others) Diazepam (Valium; Vazepam) Lorazepam (Alzapam; Ativan)	Potentiate inhibitory effects of GABA
Carboxylic acids Valproic acid (Depakene; others)	Unclear; may hyperpolarize membrane through an effect on potassium channels; higher concentrations increase CNS GABA concentrations
Dicarbamates Felbamate (Felbatol)	Unclear; may block excitatory effects of glutamate in CNS
Hydantoins Ethotoin (Peganone) Mephenytoin (Mesantoin) Phenacemide (Phenurone) Phenytoin (Dilantin)	Primary effect is to stabilize membrane by blocking sodium channels in repetitive-firing neurons; higher concentrations may also influence concentrations of other neurotransmitters (GABA, norepinephrine, others)
Iminostilbenes Carbamazepine (Tegretol)	Similar to hydantoins
Oxazolidinediones Paramethadione (Paradione) Trimethadione (Tridione)	Affect calcium channels; appear to inhibit spontaneous firing in thalamic neurons by limiting calcium entry
Succinimides Ethosuximide (Zarontin) Methsuximide (Celontin) Phensuximide (Milontin)	Similar to oxazolidinediones

GABA = gamma-aminobutyric acid.

activity is unclear. Barbiturates may have a direct effect on membrane function and may decrease synaptic excitability because of their effect on presynaptic and postsynaptic membrane fluidity and organization.

Adverse Side Effects. Sedation (primary problem), nystagmus, ataxia, folate deficiency, vitamin K deficiency, and skin problems are typical side effects. A paradoxical increase in seizures and increased hyperactivity may occur in children.

Benzodiazepines

Several members of the benzodiazepine group are effective in treating epilepsy, but most are limited because of problems with sedation and tolerance. Some agents such as diazepam and lorazepam are used in the acute treatment of status epilepticus (see "Treatment of Status Epilepticus"), but only a few are used in the long-term treatment of epilepsy. Clonazepam (Klonopin) is recommended in specific forms of absence seizures (e.g., the Lennox-Gastaut variant) and may also be useful in minor generalized seizures such as akinetic spells and myoclonic jerks. Clorazepate (Tranxene) is another benzodiazepine that is occasionally used as an adjunct in certain partial seizures.

Mechanism of Action. These drugs are known to potentiate the inhibitory effects of GABA in the brain (see Chapter 6), and their antiepileptic properties are probably exerted through this mechanism.

Adverse Side Effects. Sedation, ataxia, and behavioral changes can be observed.

Carboxylic Acids

Valproic acid (Depakene, others) is a member of this chemical class that is used primarily to treat absence seizures or as a secondary agent in generalized tonic-clonic forms of epilepsy.

Mechanism of Action. High concentrations of valproic acid are associated with increased levels of GABA in the brain, and this increase in GABA-ergic inhibition may be responsible for this drug's antiepileptic action. However, lower concentrations that are still effective in limiting seizures do not increase CNS GABA, indicating that some other mechanism must occur. Valproic acid also exerts some of its effects in a manner similar to phenytoin; that is, it limits sodium entry into rapidly firing neurons. Hence, the exact way in which this drug is effective against partial seizures remains to be determined, and valproic acid may actually work through a combination of several different molecular mechanisms.

Adverse Side Effects. Gastrointestinal distress, temporary hair loss, weight gain or loss, and impaired platelet function are documented adverse reactions.

Dicarbamates

This class contains a relatively new drug, felbamate (Felbatol), which is indicated for treatment of partial seizures in adults and children as well as generalized absence seizures (Lennox-Gastaut syndrome) in children. Because this drug has not been used on a widespread basis, it is unclear at this time exactly how this drug compares to other agents in terms of efficacy and safety, and it remains to be seen how felbamate will be incorporated into the arsenal of antiseizure drugs.

Mechanism of Action. It is not exactly clear how felbamate exerts its beneficial effects. There is some evidence that this drug blocks the excitatory effects of glutamate, but the antiseizure properties of felbamate remain to be fully determined.

Adverse Side Effects. The most common side effects associated with felbamate involve gastrointestinal problems such as anorexia, nausea, and vomiting. Other common side effects include insomnia, headache, and dizziness.

Hydantoins

This category includes phenytoin (Dilantin), mephenytoin (Mesantoin), phenacemide (Phenurone), and ethotoin (Peganone). Phenytoin is often the first drug considered in treating many types of epilepsy, and it is especially effective in treating partial seizures and generalized tonic-clonic seizures. Mephenytoin has similar properties but is somewhat more toxic. Phenacemide is recommended for use in cases of severe complex partial seizures, and ethotoin has been effective in treating absence seizures. The last three drugs are usually reserved for use if the patient has not responded to other, less toxic drugs.

Mechanism of Action. Phenytoin stabilizes neural membranes and decreases neuronal excitability by interfering with the movement of sodium across the membrane. Open and inactivated sodium channels are directly affected, and sodium entry into the cell at rest and during action potentials is decreased. Phenytoin may also decrease neuronal excitability by influencing the movement of potassium and calcium across the nerve membrane, but the effects on these other ions generally occur at drug concentrations that are higher than those used therapeutically to control seizures. Less is known about the molecular mechanisms of the other drugs in this category, but they probably work by a similar effect on the sodium channels.

Adverse Side Effects. Gastric irritation, confusion, sedation, dizziness, headache, cerebellar signs (nystagmus, ataxia, dysarthria), gingival hyperplasia, increased body and facial hair (hirsutism), and skin disorders are typical adverse effects.

Iminostilbenes

Carbamazepine (Tegretol) is included in this class because it is chemically and structurally similar to the tricyclic antidepressants but has been shown to be effective in treating all types of epilepsy except absence seizures. Carbamazepine is regarded as equivalent to phenytoin in efficacy and side effects, and may be substituted for that drug, depending on the individual patient response.

Mechanism of Action. Carbamazepine is believed to exert its primary antiepileptic effects in a manner similar to phenytoin—that is, stabilizing the neuronal membrane by impairing sodium influx through membrane channels. This drug may also inhibit the presynaptic uptake and release of norepinephrine, and this effect may contribute to its antiseizure activity.

Adverse Side Effects. Dizziness, drowsiness, ataxia, blurred vision, anemia, water retention (because of abnormal antidiuretic hormone [ADH] release), cardiac arrhythmias, and congestive heart failure can occur with use of this drug.

Oxazolidinediones

Paramethadione (Paradione) and trimethadione (Tridione) are the two members of this class, and these drugs are used exclusively in the treatment of absence seizures. These are not typically the drugs of choice, however, and they are usually reserved for patients whose seizures are poorly controlled or who do not tolerate other agents used to treat absence seizures.

Mechanism of Action. These drugs exert a number of effects on CNS synaptic activity, including inhibition of calcium entry into thalamic neurons. This decrease in calcium influx seems to prevent repetitive firing of certain thalamic neurons that are associated with absence seizures.

Adverse Side Effects. The most common side effects include sedation and vision disturbances such as blurring or glare when exposed to bright light.

Succinimides

Drugs in this category include ethosuximide (Zarontin), methsuximide (Celontin), and phensuximide (Milontin). All three drugs are primary agents in the treatment of absence (petit mal) seizures, but ethosuximide is the most commonly prescribed.

Mechanism of Action. These drugs are known to increase the seizure threshold and limit the spread of electrical activity in the brain, but their exact cellular mechanism is unknown. Some evidence suggests these drugs may exert their beneficial effects by acting like the oxazolidinediones, that is, by decreasing calcium influx in certain thalamic neurons. The spontaneous, rhythmic entry of calcium into thalamic neurons may be responsible for initiating partial seizures, and the succinimides prevent the onset of these seizures by blunting calcium influx. Further research is needed to elaborate on this theory.

Adverse Side Effects. Gastrointestinal distress (nausea, vomiting), headache, dizziness, fatigue, lethargy, movement disorders (dyskinesia, bradykinesia), and skin rashes/itching are common side effects.

SELECTION OF A SPECIFIC ANTIEPILEPTIC AGENT

It is apparent from the preceding discussion that certain drugs are often preferred when treating certain types of seizures. Table 9–3 lists some of the more common types of seizures and the primary and alternative agents used to treat each seizure type. It is important to note, however, that Table 9–3 indicates general guidelines for drug selection, but selection of the best agent must be done on a patient-by-patient basis. Some patients will understandably exhibit a better response to agents that are not typically used as the first or second choice for a specific type of seizure. Hence, some trial and error may occur before the best drug is found for a given patient, and drug selection may need to be altered periodically throughout the patient's lifetime to achieve optimal results.[8]

Thus, a fairly large number of drugs can be used to treat epileptic seizures (see Table 9–2), but certain agents are usually considered first when attempting to treat the most common seizures. These agents comprise a fairly small group consisting of five or six drugs that tend to be used most often. These commonly used drugs and their relevant pharmacologic parameters are listed in Table 9–4. Again, alternative antiseizure drugs can be used if these commonly used drugs are ineffective or poorly tolerated.

SINGLE-DRUG THERAPY IN EPILEPSY

When treating epilepsy, an effort is typically made to use only one drug (primary agent), with an additional drug (secondary agent) being added only if the epilepsy is especially resistant to management with the primary medication. Clinical experience

TABLE 9–3 Common Methods of Treating Specific Seizures

Seizure Type	Primary Agents	Alternative Agents
Generalized tonic-clonic and simple partial seizures	Carbamazepine, phenytoin	Phenobarbital, primidone, valproic acid
Absence	Ethosuximide, valproic acid	Clonazepam
Complex partial	Carbamazepine, phenytoin, valproic acid	Phenobarbital, primidone
Myoclonic	Valproic acid	Clonazepam

TABLE 9–4 Pharmacologic Parameters of Common Antiepileptic Drugs

Drug	Absorption	Half-Life (Hours)	Time to Reach Steady State (Days)	Therapeutic Range (μg/mL)
Phenytoin	Slow	10–40	5–7	10–20
Carbamazepine	Slow to moderate	8–20	3–5	4–10
Valproic acid	Rapid	8–12	2–3	50–100
Phenobarbital	Moderate	50–150	2–3 wk	10–45
Primidone	Slow to moderate	6–18	2–3	5–15
Ethosuximide	Rapid	20–60	4–10	50–100

Source: Bruni,[1] 854, with permission.

has shown that it is better to use one antiepileptic drug (monotherapy) at a relatively high dose, rather than several different drugs at smaller doses.[16,18,23] The single-drug method offers several advantages including fewer side effects, a lack of drug interactions, better ability of the patient to adhere to the drug regimen, lower cost, and better seizure control because the patient is able to tolerate a higher dose of a single agent.[1,8] Likewise, management of adverse side effects in single-drug therapy is easier because there is no question about which drug is producing the adverse effect.

Hence, the drug of choice is often initiated at a relatively low dose, and dosage is increased until either the seizures are adequately controlled or side effects become a problem.[19] If the primary agent must be switched for any reason, it is usually advisable to taper off the original drug and slowly institute the new primary agent. This procedure avoids any adverse effects from the sudden withdrawal of one drug and potential interaction as the new drug is started.[20]

PHARMACOKINETICS

When given for the long-term control of epilepsy, these drugs are normally administered orally. Daily oral doses are usually divided into three or four equal quantities, and the amount of each dose varies widely depending on the specific drug and the severity of patient seizures. Distribution within the body is fairly extensive, with all antiepileptic drugs eventually reaching the brain to exert their beneficial effects. Drug biotransformation usually occurs via liver microsomal oxidases, and this is the primary method of drug termination.

SPECIAL PRECAUTIONS DURING PREGNANCY

Evidence exists that children of epileptic mothers have an increased incidence of birth defects compared with children of nonepileptic mothers.[4,14,21] Increases in the occurrence of problems such as stillbirth, microencephaly, mental retardation, infant seizures, and congenital malformations (cleft palate, cardiac defects) have been noted in children of women with seizure disorders. There is considerable debate as to whether this is a side effect of antiepileptic drug therapy or a sequela of the epilepsy itself. Since there is at least some concern that fetal malformations may be a drug side effect, many mothers choose to discontinue drug therapy during their pregnancies.[14]

This obviously places the mother at risk for uncontrolled seizures, which may be even more harmful to the mother and unborn child. No consensus currently exists regarding this dilemma. Women taking antiepileptic drugs who wish to bear children should discuss the risks with their family members and physician, and try to arrive at a conclusion as to whether or not they will continue taking their medication.

TREATMENT OF STATUS EPILEPTICUS

Status epilepticus is a series of seizures that occur without any appreciable period of recovery between individual seizures.[6,9] Essentially the patient experiences one long, extended seizure. This may be brought on by a number of factors such as sudden withdrawal from antiepileptic drugs, cerebral infarct, systemic or intracranial infection, or withdrawal from addictive drugs including alcohol.[10,13] If untreated, status epilepticus will result in permanent damage or death, especially if the seizures are generalized tonic-clonic in nature.[9] Consequently, this event is regarded as a medical emergency that should be resolved as rapidly as possible.

Treatment begins with standard emergency procedures such as maintaining an airway, starting an IV line for blood sampling and drug administration, and so on.[1,24] The first drugs administered are usually benzodiazepines: either diazepam (Valium) or lorazepam (Ativan) given intravenously. This approach is followed by phenytoin, which is also administered intravenously. The phenytoin is given concurrently with or immediately after the benzodiazepine so that seizures are controlled when the relatively short-acting benzodiazepine is metabolized. If seizures continue despite these drugs, phenobarbital is given intravenously. If all other attempts fail, general anesthesia (e.g., halothane) may be used as a last resort. When the status epilepticus is eventually controlled, an attempt is made to begin or reinstitute chronic antiepileptic therapy.

SPECIAL CONCERNS IN REHABILITATION PATIENTS

Rehabilitation specialists must always be cognizant of their patients who have a history of seizures and who are taking antiepileptic drugs. Patients being treated for conditions unrelated to epilepsy (e.g., the outpatient with low back pain) should be identified as potentially at risk for a seizure during the therapy session. This knowledge will better prepare the therapist to recognize and deal with such an episode. This approach emphasizes the need for a thorough medical history of all patients. Also, therapists may help determine the efficacy of antiepileptic drug therapy. The primary goal in any patient taking antiepileptic drugs is maintaining the drug dosage within a therapeutic window. Dosage must be high enough to adequately control seizure activity, but not so high as to invoke serious side effects. By constantly observing and monitoring patient progress, rehabilitation specialists may help determine if this goal is being met. By noting changes in either seizure frequency or side effects, physical and occupational therapists and other rehabilitation personnel may help the medical staff arrive at an effective dosing regimen. This information can be invaluable in helping achieve optimal patient care with a minimum of adverse side effects.[2]

Some of the more frequent side effects may affect physical therapy and other rehabilitation procedures. Headache, dizziness, sedation, and gastric disturbances (nausea, vomiting) may be bothersome during the therapy session. Often these reactions can be addressed by scheduling therapy at a time of day when these problems are relatively mild. The optimal treatment time will vary from patient to patient, depending on the particular drug, dosing schedule, and age of the patient. Cerebellar side effects such as ataxia also occur frequently and may impair the patient's ability to participate in various functional activities. If ataxia persists despite efforts to alter drug dosage or substitute another agent, coordination exercises may be instituted to help resolve this problem. Skin conditions (dermatitis, rashes, etc.) are another frequent problem in long-term antiepileptic therapy. Any therapeutic modalities that might exacerbate these conditions should be discontinued.

Finally, in some patients, seizures tend to be exacerbated by environmental stimuli such as lights and sound. In such patients, conducting the therapy session in a busy, noisy clinic may be sufficient to precipitate a seizure, especially if the epilepsy is poorly controlled by drug therapy. Also, certain patients may have a history of increased seizure activity at certain times of the day, which may be related to when the antiepileptic drug is administered. Consequently, certain patients may benefit if the therapy session is held in a relatively quiet setting at a time when the chance of a seizure for that individual is minimal.

CASE STUDY

ANTIEPILEPTIC DRUGS

Brief History. F.B. is a 43-year-old man who works in the mail room of a large company. He was diagnosed in childhood as having generalized tonic-clonic epilepsy, and his seizures have been managed successfully with various drugs over the years. Most recently, he has been taking carbamazepine (Tegretol), 800 mg/day (i.e., one 200-mg tablet, QID). One month ago, he began complaining of dizziness and blurred vision, so the dosage was reduced to 600 mg/day (one tablet TID). He usually took the medication after meals. Two weeks ago, he injured his back while lifting a large box at work. He was evaluated in physical therapy as having an acute lumbosacral strain. He began to attend physical therapy each day as an outpatient. Treatment included heat, ultrasound, and manual therapy, and the patient was also being instructed in proper body mechanics and lifting technique. F.B. continued to work at his normal job, but he avoided heavy lifting. He would attend therapy on his way home from work, at about 5 PM.

Problem/Influence of Medication. F.B. arrived at physical therapy the first afternoon stating that he had had a particularly long day. He was positioned prone on a treatment table, and hot packs were placed over his low back. As the heat was applied, he began to drift off to sleep. Five minutes into the treatment, he had a seizure. Because of a thorough initial evaluation, the therapist was aware of his epileptic condition and protected him from injury during the seizure. The patient regained consciousness and rested quietly until he felt able to go home. No long-term effects were noted from the seizure.

Decision/Solution. The seizure may have been precipitated by a number of factors, including the recent decrease in drug dosage and the fact that he was nearing the end of a dosing interval. (He had taken his last dose at lunch and would take his next dose after he went home and had dinner). The fact that he was tired and fell asleep during the treatment probably played a role. He reported later that when seizures do occur, they tend to be when he is asleep. To prevent the recurrence of seizures, the therapy session was rescheduled to earlier in the day, at 8 AM (his schedule was flexible enough that he could attend therapy before going to work). Also, he would have taken his first dose of the day approximately 1 hour before arriving at physical therapy. No further seizures occurred during the course of rehabilitation, and F.B.'s lumbosacral strain was resolved after 2 weeks of physical therapy.

SUMMARY

Epilepsy is a chronic condition characterized by recurrent seizures. Causes of this disorder range from a distinct traumatic episode to obscure or unknown origins. Seizures are categorized according to the clinical and electrophysiologic manifestations that occur during the seizure. Fortunately, most individuals with epilepsy (up to 80 percent) can be treated successfully with antiepileptic drugs. Although these drugs do not cure this disorder, reduction or elimination of seizures will prevent further CNS damage. Currently a wide variety of drugs are used, with specific agents being most successful in specific types of epilepsy. As in any area of pharmacotherapeutics, these drugs are not without adverse side effects. Some of these side effects may become a problem in rehabilitation patients, so therapists should be ready to alter the time and type of treatment as needed to accommodate these side effects. Physical therapists and other rehabilitation personnel should also be alert for any behavioral or functional changes in the patient that might indicate a problem in drug therapy. Insufficient drug therapy (as evidenced by increased seizures) or possible drug toxicity (as evidenced by increased side effects) should be brought to the physician's attention so that these problems can be rectified.

REFERENCES

1. Bruni, J: Epilepsy in adolescents and adults. In Rakel, RE (ed): Conn's Current Therapy. WB Saunders, Philadelphia, 1993.
2. Collaborative Group for Epidemiology of Epilepsy: Adverse reactions to antiepileptic drugs: A follow-up study of 355 patients with chronic antiepileptic drug treatment. Epilepsia 29:787, 1988.
3. Commission on Classification and Terminology of the International League Against Epilepsy: Proposal for revised clinical and electroencephalographic classification of epileptic seizures. Epilepsia 30:389, 1989.
4. Dalessio, DJ: Current concepts: Seizure disorders and pregnancy. N Engl J Med 312:559, 1985.
5. Delgado-Escueta, AV, et al: New wave of research in the epilepsies. In Delgado-Escueta, AV, et al (eds): Basic Mechanisms of the Epilepsies: Molecular and Cellular Approaches, Advances in Neurology, Vol 44. Raven Press, New York, 1986.
6. Delgado-Escueta, AV, et al (eds): Status Epilepticus: Mechanisms of Brain Damage and Treatment, Advances in Neurology, Vol 34. Raven Press, New York, 1983.
7. Elwes, RDC, et al: The prognosis for seizure control in newly diagnosed epilepsy. N Engl J Med 311:944, 1984.
8. French, J: The long-term therapeutic management of epilepsy. Ann Intern Med 120:411, 1994.
9. Leppik, IE: Status epilepticus: The next decade. Neurology 40(suppl 2):4, 1990.
10. Lothman, E: The biochemical basis and pathophysiology of status epilepticus. Neurology 40(suppl 2):13, 1990.
11. MacDonald, RL and McLean, MJ: Anticonvulsant drugs: Mechanisms of action. In Delgado-Escueta, AV, et al (eds): Basic Mechanisms of the Epilepsies: Molecular and Cellular Approaches, Advances in Neurology, Vol 44. Raven Press, New York, 1986.

12. Martin, JH: The collective electrical behavior of cortical neurons: The electroencephalogram and the mechanisms of epilepsy. In Kandel, ER, Schwartz, JH, and Jessell, TM (eds): Principles of Neural Science, ed 3. Appleton & Lange, Norwalk, CT, 1991.
13. Ojemann, LM and Ojemann, GA: Treatment of epilepsy. Am Fam Physician 30:113, 1984.
14. Philbert, A and Pedersen, B: Treatment of epilepsy in women of child-bearing age: Patient's opinion of teratogenic potential of valproate. Acta Neurol Scand (suppl)94:35, 1983.
15. Porter, RJ and Meldrum, BS: Antiepileptic drugs. In Katzung, BG (ed): Basic and Clinical Pharmacology, ed 5. Appleton & Lange, Norwalk, CT, 1992.
16. Rall, TW and Schleifer, LS: Drugs effective in the therapy of the epilepsies. In Gilman, AG, et al (eds): The Pharmacological Basic of Therapeutics, ed 8. Pergamon Press, New York, 1990.
17. Scheuer, ML and Pedley, TA: Current concepts: The evaluation and treatment of seizures. N Engl J Med 323:1468, 1990.
18. Schmidt, D: Single drug therapy for intractable epilepsy. J Neurol 229:221, 1983.
19. Schmidt, D and Haenel, F: Therapeutic plasma levels of phenytoin, phenobarbital, carbamazepine: Individual variation in relation to seizure frequency and time. Neurology 34:1252, 1984.
20. Shorvon, SD: Medical assessment and treatment of chronic epilepsy. Br Med J 302:363, 1991.
21. Symposium (various authors): Pregnancy and teratogenesis in epilepsy. Neurology 42(suppl 5):7, 1992.
22. Symposium (various authors): Basic mechanisms of the epilepsies: Molecular and cellular approaches. Adv Neurol 44:1, 1986.
23. Theodore, WH: Recent advances in the diagnosis and treatment of seizure disorders. Trends Neurosci 8:144, 1985.
24. Treiman, DM: The role of benzodiazepines in the management of status epilepticus. Neurology 40(suppl 2):32, 1990.

CHAPTER 10

Pharmacologic Management of Parkinson's Disease

Parkinson's disease is a movement disorder characterized by resting tremor, bradykinesia, rigidity, and postural instability.[1,9,18] In Parkinson's disease, there is a slow, progressive degeneration of certain dopamine-secreting neurons in the basal ganglia.[1,11] Several theories have been proposed to explain this spontaneous neuronal degeneration, including the possibility that Parkinson's disease may be related to some type of toxic substance (see "Etiology of Parkinson's Disease: Potential Role of Toxic Substances").[2,29] However, the precise initiating factor in Parkinson's disease is still largely unknown.[11] The clinical syndrome of parkinsonism (i.e., rigidity, bradykinesia, and so on) may also be caused by other factors such as trauma, encephalitis, antipsychotic drugs, and various forms of cortical degeneration (including Alzheimer's disease).[18] However, the most frequent cause of parkinsonism is the slow, selective neuronal degeneration characteristic of Parkinson's disease itself.[1] Also, the drug management of parkinsonism caused by these other factors closely resembles the management of Parkinson's disease.[45] Consequently, this chapter will address the idiopathic onset and pharmacologic treatment of Parkinson's disease per se.

Parkinson's disease usually begins in the fifth or sixth decade, and symptoms slowly but progressively worsen over a period of 10 to 20 years. It is estimated that more than 1 percent of the U.S. population older than 60 years of age is afflicted with this illness, making Parkinson's disease one of the most prevalent neurologic disorders affecting elderly individuals.[9,18] In addition to the symptoms of bradykinesia and rigidity, the patient with advanced Parkinson's disease maintains a flexed posture and speaks in a low, soft voice (microphonia). If left untreated, the motor problems associated with this illness eventually lead to total incapacitation of the patient. Because of the prevalence of Parkinson's disease and the motor problems associated with this disorder, rehabilitation specialists are often involved in treating patients with this illness.

Fortunately, the pharmacologic management of Parkinson's disease has evolved to where the symptoms associated with this disorder can be greatly diminished in many patients. The use of levodopa (L-dopa), alone or in combination with other drugs, can improve motor function and general mobility well into the advanced stages of this disease. Drugs used in treating Parkinson's disease do not cure this condition, and motor function tends to slowly deteriorate in these patients regardless of when drug therapy is initiated.[30] However, by alleviating the motor symptoms (i.e., bradykinesia and rigidity), drug therapy can allow patients with Parkinson's disease to continue to lead relatively active lifestyles, thus improving their overall physiologic as well as psychologic well-being.

PATHOPHYSIOLOGY OF PARKINSON'S DISEASE

During the past 30 years, the specific neuronal changes associated with the onset and progression of Parkinson's disease have been established. Specific alterations in neurotransmitter balance in the basal ganglia are responsible for the symptoms associated with this disorder.[11,45] The basal ganglia are groups of nuclei located in the brain that are involved in the coordination and regulation of motor function. One such nucleus, the substantia nigra, contains the cell bodies of neurons that project to other areas such as the putamen and caudate nucleus (known collectively as the "corpus striatum"). The neurotransmitter used in this nigrostriatal pathway is dopamine. The primary neural abnormality in Parkinson's disease is that dopamine-producing cells in the substantia nigra begin to degenerate, resulting in the eventual loss of dopaminergic input into the corpus striatum.[1,11,34]

Consequently, the decrease in striatal dopamine seems to be the initiating factor in the onset of the symptoms associated with Parkinson's disease. However, it also appears that the lack of dopamine results in an increase in activity in cholinergic pathways in the basal ganglia.[1,11,39] As illustrated in Figure 10–1, there is a balance between dopaminergic and cholinergic influence in the basal ganglia under normal conditions. However, the loss of dopaminergic influence in Parkinson's disease appears to allow cholinergic influence to dominate.

The relationship between these two neurotransmitters suggests that the role of striatal dopamine may be to modulate acetylcholine release; that is, the lack of inhibitory dopaminergic influence allows excitatory acetylcholine pathways to run wild. Thus, the symptoms associated with Parkinson's disease may really be directly caused by increased cholinergic influence occurring secondary to the loss of dopamine. Current research also suggests that other imbalances involving transmitters such as gamma-aminobutyric acid (GABA), 5-hydroxytryptamine (serotonin), and endogenous opioids may also be present in the basal ganglia subsequent to the loss of dopamine.[11,34] In any event, drug therapy focuses on resolving the dopamine-acetylcholine imbalance to restore normal motor function in Parkinson's disease.

ETIOLOGY OF PARKINSON'S DISEASE: POTENTIAL ROLE OF TOXIC SUBSTANCES

As stated previously, the exact factors that initiate the loss of striatal dopamine are unknown in most patients with Parkinson's disease. However, recent evidence suggests that some sort of environmental or endogenous toxin may be responsible for accelerating the destruction of dopaminergic neurons in the substantia nigra.[20,41] Much of this evidence is based on the finding that a compound known as 1-methyl-4-phenyl-

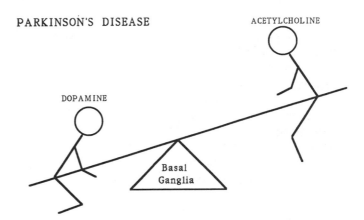

FIGURE 10–1. Schematic representation of the neurotransmitter imbalance in Parkinson's disease. Normally, a balance exists between dopamine and acetylcholine in the basal ganglia. In Parkinson's disease, decreased dopaminergic influence results in increased acetylcholine influence.

1,2,3,6-tetrahydropyridine (MPTP) appears to be selectively toxic to these neurons and can invoke parkinsonism in primates.[5,8,26,27,29]

The theory that a toxin like MPTP might cause Parkinson's disease was formulated in a rather interesting fashion. In 1982, several young adults in their 20s and 30s developed permanent, severe parkinsonism.[2] Since the onset of Parkinson's disease before age 40 is extremely rare, these individuals aroused a great deal of interest. Upon close investigation, all of these individuals were found to have experimented with synthetic heroin-like drugs. These so-called designer drugs were manufactured by drug dealers in an attempt to create an illicit supply of narcotics for sale to heroin addicts. However, the illicit narcotics contained the toxin MPTP, which was discovered to cause selective destruction of substantia nigra neurons.[2]

The discovery of toxin-induced parkinsonism in drug addicts led to the idea that idiopathic Parkinson's disease may be caused by previous exposure to some environmental toxin.[41] Exposure to such a toxin through industrial waste or certain herbicides may begin the neuronal changes that ultimately result in Parkinson's disease. Although a specific environmental factor has not been identified yet, the possible relationship between an environmental toxin and Parkinson's disease has opened up a new and exciting avenue of research that may eventually reveal more about the etiology of this disorder.

In addition, the finding that some toxin may initiate Parkinson's disease has led to the idea that other drugs may be helpful in delaying or preventing the biochemical changes induced by such a toxin. This has encouraged the use of drugs that can potentially delay the neuronal changes seen in Parkinson's disease.[33,46] A specific enzyme in the brain known as monoamine oxidase B (MAO_B) appears to be involved in the activation of some substance or substances that are ultimately responsible for accelerating the cell death that underlies Parkinson's disease. Drugs such as selegiline (Eldepryl) inhibit this enzyme and have been shown to delay the progression of Parkinson's disease.[33,37,46] The role of selegiline in the management of Parkinson's disease is discussed in more detail in "Other Drugs Used to Treat Parkinson's Disease."

THERAPEUTIC AGENTS IN PARKINSONISM

An overview of the drugs used to treat Parkinson's disease is shown in Table 10–1. The primary drug used to treat parkinsonism is levodopa. Other agents such as amantadine, anticholinergic drugs, and direct-acting dopamine agonists can be used alone or in conjunction with levodopa, depending on the needs of the patient. Each of these agents is discussed here.

Levodopa

Because the underlying problem in Parkinson's disease is a deficiency of dopamine in the basal ganglia, simple substitution of this chemical would seem a logi-

TABLE 10–1 Overview of Drug Therapy in Parkinson's Disease

Drug	Mechanism of Action	Special Comments
Levodopa	Resolves dopamine deficiency by being converted to dopamine after crossing blood-brain barrier.	Still the best drug for resolving parkinsonian symptoms; long-term use limited by side effects and decreased efficiency.
Dopamine agonists (bromocriptine, pergolide)	Directly stimulate dopamine receptors in basal ganglia.	Often used in combination with levodopa to get optimal benefits with lower dose of each drug.
Anticholinergics (see Table 10–2)	Inhibit excessive acetylcholine influence caused by dopamine deficiency.	Use in Parkinson's disease limited by frequent side effects.
Amantadine	Unclear; may stimulate release of remaining dopamine.	May be used alone during early/mild stages or added to drug regimen when levodopa loses effectiveness.
Selegiline	Inhibits the enzyme that breaks down dopamine in the basal ganglia; enables dopamine to remain active for longer periods of time.	May also have neuroprotective effects; can delay the degeneration of dopaminergic neurons.

cal course of action. However, dopamine does not cross the blood-brain barrier. Administration of dopamine either orally or parenterally will therefore be ineffective because it will be unable to cross from the systemic circulation into the brain where it is needed. Fortunately, the immediate precursor to dopamine, dihydroxyphenylalanine (dopa) (Fig. 10–2) does cross the blood-brain barrier quite readily. Dopa, or more specifically levodopa (the L-isomer of dopa), is able to cross the brain capillary endothelium intact. Upon entering the brain, levodopa is then transformed into dopamine by decarboxylation via **dopa decarboxylase** (Fig. 10–3).

Administration of levodopa often dramatically improves all of the symptoms of parkinsonism, especially bradykinesia and rigidity. In patients who respond well to this drug, the decrease in symptoms and increase in function are remarkable. As with any medication, there is a portion of the population who, for unknown reasons, do not respond well or simply cannot tolerate the drug. Also, prolonged use of levodopa is associated with some rather troublesome and frustrating side effects (see "Problems and Adverse Effects of Levodopa Therapy"). However, the use of levodopa has been the most significant advancement in the management of Parkinson's disease to date, and it remains the most effective single drug in the treatment of most patients with this disorder.[16,24,39]

Tyrosine

Tyrosine
hydroxylase

HO—⟨benzene ring⟩—CH_2—CH—NH_2
HO $COOH$

Dopa

Dopa
decarboxylase

HO—⟨benzene ring⟩—CH_2—CH_2—NH_2
HO

Dopamine

FIGURE 10–2. Synthesis of dopamine.

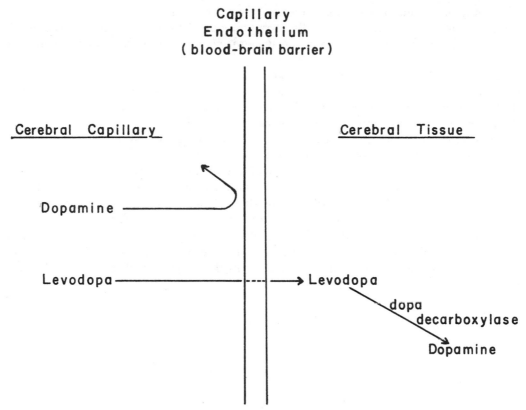

FIGURE 10–3. Selective permeability of the blood-brain barrier to levodopa.

LEVODOPA ADMINISTRATION AND METABOLISM: USE OF PERIPHERAL DECARBOXYLASE INHIBITORS

Levodopa is usually administered orally beginning with dosages of 500 to 1000 mg/day. Dosages are progressively increased until a noticeable reduction in symptoms occurs, or until side effects begin to be a problem. Maximum doses can run as high as 8 g/day. Daily titers are usually divided into two to three doses per day, and individual doses are often given with meals to decrease gastrointestinal irritation.

Following absorption from the gastrointestinal tract, levodopa is rapidly converted to dopamine by the enzyme dopa decarboxylase. This enzyme is distributed extensively throughout the body and can be found in such locations as the liver, intestinal mucosa, kidney, and skeletal muscle. Conversion of levodopa to dopamine in the periphery is rather extensive, such that only 1 to 3 percent of the administered levodopa reaches the brain in that form. This fact is significant because only levodopa will be able to cross the blood-brain barrier to be subsequently transformed into dopamine. Any levodopa that is prematurely converted to dopamine in the periphery must remain in the periphery and is essentially useless in alleviating parkinsonism symptoms.

Consequently, when given alone, rather large quantities of levodopa must be administered to ensure that enough levodopa reaches the brain in that form. This is often undesirable because the majority of the levodopa ends up as dopamine in the peripheral circulation, and these high levels of circulating dopamine can cause some unpleasant gastrointestinal and cardiovascular side effects (see the next section). An alternative method is to give levodopa in conjunction with a peripheral decarboxylase inhibitor (Fig. 10–4). The simultaneous use of a drug that selectively inhibits the dopa decarboxylase enzyme outside of the CNS enables more levodopa to reach the brain before being converted to dopamine. Carbidopa is such a drug and is given in conjunction with levodopa to prevent peripheral decarboxylation (see Fig. 10–4).[1,6] Use of carbidopa with levodopa dramatically decreases the amount of levodopa needed to achieve a desired effect, with the required levodopa dosage often being reduced by 75 to 80 percent.[3] Another decarboxylase inhibitor known as benserazide is also available outside of the United States, and this drug can also be used to prevent peripheral conversion of levodopa to dopamine.[6]

Hence, the effects of levodopa are accentuated by combining this drug with a decarboxylase inhibitor such as carbidopa; for this reason, these two drugs are often combined in the same pill and marketed under the trade name Sinemet. (Preparations of levodopa with benserazide are marketed as Madopar.) When prepared together as Sinemet, levodopa and carbidopa are combined in specific proportions, usually a fixed carbidopa-to-levodopa ratio of either 1:4 or 1:10.[6,21] The Sinemet preparation that is typically used to initiate therapy consists of tablets containing 25 and 100 mg of carbidopa and levodopa, respectively. This ratio is used to achieve a rapid and effective inhibition of the dopa decarboxylase enzyme. A 10:100- or 25:250-mg preparation of carbidopa to levodopa is usually instituted as the parkinsonism symptoms become more pronounced and there is a greater need for larger relative amounts of levodopa. The average maintenance dosage of levodopa is between 600 to 700 mg/day, but this is highly variable according to the needs of the individual patient.

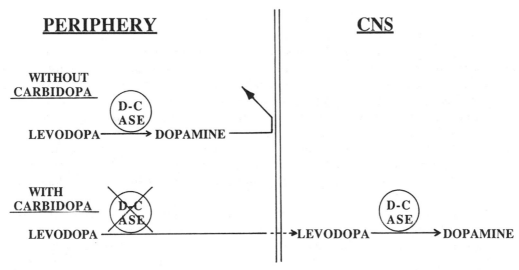

FIGURE 10–4. Use of a carbidopa, a peripheral decarboxylase inhibitor, on levodopa absorption. Without carbidopa, most of the levodopa is converted to dopamine in the periphery, rendering it unable to cross the blood-brain barrier. Carbidopa inhibits the peripheral decarboxylase (D-C ase) enzyme so that levodopa can cross the blood-brain barrier intact. Carbidopa does not cross the blood-brain barrier so that conversion of levodopa to dopamine still occurs within the CNS.

PROBLEMS AND ADVERSE EFFECTS OF LEVODOPA THERAPY

Gastrointestinal Problems. Levodopa administration is often associated with nausea and vomiting. These symptoms can be quite severe, especially during the first few days of drug use. However, the incidence of this problem is greatly reduced if levodopa is given in conjunction with a peripheral decarboxylase inhibitor such as carbidopa. The reduction in nausea and vomiting when peripheral decarboxylation of levodopa to dopamine is inhibited suggests that these symptoms may in fact be caused by excessive levels of peripheral circulating dopamine.

Cardiovascular Problems. Some problems with cardiac arrhythmias may arise in the patient taking levodopa. However, these problems are usually fairly minor unless the patient has a history of cardiac irregularity. Caution should be used in cardiac patients undergoing levodopa therapy, especially during exercise.

Postural hypotension can also be an extremely troublesome problem in the patient taking levodopa. Again, this side effect is usually diminished when peripheral decarboxylation is inhibited and peripheral dopamine levels are not allowed to increase excessively. Still, patients undergoing physical therapy or similar regimens should be carefully observed during changes in posture and should be instructed to avoid sudden postural adjustments. This factor is especially true in patients beginning levodopa therapy or in those resuming taking levodopa after a period of time without this drug.

Dyskinesias. A more persistent and challenging problem is the appearance of various movement disorders in the patient taking levodopa for prolonged periods of time. Approximately 80 percent of patients receiving chronic levodopa therapy begin to exhibit various dyskinesias such as choreoathetoid movements, ballismus, dystonia, myoclonus, and various tics and tremors.[1,18,39] The specific type of movement disorder varies from patient to patient but seems to remain constant within a given patient. The onset of dyskinetic side effects is particularly frustrating in light of the ability of levodopa to ameliorate one form of movement disorder only to institute a different motor problem.

The onset of dyskinesias usually occurs after the patient has been receiving levodopa therapy for periods ranging from 3 months to several years. These abnormal movements are probably caused by overstimulation of certain dopaminergic pathways in the basal ganglia, and management usually consists of decreasing the daily dosage of levodopa. The goal is to adjust daily dosages to a level high enough to prevent the incapacitating parkinsonism symptoms but not so high that other movement disorders begin to occur.[31] In some patients, this level may be somewhat difficult to achieve because this optimal dosage may fall into a fairly narrow range, and some of the parkinsonism side effects may appear quite similar to the dyskinetic side effects. The physician, physical therapist, patient, and other individuals who deal with the patient should make careful observations to determine if adjustments in levodopa dosage are resulting in the desired effect.

Behavioral Changes. A wide variety of mental side effects have been reported in the patient taking levodopa. Symptoms such as depression, anxiety, confusion, and hallucinations, as well as other changes in behavior, have been noted. These problems are especially prevalent in older patients or individuals who have some pre-existing psychologic disturbance.[6,18] Unlike the gastrointestinal and vascular problems described earlier, these behavioral changes appear to be exacerbated if levodopa is used in conjunction with carbidopa. This event may be caused by the greater quantities of levodopa crossing the blood-brain barrier before being converted to dopamine, and thus generating higher quantities of dopamine within the brain.

Diminished Response to Levodopa. One of the most serious problems in levodopa therapy is that this drug seems to become less effective in many patients when it is administered for prolonged periods. When used continually for periods of 3 to 4 years, the ability of levodopa to relieve parkinsonism symptoms often progressively diminishes to the point where this drug is no longer effective in treating the patient.[1,49] One explanation for this occurrence is that the patient develops tolerance to the drug. A second theory is that the decreased effectiveness of levodopa may be caused by a progressive increase in the severity of the underlying disease rather than a decrease in drug efficacy. These two theories on the decreased effectiveness of levodopa have initiated a controversy as to whether or not levodopa therapy should be started early or late in the course of Parkinson's disease (see "Clinical Course of Parkinson's Disease: When to Use Specific Drugs"). Regardless of why this occurs, the loss of levodopa efficacy can be a devastating blow to the patient who had previously experienced excellent therapeutic results from this drug.

Fluctuations in Response to Levodopa. Several distinct fluctuations in the response to levodopa are fairly common in most patients.[1,6,18] **End-of-dose akinesia** describes the phenomenon where the effectiveness of the drug simply seems to wear off prior to the next dose. This condition is usually resolved by adjusting the quantity and timing of levodopa administration (i.e., smaller doses may be given more frequently). A more bizarre and less understood fluctuation in response is the **on-off phenomenon**. Here the effectiveness of levodopa may suddenly and spontaneously decrease, resulting in the abrupt worsening of parkinsonism symptoms (off period). Remission of symptoms may then occur spontaneously or after taking a dose of levodopa (on period). This on-off pattern may repeat itself several times during the day. Although the exact reasons for this phenomenon are unclear, the off periods are directly related to diminishing plasma levels of levodopa.[35,40] These low levels may occur when the absorption of orally administered levodopa is delayed by the presence of food in the gastrointestinal tract, or if levodopa must compete with large amino acids for transport across the intestinal mucosa.[36] The off periods can be eliminated by administering levodopa continuously by intravenous infusion, thus preventing the fall in plasma levels. However, this is not a long-term solution, and alternations in the oral dosage schedule may have to be made in an attempt to maintain plasma levels at a relatively constant level.

An alternative solution that may help prevent fluctuations in plasma levels of levodopa has been the development of sustained-release preparations of this drug.[6,19,28] These preparations allow a more steady, controlled release of levodopa into the bloodstream, thus preventing the fluctuations in plasma levodopa that seem to be responsible for the on-off phenomenon and similar problems. Hence, the use of these controlled-release preparations may be helpful in patients who respond well to levodopa initially but experience fluctuations in response such as the on-off phenomenon.[31]

DRUG HOLIDAYS FROM LEVODOPA

Drug holidays are sometimes used in the patient who has become refractory to the beneficial effects of levodopa or has had a sudden increase in adverse side effects.[1] During this period, the patient is gradually removed from all antiparkinson medication for 3 days to 3 weeks while under close medical supervision. The purpose of the holiday is to allow the body to recover from any toxicity or tolerance that may have developed because of prolonged use of levodopa at relatively high dosages. Drug holidays are done with the hope that levodopa can eventually be resumed at a lower dosage and with better results. Drug holidays do appear to be successful in some patients with Parkinson's disease. Beneficial effects may be achieved at only half the preholiday dosage, and the incidence of side effects (such as dyskinesias, confusion, and the on-off phenomenon) may be markedly reduced.[48] However, drug holidays are only successful in a limited number of patients with Parkinson's disease, and there is no way of predicting which patients will benefit from such a holiday.[1,23] Also, there is no guarantee of how long the success will last, and the patient may return to the preholiday condition fairly quickly. Drug holidays have also been criticized lately because there is a certain amount of risk to the patient, and deaths have occurred when antiparkinson medications are suddenly discontinued.[6] Hence, drug holidays may still be used in some patients with Parkinson's disease, but the continued use of this intervention remains somewhat uncertain at the present time.

Other Drugs Used to Treat Parkinson's Disease

DOPAMINE AGONISTS

Because the basic problem in Parkinson's disease is a deficiency of striatal dopamine, it would seem logical that drugs similar in function to dopamine would be effective in treating this problem. However, many dopamine agonists have serious side effects that prevent their clinical use. Two exceptions are bromocriptine (Parlodel) and pergolide (Permax), which have been shown to be effective in treating parkinsonism without excessive adverse effects.[6,18] These dopamine agonists are typically used in conjunction with levodopa, especially in patients who have begun to experience a decrease in levodopa effects, or in those who experience problems such as end-of-dose akinesia and the on-off effect.[17,47] Simultaneous administration of levodopa with a dopamine agonist permits optimal results with relatively smaller doses of each drug. Low doses of bromocriptine or pergolide may also be used alone in the early stages of mild-to-moderate parkinsonism, thus providing an alternative if other antiparkinson drugs (including levodopa) are poorly tolerated.[43,44] However, neither bromocriptine nor pergolide has been shown to be superior to levodopa, which remains the drug of choice for treatment in the early stages of Parkinson's disease.[16]

When dopamine agonist therapy is initiated, adverse side effects such as nausea and vomiting may occur. Postural hypotension is also a problem in some patients. With prolonged use, bromocriptine and pergolide may cause CNS-related side effects such as confusion and hallucinations.

ANTICHOLINERGIC DRUGS

As mentioned previously, the deficiency of striatal dopamine results in excessive activity in certain cholinergic pathways in the basal ganglia. Consequently, drugs that limit acetylcholine transmission are used to help alleviate the symptoms of Parkinson's disease, especially the tremor and rigidity associated with this disorder. Various **anticholinergic** agents are available for this purpose, and the choice of drug usually depends on which one works best for a given patient (Table 10-2). When used alone, anticholinergics are usually only mildly to moderately successful in reducing symp-

TABLE 10-2 Anticholinergic Drugs Used in Treating Parkinsonism

Generic Name	Trade Name	Usual Daily Dose (mg)
Benztropine mesylate	Cogentin	0.5-6.0
Biperiden	Akineton	6.0-8.0
Ethopropazine	Parsidol	50-600
Procyclidine	Kemadrin	7.5-20.0
Trihexyphenidyl	Artane	6.0-10.0
Orphenadrine	Disipal	150-250
Diphenhydramine*	Benadryl	75-200

*Antihistamine drugs with anticholinergic properties.

toms and are often used in conjunction with levodopa or other antiparkinson drugs to obtain optimal results.

Anticholinergics are associated with many troublesome side effects including mood changes, confusion, hallucinations, drowsiness, and cardiac irregularities.[18] In addition, blurred vision, dryness of the mouth, nausea/vomiting, constipation, and urinary retention are fairly common. Antihistamine drugs with anticholinergic properties are also occasionally used (Table 10-2). These drugs tend to be somewhat less effective in treating parkinsonism, but appear to have milder side effects than their anticholinergic counterparts.

AMANTADINE

Amantadine (Symmetrel) was originally developed as an antiviral drug, and its ability to reduce parkinsonian symptoms was discovered by chance.[15] Amantadine was being used to treat influenza in a patient with Parkinson's disease, and a noticeable improvement in the patient's tremor and rigidity was also observed. Since that time, amantadine has been approved for use in patients with Parkinson's disease and is usually given along with levodopa or anticholinergic drugs. The exact mechanism of amantadine's antiparkinson activity remains unclear, although it is believed to facilitate the release of dopamine from synaptic storage sites in the basal ganglia.

The primary adverse effects associated with amantadine are orthostatic hypotension, CNS disturbances (depression, confusion, hallucinations), and patches of skin discoloration on the lower extremities (livedo reticularis). However, these side effects are relatively mild compared to those of the other antiparkinson drugs and are usually reversed by altering the drug dosage.

SELEGILINE

Selegiline (deprenyl, Eldepryl) is a drug that potently and selectively inhibits the monoamine oxidase type B (MAO_B) enzyme. This enzyme is responsible for breaking down dopamine. By inhibiting this enzyme, selegiline prolongs the local effects of dopamine at CNS synapses. Thus, selegiline may serve as a useful adjunct to levodopa therapy. Administering selegiline along with levodopa potentiates the motor effects of levodopa in Parkinson's disease.[22] Selegiline prolongs the action of levodopa and allows the dosage of levodopa to be reduced by 10 to 25 percent.[4,18]

Selegiline may actually slow the progression of Parkinson's disease.[37,46] As discussed previously, cell death in the substantia nigra may be caused by some type of toxic substance. In particular, the generation of free radicals may produce harmful effects that accelerate cell death in the basal ganglia. Free radicals are chemical products that exist in a highly reactive state because of a single, unpaired electron in their outer orbit.[25] These free radicals often initiate chemical reactions that can be harmful to various other cells including dopamine-producing cells in the substantia nigra.[6] It is currently believed that selegiline can limit free radical production by inhibiting dopamine oxidation, thus producing a neuroprotective effect in patients with Parkinson's disease.[6] A growing body of evidence supports the idea that administering selegiline early in the course of Parkinson's disease can delay the onset of the more severe motor problems associated with this disease.[12,33,37,46] Hence, selegiline represents the first pharmacologic method that may help alter the course of Parkinson's disease, and this drug will hopefully continue to show clinical benefits in slowing the progressive nature of this illness.

Selegiline appears to be relatively safe in terms of adverse side effects. With some MAO inhibitors, there is frequently a sudden, large increase in blood pressure if the patient ingests foods containing tyramine (see Chapter 7). However, selegiline does not appear to cause a hypertensive crisis even when such tyramine-containing foods are eaten.[18,22] Consequently, selegiline appears to be a valuable adjunct to levodopa therapy and may help improve the management of Parkinson's disease.

CLINICAL COURSE OF PARKINSON'S DISEASE: WHEN TO USE SPECIFIC DRUGS

Considerable controversy exists as to when specific antiparkinson drugs should be employed in treating this disease.[1,6,7,24] Much of the debate focuses on when levodopa therapy should be initiated. As mentioned previously, the effectiveness of this drug seems to diminish after several years of use. Consequently, some practitioners feel that levodopa therapy should be withheld until the parkinsonian symptoms become severe enough to truly impair motor function. In theory, this saves the levodopa for more advanced stages of this disease when it would be needed the most.[13,42] In the milder stages of Parkinson's disease, other medications such as amantadine, anticholinergics, selegiline, or bromocriptine could be prescribed. Other physicians feel that the decreased effectiveness of levodopa is simply the result of an increase in the severity of the disease itself. Consequently, there may be no advantage in delaying the start of levodopa, and it should be instituted as soon as the symptoms become obvious.[30,32] At present, the issue of when to begin levodopa remains largely unresolved, and the choice is ultimately left to the discretion of the physician.[6]

TISSUE TRANSPLANTS IN PARKINSON'S DISEASE

A great deal of attention and controversy have centered on the idea of using tissue transplants in the long-term management of patients with Parkinson's disease.[6] The basic idea of this treatment is to surgically implant dopamine-producing cells into the substantia nigra to replace the cells that have been destroyed by the disease process.

This strategy is impeded by several issues, including how to get a supply of viable cells. A potential source of these cells has been from fetal mesenchymal tissues, but this approach has generated considerable concern about the ethical use of fetal tissues for medical research and treatment. Likewise, there are some practical limitations associated with implanting a sufficient number of these cells into a small area deep in the brain and then keeping these cells alive and producing dopamine. Patients who would benefit from such transplants are typically older and somewhat debilitated with a possible reduction in blood flow and oxygenation of tissues deep in the brain. These facts, combined with the presence of the original pathologic process that caused Parkinson's disease in the first place, may limit the chances for survival of the transplanted tissues.

Hence, tissue transplants have not shown overwhelming clinical success, and the future of this technique as an effective and widely used method of treating Parkinson's disease remains doubtful at the present time. It may be possible that new developments, including the use of cell cultures as a source of dopamine-producing cells and the use of drugs to prolong the survival of transplanted tissues, may improve the clinical outcome of this technique. Still, it remains to be seen whether tissue transplants will ever be a practical and routine method of treating the rather large number of patients who are afflicted with Parkinson's disease.

SPECIAL CONSIDERATIONS FOR REHABILITATION

Therapists who are treating patients with Parkinson's disease usually wish to coordinate the therapy session with the peak effects of drug therapy. In patients receiving levodopa, this usually occurs approximately 1 hour after a dose of the medication has been taken. If possible, scheduling the primary therapy session after the breakfast dose of levodopa often yields optimal effects from the standpoint of both maximal drug efficacy and low fatigue levels in these elderly patients.

Many therapists working in hospitals and other institutions are faced with the responsibility of treating patients who are on a drug holiday. As discussed previously, during those several days the patient is placed in the hospital and all antiparkinson medication is withdrawn so that the patient may recover from the adverse effects of prolonged levodopa administration. During the drug holiday, the goal of physical therapy is to maintain patient mobility as much as possible. Obviously, without antiparkinson drugs, this task is often quite difficult. Many patients are well into the advanced stages of this disease, and even a few days without medication can produce profound debilitating effects. Consequently, any efforts to maintain joint range of motion and cardiovascular fitness during the drug holiday are crucial in helping the patient resume activity when medications are reinstated.

Therapists should also be aware of the need to monitor blood pressure in patients receiving antiparkinson drugs. Most of these drugs cause orthostatic hypotension, especially during the first few days of drug treatment. Dizziness and syncope often occur because of a sudden drop in blood pressure when the patient stands up. Since patients with Parkinson's disease are susceptible to falls anyway, this problem is only increased by the chance of orthostatic hypotension. Consequently, therapists must be especially careful to guard against falls by the patient taking antiparkinson drugs.

Finally, rehabilitation specialists should recognize that they can have a direct and positive influence on the patient's health and need for drug treatment. There is consensus that an aggressive program of gait training, balance activities, and other appropriate exercises can be extremely helpful in promoting optimal health and function in patients with Parkinson's disease.[10,14,38] Using nonpharmacologic methods to maintain motor function can diminish the patient's need for antiparkinson drugs. The synergistic effects of physical rehabilitation and the judicious use of antiparkinson drugs will ultimately provide better results than either intervention used alone.

CASE STUDY

ANTIPARKINSON DRUGS

Brief History. M.M. is a 67-year-old woman who was diagnosed with Parkinson's disease 6 years ago, at which time she was treated with anticholinergic drugs (i.e., benztropine mesylate, diphenhydramine). After approximately 2 years, the bradykinesia and rigidity associated with this disease began to be more pronounced, so she was started on a combination of levodopa-carbidopa. The initial levodopa dosage was 400 mg/day. She was successfully maintained on levodopa for the next 3 years, with minor adjustments in the dosage being made from time to time. During that time, M.M. had been living at home with her husband. During the past 12 months, her husband noted that her ability to get around seemed to be declining, so the levodopa dosage was progressively increased to 600 mg/day. The patient was also referred to physical therapy on an outpatient basis in an attempt to maintain mobility and activities of daily living (ADL) skills. She began attending physical therapy three times per week, and a regimen designed to maintain musculoskeletal flexibility, posture, and balance was initiated.

Problem/Influence of Medication. The patient was seen by the therapist three mornings each week. After a few sessions, the therapist observed that there were certain days when the patient was able to actively and vigorously participate in the therapy program. On other days, the patient was essentially akinetic, and her active participation in exercise and gait activities was virtually impossible. There was no pattern to her good and bad days, and the beneficial effects of the rehabilitation program seemed limited by the rather random effects of her levodopa medication. The patient stated that these akinetic episodes sometimes occurred even on nontherapy days.

Decision/Solution. After discussions with the patient and her husband, the therapist realized that the morning dose of levodopa was sometimes taken with a rather large breakfast. On other days, the patient consumed only a light breakfast. In retrospect, the akinetic episodes usually occurred on days when a large morning meal was consumed. The therapist surmised that this probably occurred because the large breakfast was impairing absorption of levodopa from the gastrointestinal tract. The patient was probably exhibiting the on-off phenomenon sometimes seen in patients receiving long-term levodopa therapy, which was brought on by the impaired absorption of the drug. This problem was resolved by having the patient consistently take the morning dose with a light breakfast. On mornings when the patient was still hungry, she waited 1 hour before consuming additional food to allow complete absorption of the medication.

SUMMARY

The cause of Parkinson's disease remains unknown. However, the neuronal changes that produce the symptoms associated with this movement disorder have been identified. Degeneration of dopaminergic neurons in the substantia nigra results in a deficiency of dopamine and subsequent overactivity of acetylcholine in the basal ganglia. Pharmacologic treatment attempts to rectify this dopamine-acetylcholine imbalance. Although no cure is currently available, drug therapy can dramatically improve the clinical picture in many patients by reducing the incapacitating symptoms of parkinsonism.

The use of levodopa and several other medications has allowed many patients with Parkinson's disease to remain active despite the steadily degenerative nature of this disease. Levodopa, currently the drug of choice in treating parkinsonism, often produces remarkable improvements in motor function. However, levodopa is associated with several troublesome side effects, and the effectiveness of this drug tends to diminish with time. Other agents, such as dopamine agonists, amantadine, selegiline, and anticholinergic drugs, can be used alone or in combination with levodopa or with each other to prolong the functional status of the patient. Physical therapists and other rehabilitation specialists can maximize the effectiveness of their treatments by coordinating therapy sessions with drug administration. Therapists also play a vital role in maintaining function in the patient with Parkinson's disease when the efficacy of these drugs begins to diminish.

REFERENCES

1. Aminoff, MJ: Pharmacologic management of parkinsonism and other movement disorders. In Katzung, BG (ed): Basic and Clinical Pharmacology, ed 5. Appleton & Lange, Norwalk, CT, 1992.
2. Ballard PA, Tetrud, JW, and Langston, JW: Permanent human parkinsonism due to 1-methyl-4-phenyl-1,2,3,6-tetrahydropyridine (MPTP): Seven cases. Neurology 35:949, 1985.
3. Bianchine, JR: Drug therapy of parkinsonism. N Engl J Med 295:814, 1976.
4. Birkmayer, W, et al: MBH: (-) Deprenyl leads to prolongation of L-dopa efficacy in Parkinson's disease. Mod Probl Pharmacopsychiatry 19:170, 1983.
5. Burns, RS, et al: A primate model of parkinsonism: Selective destruction of dopaminergic neurons in pars compacta of the substantia nigra by N-methyl-4-phenyl-1,2,3,6-tetrahydropyridine. Proc Natl Acad Sci USA 80:4546, 1983.
6. Calne, DB: Drug therapy: Treatment of Parkinson's disease. N Engl J Med 329:1021, 1993.
7. Calne, DB: Progress in Parkinson's disease. N Engl J Med 310:523, 1984.
8. Calne, DB and Langston, JW: The aetiology of Parkinson's disease. Lancet II(8365/6):1457, 1983.
9. Cedarbaum, JM and Schleifer, LS: Drugs for Parkinson's disease, spasticity, and acute muscle spasms. In Gilman, AG, et al (eds): The Pharmacological Basis of Therapeutics, ed 8. Pergamon Press, New York, 1990.
10. Comela, CL, et al: Physical therapy and Parkinson's disease: A controlled clinical trial. Neurology 44:376, 1994.
11. Cote, L and Crutcher, MD: The basal ganglia. In Kandel, ER, Schwartz, JH, and Jessell, TM (eds): Principles of Neural Science, ed 3. Appleton & Lange, Norwalk, CT, 1991.
12. Elizan, TS, Moros, DA, and Yahr, MD: Early combination of selegiline and low-dose levodopa as initial symptomatic therapy in Parkinson's disease: Experience in 26 patients receiving combined therapy for 26 months. Arch Neurol 48:31, 1991.
13. Fahn, S and Bressman, SB: Should levodopa therapy for parkinsonism be started early or late? Evidence against early treatment. Can J Neurol Sci 11 (suppl):200, 1984.
14. Formisano, R, et al: Rehabilitation and Parkinson's disease. Scand J Rehabil Med 24:157, 1992.
15. Forssman, B, Kihlstrand, S, and Larsson LE: Amantadine therapy in parkinsonism. Acta Neurol Scand 48:1, 1972.
16. Hely, MA, et al: The Sydney multicentre study of Parkinson's disease: A report on the first 3 years. J Neurol Neurosurg Psychiatry 52:324, 1989.

17. Hoehn, MMM and Elton, RL: Low doses of bromocriptine added to levodopa in Parkinson's disease. Neurology 35:199, 1985.
18. Hubble, JP and Koller, WC: Parkinson's disease. In Rakel, RE (ed): Conn's Current Therapy. WB Saunders, Philadelphia, 1993.
19. Hutton, JT and Morris, JL: Long-acting carbidopa-levodopa in the management of moderate and advanced Parkinson's disease. Neurology 42(suppl 1):51, 1992.
20. Jenner, P, Schapira, AHV, and Marsden, CD: New insights into the cause of Parkinson's disease. Neurology 42:2241, 1992.
21. Kaakkola, S, Mannisto, PT, and Nissinen, E: The effect of an increased ratio of carbidopa to levodopa on the pharmacokinetics of levodopa. Acta Neurol Scand 72:385, 1985.
22. Knoll, J: Role of B-type monamine oxidase inhibition in the treatment of Parkinson's disease. In Shah, NS and Donald, AG (eds): Movement Disorders. Plenum, New York, 1986.
23. Kofman, OS: Are levodopa "drug holidays" justified? Can J Neurol Sci 11(suppl):206, 1984.
24. Koller, WC: Initiating treatment of Parkinson's disease. Neurology 42(suppl 1):33, 1992.
25. Kumar, V, Cotran, RS, and Robbins, SL: Basic Pathology, ed 5. WB Saunders, Philadelphia, 1992.
26. Langston, JW: MPTP and Parkinson's disease. Trends Neurosci 8:79, 1985.
27. Langston, JW, et al: Selective nigral toxicity after systemic administration of 1-methyl-4-phenyl-1,2,5,6-tetrahydropyridine (MPTP) in the squirrel monkey. Brain Res 292:390, 1984.
28. LeWitt, PA: Clinical studies with and pharmacokinetic consideration of sustained-released levodopa. Neurology 42(suppl 1):29, 1992.
29. Markey, SP, et al (eds): MPTP: A Neurotoxin Producing a Parkinsonian Syndrome. Academic Press, New York, 1986.
30. Markham, CH and Diamond, SG: Long-term follow up of early DOPA treatment in Parkinson's disease. Ann Neurol 19:365, 1986.
31. Montgomery, EB: Pharmacokinetics and pharmacodynamics of levodopa. Neurology 42(suppl 1):17, 1992.
32. Muenter, MD: Should levodopa therapy be started early or late? Can J Neurol Sci 11(suppl):295, 1984.
33. Myllyla, VV, et al: Selegiline as initial treatment in de novo parkinsonian patients. Neurology 42:339, 1992.
34. Newman, RP and Calne, DB: Parkinsonism: Physiology and pharmacology. In Shah, NS and Donald, AG (eds): Movement Disorders. Plenum, New York, 1986.
35. Nutt, JG, et al: Effect of long-term therapy on the pharmacodynamics of levodopa: Relation to on-off phenomenon. Arch Neurol 49:1123, 1992.
36. Nutt, JG, et al: The "on-off" phenomenon in Parkinson's disease. N Engl J Med 310:483, 1984.
37. Parkinson Study Group: Effects of tocopherol and deprenyl on the progression of disability in early Parkinson's disease. N Engl J Med 328:176, 1993.
38. Pfeiffer, R: Optimization of levodopa therapy. Neurology 42(suppl 1):39, 1992.
39. Quinn, NP: Anti-parkinsonian drugs today. Drugs 28:236, 1984.
40. Quinn, N, Parkes, JD, and Marsden, CD: Control of on/off phenomenon by continuous infusion of levodopa. Neurology 34:1131, 1984.
41. Rajput, AH: Environmental causation of Parkinson's disease. Arch Neurol 50:651, 1993.
42. Rajput, AH, Stern, W, and Laverty, WH: Chronic low-dose levodopa therapy in Parkinson's disease: An argument for delaying levodopa treatment. Neurology 34:991, 1984.
43. Rascol, A, Montastruc, JL, and Rascol, O: Should dopamine agonists be given early or late in the treatment of Parkinson's disease? Can J Neurol Sci 11(suppl):229, 1984.
44. Staal-Schreinemachers, AL, Wesseling, H, and Kamphuis, DJ: Low-dose bromocriptine therapy in Parkinson's disease: Double-blind, placebo-controlled study. Neurology 36:291, 1986.
45. Stahl, SM: Neuropharmacology of movement disorders: Comparison of spontaneous and drug-induced movement disorders. In Shah, NS and Donald, AG (eds): Movement Disorders. Plenum, New York, 1986.
46. Tetrud, JW and Langston, JW: The effect of deprenyl (selegiline) on the natural history of Parkinson's disease. Science 245:519, 1989.
47. Toyokura, Y, et al: Effects of bromocriptine on parkinsonism: A nationwide double-blind study. Acta Neurol Scand 72:157, 1985.
48. Weiner, WJ, et al: Drug holiday and the management of Parkinson's disease. Neurology 30:1257, 1980.
49. Yahr, MD: Limitations of long-term use of antiparkinson drugs. Can J Neurol Sci 11(suppl):191, 1984.

CHAPTER 11

General Anesthetics

The discovery and development of anesthetic agents has been one of the most significant contributions in the advancement of surgical technique. Before the use of anesthesia, surgery was used only as a last resort and was often performed with the patient conscious, but physically restrained by several large "assistants." During the past century, general and local anesthetic drugs have been used to allow surgery to be performed in a manner that is both safer and much less traumatic to the patient, and that permits lengthier and more sophisticated surgical procedures.

Anesthetics are categorized as general or local, depending on whether or not the patient remains conscious when the anesthetic is administered. General anesthetics are usually administered during the more extensive surgical procedures. Local anesthetics are given when analgesia is needed in a relatively small, well-defined area, or when the patient should remain conscious during surgery. The use of general anesthesia and general anesthetic agents is presented in this chapter; local anesthetics are dealt with in Chapter 12.

Most physical therapists and other rehabilitation specialists are not usually involved in working with patients while general anesthesia is actually being administered. However, knowledge of how these agents work will help the therapist understand some of the residual effects that may occur when the patient is recovering from the anesthesia. This knowledge will help the therapist understand how these effects may directly influence the therapy sessions that take place during the first few days after procedures in which general anesthesia was used.

GENERAL ANESTHESIA: REQUIREMENTS

During major surgery (such as laparotomy, thoracotomy, joint replacement, amputation), the patient should be unconscious throughout the procedure and, upon awakening, have no recollection of what occurred during the surgery. An ideal anesthetic agent must be able to produce each of the following conditions:

1. Loss of consciousness and sensation.
2. Amnesia (i.e., no recollection of what occurred during the surgery).

3. Skeletal muscle relaxation (this requirement is currently met with the aid of skeletal muscle blockers used in conjunction with the anesthetic [see "Neuromuscular Blockers"]).
4. Inhibition of sensory and autonomic reflexes.
5. A minimum of toxic side effects (i.e., be relatively safe).
6. Rapid onset of anesthesia; easy adjustment of the anesthetic dosage during the procedure; and rapid, uneventful recovery after administration is terminated.

Current general anesthetics meet these criteria quite well, providing that the dosage is high enough to produce an adequate level of anesthesia but not so high that problems occur. The relationship between dosage and level or plane of anesthesia is discussed in the next section, "Stages of General Anesthesia."

STAGES OF GENERAL ANESTHESIA

During general anesthesia, the patient goes through a series of stages as the anesthetic dosage and the amount of anesthesia reaching the brain progressively increase. Four stages of anesthesia are commonly identified[23]:

Stage I. Analgesia. The patient begins to lose somatic sensation but is still conscious and somewhat aware of what is happening.

Stage II. Excitement (Delirium). The patient is unconscious and amnesiac but appears agitated and restless. This paradoxical increase in the level of excitation is highly undesirable because patients may injure themselves while thrashing about. Thus, an effort is made to move as quickly as possible through this stage and on to stage III.

Stage III. Surgical Anesthesia. As the name implies, this level is desirable for the surgical procedure and begins with the onset of regular, deep respiration. Some texts subdivide this stage into several planes, according to respiration rate and reflex activity.[15]

Stage IV. Medullary Paralysis. This stage is marked by the cessation of spontaneous respiration because respiratory control centers located in the medulla oblongata are inhibited by excessive anesthesia. The ability of the medullary vasomotor center to regulate blood pressure is also affected, and cardiovascular collapse ensues. If this stage is inadvertently reached during anesthesia, respiratory and circulatory support must be provided or the patient will die.[23]

Consequently, the goal of the anesthetist is to bring the patient to stage III as rapidly as possible and to maintain the patient at that stage for the duration of the surgical procedure. This goal is often accomplished by using both an intravenous and an inhaled anesthetic agent (see "General Anesthetic Agents: Classification and Use According to Route of Administration"). Finally, the anesthetic should not be administered for any longer than necessary, or recovery will be delayed. This state is often accomplished by beginning to taper off the dosage toward the end of the surgical procedure, so that the patient is already recovering as the surgery is completed.

GENERAL ANESTHETIC AGENTS: CLASSIFICATION AND USE ACCORDING TO ROUTE OF ADMINISTRATION

Specific agents are classified according to the two primary routes of administration—intravenous or inhaled.[13,23] Intravenously injected anesthetics offer the advantage of a rapid onset, thus allowing the patient to pass through the first two stages of anesthesia very quickly. The primary disadvantage is that there is a relative lack of control over the level of anesthesia if too much of the drug is injected. Inhaled anesthetics provide an easier method of making adjustments in the dosage during the procedure, but it takes a relatively long time for the onset of the appropriate level of anesthesia when administered through inhalation. Consequently, a combination of injected and inhaled agents is often used sequentially during the lengthier surgical procedures. The intravenous drug is injected first to quickly get the patient to stage III, and an inhaled agent is then administered to maintain the patient in a stage of surgical anesthesia. Ultimately, the selection of exactly which agents will be used depends on the type and length of the surgical procedure and any possible interactions with other anesthetics or medical problems of the patient. Specific injected and inhaled anesthetics are presented here.

GENERAL ANESTHETICS: SPECIFIC AGENTS

Inhalation Anesthetics

Anesthetics administered by this route exist either as gases or as volatile liquids that can be easily mixed with air or oxygen and then inhaled by the patient. When administered to the patient, a system of tubing and valves is usually employed to deliver the anesthetic drug directly to the patient through an endotracheal tube or a mask over the patient's face (Fig. 11–1). This delivery system offers the obvious benefit of focusing the drug on the patient without anesthetizing everyone else in the room. These systems also allow for easy adjustment of the rate of delivery and concentration of the inhaled drug.

Inhaled anesthetics currently in use include halogenated volatile liquids such as halothane, enflurane, isoflurane, and methoxyflurane (Table 11–1). The only gaseous anesthetic currently in widespread use is nitrous oxide, which is usually reserved for relatively short-term procedures (e.g., tooth extractions). Earlier inhaled anesthetics, such as ether, chloroform, and cyclopropane, are not currently used because they are

FIGURE 11–1. Schematic diagram of a closed anesthesia system. (1) Vaporizer for volatile liquid anesthetics. (2) Compressed gas source. (3) Inhalation unidirectional valve. (4) Mask. (5) Unidirectional exhalation valve. (6) Rebreathing bag. (7) Carbon dioxide absorption chamber. (From Brown, BR: Pharmacology of general anesthesia. In Clark, WG, Brater, DC, and Johnson, AR: Goth's Medical Pharmacology, ed. 13. CV Mosby, St. Louis, 1992, p 385, with permission.)

TABLE 11-1 General Anesthetics

Anesthetic	Representative Structure
Inhaled Anesthetics	

Volatile liquids
  Enflurane (Ethrane)
  Halothane (Fluothane)
  Isoflurane (Forane)
  Methoxyflurane (Penthrane)
	Halothane

Gas Nitrous oxide (nitrogen monoxide)	Nitrous oxide
Intravenous Anesthetics	

Barbiturates
  Methohexital (Brevital sodium)
  Thiamylal (Surital)
  Thiopental (Pentothal)
	Thiopental

Benzodiazepines
  Diazepam (Valium)
  Lorazepam (Ativan)
  Midazolam (Versed)
	Diazepam

Opioids
  Fentanyl (Sublimaze)
  Meperidine (Demerol)
  Morphine
	Meperidine

Ketamine (Ketaject, Ketalar)	Ketamine

explosive in nature or they produce toxic effects that do not occur with the more modern anesthetic agents.

Intravenous Anesthetics

When given in appropriate doses, several categories of CNS depressants can serve as general anesthetics (see Table 11–1).[21] The most widely used are the barbiturate drugs (thiopental, methohexital, thiamylal). Barbiturates are noted for their fast onset (when administered intravenously) and relative safety when used appropriately. Several other types of drugs including benzodiazepines (diazepam, lorazepam, midazolam) and opioid analgesics (fentanyl, morphine, meperidine) have also been used to induce or help maintain general anesthesia. For the most part, these other agents are used as preoperative sedatives, but larger doses have been used occasionally to produce anesthesia in short surgical or diagnostic procedures or where other general anesthetics may be contraindicated (e.g., cardiovascular disease).

Another intravenous general anesthetic is ketamine (Ketalar). This agent produces a somewhat different type of condition known as *dissociative anesthesia*.[23] This term is used because of the clinical observation that the patient appears detached or dissociated from the surrounding environment. The patient appears awake but is sedated and usually unable to recall events that occurred when the ketamine was in effect. Dissociative anesthesia is useful during relatively short diagnostic or surgical procedures (e.g., endoscopy) or during invasive procedures in children.[22,23] A similar type of anesthesia is produced by combining the opioid fentanyl with the antipsychotic drug droperidol. The combination of these two agents produces a condition known as *neuroleptanalgesia*, which is also characterized by dissociation of the patient from what is happening around him or her with or without loss of consciousness. An inhaled anesthetic such as nitrous oxide can also be added to convert neuroleptanalgesia to neuroleptanesthesia.[13] Neuroleptanalgesia and neuroleptanesthesia are typically used for short surgical procedures, including endoscopy or burn dressings, or for patients who are seriously ill and may not tolerate general anesthesia using more conventional methods.

Finally, newer intravenous anesthetics such as etomidate (Amidate) and propofol (Diprivan) are available. Etomidate is a hypnotic-like drug that causes a rapid onset of general anesthesia with a minimum of cardiopulmonary side effects. Hence, this drug may be useful in patients with compromised cardiovascular or respiratory function. Propofol is a short-acting hypnotic that is useful as a general anesthetic in some short invasive procedures, or this drug can be used as an adjunct to other general anesthetics in longer procedures. Recovery from propofol may also be more rapid than with other anesthetics, making this drug useful when early mobilization of the patient is desirable.

PHARMACOKINETICS

Following either injection or inhalation administration, general anesthetics become widely and uniformly distributed throughout the body, largely because of their high degree of lipid solubility. As a result, a great deal of the anesthetic may become temporarily stored in adipose tissues and may slowly wash out of these tissues when the patient is recovering from surgery. If the person was anesthetized for an extended period of time and has large deposits of fat, this washout may take quite some time.[3] During this period, symptoms such as confusion, disorientation, and lethargy may occur, presumably because the drug is being redistributed to the CNS. The patient's age also influences anesthetic requirements and distribution, with older individuals usually requiring less anesthetic for a given procedure.[11] Since older people need smaller concentrations of anesthetic, the chance that, during surgery, more anesthetic may be administered than is needed is increased and recovery will be somewhat delayed.

Depending on the individual drug, elimination occurs through excretion of the drug from the lungs, biotransformation in the liver, or a combination of these two methods.[4,5] If the patient has any pulmonary or hepatic dysfunction, elimination of the anesthetic will be further delayed.

MECHANISMS OF ACTION

Actions of Inhaled Anesthetics

A great deal of debate still exists as to how the inhaled general anesthetics work. Clearly these drugs are able to inhibit the neuronal activity within all levels of the CNS, and generally they decrease the level of consciousness in the brain through an effect on neurons in the reticular activating system. However, the exact way in which these drugs affect these neurons remains speculative. The two primary schools of thought are that (1) the anesthetic exerts a general effect on membrane structure and function (general perturbation theory) or (2) the drug binds to a specific receptor on the neuron (specific receptor theory).[10,12] The major features of each theory are presented here.

1. General Perturbation Theory. The major premise of this theory is that general anesthetic molecules become dissolved directly in the lipid bilayer of the nerve membrane and serve to generally perturb membrane function by increasing membrane fluidity and disrupting the phospholipid environment that surrounds the protein channel.[8-10,19] Presence of the anesthetic apparently causes changes in the physicochemical properties of the lipids that are adjacent to the protein channels, thereby disrupting channel function.[12] Membrane excitability is decreased because ion channels, including the sodium channels, are unable to open and allow the influx of sodium needed to initiate an action potential (Fig. 11–2). A variation on this idea (which may be somewhat of an oversimplification) is that anesthetic molecules simply crowd into the lipid bilayer and cause it to swell, thus squeezing sodium ion channels shut. In any event, this theory proposes that the major site of anesthetic action is directly on the lipid bilayer rather than on some specific binding site on the protein channel.

The primary support for the membrane perturbation theory is that there is a direct correlation between anesthetic potency and lipid solubility,[12] meaning that the more easily the drug can become dissolved in the bilayer, the less drug is needed to achieve a given level of anesthesia. This theory is further supported by the fact that general anesthetics all produce a similar effect, even though they have quite diverse chemical structures (see Table 11–1). Presumably, if drugs bind to some type of receptor, they should share some structural similarities. Different classes of general anesthetics seem to have only lipid solubility as a common denominator.

2. Specific Receptor Theory. Some evidence now exists to show that membrane

No Drug
(Na⁺ channel shown open)

Anesthetized
(Na⁺ channel closed)

A. General Perturbation Theory

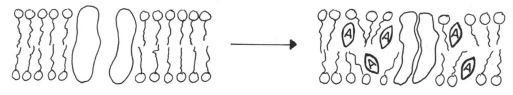

B. Specific Receptor Theory

FIGURE 11–2. Schematic illustration of two possible ways in which general anesthetics may act on the nerve membrane. In the general perturbation theory, anesthetic molecules lodge in the lipid bilayer and inhibit sodium channel function by disrupting membrane structure. In the specific receptor therapy, anesthetics inhibit opening of the sodium channel by binding directly to the channel protein.

proteins rather than the lipid bilayer may be the target site for general anesthetics.[6,7,10,12,18] This notion suggests the more traditional approach of an anesthetic molecule binding to a specific cellular component, such as a receptor on the sodium channel protein. In this scenario, the anesthetic molecule binds directly to the receptor, which in turn inactivates the sodium channel (see Fig. 11–2). This theory has not been as widely accepted as the general perturbation theory, mainly because of the diverse chemical structures of the different agents and the failure to demonstrate a definite binding site on membrane proteins. However, some evidence suggests that proteins in the nerve membrane may have a rather nonspecific pocket that accepts diverse general anesthetics, and that these drugs exert their effects by occupying this pocket rather than simply being dissolved in the bilayer.[6] The high correlation between lipid solubility and anesthetic potency discussed earlier does not necessarily rule out the specific receptor theory, but may in fact indicate that the drug must first become dissolved in the lipid bilayer in order to reach the target site on the membrane receptor.

Consequently, the exact way that inhaled anesthetics affect cellular function remains unclear. The preponderance of evidence, however, suggests that some form of structural or functional change in membrane behavior takes place. Additional research is required to discover if these anesthetics mediate this change by a direct effect on membrane receptors, by a more general effect on the lipid bilayer, or by some other, as yet unidentified, mechanism.

Actions of Intravenous Anesthetics

Injected anesthetics work by neurophysiologic mechanisms that typically involve a specific CNS receptor and the neurotransmitter associated with that receptor. For instance, the barbiturates and the benzodiazepines work by binding to CNS chloride ion channels and thereby enhancing the inhibitory effects of gamma-aminobutyric acid (GABA). The cellular action of these drugs is discussed in detail in Chapter 6. As discussed in Chapter 14, opioids decrease transmission in nociceptive pathways by binding to specific neuronal receptors in the brain and spinal cord. Ketamine appears to work by binding to the N-methyl-D-aspartate (NMDA) receptor in the brain and thus inhibiting the excitatory effects of glutamate.[23] Etomidate seems to work by mimicking the inhibitory effects of GABA, whereas the mechanism of propofol remains unknown.

ADJUVANTS IN GENERAL ANESTHESIA

Preoperative Medications

Frequently a preoperative sedative is given to the patient 1 to 2 hours before the administration of general anesthesia.[14,16] Sedatives are usually administered via intramuscular injection and are given while the patient is still in his or her room. This approach serves to relax the patient and reduce anxiety when the patient arrives at the operating room. Frequently used preoperative sedatives include barbiturates (secobarbital, pentobarbital), opioids (morphine, meperidine), and benzodiazepines (diazepam, lorazepam) (Table 11–2). Different sedatives are used depending on the patient, the type of general anesthesia used, and the preference of the physician.

A number of other medications may be used preoperatively to achieve various goals (see Table 11–2).[16] Antihistamines (promethazine, hydroxyzine) offer the dual advantage of producing sedation and reducing vomiting (antiemesis). Antacids and other drugs that increase gastric pH are sometimes used to decrease stomach acidity and thus reduce the risk of serious lung damage if gastric fluid is aspirated during general surgery. In the past, anticholinergics (atropine, scopolamine) were often administered to help reduce bronchial secretions and aid in airway intubation. However, anesthetics currently in use do not produce excessive airway secretions (as did prior agents), so the preoperative use of anticholinergics is no longer critical.[14,16]

Neuromuscular Blockers

Skeletal muscle paralysis is essential during surgical procedures. The patient must be relaxed to allow proper positioning on the operating table and to prevent spontaneous muscle contractions from hampering the surgery.[2,20] Imagine the disastrous effects that a muscular spasm in the arm would have on a delicate procedure such as nerve repair or limb reattachment. Most currently used general anesthetics produce skeletal muscle relaxation, but it takes a larger dose of the anesthetic to produce ade-

TABLE 11–2 Drugs and Doses Used for Preoperative Premedication

Classification	Drug	Typical Adult Dose (mg)	Route of Administration (Oral, IM*)
Barbiturates	Secobarbital	50–150	Oral, IM
	Pentobarbital	50–150	Oral, IM
Opioids	Morphine	5–15	IM
	Meperidine	50–100	IM
Benzodiazepines	Diazepam	5–10	Oral
	Lorazepam	2–4	Oral, IM
Antihistamines	Diphenhydramine	25–75	Oral, IM
	Promethazine	25–50	IM
	Hydroxyzine	50–100	IM
Anticholinergics	Atropine	0.3–0.6	IM
	Scopolamine	0.3–0.6	IM
	Glycopyrrolate	0.1–0.3	IM
Antacids	Particulate	15–30 mL	Oral
	Nonparticulate	15–30 mL	Oral

*IM—intramuscular.
Source: Modified from Stoelting, RK: Psychological preparation and preoperative medication. In Stoelting, RK and Miller, RD (eds): Basics of Anesthesia. Churchill Livingstone, New York, 1984, p 381, with permission.

quate muscular relaxation than is needed to produce unconsciousness and amnesia; that is, the patient must be well into stage III and almost into stage IV before muscle paralysis is complete. Consequently, a drug that blocks the skeletal neuromuscular junction is given in conjunction with the general anesthetic to allow a lower dose of anesthetic to be used while still ensuring skeletal muscle paralysis. These drugs work by blocking the postsynaptic acetylcholine receptor located at the skeletal neuromuscular junction.

Several different neuromuscular blockers are currently available, and the choice of a specific agent depends primarily on the desired length of action and the potential side effects of each agent (Table 11–3).[17] The paralytic effects of these agents should disappear by the end of the surgical procedure. However, complications such as prolonged paralysis, hyperkalemia, and muscle rigidity may occur, especially if the patient has a concurrent neuromuscular condition such as a spinal cord injury, peripheral neuropathies, intracranial lesions, or muscle pathologies.[1]

Discussed here are the two general types of neuromuscular blockers, which are classified according to whether or not they depolarize the skeletal muscle cell when binding to the cholinergic receptor.[17]

Nondepolarizing Blockers. These drugs act as competitive antagonists of the postsynaptic receptor; that is, they bind to the receptor but do not activate it (see Chapter 4). This binding prevents the agonist (acetylcholine) from binding to the receptor, and paralysis of the muscle cell results. These drugs all share a structural similarity, which apparently explains their affinity and relative selectivity for the cholinergic receptor at the skeletal neuromuscular junction. Specific agents and their onset and duration of action are listed in Table 11–3.

Depolarizing Blockers. Although these drugs also inhibit transmission at the skeletal neuromuscular junction, their mechanism is different from that of the nonde-

TABLE 11–3 Neuromuscular Junction Blockers

Drug	Onset of Initial Action* (min)	Time to Peak Effects (min)	Duration of Peak Effect (min)
Nondepolarizing blockers			
Atracurium	Within 2	3–5	20–35
Gallamine	1–2	3–5	15–30
Metocurine	1–4	1.5–10	35–60
Pancuronium	Within 0.75	4.5	35–45
Tubocurarine	Within 1	2–5	20–40
Vecuronium	1	3–5	25–30
Depolarizing blockers			
Succinylcholine	0.5–1	1–2	4–10

*Reflects usual adult intravenous dosage.

Source: Copied from *USP DI®*, *14th Edition* Copyright 1994. The USP Convention, Inc. Permission granted. The USP is not responsible for any inaccuracy of quotation nor for any false or misleading implication that may arise due to the text used or due to the quotation of information subsequently changed in later editions.

polarizing agents. These drugs initially act like acetylcholine by binding to and stimulating the receptor, resulting in depolarization of the muscle cell. However, the enzymatic degradation of the drug is not as rapid as the destruction of acetylcholine, so the muscle cell remains depolarized for a prolonged period of time. While depolarized, the muscle is unresponsive to further stimulation. The cell must become repolarized or reprimed before the cell will respond to a second stimulus. This event is often referred to as phase I blockade.[17] If the depolarizing blocker remains at the synapse, the muscle cell does eventually repolarize but remains unresponsive to stimulation by acetylcholine. This occurrence is referred to as phase II blockade and is believed to occur because the drug exerts some sort of modification on the receptor. This modification could be in the form of a temporary conformational change on the receptor. Clinically, when these drugs are first administered, they are often associated with a variable amount of muscle tremor and fasciculation (because of the initial depolarization), but this is followed by a period of flaccid paralysis. Although several drugs that act as depolarizing blockers are available, the only agent currently in clinical use is succinylcholine (see Table 11–3).

SPECIFIC CONCERNS IN REHABILITATION

The major problems that a physical therapist may encounter occur when the patient is not quite over the effects of the anesthesia. Dealing with a patient the day after surgery or possibly even the same day as surgery may be difficult because the patient is woozy. Some anesthetics may produce confusion or psychoticlike behavior during the recovery period. Muscle weakness may also be present for a variable amount of time, especially if a neuromuscular blocker was used during the surgical procedure. Of course, patients who are in relatively good general health and who have had relatively short or minor surgeries will have minimal residual effects. However, patients who are debilitated or who have other medical problems that impair drug elimination may continue to show some anesthesia aftereffects for several days. These problems should disappear with time, so the therapist must plan activities accordingly until recovery from the anesthetic effects is complete.

Another problem that therapists frequently deal with is the tendency for bronchial secretions to accumulate in the lungs of patients recovering from general anesthesia. General anesthetics depress mucociliary clearance in the airway, leading to pooling of mucus, which may produce respiratory infections and atelectasis. Therapists play an important role in preventing this accumulation by encouraging early mobilization of the patient and by implementing respiratory hygiene protocols (i.e., breathing exercises and postural drainage).

CASE STUDY

GENERAL ANESTHETICS

Brief History. B.W., a 75-year-old woman, fell at home and experienced a sudden sharp pain in her left hip. She was unable to walk and was taken to a nearby hospital where x-ray examination showed an impacted fracture of the left hip. The patient was alert and oriented at the time of admission. She had a history of arteriosclerotic cardiovascular disease and diabetes mellitus, but her medical condition was stable. The patient was relatively obese, and a considerable amount of osteoarthritis was present in both hips. Two days after admission, a total hip arthroplasty was performed under general anesthesia. Meperidine (Demerol) was given intramuscularly as a preoperative sedative. General anesthesia was induced by intravenous administration of thiopental (Pentothal) and sustained by inhalation of halothane (Fluothane). The surgery was completed successfully, and physical therapy was initiated at the patient's bedside on the subsequent day.

Problem/Influence of Medication. At the initial therapy session, the therapist found the patient to be extremely lethargic and disoriented. She appeared confused about recent events and was unable to follow most commands. Apparently, she was experiencing some residual effects of the general anesthesia.

Decision/Solution. The patient's confusion and disorientation precluded any activities that required her cooperation, including any initial attempts at weight-bearing activities. The therapist limited the initial session to passive and active-assisted exercises of both lower extremities. Active upper-extremity exercises were encouraged within the limitations of the patient's ability to follow instructions. These upper-extremity exercises were instituted to help increase metabolism and excretion of the remaining anesthesia. The patient was also placed on a program of breathing exercises in an effort to facilitate excretion of the anesthesia, as well as to maintain respiratory function and prevent the accumulation of mucus in the airways. As the patient's mental disposition gradually improved, partial weight bearing in the parallel bars was initiated. From there, the patient progressed to a walker and was soon able to ambulate independently with that device. Within 1 week after the surgery, no overt residual effects of the anesthesia were noted, and the remainder of the hospital stay was uneventful.

SUMMARY

General anesthesia has been used for some time to permit surgical procedures of various types and durations to be performed. Several different effective agents are currently available and are relatively safe in producing a suitable anesthetic condition in the patient. General anesthetics are classified according to their two primary routes of administration: by inhalation and by intravenous infusion. Specific anesthetic agents and anesthetic adjuvants (preoperative sedatives, neuromuscular blockers, etc.) are selected primarily according to the type of surgical procedure being performed and the overall condition of the patient. Health professionals should be cognizant of the fact that their patients may take some time to fully recover from the effects of general anesthesia and should adjust their postoperative care of the patient accordingly.

REFERENCES

1. Azar, I: Complications of neuromuscular blockers. Interaction with concurrent diseases. Anesthesiol Clin North Am 11:409, 1993.
2. Brull, SJ and Silverman, DG: Intraoperative use of muscle relaxants. Anesthesiol Clin North Am 11:325, 1993.
3. Carpenter, RL, Eger, EI, and Johnson, BH: Pharmacokinetics of inhaled anesthetics in humans: Measurements during and after the simultaneous administration of enflurane, halothane, isoflurane, methoxyflurane and nitrous oxide. Anesth Analg 65:572, 1986.
4. Carpenter, RL, et al: The extent of metabolism of inhaled anesthetics in humans. Anesthesiology 65:201, 1986.
5. Davis, PJ and Cook, DR: Clinical pharmacokinetics of the newer intravenous anesthetic agents. Clin Pharmacokinet 11:18, 1986.
6. Franks, NP and Lieb, WR: Mapping of general anesthetic target sites provides a molecular basis for cutoff effects. Nature 316:349, 1985.
7. Franks, NP and Lieb, WR: Do general anesthetics act by competitive binding to specific receptors? Nature 310:599, 1984.
8. Godin, DV and McGinn, P: Perturbational actions of barbiturate analogs on erythrocyte and synaptosomal membranes. Can J Physiol Pharm 63:937, 1985.
9. Goldstein, DB: The effects of drugs on membrane fluidity. Annu Rev Pharmacol Toxicol 24:43, 1984.
10. Hille, B: Theories of anesthesia: General perturbations versus specific receptors. In Fink, BR (ed): Progress in Anesthesia, Vol 2, Molecular Mechanisms of Anesthesia. Raven Press, New York, 1980.
11. Homer, TD and Stanski, DR: The effect of increasing age on thiopental disposition and anesthetic requirement. Anesthesiology 62:714, 1985.
12. Koblin, DD: Mechanisms of action. In Miller, RD (ed): Anesthesia, Vol 1, ed 3. Churchill Livingstone, New York, 1990.
13. Marshall, BE and Longnecker, DE: General anesthetics. In Gilman, AG, et al (eds): The Pharmacological Basis of Therapeutics, ed 8. Pergamon Press, New York, 1990.
14. Mirakhur, RK: Preanesthetic medication: A survey of current usage. J Royal Soc Med 84:481, 1991.
15. Moraca-Sawicki, AM: Drugs in anesthesia. In Kuhn, MA (ed): Pharmacotherapeutics: A Nursing Process Approach, ed 3. FA Davis, Philadelphia, 1994.
16. Moyers, JR: Preoperative medication. In Barash, PG, Cullen, BF, and Stoelting, RK (eds): Clinical Anesthesia. JB Lippincott, Philadelphia, 1989.
17. Ramsey, FM: Basic pharmacology of the neuromuscular blocking agents. Anesthesiol Clin North Am 11:219, 1993.
18. Richards, CD, et al: Degenerate perturbations of protein structure as the mechanism of anaesthetic action. Nature 276:775, 1978.
19. Rosenberg, PH and Alila, A: GABA inhibits inhalation anesthetic-induced membrane fluidization: A spin label study in synaptic and phospholipid membranes. Acta Pharmacol Toxicol 57:154, 1985.
20. Shanks, CA: Pharmacokinetics of the nondepolarizing neuromuscular relaxants applied to calculation of bolus and infusion dosage regimens. Anesthesiology 64:72, 1986.
21. Stoelting, RK: Pharmacology and Physiology in Anesthetic Practice, ed 2. JB Lippincott, Philadelphia, 1991.
22. Tobias, JD, et al: Oral ketamine premedication to alleviate the distress of invasive procedures in pediatric oncology patients. Pediatrics 90:537, 1992.
23. Trevor, AJ and Miller, RD: General anesthetics. In Katzung, BG (ed): Basic and Clinical Pharmacology, ed 5. Appleton & Lange, Norwalk, CT, 1992.

CHAPTER 12

Local Anesthetics

Local anesthesia is used to produce loss of sensation in a specific body part or region. Frequently this application occurs when a relatively minor surgical procedure is to be performed. This approach involves introducing an anesthetic drug near the peripheral nerve that innervates the area in question. The basic goal is to block afferent neural transmission along the peripheral nerve so that the procedure can be performed painlessly. When the local anesthetic is introduced in the vicinity of the spinal cord, transmission of impulses may be effectively blocked at a specific level of the cord to allow more extensive surgical procedures to be performed (e.g., caesarean delivery) because a larger region of the body is being anesthetized. This approach, however, is still considered a form of local anesthesia because the drug acts locally at the spinal cord and the patient remains conscious during the surgical procedure.

Using a local anesthetic during a surgical procedure offers several advantages over the use of general anesthesia, including the relatively rapid recovery and lack of residual effects from the local anesthetic.[4] There is a virtual absence of the postoperative confusion and lethargy often seen after general anesthesia. In most cases of minor surgery, patients are able to leave the practitioner's office or the hospital virtually as soon as the procedure is completed. In more extensive procedures, local anesthesia offers the advantage of not interfering with cardiovascular, respiratory, and renal function. This fact can be important in patients with problems in these physiologic systems. During childbirth, local (spinal) anesthesia imposes less of a risk to the neonate than does general anesthesia.[32] The primary disadvantages of local anesthesia are the length of time required to establish an anesthetic effect and the risk that analgesia will be incomplete or insufficient for the respective procedure.[4] The latter problem can usually be resolved by administering more local anesthesia if the procedure is relatively minor, or by switching to a general anesthetic during a major procedure in the event of an emergency arising during surgery.

Local anesthetics are sometimes used to provide analgesia in nonsurgical situations. These drugs may be used for short-term pain relief in conditions such as musculoskeletal and joint pain (e.g., bursitis, tendinitis), or in more long-term situations such as pain relief in cancer. Also, local anesthetics may be used to block efferent sympathetic activity in conditions such as reflex sympathetic dystrophy syndrome. During these nonsurgical applications, physical therapists and other rehabilitation personnel often are directly involved in treating the patient while the local anesthetic is in effect. If prescribed by the physician, the local anesthetic may actually be administered by the physical therapist via phonophoresis or iontophoresis. Consequently, these individuals should have an adequate knowledge of the pharmacology of local anesthetic agents.

TYPES OF LOCAL ANESTHETICS

Commonly used local anesthetics are listed in Table 12–1. These drugs share a common chemical strategy consisting of both a lipophilic and a hydrophilic group that

TABLE 12–1 Common Local Anesthetics

Generic Name	Trade Name	Relative Onset* of Action	Relative Duration* of Action	Principal Use(s)
Benzocaine	Americaine	—	—	Topical
Bupivacaine	Marcaine	Slow–medium	Long	Infiltration
				Peripheral nerve block
				Epidural
				Spinal
				Sympathetic block
Butamben	Butesin Picrate	—	—	Topical
Chloroprocaine	Nesacaine	Rapid	Short	Infiltration
				Peripheral nerve block
				Epidural
Dibucaine	Nupercainal	—	—	Topical
Etidocaine	Duranest	Rapid	Long	Infiltration
				Peripheral nerve block
				Epidural
Lidocaine	Xylocaine	Rapid	Intermediate	Infiltration
				Peripheral nerve block
				Epidural
				Spinal
				Transdermal
				Topical
				Sympathetic block
Mepivacaine	Carbocaine	Medium–rapid	Intermediate	Infiltration
				Peripheral nerve block
				Epidural
Pramoxine	Tronothane	—	—	Topical
Prilocaine	Citanest	Rapid	Intermediate	Infiltration
				Peripheral nerve block
Procaine	Novocain	Slow	Short	Infiltration
				Peripheral nerve block
				Spinal
Tetracaine	Pontocaine	Rapid	Intermediate–long	Topical
				Spinal

*Values for onset and duration refer to use during injection. Relative durations of action are as follows: short = 30–60 min; intermediate = 1–3 hr; and long = 3–10 hr of action.

Source: Copied from *USP DI®*, *14th Edition* Copyright 1994. The USP Convention, Inc. Permission granted. The USP is not responsible for any inaccuracy of quotation nor for any false or misleading implication that may arise due to the text used or due to the quotation of information subsequently changed in later editions.

Lidocaine

FIGURE 12-1. Structure of lidocaine. The basic structure of a lipophilic and hydrophilic group connected by an intermediate chain is common to the local anesthetics.

| Lipophilic Group | Intermediate Chain | Hydrophilic Group |

are connected by an intermediate chain (Fig. 12–1). The choice of a specific local anesthetic is made depending on factors such as (1) the operative site and nature of the procedure, (2) the type of regional anesthesia desired (such as single peripheral nerve block or spinal anesthesia), (3) the patient's size and general health, and (4) the duration of action of the anesthetic.[26]

Local anesthetics can usually be identified by their "-caine" suffix (lidocaine, procaine, etc.). Cocaine was identified as the first clinically useful local anesthetic in 1884. However, its tendency for abuse and its high incidence of addiction and systemic toxicity initiated the search for safer local anesthetics such as those listed in Table 12–1. One should note that cocaine abuse occurs because of its effects on the brain, not because of its local anesthetic effects. Cocaine is believed to produce intense feelings of euphoria and excitement through increased synaptic transmission in the brain. This fact explains why cocaine abusers inject this drug or apply it to the nasal mucous membranes (i.e., "snorting," so that it is absorbed through those membranes and into the systemic circulation, from which it ultimately reaches the brain).

PHARMACOKINETICS

Local anesthetics are administered through a variety of routes and techniques depending on the specific clinical situations (see "Clinical Use of Local Anesthetics"). In local anesthesia, the drug should remain at the site of administration. For instance, procaine (Novocain) injected into the area of the trigeminal nerve during a dental procedure will be more effective if it is not washed away from the site of administration by the blood flow through that region. Likewise, injection of a local anesthetic into the area surrounding the spinal cord (e.g., epidural or spinal injection, see "Clinical Use of Local Anesthetics") will be more effective if the drug remains near the administration site.[1] Consequently, a vasoconstricting agent (e.g., epinephrine) is often administered simultaneously to help prevent washout from the desired site. Preventing the anesthetic from reaching the bloodstream is also beneficial since local anesthetics can cause toxic side effects when sufficient amounts reach the systemic circulation (see "Systemic Effects of Local Anesthetics"). This occurrence is usually not a problem in most cases of a single dose of regional anesthesia, but the buildup of the local anesthetic in the bloodstream should be monitored if repeated doses are administered.[17]

Local anesthetics are usually eliminated by hydrolyzing or breaking apart the drug molecule. This metabolic hydrolysis is catalyzed by hepatic enzymes or enzymes circulating in the plasma (e.g., the plasma cholinesterase). Once metabolized, the polar drug metabolites are excreted by the kidney.

CLINICAL USE OF LOCAL ANESTHETICS

The primary clinical uses of local anesthetics according to their method of administration and specific indications are presented here.

1. *Topical administration:*   Local anesthetics can be applied directly to the surface of the skin, mucous membranes, cornea, and other regions to produce analgesia. This is usually done for the symptomatic relief of minor surface irritation and injury (minor burns, abrasions, inflammation). Local anesthetics can also be applied topically to reduce pain prior to minor surgical procedures such as wound cleansing, myringotomy, and circumcision.[14,18,30] Topical anesthesia can be produced in these situations by applying either a single agent or a mixture of two or more local anesthetics (e.g., lidocaine and prilocaine).[3,19]

    Topical anesthesia has also been used to improve motor function in some patients with skeletal muscle hypertonicity that resulted from a cerebrovascular accident (CVA) or head trauma.[24] In this situation, a local anesthetic (e.g., 20 percent benzocaine) can be sprayed on the skin that overlies hypertonic muscles, and then various exercises and facilitation techniques can be performed to increase and improve mobility in the affected limbs. The rationale of this treatment is to temporarily decrease abnormal or excessive excitatory feedback of cutaneous receptors on efferent motor pathways so that normal integration and control of motor function can be re-established. Preliminary evidence has suggested that repeated applications of this technique may produce fairly long-lasting improvements in joint mobility and gait characteristics in patients with hypertonicity caused by various CNS disorders.[24]

2. *Transdermal administration:*   The drug is applied to the surface of the skin or other tissues with the intention that the drug will be absorbed into underlying tissues. Transdermal administration of some local anesthetics may be enhanced by the use of electrical current (iontophoresis) or ultrasound (phonophoresis) (see Appendix A).[6,28] These approaches offer the advantage of treating painful subcutaneous structures (bursae, tendons, other soft tissues) without breaking the skin.

3. *Infiltration anesthesia:*   The drug is injected directly into the selected tissue and allowed to diffuse to sensory nerve endings within that tissue. This technique is used to saturate an area such as a skin laceration so that surgical repair (suturing) can be performed.

4. *Peripheral nerve block:*   The anesthetic is injected close to the nerve trunk so that transmission along the peripheral nerve is interrupted. This type of local anesthesia is very common in dental procedures (restorations, tooth extractions, etc.) and can also be used to block other peripheral nerves to allow certain surgical procedures or to reduce pain and improve function in chronic conditions such as rheumatoid arthritis.[9] Nerve blocks can be classified as minor, when only one distinct nerve

(e.g., ulnar, median) is blocked, or major, when several peripheral nerves or a nerve plexus (brachial, lumbosacral) is involved.

5. *Central neural blockage:*   The anesthetic is injected within the spaces surrounding the spinal cord (Fig. 12–2). Specifically, the term **epidural nerve blockade** refers to injection of the drug into the epidural space—that is, the space between the bony vertebral column and the dura mater. A variation of epidural administration known as a "caudal block" is sometimes performed by injecting the local anesthetic into the lumbar epidural space via the sacral hiatus (see Fig. 12–2). **Spinal nerve blockade** refers to injection within the subarachnoid space—that is, the space between the arachnoid membrane and the pia mater. Spinal blockade is also referred to as "intrathecal anesthesia" because the drug is injected within the tissue sheaths that surround the spinal cord (*intrathecal* means "within a sheath"; see Chapter 2).

     In theory, epidural and spinal blocks can be done at any level of the cord, but

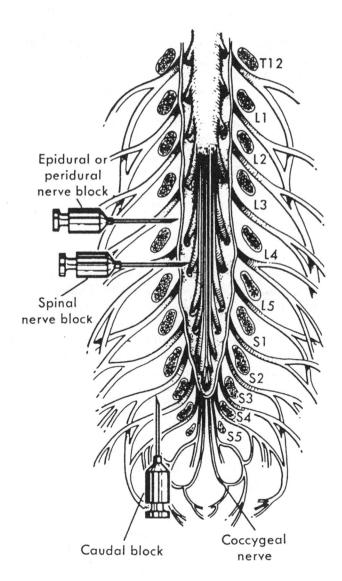

FIGURE 12–2. Sites of epidural and spinal administration of local anesthetics. Caudal block represents epidural administration via the sacral hiatus. (From Clark, JB, Queener, SF, and Karb, VB: Pharmacological Basis of Nursing Practice, ed 4, St. Louis, CV Mosby, 1993, p 688, with permission.)

Epidural or peridural nerve block

Spinal nerve block

Caudal block

T12
L1
L2
L3
L4
L5
S1
S2
S3
S4
S5
Coccygeal nerve

they are usually administered at the L3-4 or L4-5 vertebral interspace (i.e., caudal to the L-2 vertebral body, which is the point where the spinal cord ends). Epidural anesthesia is somewhat easier to perform than spinal blockade because the epidural space is larger and more accessible than the subarachnoid space. However, spinal anesthesia usually creates a more effective or solid block. These forms of local anesthesia are used whenever analgesia is needed in a large region, and they are frequently used during obstetric procedures including caesarean delivery. The epidural and intrathecal routes have also been used to administer anesthetics and narcotic analgesics for relief of acute and chronic pain. In these instances, an indwelling catheter is often left implanted in the epidural or subarachnoid space to allow repeated delivery of the anesthetic to the patient. The use of implanted drug delivery systems in managing chronic and severe pain is discussed further in Chapters 14 and 17.

6. *Sympathetic ganglion injection:*   Although blockade of sympathetic function usually occurs during peripheral and central nerve blocks, sometimes the selective interruption of sympathetic efferent discharge is desirable. In cases of reflex sympathetic dystrophy syndrome (RSDS), injection of the local anesthetic into the area surrounding a specific sympathetic chain ganglion is used to interrupt sympathetic discharge to the affected extremity.[21,29] If the upper extremity is involved, injection near the stellate ganglion is performed. Injections around the sympathetic ganglion at the L-2 vertebral level are used for lower-extremity RSDS. Usually a series of five injections on alternate days is necessary to attenuate the sympathetic discharge and to provide remission from the RSDS episode. The function of the anesthetic drug in this situation is not to provide analgesia but rather to impair efferent sympathetic outflow to the affected extremity.

MECHANISM OF ACTION

Local anesthetics work by blocking action potential propagation along neuronal axons, which is believed to result from the anesthetic molecule inhibiting the opening of membrane sodium channels.[16,23,27] The sudden influx of sodium into the neuron through open (activated) ion channels depolarizes the neuron during impulse propagation. If the sodium ion channels are inhibited from opening along a portion of the axon, the action potential will not be propagated past that point. If the neuron is sensory in nature, this information will not reach the brain, and anesthesia of the area innervated by that neuron will result.

Exactly how the anesthetic inhibits sodium channel opening has been the subject of much debate. Although several theories exist, the current consensus is that local anesthetics temporarily attach to a binding site or receptor located on or within the sodium channel.[5,13,15,16,27] These receptors probably control the opening of the channel, and when bound by the anesthetic molecule, the sodium channel is maintained in a closed, inactivated position. Two possible sites for local anesthetic binding have been proposed (Fig. 12–3).[27] One site appears to be at the interface between the channel protein and the surrounding lipid matrix. When bound by a local anesthetic molecule, this receptor site may effectively lock the sodium channel (much in the same way that the appropriate key fitting into a door keyhole is able to lock a door). Local anesthetics that are especially lipophilic may bind preferentially to this site.[27] A second site ap-

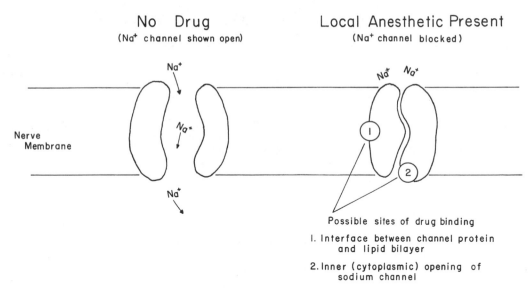

FIGURE 12–3. Schematic diagram showing mechanism of action of local anesthetics on the nerve membrane. Local anesthetics appear to inhibit channel opening by binding to one of the sites indicated.

pears to be located somewhere within the lumen or pore of the channel itself, possibly at the inner, cytoplasmic opening of the channel.[5,15,16,27] This site seems to be occupied primarily by polar, hydrophilic local anesthetic molecules. When bound by the anesthetic, this site may also lock the channel in a closed, inactivated position.

Consequently, the specific location and configuration of local anesthetic receptor/binding sites remain unclear. Possibly several potential binding sites on the channel protein may be receptive to different types of local anesthetics.

DIFFERENTIAL NERVE BLOCK

Differential nerve block refers to the ability of a given local anesthetic dose to block specific nerve fiber groups and not others, depending on the size (diameter) of the nerve fibers.[22,26] In general, smaller-diameter fibers seem to be the most sensitive to anesthetic effects, with progressively larger fibers being affected as anesthetic concentration increases.[8,11,20] This point is significant because different-diameter fibers transmit different types of information (Table 12–2). Thus, information transmitted by the smallest fibers will be lost first, with other types of transmission being successively lost as the local anesthetic effect increases. The smallest-diameter (type C) fibers that transmit pain are usually the first sensory information blocked as the anesthetic takes effect. Type C fibers also transmit postganglionic autonomic information, including the sympathetic vasomotor control of the peripheral vasculature, and are also most susceptible to block by local anesthetics. Other sensory information such as temperature, touch, and proprioception are successively lost as the concentration and effect of the anesthetic increase. Finally, skeletal motor function is usually last to disappear, since

TABLE 12–2 Relative Size and Susceptibility to Block of
Types of Nerve Fibers

Fiber Type*	Function	Diameter (μm)	Myelination	Conduction Velocity (m/s)	Sensitivity to Block
Type A					
Alpha	Proprioception, motor	12–20	Heavy	70–120	+
Beta	Touch, pressure	5–12	Heavy	30–70	++
Gamma	Muscle spindles	3–6	Heavy	15–30	++
Delta	Pain, temperature	2–5	Heavy	12–30	+++
Type B	Preganglionic autonomic	<3	Light	3–15	++++
Type C					
Dorsal root	Pain	0.4–1.2	None	0.5–2.3	++++
Sympathetic	Postganglionic	0.3–1.3	None	0.7–2.3	++++

*Fiber types are classified according to the system established by Gasser and Erlanger.[11] (Reproduced with permission from Katzung, BG: Basic and Clinical Pharmacology; fifth edition. Appleton & Lange, 1992.)

efferent impulses to the skeletal muscle are transmitted over the large, type A–alpha fibers.

The exact reason for the differential susceptibility of nerve fibers based on their axonal diameter is not known. One possible suggestion is that the anesthetic is simply able to diffuse more rapidly and completely around the thinner fibers, thus inactivating them first.[31] In fact, some evidence suggests that it is actually the largest (type A) fibers that are the most susceptible to various types of stress, including that of local anesthetic drugs.[12] However, the larger fibers are the last ones affected because of a relatively poor ability of the drug to reach them. Myelination, which is found more extensively in larger-diameter fibers, may also play a role in differential nerve block, although exactly how myelination affects anesthetic efficacy is complex and somewhat unclear. In any event, from a clinical perspective the smaller-diameter fibers appear to be affected first, although the exact reasons for this phenomenon remain to be determined.

The clinical importance of a differential nerve block is that certain sensory modalities may be blocked without the loss of motor function. Fortunately the most susceptible modality is pain since analgesia is usually the desired effect. If the dosage and administration of the anesthetic are optimal, analgesia will be produced without any significant loss of skeletal muscle function. This fact may be advantageous if motor function is required, such as during labor and delivery.[32] If local anesthetics are used to produce sympathetic blockade, postganglionic type C fibers are fortunately the first to be blocked, thus producing the desired effect at the lowest anesthetic concentration.

SYSTEMIC EFFECTS OF LOCAL ANESTHETICS

The intent of administering a local anesthetic is to produce a regional effect on specific neurons. However, these drugs may occasionally be absorbed into the general circulation and exert various effects on other organs and tissues. The most important systemic effects involve the CNS and the cardiovascular system.[25] Virtually all local anesthetics stimulate the brain initially, and symptoms such as somnolence, confusion, agitation, excitation, and seizures can occur if sufficient amounts of local anesthetic reach the brain via the bloodstream.[10,25] Central excitation is usually followed by a period of CNS depression. This depression may result in impaired respiratory function, and death may occur because of respiratory depression. The primary cardiovascular effects associated with local anesthetics include decreased cardiac excitation, decreased heart rate, and decreased force of contraction. Again, this general inhibitory effect on the myocardium may produce serious consequences if sufficient amounts of the local anesthetic reach the general circulation.[25]

The chance of systemic effects developing depends on the type of local anesthetic administered, the amount of drug administered, and the route and method of administration.[26] Therapists and other health-care professionals should always be alert for signs of the systemic effects of local anesthetics in patients receiving these drugs. Early recognition of symptoms such as restlessness or cardiac depression may help avert fatalities caused by the systemic effects of these drugs.

SIGNIFICANCE IN REHABILITATION

Because of the various clinical applications of local anesthetics, physical therapists may encounter the use of these agents in several patient situations. Therapists may be directly involved in the topical or transdermal administration of local anesthetics. As discussed previously, repeated topical application of local anesthetics may help produce long-term improvements in motor function in patients with skeletal muscle hypertonicity, so therapists may want to consider incorporating topical anesthetics into the treatment of certain patients with CNS dysfunction. Therapists may also administer local anesthetics transdermally using the techniques of iontophoresis and phonophoresis. Agents such as lidocaine can be administered through this method for the treatment of acute inflammation in bursitis, tendinitis, and so on.

Therapists may also be working with patients who are receiving local anesthetic injections for the treatment of RSDS. These patients often receive a series of anesthetic injections, so therapists may want to schedule the rehabilitation session immediately after each injection so that exercises and other rehabilitation techniques are performed while the anesthetic is still in effect. This strategy may help re-establish normal sympathetic function and blood flow to the affected extremity so that optimal results are obtained from the sympathetic blockade.

Finally, therapists may work with patients who are receiving central neural blockade in the form of an epidural or spinal injection. These procedures are common during natural and caesarean childbirth and in some other surgical procedures. Administration of local anesthetics into the spaces around the spinal cord may also be used to treat individuals with severe and chronic pain—that is, patients recovering from extensive surgery, patients who have cancer, or patients with other types of intractable pain. In these situations, therapists may notice that an indwelling catheter has been placed in the patient's epidural or subarachnoid space to allow repeated or sustained administration of the spinal anesthesia.

In situations where central neural blockade is used, therapists should be especially aware that sensation may be diminished below the level of epidural or spinal administration. Decreased sensation to thermal agents and electrical stimulation can occur when the central block is in effect.[2] Likewise, motor function may be affected in the lower extremities when local anesthetics are administered spinally or epidurally.[7] Hence, therapists should test sensation and motor strength before applying any physical agents or attempting ambulation with patients who have received some type of central neural blockade using a local anesthetic.

CASE STUDY

LOCAL ANESTHETICS

Brief History. R.D. is a 35-year-old man who developed pain in his right shoulder after spending the weekend chopping firewood. He was examined by a physical therapist and evaluated as having supraspinatus tendinitis. Apparently this tendinitis recurred intermittently, usually after extensive use of the right shoulder. During past episodes, the tendinitis was resistant to treatment and usually took several months to resolve.

Decision/Solution. The therapist began an aggressive rehabilitation program consisting of daily heat, ultrasound, soft-tissue massage, and exercise. Soft-tissue massage consisted of transverse-friction techniques applied to the supraspinatus tendon. In order to improve the patient's tolerance to this technique, 5 percent lidocaine (Xylocaine) ointment was administered via phonophoresis during the ultrasound treatment. This approach allowed both the massage technique and subsequent exercises to be performed more aggressively by the therapist and patient, respectively. Under this regimen, the supraspinatus tendinitis was resolved and the patient had full, pain-free use of the right shoulder within 3 weeks.

SUMMARY

Local anesthetics are frequently used when a limited, well-defined area of anesthesia is required, as is the case for most minor surgical procedures. Depending on the method of administration, local anesthetics can be used to temporarily block transmission in the area of peripheral nerve endings, along the trunk of a single peripheral nerve, along several peripheral nerves or plexuses, or at the level of the spinal cord. Local anesthetics may also be used to block efferent sympathetic activity. Although the exact way in which these drugs block transmission is unclear, they appear to bind to receptors associated with membrane sodium channels and to prevent the channels from opening during neuronal excitation. Physical therapists may frequently encounter the use of these agents in their patients for both short-term and long-term control of pain, as well as in the management of sympathetic hyperactivity.

REFERENCES

1. Batra, MS: Adjuvants in epidural and spinal anesthesia. Anesthesiol Clin North Am 10:13, 1992.
2. Brennum, J, et al: Quantitative sensory examination in human epidural anaesthesia and analgesia: Effects of lidocaine. Pain 51:27, 1992.

3. Buckley, MM and Benfield, P: Eutectic lidocaine/prilocaine cream: A review of the topical anaesthetic analgesic efficacy of a eutectic mixture of local anaesthetics (EMLA). Drugs 46:126, 1993.
4. Buist, RJ: A survey of the practice of regional anesthesia. J R Soc Med 83:709, 1990.
5. Cahalan, M, Shapiro, BI, and Almers, W: Relationship between inactivation of sodium channels and block by quaternary derivatives of local anesthetics and other compounds. In Fink, BR (ed): Progress in Anesthesiology, Vol 2, Molecular Mechanisms of Anesthesia. Raven Press, New York, 1980.
6. Ciccone, CD: Iontophoresis. In Robinson, AJ and Snyder-Mackler, L (eds): Clinical Electrophysiology, ed 2. Williams & Wilkins, Baltimore, 1994.
7. Cohen, S, et al: Adverse effects of epidural 0.03 percent bupivacaine during analgesia after cesarean section. Anesth Analg 75:753, 1992.
8. Franz, DN and Perry, RS: Mechanisms for differential nerve block among similar myelinated and non-myelinated axons by procaine. J Physiol 236:193, 1974.
9. Gado, K and Emery, P: Modified suprascapular nerve block with bupivacaine alone effectively controls chronic shoulder pain in patients with rheumatoid arthritis. Ann Rheum Dis 52:215, 1993.
10. Garfield, JM and Gugino, L: Central effects of local anesthetic agents. In Strichartz, GR (ed): Handbook of Experimental Pharmacology, Vol 81, Local Anesthetics. Springer-Verlag, New York, 1987.
11. Gasser, HS and Erlanger, J: Role of fiber size in the establishment of nerve block by pressure or cocaine. Am J Physiol 88:581, 1929.
12. Gissen, AJ, Covino, BG, and Gregus, J: Differential sensitivities of mammalian nerve fibers to local anesthetic agents. Anesthesiology 53:467, 1980.
13. Grima, M, et al: ^{3}H-tetracaine binding on rat synaptosomes and sodium channels. Br J Pharmacol 86:125, 1985.
14. Hansson, C, et al: Repeated treatment with lidocaine prilocaine cream (EMLA) as a topical anaesthetic for the cleansing of venous leg ulcers: A controlled study. Acta Derm Venereol 73:231, 1993.
15. Hille, B: Theories of anesthesia: General perturbations versus specific receptors. In Fink, BR (ed): Progress in Anesthesia, Vol 2, Molecular Mechanisms of Anesthesia. Raven Press, New York, 1980.
16. Hille, B: Local anesthetics: Hydrophilic and hydrophobic pathways for the drug-receptor reaction. J Gen Physiol 69:497, 1977.
17. Inoue, R, et al: Plasma concentrations of lidocaine and its principle metabolites during intermittent epidural anesthesia. Anesthesiology 63:304, 1985.
18. Koren, G: Use of the eutectic mixture of local anesthetics in young children for procedure-related pain. J Pediatr 122(suppl 5, part 2):S30, 1993.
19. Lycka, BAS: EMLA: A new and effective topical anesthetic. J Derm Surg Oncol 18:859, 1992.
20. Nathan, PW and Sears, TA: Some factors concerned in differential nerve block by local anesthetics. J Physiol 157:565, 1961.
21. Owenfalkenberg, A and Olsen, KS: Continuous stellate ganglion blockade for reflex sympathetic dystrophy. Anesth Analg 75:1041, 1992.
22. Raymond, SA and Gissen, AJ: Mechanisms of differential nerve block. In Strichartz, GR (ed): Handbook of Experimental Pharmacology, Vol 81, Local Anesthetics. Springer-Verlag, New York, 1987.
23. Ritchie, JM and Greene, NM: Local anesthetics. In Gilman AG, et al (eds): The Pharmacological Basis of Therapeutics, ed 8. Pergamon Press, New York, 1990.
24. Sabbahi, MA and De Luca, CJ: Topical anesthetic–induced improvements in the mobility of patients with muscular hypertonicity: Preliminary results. J Electromyogr Kinesiol 1:41, 1991.
25. Scott, DB: Toxicity caused by local anesthetic drugs. Br J Anaesth 53:553, 1981.
26. Strichartz, GR and Covino, BG: Local anesthetics. In Miller, RD (ed): Anesthesia, Vol 1, ed 3. Churchill Livingstone, New York, 1990.
27. Strichartz, GR and Ritchie, JM: The action of local anesthetics on ion channels in excitable tissues. In Strichartz, GR (ed): Handbook of Experimental Pharmacology, Vol 81, Local Anesthetics. Springer-Verlag, New York, 1987.
28. Tachibana, K and Tachibana, S: Use of ultrasound to enhance the local anesthetic effect of topically applied aqueous lidocaine. Anesthesiology 78:1091, 1993.
29. Van Wyngarden, TM and Bleyaert, AL: Reflex sympathetic dystrophy: Objective clinical signs in diagnosis and treatment. J Am Podiatr Assoc 81:580, 1991.
30. Weatherstone, KB, et al: Safety and efficacy of topical anesthetic for neonate circumcision. Pediatrics 92:710, 1993.
31. Wildsmith, JAW: Peripheral nerve and local anesthetic drugs. Br J Anaesth 58:692, 1986.
32. Writer, D: Epidural anesthesia for labor. Anesthesiol Clin North Am 10:59, 1992.

SECTION III

Drugs Affecting Skeletal Muscle

CHAPTER 13

Skeletal Muscle Relaxants

Skeletal muscle relaxants are used to treat conditions associated with hypertonic skeletal muscle—specifically, spasticity and muscle spasms. Although these two terms are often used interchangeably, spasticity and muscle spasms represent two distinct abnormalities. The use of relaxant drugs, however, is similar in each condition because the ultimate goal is a decrease in muscle hypertonicity without a profound decrease in muscle function. Considering the number of rehabilitation patients with muscle hypertonicity caused by either spasm or spasticity, skeletal muscle relaxants represent an important class of drugs to the rehabilitation specialist.

Drugs discussed in this chapter are used to decrease muscle excitability and contraction via an effect at the spinal cord level (centrally acting relaxants) or on the muscle cell itself (direct-acting relaxants). Some texts also classify neuromuscular junction blockers such as curare and succinylcholine as skeletal muscle relaxants. These drugs are more appropriately classified as skeletal muscle *paralytics* because they eliminate muscle contraction by blocking transmission at the myoneural synapse. This type of skeletal muscle paralysis is used primarily during general anesthesia; using neuromuscular blockers as an adjunct in surgery was discussed in Chapter 11. Skeletal muscle relaxants do not prevent muscle contraction; they only attempt to normalize muscle excitability to decrease pain and improve motor function.

INCREASED MUSCLE TONE: SPASTICITY VERSUS MUSCLE SPASMS

Much confusion and consternation often arise from the erroneous use of the terms "spasticity" and "spasm." These terms represent different types of increased tone, which result from different underlying pathologies. *Spasticity* is characterized primarily by an exaggerated muscle stretch reflex (Fig. 13–1).[7,11,14] This abnormal reflex activity is velocity-dependent, with a rapid lengthening of the muscle invoking a strong contraction in the stretched muscle. The neurophysiologic mechanisms underlying spasticity are complex, but this phenomenon occurs when supraspinal inhibition or control is lost because of some lesion in the spinal cord or brain.[5,15] Presumably, specific upper motor neuron lesions interrupt the cortical control of stretch reflex and al-

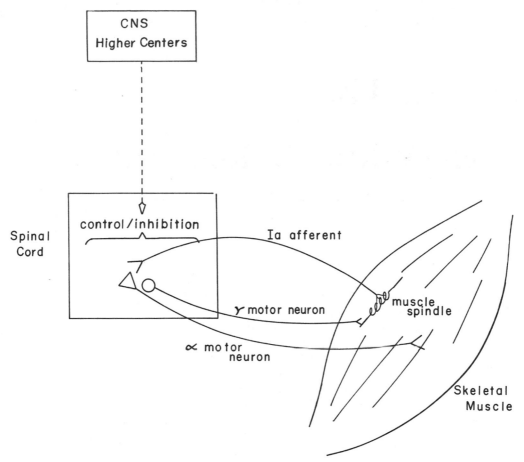

FIGURE 13–1. Schematic illustration of the basic components of the stretch reflex. Normally, higher CNS centers control the sensitivity of this reflex by inhibiting synaptic connections within the spinal cord. Spasticity is thought to occur when this higher center influence is lost because of cerebral trauma or damage to descending pathways in the spinal cord.

pha motor neuron excitability. Spasticity, therefore, is not in itself a disease but rather the motor sequela to such pathologies as cerebral vascular accident (CVA), cerebral palsy, multiple sclerosis (MS), and traumatic lesions to the brain and spinal cord (including quadriplegia and paraplegia).

Skeletal muscle *spasms* are used to describe the increased tension often seen in skeletal muscle after certain musculoskeletal injuries and inflammation (muscle strains, nerve root impingements, etc.).[3,28] This tension is involuntary, so the patient is unable to relax the muscle. Spasms are different from spasticity because spasms involve the afferent nociceptive input from the damaged tissue, which excites the outflow of alpha motor neuron to the muscle. This results in a tonic contraction of the affected muscle, which is quite painful because of the buildup of pain-mediating metabolites (e.g., lactate). In effect, a vicious cycle is created, with the increased pain caused by the spasm causing more nociceptive input, which further excites the alpha motor neuron to cause more spasms, and so on.[28]

Consequently, various skeletal muscle relaxants attempt to decrease skeletal muscle excitation and contraction in cases of spasticity and spasm. Specific drugs and their mechanisms of action are discussed here.

SPECIFIC AGENTS USED TO PRODUCE SKELETAL MUSCLE RELAXATION

Skeletal muscle relaxants can be divided into two general categories: centrally acting and direct-acting agents (Table 13–1). Centrally acting drugs exert their primary effects by decreasing excitation of the alpha motor neuron within the spinal cord. Direct-acting drugs affect the skeletal muscle cell itself.

CENTRALLY ACTING AGENTS

Baclofen

The chemical name of baclofen is beta-(p-chlorophenyl)-GABA. As this name suggests, baclofen is a derivative of the central inhibitory neurotransmitter gamma-aminobutyric acid (GABA). There appear to be some differences between baclofen and GABA. Baclofen seems to bind only to certain GABA receptors, which have been classified as $GABA_b$ receptors (as opposed to $GABA_a$ receptors).[1,22] Preferential binding to $GABA_b$ receptors enables baclofen to act as a GABA agonist in that it inhibits transmission within the spinal cord at specific synapses.[4,10,24] To put this in the context of its use as a muscle relaxant, baclofen appears to have an inhibitory effect on alpha motor neuron activity within the spinal cord. Whether this inhibition is by an effect on the alpha motor neuron itself (postsynaptic inhibition), through inhibition of other excitatory neurons that synapse with the alpha motor neuron (presynaptic inhibition), or through a combination of presynaptic and postsynaptic inhibition is unclear.[33] In any event, the re-

TABLE 13–1 Skeletal Muscle Relaxants

Generic Name	Trade Name	Clinical Use	
		Spasticity	Muscle Spasms
Centrally Acting Relaxants			
Baclofen	Lioresal	X	
Carisoprodol	Soma, Rela, others		X
Chlorphenesin carbamate	Maolate		X
Chlorzoxazone	Parafon Forte, Paraflex		X
Cyclobenzaprine hydrochloride	Flexeril		X
Diazepam	Valium	X	X
Metaxalone	Skelaxin		X
Methocarbamol	Robaxin, Robomol, others		X
Orphenadrine	Norflex, Norgesic, others		X
Direct-Acting Relaxants			
Dantrolene sodium	Dantrium	X	

sult is decreased firing of the alpha motor neuron, with a subsequent relaxation of the skeletal muscle.

Uses. Baclofen is used to treat spasticity associated with lesions of the spinal cord including traumatic injuries resulting in paraplegia or quadriplegia and spinal cord demyelination resulting in MS.[4] Baclofen appears to be particularly useful in reducing muscle spasticity associated with MS, and 80 percent of patients with MS probably benefit from baclofen therapy.[2] There is also a remarkable lack of adverse side effects when this drug is used in patients with MS.[9] Baclofen does not produce as much generalized muscle weakness as direct-acting relaxants such as dantrolene, which can be a major advantage of baclofen treatment in many patients with MS.[20] Baclofen appears to produce few side effects when used appropriately to reduce spasticity secondary to traumatic spinal cord lesions, thus providing a relatively safe and effective form of treatment.[33] Baclofen is less effective in treating spasticity associated with supraspinal lesions (stroke, cerebral palsy), because these patients are more prone to the adverse side effects of this drug.

Adverse Effects. When initiating baclofen therapy, the most common side effect is transient drowsiness, which usually disappears within a few days. When given to patients with spinal cord lesions, there are usually few other adverse effects. When given to patients who have had a CVA or to elderly individuals, there is sometimes a problem with confusion and hallucinations. Other side effects, occurring on an individual basis, include fatigue, nausea, dizziness, muscle weakness, and headache.

Intrathecal Baclofen

Baclofen is administered orally in most patients (Table 13–2). Baclofen can, however, be administered intrathecally in patients with severe, intractable spasticity. In-

TABLE 13–2 Antispasticity Drugs

Drug	Oral Dosage	Comments
Baclofen (Lioresal)	*Adult*: 5 mg TID initially; increase by 15 mg/day at 3-day intervals as required; maximum recommended dosage is 80 mg/day.	More effective in treating spasticity resulting from spinal cord lesions (versus cerebral lesions).
Dantrolene sodium (Dantrium)	*Adult*: 25 mg/day initially; increase up to 100 mg 2, 3, 4 times per day as needed; maximum recommended dose is 400 mg/day. *Children* (older than 5 yr of age): initially, 0.5 mg/kg body weight BID; increase total daily dosage by 0.5 mg/kg every 4–7 days as needed, and give total daily amount in 4 divided doses; maximum recommended dose in 400 mg/day.	Exerts an effect directly on the muscle cell; may cause generalized weakness in all skeletal musculature.
Diazepam (Valium)	*Adult*: 2–10 mg TID or QID. *Children* (older than 6 mo of age): 1.0–2.5 mg TID or QID (in both adults and children, begin at lower end of dosage range and increase gradually as tolerated and/or needed).	Produces sedation at dosages that decrease spasticity.

trathecal administration is the delivery of a drug directly into the subarachnoid space surrounding a specific level of the spinal cord. This places the drug very close to the spinal cord, thus allowing increased drug effectiveness with much smaller doses of the drug. Likewise, fewer systemic side effects occur because the drug tends to remain in the area of the cord rather than circulating in the bloodstream and causing adverse effects on other tissues.

When baclofen is administered intrathecally for the long-term treatment of spasticity, a small catheter is usually implanted surgically so that the open end of the catheter is located in the subarachnoid space and the other end of the catheter is attached to some type of programmable pump. The pump is implanted subcutaneously in the abdominal wall and is adjusted to deliver the drug at a slow, continuous rate. The rate of infusion is titrated over time to achieve the best clinical reduction in spasticity.

Intrathecal baclofen delivery using implantable pumps has been used in a variety of patients with spasticity of spinal origin. Studies involving these patients have typically noted a substantial decrease in rigidity with an increase in ability to perform functional activities including activities of daily living.[6,19,25] Muscle function also increased in some patients where voluntary motor control was being masked by hypertonicity.[16,18,25]

Despite these benefits, intrathecal baclofen is associated with a number of potential complications. Primary among these is the possibility of a disruption in the delivery system; that is, a pump malfunction or a displacement or blocking of the delivery catheter can occur. Such disruptions could cause overdose if too much drug is delivered or withdrawal if the drug is suddenly stopped.[19,25] A second major concern is the possibility that tolerance could develop with long-term, continuous baclofen administration. Tolerance is the need for more drug to achieve a beneficial effect when the drug is used for prolonged periods. Several studies have reported that doses must indeed be increased progressively when intrathecal baclofen systems are used for periods of several months to several years.[6,19,25] However, at the present time, it is not clear whether tolerance will develop to such an extent that intrathecal baclofen will become ineffective.

Hence, intrathecal baclofen offers a means of treating certain patients with severe spasticity who have not responded to more conventional means of treatment including oral baclofen. Additional research will help determine if intrathecal baclofen can be used safely for prolonged periods in a wider variety of patients. Further improvements in the technologic and mechanical aspects of intrathecal delivery, including better pumps and catheter systems, will also make this a safer and more practical method of treating these patients.

Diazepam

The effect of diazepam (Valium) on the CNS and its use as an antianxiety drug are discussed in Chapter 6. Basically, diazepam and other benzodiazepines work by increasing the central inhibitory effects of GABA; that is, diazepam binds to receptors located at GABA-ergic synapses and increases the GABA-induced inhibition at that synapse. Diazepam appears to work as a muscle relaxant through this mechanism, potentiating the inhibitory effect of GABA on alpha motor neuron activity in the spinal cord.[17,33] Diazepam also exerts some supraspinal sedative effects; in fact, some of its muscle relaxant properties may derive from the drug's ability to produce a more generalized state of sedation.[8,20,23]

Uses. Diazepam is used in patients with spasticity resulting from cord lesions and is sometimes effective in patients with cerebral palsy. Diazepam has also seen extensive use in treating muscle spasms associated with musculoskeletal injuries such as acute low-back strains.

Adverse Effects. The primary problem with diazepam is that dosages successful in relaxing skeletal muscle also produce sedation.[17,20] This effect may not be a problem and may actually be advantageous for the patient recovering from an acute musculoskeletal injury. However, the patient with spasticity who does not want a decrease in mental alertness will not tolerate diazepam therapy as well. Extended use of diazepam has also been associated with tolerance and physical dependence, limiting its use in the long-term treatment of spasticity.

Other Central Relaxants

A variety of other compounds have been used in an attempt to enhance muscle relaxation (see Table 13–1). Some examples are carisoprodol (Soma, Rela), chlorphenesin carbamate (Maolate), chlorzoxazone (Parafon Forte, Paraflex), cyclobenzaprine hydrochloride (Flexeril), metaxalone (Skelaxin), methocarbamol (Robaxin, Robomol), and orphenadrine (Norflex, Norgesic). The mechanism of action of these drugs is not well defined. Research in animals has suggested that some of these drugs may decrease polysynaptic reflex activity in the spinal cord, leading to a selective decrease in the excitation of the alpha motor neuron. However, these compounds all have some general depressant activity on the CNS, and the consensus is that any muscle relaxant effect of these drugs stems from their ability to produce a general state of sedation.[8] The ability of these compounds to selectively relax skeletal muscle in humans has not been demonstrated conclusively.

Hence, the muscle relaxant properties of these other central relaxants may simply be because of their more general sedative effects.[4] This observation is not to say that they are ineffective, since clinical research has shown these drugs to be superior to a placebo in producing subjective muscle relaxation.[8] However, the specific ability of these drugs to relax skeletal muscle remains doubtful, and it is generally believed that their muscle relaxant properties are secondary to a nonspecific CNS sedation.

Uses. These drugs are typically used "as adjuncts to other measures, such as rest and physical therapy, for the relief of muscle spasms associated with acute, painful musculoskeletal conditions."[29] When used to treat spasms, these compounds are sometimes incorporated into the same tablet with an analgesic such as acetaminophen or aspirin. For instance, Parafon Forte is the trade name for chlorzoxazone combined with acetaminophen, and Norgesic is orphenadrine combined with aspirin (and caffeine). Such combinations have been reported to be more effective than the individual components given separately.[8] These drugs are not effective in the treatment of spasticity.

Adverse Effects. Because of their sedative properties, the primary side effects of these drugs are drowsiness and dizziness. A variety of additional adverse effects, including nausea, light-headedness, vertigo, ataxia, and headache, may occur depending on the patient and the specific drug administered.

DIRECT-ACTING RELAXANTS

Dantrolene Sodium

The only available muscle relaxant that exerts its effect directly on the skeletal muscle cell is dantrolene sodium (Dantrium). This drug works by impairing the release of calcium from the sarcoplasmic reticulum within the muscle cell during excitation (Fig. 13–2).[7,30,33] In response to an action potential, the release of calcium from sarcoplasmic storage sites initiates myofilament cross-bridging and subsequent muscle contraction. By inhibiting this release, dantrolene attenuates muscle contraction and therefore enhances relaxation.

Uses. Dantrolene is effective in treating severe spasticity, regardless of the underlying pathology.[21,33] Patients with traumatic cord lesions, advanced MS, cerebral palsy, or CVAs will probably experience a reduction in spasticity with this drug. Dantrolene is not prescribed to treat muscle spasms caused by musculoskeletal injury.

Adverse Effects. The most common side effect of dantrolene is generalized muscle weakness; this makes sense considering that dantrolene impairs sarcoplasmic calcium release in skeletal muscles throughout the body, not just in the hypertonic tissues. Thus, the use of dantrolene is sometimes counterproductive because the increased motor function that occurs when spasticity is reduced may be offset by the generalized motor weakness.[4] This drug may also cause severe hepatotoxicity, and cases of fatal hepatitis have been reported.[4] The risk of toxic effects on the liver seems to be greater in women, in patients older than 35 years of age, and in individuals receiving drugs such as estrogen.[33] Other, less serious side effects that sometimes occur during the first few days of dantrolene therapy include drowsiness, dizziness, nausea, and diarrhea, but these problems are usually transient.

FIGURE 13–2. Possible mechanism of action of dantrolene sodium (Dantrium). Dantrolene blocks channels in the sarcoplasmic reticulum, thus interfering with calcium release onto the contractile (actin, myosin) filaments. Muscle contraction is reduced because less calcium is available to initiate cross-bridge formation between actin and myosin filaments.

OTHER MUSCLE RELAXANTS

Botulinum Toxin

Injection of botulinum toxin (Botox) is a relatively new method of treating conditions such as spasmodic torticollis, blepharospasm, laryngeal dystonia, strabismus, and several other types of focal dystonias.[12,13,26,27] Botulinum toxin binds strongly to presynaptic acetylcholine vesicles at the skeletal neuromuscular junction and disrupts synaptic activity by preventing these vesicles from releasing acetylcholine into the synaptic cleft.[13] When used therapeutically, small amounts of this toxin are injected directly into the muscles responsible for producing the dystonia, and relaxation of these muscles typically occurs within a few days to 1 week. This technique appears to be fairly safe and effective in many patients, but relief may only be temporary. Symptoms often return 2 to 3 months after each injection, necessitating additional treatments.[13,27] Still, this technique represents a method of treating patients with severe, incapacitating conditions marked by focal dystonias and spasms.

Transdermal Clonidine

Clonidine is classified as an alpha-2 adrenergic agonist, meaning that this drug binds selectively to the alpha-2 receptors in the CNS and stimulates these receptors. This drug is typically used as an antihypertensive agent because it can decrease sympathetic nervous system activity in the brainstem (see Chapter 21). Preliminary reports further indicate that clonidine may also be useful in reducing the spasticity that occurs following spinal cord injury.[31,32] When used to treat spasticity, clonidine can be administered transdermally by applying patches that are impregnated with this drug. These patches adhere to the surface of the skin and allow a slow, continuous infusion of the drug through the skin and into the bloodstream. This provides an effective way of delivering the drug so that the plasma concentration of the drug is maintained at a fairly constant level for an indefinite period of time.

Exactly why clonidine is effective in decreasing spasticity is not clear. Transdermal administration of this drug may, however, reduce or eliminate the patient's needs for other antispasticity drugs such as oral baclofen.[31,32] Hence, treatment of patients with spasticity using transdermal clonidine is still fairly experimental at present, but this procedure may become more common if clinical research continues to document the benefits of this technique.

PHARMACOKINETICS

These drugs are all absorbed fairly easily from the gastrointestinal tract, and the oral route is the most frequent method of drug administration. In cases of severe spasms, certain drugs such as methocarbamol and orphenadrine can be injected intramuscularly or intravenously to permit a more rapid effect. Likewise, diazepam and dantrolene can be injected to treat spasticity if the situation warrants a faster onset. As discussed earlier, continuous intrathecal baclofen administration may be used in certain patients with severe spasticity. Metabolism of muscle relaxants is usually accomplished by hepatic microsomal enzymes, and excretion of the metabolite or the intact drug is through the kidneys.

TREATMENT OF SPASTICITY

The pharmacologic reduction of spasticity is often beneficial because of increased motor function, easier self-care or nursing care, and decreased painful and harmful effects of strong spastic contractions. Drug treatment of spasticity, however, is often a trade-off. The beneficial effects of decreased muscle excitability are balanced against the side effects of the drugs used. Depending on the drug in question, problems with sedation, generalized muscle weakness, and hepatotoxicity can negate any beneficial effects from a reduction in muscle tone. Also, reducing spasticity may adversely affect the individual who has come to rely on increased muscle tone to assist in functional activities such as ambulation. Patients who have had a CVA and who use increased extensor tone in the lower extremity to support themselves when walking may begin to have episodes of falling if this muscle tone is reduced by drugs. Consequently, the ultimate goal is to find an appropriate antispasticity drug that provides optimal muscle relaxant effects with a minimum of adverse side effects or functional deficits.

The three primary agents used in the treatment of spasticity are baclofen, diazepam, and dantrolene sodium (see Table 13–2; Fig. 13–3). Baclofen is generally the drug of choice in patients with lesions in the spinal cord rather than the brain. When baclofen is given to these patients, there is usually a decrease in spasticity with a minimum of sedation and generalized muscle weakness. Diazepam appears to be as effective as baclofen in reducing spasticity in spinal as well as supraspinal lesions, but the use of diazepam is limited in many situations because of its sedative effects. Dantrolene sodium is usually very effective in reducing the spasticity that results from spinal or cerebral lesions, but this drug often produces a generalized muscle weakness. Dantrolene is best reserved for patients who will benefit from a reduction in spasticity without suffering from a decrease in voluntary muscle power (e.g., the patient with advanced MS or severe cerebral palsy). Also, because of the risk of hepatotoxicity, dantrolene should be used cautiously when administered for prolonged periods or in high doses.

TREATMENT OF MUSCLE SPASMS

The treatment of muscle spasms following musculoskeletal trauma often involves several types of pharmacologic agents as well as other therapeutic modalities. Skeletal muscle relaxants are sometimes added to opioid and nonopioid analgesics in an at-

FIGURE 13–3. Structure of three primary antispasticity drugs.

tempt to provide optimum pain relief. However, all skeletal relaxants used in this capacity have sedative properties, and their muscle relaxant effects may simply be secondary to their ability to sedate the patient. Still, this side effect may actually be helpful during the acute phase of an injury when it is desirable for the patient to rest or remain in bed. Of course, the long-term use of sedative-like drugs as muscle relaxants is not practical, and this fact emphasizes the need to use all available measures to interrupt the pain-spasm cycle so that these drugs can be discontinued as soon as possible.

Diazepam and the diverse group of centrally acting agents discussed previously (carisoprodol, chlorphenesin carbamate, others) have all been used to treat muscle spasms (Table 13–3). No drug appears to be significantly better than another in reducing spasms, and the choice of a specific agent is usually left to the preference and experience of the prescribing physician.

SPECIAL CONCERNS IN REHABILITATION PATIENTS

Because of the very nature of their use, skeletal muscle relaxants are prescribed for many patients involved in rehabilitation programs. Physical therapists and other rehabilitation professionals will encounter these drugs applied as both antispasticity and antispasm agents. When used for either purpose, these drugs can be valuable adjuncts to the therapeutic regimen. When used to reduce spasms following nerve root impingements, muscle strains, and the like, these drugs will complement the thermal, electrotherapeutic, and manual techniques used by the therapist. By reducing muscle tone in spasticity, these drugs will allow more effective passive range-of-motion and stretching activities, as well as permit neuromuscular facilitation techniques to be performed more easily and effectively.

The primary interactions between the use of muscle relaxants and physical therapy treatments involve the side effects of these drugs. Sedation, which may occur to a variable degree with all skeletal muscle relaxants, must sometimes be accommodated in the rehabilitation program. If the patient needs to be awake and alert, treatments may have to be scheduled at a time of the day when the sedative effects are minimal. A potentially more troublesome effect, with regard to the antispasticity drugs, is the de-

TABLE 13–3 Drugs Used to Treat Skeletal Muscle Spasms

Drug	Usual Adult Oral Dosage (mg)	Onset of Action (min)	Duration of Action (hr)
Carisoprodol (Soma, Rela)	350 TID and bedtime	30	4–6
Chlorphenesin carbamate (Maolate)	400 QID	—	—
Chlorzoxazone (Paraflex)	250–750 TID or QID	Within 60	3–4
Cyclobenzaprine HCl (Flexeril)	10 TID	60	12–24
Diazepam (Valium)	2–10 TID or QID	15–45	Variable
Metaxalone (Skelaxin)	800 TID or QID	60	4–6
Methocarbamol (Robaxin, Robomol)	1000 QID	Within 30	24
Orphenadrine (Norflex, Norgesic)	100 BID	Within 60	8

crease in muscle tone and general muscle weakness that sometimes occur. As described earlier, a decrease in spasticity may actually produce a functional deficit in the patient who uses increased muscle tone for support during ambulation. This loss of support from the hypertonic muscles will hopefully be replaced by a more normal form of motor function. The physical therapist may play a vital role in facilitating the substitution of normal physiologic motor control for the previously used spastic tone. For instance, patients who receive intrathecal baclofen through programmable pump systems often require a period of intensive rehabilitation to enable the patient to benefit from the decreased spasticity and increased voluntary motor function that can occur when this form of drug therapy is initiated.[19]

In cases when the muscle weakness is more general in nature (i.e., during the use of dantrolene sodium), there is often little the physical therapist can do to resolve this problem. For instance, the patient with paraplegia who requires adequate upper-extremity strength to perform transfers, wheelchair mobility, and ambulation with crutches and braces may find his or her ability to perform these activities compromised by the antispasticity drug. The role of the therapist in this situation may simply be to advise the patient that voluntary muscular power is limited and that some upper-extremity strength deficits can be expected. The therapist may also work closely with the physician in trying to find the minimum acceptable dose for that patient or in attempting to find a better drug (e.g., switching from dantrolene to baclofen).

CASE STUDY

MUSCLE RELAXANTS

Brief History. F.D. is a 28-year-old man who sustained complete paraplegia below the L-2 spinal level during an automobile accident. Through the course of rehabilitation, he was becoming independent in self-care, and he had begun to ambulate in the parallel bars and with crutches while wearing temporary long leg braces. He was highly motivated to continue this progress and was eventually fitted with permanent leg orthoses. During this period, spasticity had increased in his lower extremities to the point where dressing and self-care were often difficult. Also, the ability of the patient to put his leg braces on was often compromised by the lower-extremity spasticity. The patient was started on dantrolene (Dantrium) at an initial oral dosage of 25 mg/day. The daily dosage of dantrolene was gradually increased until he was receiving 400 mg/day.

Problem/Influence of Medication. Although the dantrolene was effective in controlling his spasticity, F.D. began to notice weakness in his arms and upper torso when he attempted to ambulate and transfer. This decrease in voluntary power in his upper extremities was caused by the generalized muscle weakness sometimes seen when this drug is used.

Decision/Solution. The therapist conferred with the patient's physician, and the decreased voluntary muscle power was noted. As an alternative, the patient was switched to baclofen (Lioresal). The dosage was adjusted until the spasticity was adequately reduced, and no further problems were noted.

SUMMARY

Skeletal muscle relaxants are used to treat the spasticity that occurs following lesions in the CNS and muscle spasms that result from musculoskeletal injuries. These drugs are classified as centrally acting if they exert their effects primarily on the spinal cord, or as direct-acting if their action is on the skeletal muscle fiber. The primary agents used in treating spasticity are baclofen, diazepam, and dantrolene. Each drug works by a somewhat different mechanism, and the selection of a specific antispasticity agent depends on the patient and the underlying CNS lesion (e.g., stroke, MS, and so on). Diazepam and a variety of other sedativelike drugs are used in the treatment of muscle spasms, but their effectiveness as muscle relaxants may be because of their nonspecific sedative properties. Physical therapists and other rehabilitation personnel will frequently work with patients taking these drugs for the treatment of either spasticity or spasms. Although there are some side effects that may be troublesome, these drugs generally facilitate the rehabilitation program by directly providing benefits (muscle relaxation) that are congruent with the major rehabilitation goals.

REFERENCES

1. Bowery, NG, Hill, DR, and Hudson, AL: Characteristics of $GABA_b$ receptor binding sites on rat whole brain synaptic membranes. Br J Pharmacol 78:191, 1983.
2. Burks, JS: Multiple sclerosis. In Rakel, RE (ed): Conn's Current Therapy. WB Saunders, Philadelphia, 1993.
3. Calliet, R: Low Back Pain Syndrome, ed 4. FA Davis, Philadelphia, 1988.
4. Cedarbaum, JM and Schleifer, LS: Drugs for Parkinson's disease, spasticity, and acute muscle spasms. In Gilman, AG, et al (eds.): The Pharmacological Basis of Therapeutics. ed 8. Pergamon Press, New York, 1990.
5. Clemente, CD: Neurophysiological mechanisms and neuroanatomic substrates related to spasticity. Neurology 28:40, 1978.
6. Coffey, RJ, et al: Intrathecal baclofen for intractable spasticity of spinal origin: Results of a long-term multicenter study. J Neurosurg 78:226, 1993.
7. Davidoff, RA: Pharmacology of spasticity. Neurology 28:46, 1978.
8. Elenbaas, JK: Centrally acting oral skeletal muscle relaxants. Am J Hosp Pharm 37:1313, 1980.
9. Feldman, RG, et al: Baclofen for spasticity in multiple sclerosis: Double blind cross-over and three year study. Neurology 28:1094, 1978.
10. Fukuda, T, Kudo, Y, and Ono, H: Effects of beta-(p-chlorophenyl)-GABA (baclofen) on spinal synaptic activity. Eur J Pharmacol 44:17, 1977.
11. Gordon, J and Ghez, C: Muscle receptors and spinal reflexes: The stretch reflex. In Kandel, ER, Schwartz, JH, and Jessell, TM (eds): Principles of Neural Science, ed 3. Appleton & Lange, Norwalk, CT, 1991.
12. Greene, P, et al: Double-blind, placebo-controlled trial of botulinum toxin injections for the treatment of spasmodic torticollis. Neurology 40:1213, 1990.
13. Jankovic, J and Brin, MF: Therapeutic uses of botulinum toxin. N Engl J Med 324:1186, 1991.
14. Lance, JW: Symposium synopsis. In Feldman, RG, Young, RR, and Koella, WP (eds): Spasticity: Disordered Motor Control. Year Book, Chicago, 1980.
15. Lance, JW and Burke, D: Mechanisms of spasticity. Arch Phys Med Rehabil 55:332, 1974.
16. Latash, ML, et al: Effects of intrathecal baclofen on voluntary motor control in spastic paresis. J Neurosurg 72:388, 1990.
17. Lossius, R, Dietrichson, P, and Lunde, PKM: Effects of diazepam and desmethyl-diazepam in spasticity and rigidity: A quantitative study of reflexes and plasma concentrations. Acta Neurol Scand 61:378, 1980.
18. Meythaler, JM, et al: Intrathecal baclofen in hereditary spastic paraparesis. Arch Phys Med Rehabil 73:794, 1992.
19. Meythaler, JM, et al: Continuous intrathecal baclofen in spinal cord spasticity: A prospective study. Arch Phys Med Rehabil 71:321, 1990.
20. Miller, RD: Skeletal muscle relaxants. In Katzung, BG (ed): Basic and Clinical Pharmacology, ed 5. Appleton & Lange, Norwalk, CT, 1992.
21. Monster, AW: Spasticity and the effect of dantrolene sodium. Arch Phys Med Rehabil 55:373, 1974.
22. Newberry, NR and Nicoll, RA: Direct hyperpolarizing action of baclofen on hippocampal pyramidal cells. Nature 308:450, 1984.

23. Ollinger, H, Gruber, J, and Singer, F: Outcomes of electromyographic investigations with muscle relaxant drugs acting primarily at a supraspinal or spinal level: Considerations on assessment, reproducibility and clinical significance. EEG EMG 16:104, 1985.
24. Pedersen, E, Alien-Soborg, P, and Mai, J: The mode of action of the GABA derivative baclofen in human spasticity. Acta Neurol Scand 50:665, 1974.
25. Penn, RD and Kroin, JS: Long-term intrathecal baclofen infusion for treatment of spasticity. J Neurosurg 66:181, 1987.
26. Shaari, CM and Sanders, I: Quantifying how location and dose of botulinum toxin injections affect skeletal muscle. Muscle Nerve 16:964, 1993.
27. Stell, R, Thompson, PD, and Marsden, CD: Botulinum toxin in spasmodic torticollis. J Neurol Neurosurg Psychiatry 51:920, 1988.
28. Travell, JG and Simons, DG: Myofascial Pain and Dysfunction: The Trigger Point Method, Vol 2. Williams & Wilkins, Baltimore, 1992.
29. USP-DI: Drug Information for the Health Care Professional, Vol 1, ed 14. The United Stated Pharmacopeial Convention, Rockville, MD, 1994.
30. VanWinkle, WB: Calcium release from skeletal muscle sarcoplasmic reticulum: Site of action of dantrolene sodium? Science 193:1130, 1976.
31. Weingarden, SI and Belen, JG: Clonidine transdermal system for treatment of spasticity in spinal cord injury. Arch Phys Med Rehabil 73:876, 1992.
32. Yablon, SA and Sipski, ML: Effect of transdermal clonidine on spinal spasticity: A case series. Am J Phys Med Rehabil 72:154, 1993.
33. Young, RR and Delwaide, PJ: Drug therapy: Spasticity (parts 1 and 2). N Engl J Med 304:28, 96, 1981.

SECTION IV

Drugs Used to Treat Pain and Inflammation

CHAPTER 14

Opioid Analgesics

Analgesic drug therapy and certain physical therapy interventions share a common goal: pain relief. Consequently, these drugs are among the most frequently taken by patients being treated in a rehabilitation setting. The vast array of drugs that are used to treat pain can be roughly divided into two categories: opioid and nonopioid **analgesics**. Nonopioid analgesics are composed of drugs such as acetaminophen, aspirin, and similar agents. These drugs are discussed in Chapter 15. **Opioid** analgesics are a group of naturally occurring, semisynthetic, and synthetic agents that are characterized by their ability to relieve moderate-to-severe pain. These drugs exert their effects by binding to specific neuronal receptors that are located primarily in the CNS. Opioid analgesics are also characterized by their potential ability to produce physical dependence, and these agents are classified as controlled substances in the United States because of their potential for abuse (see Chapter 1 for a description of controlled substance classification). Morphine (Fig. 14–1) is considered the prototypical opioid analgesic, and other drugs of this type are often compared to morphine in terms of efficacy and potency.[31]

In the past, the term "narcotic" was often applied to these compounds because they tend to have sedative or sleep-inducing side effects and high doses can produce a state of unresponsiveness and stupor. Narcotic is a misleading name, however, because it describes a side effect of these agents rather than their principal therapeutic effect. Likewise, these drugs are sometimes referred to as "opiate" analgesics because some of these compounds are derived from opium (see the next section, "Source of Opioid Analgesics"). More recently, the term "opioid" has also been instituted to represent all types of narcotic analgesiclike agents, regardless of their origin.[20,54] Hence, most sources preferentially use the term "opioid" to describe these drugs, and clinicians should recognize that this term represents all of the morphinelike medications.

SOURCE OF OPIOID ANALGESICS

As mentioned previously, opioid analgesics can be obtained from natural, synthetic, or semisynthetic sources. Synthetic agents, as the designation implies, are simply formulated from basic chemical components in the laboratory. The source of the

Morphine

FIGURE 14–1. Structure of morphine.

naturally occurring and the semisynthetic narcotic analgesics is the opium poppy.[54] When the extract from the seeds of this flower is allowed to dry and harden, the resulting substance is opium. Opium contains about 20 biologically active compounds, including morphine and codeine. Other derivatives from opium can also directly produce analgesia in varying degrees or can serve as precursors for analgesic drugs. The most notable of these precursors is thebaine, which can be modified chemically to yield compounds such as heroin. Hence, the semisynthetic narcotic analgesics are derived from these precursors. Semisynthetic opioids can also be formulated by modifying one of the other naturally occurring narcotic drugs, such as morphine.

In addition to analgesic drugs and their precursors, opium also contains compounds that do not have any analgesic properties. These compounds can actually antagonize the analgesic effects of opioid agonists such as morphine. (As defined in Chapter 4, an *agonist* stimulates its respective receptor and exerts a physiologic response, whereas an *antagonist* blocks the receptor, thus preventing the response.) The role of these opioid antagonists is discussed in "Classification of Specific Agents."

ENDOGENOUS OPIOID PEPTIDES AND OPIOID RECEPTORS

Endogenous Opioids

Neurons at specific locations within the brain and spinal cord have been identified as having receptors that serve as binding sites for morphine and other similar exogenous substances. Exogenous opioids exert their effects by binding to these receptors; the proposed mechanisms of these drug-receptor interactions are discussed in "Mechanism of Action." The discovery of these opioid receptors also suggested the existence of an endogenous opioidlike substance. Rather than isolating one such compound, the search for an "endogenous morphine" has actually revealed several groups of peptides with analgesic and other pharmacologic properties. It is now recognized that three distinct families of endogenous opioids exist: the endorphins, enkephalins, and dynorphins.[20] These peptides are manufactured and released within the body to control pain under specific conditions.[2,4,5,51] This chapter is not intended to elucidate all the known details of the endogenous opioid peptide system or how these endogenous compounds can be influenced by opioid drugs. These endogenous compounds do exert their effects, however, via the same receptors as the exogenous opioid drugs. There is obviously the possibility for a great deal of interaction between the endogenous and exogenous opioids, and research continues to investigate how exogenous drugs influence the function of the endogenous peptides, and vice versa.[1,23]

Opioid Receptors

Since their discovery, the opioid receptors have been examined in considerable detail. Studies in animals have suggested that rather than one homogeneous opioid receptor, there are at least three primary subtypes known as mu, kappa, and delta receptors (Table 14–1).[7,14,27,45,53] A fourth subtype, the sigma receptor, is also included by some investigators, but the significance of this subtype is uncertain at the present time.[20] There may actually be more than these four classes of opioid receptors; furthermore, some of the primary classes may have subclassifications (e.g., there are believed to be two types of mu receptors, usually referred to as mu_1 and mu_2).[20,29,44] At the moment, we do not know if all of these subpopulations are present in humans, or if all are important in the response to exogenous opioids. However, some specialization regarding both the location and the response of specific types of opioid receptors does exist (see Table 14–1).

Subcategories of opioid receptors seem to have different affinities for different endogenous or exogenous compounds. Specific types of opioid receptors also seem to be concentrated at certain locations within the brain and spinal cord and may each be responsible for producing a specific effect when stimulated (see Table 14–1). For instance, the analgesic effects of opioids are mediated at the supraspinal and spinal levels by the mu and kappa receptors, respectively.[34,54,56] Other side effects of opioid drugs such as sedation, respiratory depression, and mood changes (either euphoria or dysphoria) have also been attributed to one or more receptor categories.

TABLE 14–1 Opioid Receptors

Receptor Subtype	Primary CNS Location	Primary Physiologic Response	Abuse Potential
Mu	Supraspinal areas of pain modulation (periaqueductal gray, medial thalamic nuclei, hypothalamus, limbic system)	Supraspinal analgesia, euphoria, respiratory depression	High
Kappa	Dorsal horn of spinal gray matter (substantia gelatinosa); deep layers of cerebral cortex	Spinal analgesia, sedation, depressed flexor reflexes	Low
Delta	Substantia nigra, globus pallidus, corpus striatum, other limbic structures	Euphoria, sedation	Low
Sigma	Hippocampus	Dysphoria, hallucinations, cardiovascular stimulation	Low

Research on opioid receptors has also revealed that certain receptor subtypes tend to be associated with the addictive properties of these drugs more than others. Stimulation of mu receptors in particular seems to cause dependence to a greater extent than other receptors.[34,54] This fact is important because drugs that selectively avoid or even antagonize these high-abuse receptors, but still provide sufficient analgesia through other receptor subtypes, will be less likely to provoke opioid abuse. Certain mixed agonist-antagonist opioids (see the next section, "Classification of Specific Agents") are currently available that can stimulate kappa receptors while avoiding or blocking the mu receptors. These drugs tend to have fewer addictive qualities than strong mu receptor agonists such as morphine.[21,31,32,34] Drug developers will hopefully capitalize on the existence of opioid receptor subtypes, and new agents will be produced that are even more specific in relieving pain without provoking a strong tendency for abuse, addiction, or other adverse side effects.

CLASSIFICATION OF SPECIFIC AGENTS

Opioid analgesics are classified as strong agonists, mild-to-moderate agonists, mixed agonist-antagonists, and antagonists according to their interaction with opioid receptors. Some opioids in these categories are listed in Table 14–2. The basic characteristics of each category and clinically relevant examples are also discussed here.

Strong Agonists. These agents are used to treat severe pain. As the name implies, these drugs have a high affinity for certain receptors and are believed to interact primarily with mu and kappa opioid receptors in the CNS. The best-known member of this group is morphine, and the other strong agonists are similar pharmacologically. Examples of strong opioid agonists include the following:

- fentanyl (Sublimaze)
- hydromorphone (Dilaudid)
- levorphanol (Levo-Dromoran)
- meperidine (Demerol, Pethadol)
- methadone (Dolophine, Methadose)
- morphine (Duramorph, Epimorph, Roxanol, Statex, others)
- oxymorphone (Numorphan)

Mild-to-Moderate Agonists. These drugs are still considered agonists that affect mu and kappa opioid receptors, but they do not have as high an affinity or efficacy as the drugs listed previously. These drugs are more effective in treating pain of moderate intensity. Examples include the following:

- codeine
- hydrocodone (Dicodid, Hycodan)
- oxycodone (Percodan, Supeudol)
- propoxyphene (Darvon, Dolene, Novopropoxyn, others)

Mixed Agonist-Antagonists. These drugs exhibit some agonist and antagonist-like activity at the same time because of the ability of the drug to act differently at specific subpopulations of opioid receptors (Table 14–3). For instance, drugs in this category typically bind to and activate kappa and sigma receptors but often act as

TABLE 14–2 Opioid Analgesics

Drug	Route of Administration*	Onset of Action (min)	Time to Peak Effect (min)	Duration of Action (hr)
Strong Agonists				
Fentanyl	IM	7–15	20–30	1–2
(Sublimaze)	IV	1–2	3–5	0.5–1
Hydromorphone	Oral	30	90–120	4
(Dilaudid)	IM	15	30–60	4
	IV	10–15	15–30	2–3
	Sub-Q	15	30–90	4
Levorphanol	Oral	10–60	90–120	4–5
(Levo-Dromoran)	IM	—	60	4–5
	IV	—	Within 20	4–5
	Sub-Q	—	60–90	4–5
Meperidine	Oral	15	60–90	2–4
(Demerol)	IM	10–15	30–50	2–4
	IV	1	5–7	2–4
	Sub-Q	10–15	30–50	2–4
Methadone	Oral	30–60	90–120	4–6
(Dolophine)	IM	10–20	60–120	4–5
	IV	—	15–30	3–4
Morphine	Oral	—	60–120	4–5
(many trade names)	IM	10–30	30–60	4–5
	IV	—	20	4–5
	Sub-Q	10–30	50–90	4–5
	Epidural	15–60	—	Up to 24
Oxymorphone	IM	10–15	30–90	3–6
(Numorphan)	IV	5–10	15–30	3–4
	Sub-Q	10–20	—	3–6
	Rectal	15–30	120	3–6
Mild-to-Moderate Agonists				
Codeine	Oral	30–40	60–120	4
(many trade names)	IM	10–30	30–60	4
	Sub-Q	10–30	—	4
Hydrocodone	Oral	10–30	30–60	4–6
(Hycodan)				
Oxycodone	Oral	—	60	3–4
(Percodan)				
Propoxyphene	Oral	15–60	120	4–6
(Darvon, Dolene)				
Mixed Agonist-Antagonist				
Butorphanol	IM	10–30	30–60	3–4
(Stadol)	IV	2–3	30	2–4
Nalbuphine	IM	Within 15	60	3–6
(Nubain)	IV	2–3	30	3–4
	Sub-Q	Within 15	—	3–6
Pentazocine	Oral	15–30	60–90	3
(Talwin)	IM	15–20	30–60	2–3
	IV	2–3	15–30	2–3
	Sub-Q	15–20	30–60	2–3

*IM = intramuscular; IV = intravenous; sub-Q = subcutaneous.

TABLE 14–3 Effects of Opioid Classes on Certain Receptor Subtypes

Classes	Receptor Types*		
	Mu	Kappa	Sigma
Opioid agonists (e.g., morphine)	ag	ag	—
Mixed agonist-antagonists			
Butorphanol	—	ag	ag
Nalbuphine	ant	ag	ag
Pentazocine	ant	ag	ag
Narcotic antagonists (e.g., naloxone)	ant	ant	ant

*ag = agonist; ant = antagonist; — = no significant effect.

antagonists at mu receptors. Mixed agonist-antagonist opioids appear to have the advantage of producing adequate analgesia with less risk of tolerance and dependence.[32,34,54] These drugs also tend to produce less respiratory depression, and they are safer in terms of a reduced risk of fatal overdose. Consequently, these drugs are gaining popularity, especially in situations requiring the extended use of opioid drugs. Examples include the following:

- butorphanol (Stadol)
- nalbuphine (Nubain)
- pentazocine (Talwin)

Antagonists. These drugs block all opioid receptors, with a particular affinity for the mu variety. Because of their antagonistic properties, these agents will not produce analgesia but will displace opioid agonists from the opioid receptors and block any further effects of the agonist molecules. Consequently, these drugs are used primarily in the treatment of opioid overdose and addiction. Certain opioid antagonists (e.g., naloxone) can rapidly (within 1 to 2 minutes) and dramatically reverse the respiratory depression that is usually the cause of death in excessive opioid ingestion. Other antagonists (e.g., naltrexone) are used in conjunction with behavioral therapy to maintain an opioid-free state in individuals recovering from opioid addiction. Hence, the primary agents used clinically as opioid antagonists are the following:

- naloxone (Narcan)
- naltrexone (Trexan)

PHARMACOKINETICS

Some opioid analgesics can be given orally, a preferred route of administration in terms of convenience and safety. Several of these enteral drugs also come in suppository form, permitting rectal administration if nausea and vomiting prohibit the oral route. Because of poor intestinal absorption or significant first-pass inactivation, other agents must be administered parenterally, usually through subcutaneous or intramuscular injection. Intravenous administration is also sometimes used but must be done slowly and with caution. When the intravenous route is used, the narcotic is frequently diluted, and infusion pumps are used to allow the slow, controlled administration of the drug. The intravenous route or other parenteral routes (epidural and intrathecal infusion) can also be used to administer opioids during patient-controlled analgesia; this concept is addressed in Chapter 17.

The feasibility of using other relatively new methods for administering opioids has also been investigated. For instance, the intranasal route may be a suitable means of administering fentanyl, a potent and fast-acting opioid.[49,50] Other agents including morphine can be given through the transdermal route by using skin patches or iontophoresis techniques.[3] It will be interesting to see if these newer methods of administration will gain widespread acceptance in the future.

Because of different degrees of solubility, the distribution and subsequent onset of action of specific agents vary (see Table 14–2). Opioids are ultimately distributed throughout all tissues, and these agents probably exert their principal analgesic effects after they reach the CNS. Some opioid effects may also be mediated by peripheral receptors located at the site of painful inflammation (see "Mechanism of Action"). Metabolic inactivation of these drugs takes place primarily in the liver, although some degree of metabolism also occurs in other tissues such as kidneys, lungs, and CNS. The kidneys excrete the drug metabolite and, to a lesser extent, the intact drug in the urine.

MECHANISM OF ACTION

Effect of Narcotic Analgesics on the Spinal Cord

As discussed earlier, opioid receptors exist at specific locations throughout the CNS and possibly in peripheral nerve tissues as well. In the spinal cord, these receptors are concentrated on neurons located in the dorsal gray matter; stimulation of these receptors inhibits the transmission of nociceptive input to higher (supraspinal) levels.[57] This inhibitory effect is mediated by opioid receptors that are located on both presynaptic and postsynaptic membranes of pain-mediating synapses (Fig. 14–2). That is, receptors are located on the presynaptic terminals of primary (first-order) nociceptive afferents, and when bound by opioids, they directly decrease the release of pain-mediating transmitters such as substance P.[17,57] Opioid drug-receptor interactions also take place on the postsynaptic membrane of the secondary afferent neuron—that is, the second-order nociceptive afferent neuron.[16,57] When stimulated, these receptors also inhibit pain transmission by hyperpolarizing the postsynaptic neuron.

It is currently unknown which of these mechanisms is the primary way in which opioids work, or if the effects of opioids on the spinal cord are, in fact, a combination of both methods. In either case, exactly how the receptor influences cell function after it is stimulated is also unclear. Drug-receptor binding may alter potassium and calcium conductance.[14,16] Decreased calcium entry into the presynaptic terminal would explain the decreased neurotransmitter release from primary afferents because calcium influx mediates transmitter release at a chemical synapse. A relative loss of potassium from the postsynaptic cell would explain postsynaptic hyperpolarization because efflux of potassium (a cation) results in a relative increase in the negative intracellular electric potential.

Opioids have also been suggested as inhibiting the formation of intracellular second messengers such as cyclic adenosine monophosphate (cAMP), which may help explain how these drugs alter pain transmission.[14,42,53] In addition, different receptor subtypes may work through different cellular mechanisms to alter neuronal excitability.

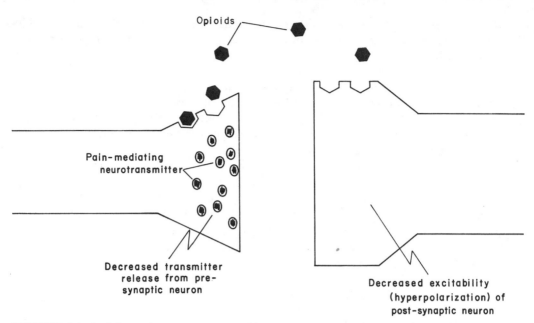

FIGURE 14–2. Schematic representation of how opioid analgesics may impair synaptic transmission in pain-mediating pathways. The drug binds to specific opioid receptors on the presynaptic and postsynaptic membranes.

For instance, mu and delta receptors appear to indirectly affect potassium channels, whereas kappa receptors act directly on calcium channels.[14] Hence, the molecular mechanisms of opioid analgesics continue to be clarified through ongoing research that will ultimately increase our knowledge of how these substances attenuate pain.

Effect of Narcotic Analgesics on the Brain

Opioid receptors have been identified in several locations of the brain that are associated with pain transmission and interpretation. These areas include the periaqueductal gray region of the spinoreticular tract, medial thalamic nuclei, hypothalamus, limbic system, and several other areas.[17,45] Opioid analgesics are believed to exert their effects on the brain by binding to these receptors and inhibiting neurons involved in pain transmission or exciting neurons involved in pain suppression. As with the spinal effects of these drugs, further details about the cellular mechanisms remain unclear. Again, evidence exists that opioids alter neuronal excitability by affecting potassium and calcium conductance or by impairing second-messenger cAMP synthesis.[14,16,42] Additional information about how these drugs work at the cellular level will surely be forthcoming.

Peripheral Effects of Opioids

Opioid receptors may exist outside the CNS, and some of the analgesic effects of opioid drugs may be mediated at peripheral sites.[46] Opioid receptors have been identified on the distal (peripheral) ends of primary afferent (sensory) neurons.[46,47] Binding of opioid agents to these peripheral receptors will provide an analgesic effect by decreasing the excitability of these sensory neurons (Fig. 14–3). This idea is supported by the fact that endogenous opioids (endorphins, enkephalins) are often produced in peripheral tissues during certain types of painful inflammation and that these endogenous substances seem to act locally on the peripheral sensory nerve terminals.[47] Likewise, results from some studies in animals and humans suggest that exogenous opioids can be administered directly into peripheral tissues (e.g., injected into an inflamed joint) and that these agents exert analgesic effects even though the drug never reaches the CNS.[22,46]

Hence, some evidence suggests that opioid receptors exist outside the CNS and that opioid drugs may help produce analgesia at these peripheral sites. However, the clinical significance of these peripheral opioid effects remains to be fully determined. For instance, these receptors may play a role in mediating only certain types of pain such as the pain associated with inflammation.[46] Nonetheless, the fact that certain types of pain might be controlled by peripherally acting opioids has important pharmacologic implications. For instance, opioids that work exclusively in the periphery would not cause CNS-mediated side effects such as sedation, respiratory depression, and tolerance. Peripheral-acting opioids could be developed by creating lipophobic compounds that are unable to cross the blood-brain barrier.[46,47] The use of these peripheral-acting drugs remains fairly experimental at the present time, and additional clinical trials will be needed to determine whether this becomes a viable means of treating certain types of pain.

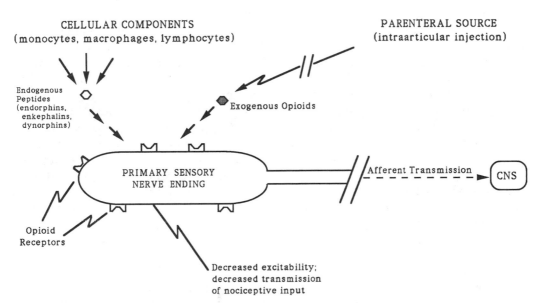

FIGURE 14–3. Putative mechanism of opioid action on peripheral nerve terminals. See text for discussion.

CLINICAL APPLICATIONS

Treatment of Pain

Opioid analgesics are most effective in treating moderate-to-severe pain that is more or less constant in duration. These drugs are not as effective in treating sharp, intermittent pain, although higher doses will also relieve this type of pain as well. Some examples of the clinical use of opioid analgesics include the treatment of acute pain following surgery, trauma, and myocardial infarction, as well as the treatment of chronic pain in patients with conditions such as cancer. Because of the potential for tolerance and addiction, these drugs should be used only when necessary, and the dose should be titrated according to the patient's pain. Generally, oral administration of a mild-to-moderate opioid agonist should be used first, with stronger agonists being instituted orally and then parenterally if needed. In cases of chronic pain (e.g., terminal cancer), pain control by nonopioid drugs should be attempted first. However, opioid analgesics should be instituted when the improvement in the quality of life offered to the patient with a terminal disease clearly outweighs the potential risks of these drugs.[30]

Opioid analgesics often produce a rather unique form of analgesia as compared to the nonopioid agents. Opioids often alter the perception of pain rather than eliminating the painful sensation entirely. The patient may still be aware of the pain, but it is no longer the primary focus of his or her attention. In a sense, the patient is no longer preoccupied by the pain. This type of analgesia is also often associated with euphoria and a sensation of floating. These sensations may be caused by the stimulation of specific types of opiate receptors within the limbic system (i.e., delta receptors).

The route of opioid administration appears to be important in providing effective pain relief.[31] Although the oral route is the easiest and most convenient, parenteral routes may be more effective in chronic or severe, intractable pain. In particular, spinal administration of the opioid—that is, administration directly into the epidural or intrathecal space—has been suggested as being optimal in relieving pain following certain types of surgery or in terminal cancer.[8,11,25,35,36,52,55,58] Since reinsertion of a needle every time the drug is needed is impractical, indwelling catheters are often implanted surgically so that the tip of the catheter lies in the epidural or intrathecal space. The free end of the catheter can be brought out through the patient's skin and used to administer the opioid directly into the area surrounding the spinal cord. Alternatively, the catheter can be connected to some sort of a drug reservoir or pump that contains the opioid drug. Such devices can be located outside the patient's body or implanted surgically beneath the patient's skin (e.g., in the abdominal wall), and these pumps are programmed to deliver the drug at a fixed rate into the indwelling catheter.[13] Although these programmable drug delivery systems do have some risks, they appear to be an effective way of treating severe, chronic pain in selected patients such as those with terminal cancer.[11,25,35,41,52]

The effectiveness of opioid analgesics also appears to be influenced by the dosing schedule. The current consensus is that orally administered opioids are more effective when given at regularly scheduled intervals rather than when the patient feels the need for the drug.[43] This may be because with regularly scheduled dosages, plasma concentrations may be maintained within a therapeutic range, rather than allowing the large plasma fluctuations that may occur if the drugs are given at sporadic intervals. Consistent with this hypothesis is the finding that continuous infusion of the opioid (either intravenously or spinally) provides optimal pain relief postoperatively or in chronic, intractable pain.[11,25,35,52] Continuous infusion is associated with certain side effects, especially nausea and constipation, as well as the potential for disruption of the drug delivery system.[35,52,55] Problems with tolerance have also been reported during continuous administration,[28,33] but it is somewhat controversial whether tolerance really develops when these drugs are used appropriately in the clinical management of pain (see "Concepts of Addiction, Tolerance, and Physical Dependence"). Hence, the benefit-to-risk ratio for continuous infusion is often acceptable in patients with severe pain. This method of opioid administration continues to gain acceptance.[52]

Use of Opioids in Patient-Controlled Analgesia

Finally, some rather innovative techniques have been employed whereby the patient is able to control the delivery of the analgesic.[9,18,26] These techniques are collectively known as patient-controlled analgesia (PCA) because the patient is able to periodically administer a specific dose of the drug (by pushing a button or some other device). PCA systems have some distinct advantages over conventional administration, and PCAs are often used in the treatment of severe, chronic pain as well as following various types of surgery.[9,18,26] The use of opioids and other drugs in PCA systems is discussed in Chapter 17.

Other Opioid Uses

Opioids have several other clinical applications. These agents can be used as an anesthetic premedication or as an adjunct in general anesthesia. Opioids are effective in cough suppression, and the short-term use of codeine in this regard is quite common. Opioid agonists decrease gastrointestinal motility and can be used to control cases of severe diarrhea. This effect is probably mediated indirectly through an effect on the CNS as well as through a direct effect on the intestine. Finally, opioid agonists are used as an adjunct in cases of acute pulmonary edema. These drugs probably do not directly improve ventilatory capacity, but they do serve to reduce feelings of intense panic and anxiety associated with the dyspnea inherent to this disorder. Patients feel they can breathe more easily following opioid administration.

PROBLEMS AND ADVERSE EFFECTS

Opioid analgesics produce a number of central and peripheral side effects. Virtually all of these drugs have sedative properties and induce some degree of mental slowing and drowsiness. Patients taking opioids for the relief of pain may also become somewhat euphoric, although the manner and degree of such mood changes vary from individual to individual. One of the more potentially serious side effects is the respiratory depression often seen after narcotic administration.[24] Within a few minutes after administration, these drugs cause the breathing rate to slow down, which can last for several hours. Although not usually a major problem when therapeutic doses are given to relatively healthy individuals, respiratory depression can be severe or even fatal in seriously ill patients, in patients with pre-existing pulmonary problems, or in cases of overdose. Some cardiovascular problems such as orthostatic hypotension may also occur immediately after opioids are administered, especially when parenteral routes are used. Finally, gastrointestinal distress in the form of nausea and vomiting is quite common with many of the narcotic analgesics. Because of their antiperistaltic action, these drugs can also cause constipation.

CONCEPTS OF ADDICTION, TOLERANCE, AND PHYSICAL DEPENDENCE

When used inappropriately, opioid drugs can produce addiction. The term *addiction* is now used to refer to situations in which certain individuals repeatedly seek out and ingest certain substances for mood-altering and pleasurable experiences, such as the heroin addict who takes this drug illicitly to achieve an opioid "high." In this sense, addiction is a very complex phenomenon that has strong psychologic implications regarding why certain chemicals cause this behavior in certain people. This concept of addiction is often separated from the physiologic changes that can accompany prolonged opioid use, namely tolerance and physical dependence.

Tolerance is the need for more drug to achieve a given effect, and **physical dependence** is the onset of withdrawal symptoms if a drug is suddenly discontinued. Tolerance and physical dependence are also rather complex phenomena, and a complete discussion of the factors involved in producing these occurrences is not possible at this time. The primary characteristics of tolerance and physical dependence will be briefly discussed here as they relate to opioid usage.

Tolerance

Tolerance is defined as the need for more drug to achieve the same effect when the drug is used for prolonged periods. When used for the treatment of pain, the dosage of the opioid may need to be increased periodically to continue to provide adequate relief. The physiologic reasons for tolerance are somewhat unclear but probably involve changes in drug receptor number and sensitivity and a disturbance in the balance between specific central neurotransmitters.[19,37-39] Tolerance actually begins after the first dose of the narcotic, but the need for increased amounts of the drug usually becomes obvious after 2 to 3 weeks of administration. Tolerance seems to last approximately 1 to 2 weeks after the drug is removed. This does not mean that the patient no longer has any desire for the drug, but that the patient will again respond to the initial dosage after 14 days or so. Other factors may influence the individual's desire for the drug long after any physiologic effects have disappeared (see "Physical Dependence").

Physical Dependence

Physical dependence is usually defined as the onset of withdrawal symptoms when the drug is abruptly removed. **Withdrawal syndrome** from opioid dependence is associated with a number of obvious and unpleasant symptoms (Table 14–4). In severe dependence, withdrawal symptoms become evident within 6 to 10 hours after the last dose of the drug and reach their peak in the second or third day after the drug has

TABLE 14-4 Abstinence Syndromes:
Symptoms of Narcotic Withdrawal

Body aches	Runny nose
Diarrhea	Shivering
Fever	Sneezing
Gooseflesh	Stomach cramps
Insomnia	Sweating
Irritability	Tachycardia
Loss of appetite	Uncontrollable yawning
Nausea/vomiting	Weakness/fatigue

been stopped. Withdrawal symptoms last approximately 5 days. This does not necessarily mean that the individual no longer desires the drug, only that the physical symptoms of withdrawal have ceased. Indeed, an addict may continue to crave the drug after months or years of abstinence.

Physical dependence must therefore be differentiated from the more intangible concepts of addiction and psychologic dependence. Psychologic dependence seems to be related to pleasurable changes in mood and behavior evoked by the drug. The individual is motivated to continually reproduce these pleasurable sensations because of the feelings of well-being, relaxation, and so on. Psychologic dependence seems to create the drug-seeking behavior that causes the addict to relapse into use of the drug long after the physiologic effects have disappeared.

Tolerance and Dependence During Therapeutic Opioid Use

Although tolerance and dependence can occur whenever opioid drugs are used for prolonged periods, there is some debate as to whether these phenomena must always accompany the therapeutic use of opioid drugs for the treatment of chronic pain. Some experts feel that tolerance and physical dependence will not occur even when these drugs are used indefinitely, providing that the dosage is carefully adjusted to meet the patient's needs.[31,41] It is believed that when the opioid dose exactly matches the patient's need for pain control, there is no excess drug that will stimulate the drug-seeking behavior commonly associated with opioid addiction. The opioid is essentially absorbed by the patient's pain. Of course, patients with chronic pain may still need to have the dosage increased periodically. This observation would be explained by the fact that the pain has increased because the patient's condition has worsened (e.g., the cancer has increased) rather than the idea that the patient developed pharmacologic tolerance to the drug.[10,41]

Thus, many practitioners feel that problems with addiction, tolerance, and dependence are minimized when opioid drugs are used therapeutically. These agents are essentially being used for a specific reason, treatment of pain, rather than for the pleasure-seeking purpose associated with the recreational use of these drugs. These drugs must, of course, be used carefully and with strict regard to using the lowest effective dose. Hence, there is consensus that opioids are very effective and important analgesic agents and should be used under appropriate therapeutic conditions without excessive fear of the patient developing addiction or becoming especially tolerant to the drug's effects.

Use of Methadone to Treat Opioid Addiction

The illegal use and abuse of narcotics such as heroin is a major problem in many countries. The narcotic agonist methadone is often used to treat heroin addicts. Methadone is a strong narcotic agonist, similar in potency and efficacy to morphine. While giving an opioid to treat opioid addiction may at first appear odd, methadone offers several advantages, such as milder withdrawal symptoms. Methadone is essentially substituted for the heroin and then slowly withdrawn as various methods of counseling are employed to discourage further drug abuse. For a detailed discussion on the use of methadone in heroin addiction, the reader is referred to several sources listed at the end of this chapter.[12,15,48]

SPECIAL CONCERNS IN REHABILITATION PATIENTS

Physical therapists will encounter the use of opioid analgesics in patients requiring acute pain relief (following surgery, trauma, etc.) and chronic analgesia (for patients with terminal cancer and other types of severe pain). The usual side effects of sedation and gastrointestinal discomfort may be bothersome during some of the therapy sessions. However, the relief of pain afforded by these drugs may be helpful in allowing a relatively more vigorous and comprehensive rehabilitation regimen. The benefits of pain relief usually outweigh side effects such as sedation. Scheduling therapy when these drugs reach their peak effects may be advantageous (see Table 14–2). One side effect that should be taken into account during therapy is the tendency of these drugs to produce respiratory depression. Opioids tend to make the medullary chemoreceptors less responsive to carbon dioxide, thus slowing down respiratory rate and inducing a relative hypoxia and hypercapnia.[6] This fact should be considered if any exercise is instituted as part of the rehabilitation program. The respiratory response to this exercise may be blunted.[40]

Therapists may also be working with patients who are experiencing withdrawal symptoms from opioid drugs. Such patients may be in the process of being weaned off the therapeutic use of these agents, or they may be heroin addicts who have been hospitalized for other reasons (e.g., trauma, surgery). If not on some type of methadone maintenance, the addict may be experiencing a wide variety of physical symptoms including diffuse muscle aches. The therapist should be aware that these aches and pains may be caused by opioid withdrawal rather than an actual somatic disorder. Therapists may, however, help the patient cope with opioid withdrawal by using various physical agents (heat, electrotherapy) and manual techniques (massage, relaxation techniques) to alleviate these somatic symptoms.

CASE STUDY

OPIOID ANALGESICS

Brief History: N.P., a 45-year-old woman, was involved in an automobile accident approximately 6 months ago. She received multiple contusions from the accident, but no major injuries were sustained. Two months later, she began to develop pain in the right shoulder. This pain progressively increased, and she was treated for bursitis using anti-inflammatory drugs. Her shoulder motion became progressively more limited, however; any movement of her glenohumeral joint caused rather severe pain. She was re-evaluated and a diagnosis of adhesive capsulitis was made. The patient was admitted to the hospital, and while she was under general anesthesia, a closed manipulation of the shoulder was performed. When the patient recovered from the anesthesia, meperidine (Demerol) was prescribed for pain relief. This drug was given orally at a dosage of 75 mg every 4 hours. Physical therapy was also initiated the afternoon following the closed manipulation. Passive range-of-motion exercises were used to maintain the increased joint mobility achieved during the manipulative procedure.

Relevance to Therapy/Clinical Decision. The therapist arranged the treatment schedule so that the meperidine was reaching peak effects during the therapy session. The patient was seen approximately 1 hour following the oral administration of the drug. The initial session was scheduled at the patient's bedside because the patient was still woozy from the anesthesia. On the following day, therapy was continued in the physical therapy department. However, the patient was brought to the department on a stretcher to prevent an episode of dizziness brought on by orthostatic hypotension. On the third day, the patient's medication was changed to oxycodone (Percodan), a mild-to-moderate opioid agonist. By this time, the patient was being transported to physical therapy in a wheelchair, and the therapy session also included active exercise. The patient was discharged on the fourth day after the manipulative procedure. She continued to attend therapy as an outpatient, and full function of her right shoulder was ultimately restored.

SUMMARY

Opioid analgesics represent some of the most effective methods of treating moderate-to-severe pain. When used properly, these agents can alleviate acute and chronic pain in a variety of situations. The use of these drugs is sometimes tempered with their tendency to produce tolerance and physical dependence, and with their potential for abuse. Opioid drugs do, however, represent the most effective pharmacologic means of helping patients deal with moderate-to-severe pain. The analgesic properties of these drugs often provide a substantial benefit in patients involved in rehabilitation. Physical therapists should be aware of some of the side effects such as sedation and respiratory depression and should be cognizant of the impact of these effects during the rehabilitation session.

REFERENCES

1. Adams, ML, et al: The role of endogenous peptides in the action of opioid analgesics. Ann Emerg Med 15:1030, 1986.
2. Akil, H, et al: Endogenous opioids: Biology and function. Annu Rev Neurosci 7:223, 1984.
3. Ashburn, MA, et al: Iontophoretic delivery of morphine for postoperative analgesia. J Pain Symptom Management 7:27, 1992.
4. Basbaum, AI and Fields, HL: Endogenous pain control systems: Brainstem spinal pathways and endorphin circuitry. Annu Rev Neurosci 7:309, 1984.

5. Bloom, FE: The endorphins: A growing family of pharmacologically pertinent peptides. Annu Rev Pharmacol Toxicol 23:151, 1983.
6. Camporesi, EM, et al: Ventilatory CO_2 sensitivity after intravenous and epidural morphine in volunteers. Anesth Analg 62:633, 1983.
7. Chang, K-J and Cuatrecasas, P: Heterogeneity and properties of opiate receptors. Fed Proc 40:2729, 1981.
8. Chaplan, SR, et al: Morphine and hydromorphone epidural analgesia: A prospective, randomized comparison. Anesthesiology 77:1090, 1992.
9. Citron, ML, et al: Patient-controlled analgesia for severe cancer pain. Arch Intern Med 146:734, 1986.
10. Collin, E, et al: Is disease progression the major factor in morphine tolerance in cancer pain treatment. Pain 55:319, 1993.
11. Coombs, DW, et al: Relief of continuous chronic pain by intraspinal narcotics infusion via an implanted reservoir. JAMA 250:2336, 1983.
12. Cooper, JR, et al (eds): Research on the Treatment of Narcotic Addiction: State of the Art. National Institute on Drug Abuse Treatment Research Monograph Series, Dept. of Health and Human Services Publication No. 83-1281, U.S. Government Printing Office, Washington, DC, 1983.
13. Crawford, ME, et al: Pain treatment on out-patient basis utilizing extradural opiates. A Danish multicentre study comprising 105 patients. Pain 16:41, 1983.
14. Dickenson, AH: Mechanisms of the analgesic actions of opiates and opioids. Br Med J 47:690, 1991.
15. Dole, VP: Implications of methadone maintenance for theories of narcotic addiction. JAMA 260:3025, 1988.
16. Duggan, AW and North, RA: Electrophysiology of the opioids. Pharmacol Rev 35:219, 1983.
17. Goodman, RR and Pasternak, GW: Visualization of mu_1 opiate receptors in the rat brain by using a computerized autoradiographic subtraction technique. Proc Natl Acad Sci 82:6667, 1985.
18. Graves, DA, et al: Patient-controlled anesthesia. Ann Intern Med 99:360, 1983.
19. Henriksen, SJ: Neurophysiological investigations of opiate tolerance and dependence in the central nervous system. NIDA Res Monogr Ser 54:239, 1984.
20. Jaffe, JH and Martin, WR: Opioid analgesics and antagonists. In Gilman, AG, et al (eds): The Pharmacological Basis of Therapeutics, ed 8. Pergamon Press, New York, 1990.
21. Jasinski, DR: Human pharmacology of narcotic antagonists. Br J Clin Pharmacol 7:287S, 1979.
22. Joshi, GP, et al: Intra-articular morphine for pain relief after knee arthroscopy. J Bone Joint Surg 74B:749, 1992.
23. Kachur, JF, et al: Comparison of the ability of opioid analgesics to increase endogenous opioid-like activity in the cerebrospinal fluid of rabbits. Life Sci 37:2549, 1985.
24. Keats, AS: The effect of drugs on respiration in man. Annu Rev Pharmacol Toxicol 25:41, 1985.
25. Krames, ES, et al: Continuous infusion of spinally administered narcotics for the relief of pain due to malignant disorders. Cancer 56:696, 1986.
26. Lehmann, KA, Gordes, B, and Hoeckle, W: Patient-controlled analgesia for the treatment of postoperative pain. Anaesthesist 34:494, 1985.
27. Lutz, RA and Pfister, HP: Opioid receptors and their pharmacological profiles. J Recept Res 12:267, 1992.
28. Marshall, HUW, et al: Relief of pain by infusion of morphine after operation: Does tolerance develop? Br Med J 291:19, 1985.
29. Martin, WR: Pharmacology of opioids. Pharmacol Rev 35:283, 1983.
30. McGivney, WT and Crooks, GM: The care of patients with severe chronic pain in terminal illness. JAMA 251:1182, 1984.
31. McQuay, HJ: Opioid clinical pharmacology and routes of administration. Br Med Bull 47:703, 1991.
32. Millan, MJ: K-opioid receptors and analgesia. Trends Pharmacol Sci 11:70, 1990.
33. Milne, B, et al: Analgesia and tolerance to intrathecal morphine and norepinephrine infusion via implanted miniosmotic pumps in the rat. Pain 22:165, 1985.
34. Offermeier, J and VanRooyen, JM: Opioid drugs and their receptors: A summary of the present state of knowledge. S Afr Med J 66:299, 1984.
35. Ohlsson, L, et al: Cancer pain relief by continuous administration of epidural morphine in a hospital setting and at home. Pain 48:349, 1992.
36. Ray, CD and Bagley, R: Indwelling epidural morphine for control of postlumbar spinal surgery pain. Neurosurgery 13:388, 1983.
37. Redmond, DE and Krystal, JH: Multiple mechanisms of withdrawal from opioid drugs. Annu Rev Neurosci 7:443, 1984.
38. Rogers, NF and El-Fakahany, EE: Morphine-induced opioid receptor down-regulation detected in intact adult rat brain cells. Eur J Pharmacol 124:221, 1986.
39. Rothman, DB, et al: Morphine tolerance increases noncompetitive binding sites. Eur J Pharmacol 124:113, 1986.
40. Santiago, TV, et al: Effects of morphine on ventilatory response to exercise. J Appl Physiol 47:112, 1979.
41. Schultheiss, R, et al: Dose changes in long-term and medium-term intrathecal morphine therapy of cancer pain. Neurosurgery 31:664, 1992.
42. Simon, EJ and Hiller, JM: The opiate receptors. Annu Rev Pharmacol Toxicol 18:371, 1978.
43. Slattery, PJ and Boas, RA: Newer methods of delivery of opiates for relief of pain. Drugs 30:539, 1985.
44. Snyder, SH: Neuronal receptors. Annu Rev Physiol 48:461, 1986.

45. Snyder, SH: Drug and neurotransmitter receptors in the brain. 224:22, 1984.
46. Stein, C: Peripheral mechanisms of opioid analgesia. Anesth Analg 76:182, 1993.
47. Stein, C, et al: Local anesthetic effect of endogenous opioid peptides. Lancet 342:321, 1993.
48. Strain, EC, et al: Dose-response effects of methadone in the treatment of opioid dependence. Ann Intern Med 119:23, 1993.
49. Streibel, HW, Koenigs, D, and Kramer, J: Postoperative pain management by intranasal demand-adapted fentanyl titration. Anesthesiology 77:281, 1992.
50. Streibel, HW, Pommerening, J, and Rieger, A: Intranasal fentanyl titration for postoperative pain management in an unselected population. Anaesthesia 48:753, 1993.
51. Terenius, L: Endogenous peptides and analgesia. Annu Rev Pharmacol Toxicol 18:189, 1978.
52. Vandongen, RTM, Crul, BJP, and Debock, M: Long-term intrathecal infusion of morphine and morphine bupivacaine mixtures in the treatment of cancer pain: A retrospective analysis of 51 cases. Pain 55:119, 1993.
53. Way, EL: Sites and mechanisms of basic narcotic receptor function based on current research. Ann Emerg Med 15:1021, 1986.
54. Way, WL and Way, EL: Opioid analgesics and antagonists. In Katzung, BG (ed): Basic and Clinical Pharmacology, ed 5. Appleton & Lange, Norwalk, CT, 1992.
55. White, MJ, et al: Side effects during continuous epidural infusion of morphine and fentanyl. Can J Anaesth 39:576, 1992.
56. Wood, PL, Rackham, A, and Richard, J: Spinal analgesia: Comparison of the mu agonist morphine and kappa agonist ethylketazocine. Life Sci 28:2119, 1981.
57. Yaksh, TL and Noueihed, R: The physiology and pharmacology of spinal opiates. Annu Rev Pharmacol Toxicol 25:433, 1985.
58. Zenz, M, Piepenbrock, S, and Tryba, M: Epidural opiates: Long term experiences in cancer pain. Klin Wochenschr 63:225, 1985.

CHAPTER 15

Nonsteroidal Anti-Inflammatory Drugs

This chapter discusses a chemically diverse group of substances that exert several distinct pharmacologic properties. These properties include (1) the ability to decrease inflammation, (2) the ability to relieve mild-to-moderate pain (**analgesia**), (3) the ability to decrease the elevated body temperature associated with fever (**antipyresis**), and (4) the ability to decrease blood clotting by inhibiting platelet aggregation (**anticoagulation**). These drugs are commonly referred to as nonsteroidal anti-inflammatory drugs (NSAIDs) to distinguish them from the corticosteroids (i.e., the other main group of drugs used to treat inflammation). Obviously the term NSAIDs does not fully describe the pharmacologic actions of these agents, and a more inclusive terminology should also mention the analgesic, antipyretic, and anticoagulant effects of these drugs. However, these drugs are typically referred to as NSAIDs, and this terminology is used throughout this chapter.

Because of their analgesic and anti-inflammatory effects, NSAIDs are often taken by patients receiving physical therapy for any number of problems. These drugs are a mainstay in the treatment of many types of mild-to-moderate pain, and NSAIDs are especially useful in treating pain and inflammation that occur in acute and chronic musculoskeletal disorders. Other patients are given NSAIDs to treat fever or to prevent excessive blood clotting. Consequently, physical therapists and other rehabilitation specialists will see these drugs used quite frequently in their patient population, with the specific therapeutic goal being related to the individual needs of each patient.

ASPIRIN AND OTHER NSAIDS: GENERAL ASPECTS

The best representative of the NSAIDs is aspirin (acetylsalicylic acid) (Fig. 15–1). Other newer NSAIDs are usually compared to aspirin in terms of efficacy and safety. Acetaminophen is another agent that is similar to aspirin and other NSAIDs in its ability to decrease pain and fever. Acetaminophen, however, is not considered one of the NSAIDs because it lacks anti-inflammatory and anticoagulant properties. For a discus-

$$COOH$$
$$OCOCH_3$$

Aspirin
(acetylsalicylic acid)

FIGURE 15-1. Structure of aspirin.

sion of the comparative effects of aspirin, newer NSAIDs, and acetaminophen, see "Comparison of Aspirin to Other NSAIDs."

For years it was a mystery how a drug like aspirin could exert such a diverse range of therapeutic effects; that is, how could one drug influence so many different systems to effectively alleviate pain and inflammation, decrease fever, and even affect blood clotting? This issue was essentially resolved in the early 1970s when aspirin was found to inhibit the synthesis of a group of endogenous compounds known collectively as the "prostaglandins." We now know that aspirin and the other NSAIDs exert most, if not all, of their therapeutic effects by interfering with the biosynthesis of prostaglandins and other related compounds.[10,21,48,85,99,100] To understand the way in which these drugs work, a brief discussion of prostaglandins and similar endogenously produced substances is presented here.

PROSTAGLANDINS, THROMBOXANES, AND LEUKOTRIENES

Prostaglandins are a group of lipidlike compounds that exhibit a wide range of pharmacologic activities.[14,41,75,86,88] With the exception of the red blood cell, virtually every type of living cell in the human body has been identified as being able to produce prostaglandins. These compounds appear to be hormones that act locally to help regulate cell function under normal and pathologic conditions. Other biologically active compounds known as the "thromboxanes" and "leukotrienes" have been discovered that are derived from the same precursor as the prostaglandins.[5,11,59,70,81] Together, the prostaglandins, thromboxanes, and leukotrienes are often referred to as **eicosanoids** because they all are derived from 20-carbon fatty acids that contain several double bonds.[41] (The term *eicosanoid* is derived from *eicosa*, meaning "20-carbon," and *enoic*, meaning "containing double bonds.")

Eicosanoid Biosynthesis

The biosynthetic pathway of prostaglandins and other eicosanoids is outlined in Figure 15-2. Basically these compounds are derived from a 20-carbon essential fatty

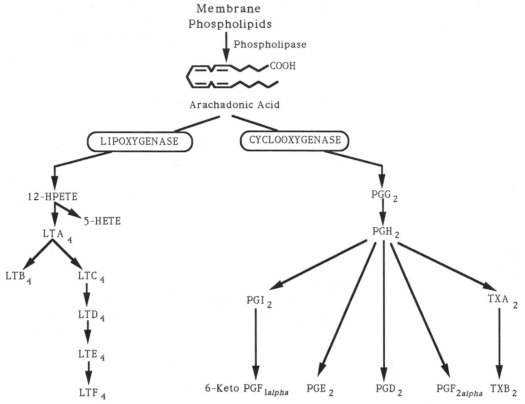

FIGURE 15–2. Eicosanoid biosynthesis. PG = prostaglandin; TX = thromboxane; LT = leukotriene.

acid. In humans, this fatty acid is usually arachidonic acid.[5,14,86] Arachidonic acid is ingested in the diet and stored as a phospholipid in the cell membrane. Thus, the cell has an abundant and easily accessible supply of this precursor. When needed, arachidonic acid is cleaved from the cell membrane by a phospholipase enzyme (i.e., phospholipase A_2). The 20-carbon fatty acid can then be used by two major enzyme systems: the cyclooxygenase enzyme and the lipoxygenase enzyme. The prostaglandins and thromboxanes are ultimately synthesized from the cyclooxygenase pathway, and the leukotrienes come from the lipoxygenase system (see Fig. 15–2).[14,59,62,75,86] Exactly which pathway is used in any particular cell depends on the type and quantity of enzymes in that cell, as well as the physiologic status of the cell. The end products within a given pathway (i.e., exactly which prostaglandins, thromboxanes, or leukotrienes will be formed) also depend on the individual cell. Any drug that inhibits one of these enzymes will also inhibit the formation of all of the subsequent products of that particular pathway. A drug that blocks the cyclooxygenase will essentially eliminate all prostaglandin and thromboxane synthesis in that cell. As this chapter will later discuss, aspirin and the other NSAIDs are cyclooxygenase inhibitors, and this is the way that these drugs exert their therapeutic effects (see "Mechanism of NSAID Action: Inhibition of Prostaglandin and Thromboxane Synthesis").

Role of Eicosanoids in Health and Disease

The prostaglandins, thromboxanes, and leukotrienes have been shown to have a variety of effects on virtually every major physiologic system. Studies have indicated that these compounds can influence cardiovascular, respiratory, renal, gastrointestinal, nervous, and reproductive function.[14,41,70,75,88] The biologic effects of the various eicosanoids cannot be generalized. Different classes of eicosanoids and even different members within the same class may exert different effects on the same system.[103] For instance, certain prostaglandins such as the PGAs and PGEs tend to produce vasodilation in most vascular beds, whereas other prostaglandins (e.g., $PGF_{2\alpha}$) and the thromboxanes are often vasoconstrictors.[70] Some of the major effects of the eicosanoids are summarized in Table 15–1.

All of the effects of different prostaglandins, thromboxanes, and leukotrienes on various systems in the body cannot be reviewed in this chapter. Besides, this issue has been reviewed extensively elsewhere.[14,41,70,75,86] Of greater interest in this chapter is the role of prostaglandins and related substances in pathologic conditions. In general, cells that are subjected to various types of trauma or disturbances in homeostasis tend to increase the production of prostaglandins.[6,67] This finding suggests that prostaglandins and other eicosanoids may be important in the protective response to cellular injury. In addition, prostaglandins are important in mediating some of the painful effects of injury and inflammation, as well as the symptoms of other pathologic conditions. Some of the better documented conditions associated with excessive prostaglandin synthesis are listed here.

Inflammation. Increased prostaglandin synthesis is usually detected at the site of local inflammation.[56,70,86] Certain prostaglandins, such as PGE_2, are thought to help mediate the local erythema and edema associated with inflammation by increasing local blood flow, increasing capillary permeability, and potentiating the permeability effects of histamine and bradykinin.[56,62] Leukotrienes, particularly LTB_4, also contribute to the inflammatory response by increasing vascular permeability, and LTB_4 has a potent chemotactic effect on polymorphonuclear leukocytes.[5,11,56,59,81,87]

Pain. Prostaglandins appear to help mediate painful stimuli in a variety of conditions (including inflammation). The compounds do not directly produce pain but are believed to increase the sensitivity of pain receptors to the effects of other pain-producing substances such as bradykinin.[67]

Fever. Prostaglandins appear to be pyretogenic; that is, they help produce the elevated body temperature during fever. Although the details are somewhat unclear, increased prostaglandin production may help alter the thermoregulatory set-point within the hypothalamus so that body temperature is maintained at a higher level.[28,69]

Dysmenorrhea. The painful cramps that accompany menstruation in some women have been attributed at least in part to excessive prostaglandin production in the endometrium of the uterus.[18,74]

Thrombus Formation. The thromboxanes, especially TXA_2, cause platelet aggregation resulting in blood clot formation[17,71,103] Whether excessive thrombus formation (as in deep vein thrombosis) is initiated by abnormal thromboxane production is unclear. Certainly, inhibition of thromboxane synthesis will help prevent thrombus formation in individuals who are prone to specific types of excessive blood clotting.[64,68,69,71,104]

Other Pathologies. Because of their many varied physiologic effects, the eicosanoids are involved in a number of other pathologic conditions. Prostaglandins

TABLE 15–1 Primary Physiologic Effects of the Major Classes of Prostaglandins, Thromboxanes, and Leukotrienes

Class	Vascular Smooth Muscle	Airway Smooth Muscle	Gastrointestinal Smooth Muscle	Gastrointestinal Secretions	Uterine Muscle (Nonpregnant)	Platelet Aggregation
PGAs	Vasodilation	—	—	Decrease	Relaxation	—
PGEs	Vasodilation	Bronchodilation	Contraction	Decrease	Relaxation	Variable
PGI$_2$	Vasodilation	—	Relaxation	Decrease	—	Decrease
PGFs	Variable	Bronchoconstriction	Contraction	—	Contraction	—
TXA$_2$	Vasoconstriction	Bronchoconstriction	—	—	—	Strong, increase
LTs	Vasoconstriction	Bronchoconstriction	Contraction	—	—	—

have been implicated in cardiovascular disorders (hypertension), respiratory dysfunction (asthma), neurologic disorders (multiple sclerosis, allergic encephalomyelitis), endocrine dysfunction (Bartter's syndrome, diabetes mellitus), and a variety of other problems.[6,31,38,70] The exact role of prostaglandins and the other eicosanoids in various diseases continues to be evaluated, and the role of these compounds in health and disease has become clearer with ongoing research.

MECHANISM OF NSAID ACTION: INHIBITION OF PROSTAGLANDIN AND THROMBOXANE SYNTHESIS

Aspirin and the other NSAIDs are all potent inhibitors of the cyclooxygenase enzyme.[10,12,21,48,52,99] Since cyclooxygenase represents the first step in the synthesis of prostaglandins and thromboxanes, these drugs will essentially eliminate all prostaglandin and thromboxane production in every cell that they reach. Considering that prostaglandins and thromboxanes are implicated in producing pain, inflammation, fever, and excessive blood clotting, virtually all of the therapeutic effects of aspirin and similar drugs can be explained by their ability to inhibit the synthesis of these two eicosanoid classes.[99]

Aspirin and other NSAIDs do not appear to directly inhibit the lipoxygenase enzyme and thus do not appreciably decrease leukotriene synthesis.[44,85,86] In fact, some evidence exists that leukotriene production may actually increase in the cyclooxygenase-inhibited cell, because of a direct stimulatory effect of certain NSAIDs on the lipoxygenase or the availability of more arachidonic acid for the lipoxygenase enzyme when the cyclooxygenase is inhibited.[43] Since leukotrienes are also pro-inflammatory, inhibition of this enzyme system is desirable in conditions that have an inflammatory component. For instance, drugs that inhibit the lipoxygenase are currently being developed, and preliminary evidence has indicated that these drugs may be helpful in treating inflammatory-based diseases such as asthma and allergic rhinitis.[49,55] Other new drugs are being developed that antagonize (block) leukotriene receptors on peripheral tissues, and these agents have also shown promise in attenuating leukotriene-induced responses.[63] Hence, drugs that inhibit leukotriene synthesis or block leukotriene effects will hopefully be available for widespread clinical use in the future. These agents will be a welcome addition to the prostaglandin inhibitors that are currently available.[59]

ASPIRIN: PROTOTYPICAL NSAID

Acetylsalicylic acid, or aspirin as it is commonly known (see Fig. 15–1), represents the major form of a group of drugs known as the **salicylates**. Other salicylates (sodium salicylate, choline salicylate) are also used clinically, but aspirin is the most frequently used and appears to have the widest range of therapeutic effects of the salicylate drugs. Because aspirin has been used clinically for almost 100 years, is inexpensive, and is readily available without prescription, many individuals may be under the impression that this drug is only a marginally effective therapeutic agent. On the contrary, aspirin is a very powerful and effective drug that should be considered a major medicine.[57,76] As discussed previously, aspirin is a potent inhibitor of cyclooxygenase activity in all cells, and thus it has the potential to affect a number of conditions that involve excessive prostaglandin and thromboxane production.

As indicated previously, aspirin is the oldest and most widely used NSAID, and other NSAIDs are compared to aspirin in terms of efficacy and safety. Hence, this discussion focuses primarily on the clinical applications of aspirin and the problems typically associated with aspirin. For the most part, these applications and problems can also be applied to the nonaspirin NSAIDs. The major similarities and differences between aspirin and the other NSAIDs are discussed in "Comparison of Aspirin to Other NSAIDs."

CLINICAL APPLICATIONS OF ASPIRIN-LIKE DRUGS

Treatment of Pain and Inflammation

Aspirin and other NSAIDs are effective in treating mild-to-moderate pain of various origins including headache, toothache, and diffuse muscular aches and soreness. Aspirin appears to be especially useful in treating pain and inflammation in musculoskeletal and joint disorders.[66,102] The safe and effective use of aspirin in both rheumatoid arthritis and osteoarthritis is well documented (see Chapter 16).[9,40,46,80] Aspirin is also recommended for treating pain and cramping associated with primary dysmenorrhea.[18,74]

Aspirin and aspirin-like drugs are also used to manage pain following certain types of surgery including arthroscopic surgery.[77,83] These drugs can serve as the primary analgesic following other types of minor or intermediate surgery, and they can also be used after extensive surgery to decrease the need for high doses of other drugs such as the opioids.[15,16,72,84] Ketorolac tromethamine (Toradol) is a relatively new NSAID that has shown exceptional promise in treating postoperative pain. This drug can be given orally or by intramuscular injection, and it has been reported to provide analgesic effects similar to opioid drugs (morphine) but without the side effects and risks associated with opioid analgesics.[27,73,84,106] Hence, ketorolac tromethamine provides a reasonable alternative for nonopioid management of postoperative pain and may be especially valuable in situations where opioid side effects (sedation, respiratory depression) are harmful or undesirable.[61,65,84]

Treatment of Fever

Although the use of aspirin in treating fever in children is contraindicated (because of the association with Reye's syndrome; see "Problems and Adverse Effects of Aspirin-like Drugs"), aspirin remains the primary NSAID used in treating fever in adults.[28] Ibuprofen is also used frequently as a nonprescription antipyretic NSAID.

Treatment of Vascular Disorders

As discussed previously, aspirin inhibits platelet-induced thrombus formation through its ability to inhibit thromboxane biosynthesis. Aspirin has therefore been used to prevent deep vein thrombosis following surgical procedures such as hip arthroplasty.[64] More importantly, there is conclusive evidence that daily doses of aspirin may help prevent the onset or recurrence of heart attacks in some individuals by inhibiting thrombus formation in the coronary arteries.[3,58,71,92] Similarly, daily aspirin use may help prevent transient ischemic attacks and stroke by preventing cerebral infarction in certain patients.[3,32,35] The role of aspirin in treating coagulation disorders is discussed in more detail in Chapter 25.

Prevention of Cancer

There is now considerable evidence that regular aspirin use decreases the risk of colon cancer and possibly other types of gastrointestinal cancer.[60,93,98] It has been estimated, for example, that people who use aspirin on a regular basis have a 40 to 50 percent lower risk of fatal colon cancer as compared to people who do not use aspirin.[96,97] The exact reasons for this apparent protective effect are unclear, but these findings have generated a great deal of interest in a potential role for aspirin and aspirin-like drugs in preventing certain forms of cancer. It will be interesting to see if these drugs are prescribed routinely in the future, especially in individuals who are at an increased risk for developing colon cancer.[98]

PROBLEMS AND ADVERSE EFFECTS OF ASPIRIN-LIKE DRUGS

Gastrointestinal Problems

The primary problem with all of the NSAIDs including aspirin is gastrointestinal damage. Problems ranging from minor stomach discomfort to variable amounts of upper gastrointestinal hemorrhage and ulceration are fairly common.[1,45,50,51] These effects may be caused by aspirin directly irritating the gastric mucosa or by the loss of protective prostaglandins from the mucosal lining (i.e., aspirin may locally inhibit the formation of prostaglandins that protect the stomach from the acidic gastric juices).[53] Certain patients are more susceptible to gastrointestinal injury from aspirin-like drugs, and factors such as increased age and a history of ulcers appear to increase the risk of serious gastrointestinal damage.[26,89]

Several pharmacologic and nonpharmacologic strategies have been employed to manage the gastrointestinal problems associated with the aspirin-like drugs. One strategy has been to coat the aspirin tablet so that dissolution and release of the drug is delayed until it reaches the small intestine. These so-called enteric-coated forms of aspirin will spare the stomach from irritation, but the duodenum and upper small intestine may still be subjected to damage.[1,50] Enteric-coated aspirin also has the disadvantage of delaying the onset of analgesic effects, so that relief from acute pain may also be delayed. Other methods such as buffering the aspirin tablet have also been used to help decrease stomach irritation. The rationale here is that including a chemical buffer helps blunt the acidic effects of the aspirin molecule on the stomach mucosa. It is questionable, however, whether sufficient buffer is added to commercial aspirin preparations to actually make a difference in stomach irritation. During chronic aspirin therapy (e.g., treatment of arthritis), taking aspirin with meals may help decrease gastrointestinal irritation because the food in the stomach will offer some direct protection of the gastric mucosa.[9] The presence of food, however, will also delay drug absorption, which may decrease the peak levels of drug that reach the bloodstream.

A great deal of attention has been focused recently on other drugs that can prevent or treat the gastrointestinal side effects associated with aspirin and the other NSAIDs. Misoprostol (Cytotec) is a prostaglandin E_1 analog that inhibits gastric acid secretion and prevents gastric damage.[91,101] This drug has been beneficial in decreasing aspirin-induced irritation, but the clinical use of misoprostol is limited somewhat by side effects such as diarrhea.[101] Drugs that antagonize certain histamine receptors—that is, the H_2 receptor blockers—have also been used to decrease gastrointestinal damage.[13,91] As indicated in Chapter 27, histamine receptor (H_2) blockers such as cimetidine (Tagamet) and ranitidine (Zantac) inhibit gastric acid secretion by antagonizing histamine receptors in the gastric mucosa. These drugs are tolerated quite well and are used to treat various forms of gastrointestinal ulceration including the gastric and duodenal damage produced by aspirin and other NSAIDs.

Hence, several drugs are currently available that can be used to prevent or treat gastrointestinal damage in patients taking aspirin and other NSAIDs. These protective agents are not usually prescribed on a routine basis to every person taking aspirin-like drugs, but are typically reserved for people who exhibit symptoms of gastrointestinal irritation or who are at risk for developing ulceration while undergoing NSAID therapy.[13,26,91,101]

Other Side Effects

Aspirin and similar NSAIDs can cause other toxic side effects if used improperly or if taken by patients who have pre-existing diseases. For instance, serious hepatotoxicity is rare with normal therapeutic use, but high doses of aspirin-like drugs can produce adverse changes in hepatic function in patients with liver disease.[8,37,82] Likewise, aspirin does not seem to cause renal disease in an individual with normal kidneys,[33] but problems such as nephrotic syndrome, acute interstitial nephritis, and even acute renal failure have been observed when aspirin is given to patients with impaired renal function.[22,30,34,54,78] This occurrence is due to aspirin inhibiting the synthesis of renal prostaglandins, which serve a protective role in maintaining renal blood flow and glomerular filtration rate during various forms of renal dysfunction.[29,30,34] These protective renal prostaglandins appear to be important in sustaining adequate renal function in other situations in which renal blood flow and perfusion pressure become compromised. Consequently, aspirin and aspirin-like drugs may create problems in other conditions such as hypovolemia, shock, hepatic cirrhosis, congestive heart failure, and hypertension.[20,30,34]

In cases of aspirin overdose, a condition known as aspirin intoxication or poisoning may occur. This event is usually identified by a number of symptoms including headache, tinnitus, difficulty in hearing, confusion, and gastrointestinal distress. More severe cases also result in metabolic acidosis and dehydration, which are the life-threatening aspects of aspirin overdose. In adults, a dose of 10 to 30 g of aspirin is sometimes fatal, although much higher doses (130 g in one documented case) have been ingested without causing death.[48] Of course, much smaller doses can produce fatalities in children.

Evidence has suggested that aspirin may also be associated with a relatively rare condition known as Reye's syndrome.[24] This condition occurs in children and teenagers, usually following a bout of influenza or chickenpox. Reye's syndrome is marked by a high fever, vomiting, liver dysfunction, and increasing unresponsiveness, often progressing rapidly and leading to delirium, convulsions, coma, and possibly death. Although no definitive link between aspirin and Reye's syndrome has been established, it is generally recommended that aspirin and all other aspirin-like NSAIDs (ibuprofen, naproxen, etc.) should not be used to treat fever in children and teenagers. Non-NSAID antipyretics such as acetaminophen are not associated with Reye's syndrome, so products containing acetaminophen are preferred for treating fever in children and teenagers.[95]

There is a small group of individuals (approximately 1 percent of the general population) who exhibit aspirin intolerance or supersensitivity.[4] These patients will display allergic-like reactions including acute bronchospasm, urticaria, and severe rhinitis within a few hours after taking aspirin and aspirin-like NSAIDs.[90,94] These reactions may be quite severe in some individuals, and cardiovascular shock may occur. Consequently, the use of all NSAIDs is contraindicated in these individuals.

Finally, there is preliminary evidence from animal and in vitro studies that aspirin-like drugs may actually delay certain types of tissue healing. Aspirin and some of the other commonly used NSAIDs have been shown to inhibit the synthesis and transport of connective tissue components such as proteoglycans.[7,23,25,42,47] This finding has implications concerning the healing of cartilage, tendons, ligaments, and bone. It is unclear at the present time, however, whether aspirin-like drugs will cause a meaningful decrease in tissue healing when these drugs are used clinically in humans. Additional research will be needed to determine the extent that aspirin and other NSAIDs can affect the healing process of articular cartilage and other tissues.

COMPARISON OF ASPIRIN TO OTHER NSAIDS

A number of drugs that bear a functional similarity to aspirin have been developed during the past several decades, and a comprehensive list of currently available NSAIDs is shown in Table 15–2. These newer NSAIDs are like aspirin in that they all inhibit the cyclooxygenase enzyme and exert their primary effects by inhibiting prostaglandin and thromboxane synthesis. Although specific approved uses of individual members of this group vary, these drugs are used much in the same way as aspirin; that is, they are administered primarily for their analgesic and anti-inflammatory effects, with some members also used as antipyretic and anticoagulant agents. Dosages commonly used to achieve analgesic or anti-inflammatory effects with some of the more common NSAIDs are listed in Table 15–3.

The rationale for the development of the newer NSAIDs was twofold: to develop a drug that had greater therapeutic efficacy than aspirin but that lacked aspirin's adverse side effects. With respect to therapeutic effects, there is no clear evidence that any of the newer NSAIDs are markedly better than aspirin as anti-inflammatory analgesics.[12,40,104] The primary differences between aspirin and the newer drugs are related to the side effects and safety profile of each agent (see Table 15–2).[105] As a group, the newer drugs tend to be associated with less gastrointestinal discomfort than plain aspirin.[40] All the NSAIDs are still associated with some degree of stomach discomfort, however, and none of the newer agents is devoid of upper gastrointestinal side effects (Table 15–4). Likewise, certain NSAIDs may offer an advantage because they are less toxic to certain organs. Ibuprofen, for instance, does not affect liver function as much as aspirin,[37] and sulindac (Clinoril) is described as a renal-sparing NSAID because it does not have any appreciable effect on kidney function.[19,34] Some of the other

TABLE 15–2 Common Nonsteroidal Anti-inflammatory Drugs

Generic Name	Trade Name(s)	Specific Comments— Comparison to Other NSAIDs
Aspirin	Many trade names	Most widely used NSAID for analgesic and anti-inflammatory effects; also used frequently for antipyretic and anticoagulant effects.
Diclofenac	Voltaren	Substantially more potent than naproxen and several other NSAIDs; adverse side effects occur in 20% of patients.
Diflunisal	Dolobid	Has potency 3–4 times greater than aspirin in terms of analgesic and anti-inflammatory effects but lacks antipyretic activity.
Etodolac	Lodine	Effective as analgesic/anti-inflammatory agent with fewer side effects than most NSAIDs; may have gastric-sparing properties.
Fenoprofen	Nalfon	GI side effects fairly common but usually less intense than those occurring with similar doses of aspirin.
Flurbiprofen	Ansaid	Similar to aspirin's benefits and side effects; also available as topical ophthalmic preparation (Ocufen).
Ibuprofen	Motrin, Rufen, others	First nonaspirin NSAID also available in nonprescription form; fewer GI side effects than aspirin but GI effects still occur in 5–15% of patients.
Indomethacin	Indameth, Indocin	Relative high incidence of dose-related side effects; problems occur in 25–50% of patients.
Ketoprofen	Orudis	Similar to aspirin's benefits and side effects but has relatively short half-life (1–2 hours).
Ketorolac	Toradol	Can be administered orally or by intramuscular injection; parenteral doses provide postoperative analgesia equivalent to opioids.
Meclofenamate	Meclofen, Meclomen	No apparent advantages or disadvantages compared to aspirin and other NSAIDs.
Mefenamic acid	Ponstel	No advantages; often less effective and more toxic than aspirin and other NSAIDs.
Nabumetone	Relafen	Effective as analgesic/anti-inflammatory agent with fewer side effects than most NSAIDs.
Naproxen	Anaprox, Naprosyn	Similar to ibuprofen in terms of benefits and adverse effects.
Oxaprozin	Daypro	Analgesic and anti-inflammatory effects similar to aspirin; may produce fewer side effects than other NSAIDs.
Phenylbutazone	Butazolidin, others	Potent anti-inflammatory effects but long-term use limited by high incidence of side effects (10–45% of patients).
Piroxicam	Feldene	Long half-life (45 hours) allows once-daily dosing; may be somewhat better tolerated than aspirin.
Sulindac	Clinoril	Relatively little effect on kidneys (renal-sparing), but may produce more GI side effects than aspirin.
Tolmetin	Tolectin	Similar to aspirin's benefits and side effects but must be given frequently (QID) because of short half-life (1 hr).

TABLE 15–3 Dosages of Common Oral NSAIDs

| Classes | Dosages (According to Desired Effect) | |
	Analgesia	Anti-inflammation
Aspirin (many trade names)	325–650 mg every 4 hr	3.6–5.4 g/day in divided doses
Diclofenac (Voltaren)	—	150–200 mg/day in 2–4 divided doses
Diflunisal (Dolobid)	1 g initially; 500 mg every 8–12 hr as needed	250–500 mg BID
Fenoprofen (Nalfon)	200 mg every 4–6 hr	300–600 mg TID or QID
Flurbiprofen (Ansaid)	—	200–300 mg/day in 2–4 divided doses
Ibuprofen (Advil, Amersol, Motrin, Nuprin, Rufen)	200–400 mg every 4–6 hr as needed	1.2–3.2 g/day in 3–4 divided doses
Indomethacin (Indameth; Indocin)	—	25–50 mg 2–4 times each day initially; can be increased up to 200 mg/day as tolerated
Ketoprofen (Orudis)	50 mg every 6–8 hr	150–300 mg/day in 3–4 divided doses
Meclofenamate (Meclofen, Meclomen)	50 mg every 4–6 hr	200–400 mg/day in 3–4 divided doses
Mefenamic acid (Ponstel)	500 mg initially; 250 mg every 6 hr as needed	—
Naproxen (Naprosyn)	500 mg initially; 250 mg every 6–8 hr	250, 375, or 500 mg BID
Naproxen sodium (Anaprox)	550 mg initially; 275 mg every 6–8 hr	275 mg BID
Phenylbutazone (Butazolidin, Butazone)	—	300–600 mg/day in 3–4 divided doses initially; 100 mg 1–4 times each day for maintenance
Piroxicam (Feldene)	—	20 mg/day single dose; or 10 mg BID
Sulindac (Clinoril)	—	150 or 200 mg BID
Tolmetin (Tolectin)	—	400 mg TID initially; 600 mg–1.8 g/day in 3–4 divided doses

NSAIDs, however, may produce more serious toxic renal and hepatic effects than aspirin.[105] Hence, it cannot be generalized that the newer NSAIDs are significantly better or worse than plain aspirin in terms of either therapeutic or adverse effects.

The primary difference between aspirin and the newer NSAIDs is cost. Most of the NSAIDs still require a physician's prescription for their use. The cost of these prescription NSAIDs can be anywhere between 10 and 20 times more expensive than an equivalent supply of plain aspirin. NSAIDs that are available in nonprescription form (e.g., ibuprofen) can still cost up to five times as much as aspirin.

Consequently, the newer NSAIDs have not always been shown to be clinically superior to aspirin, but some agents may provide better effects in some patients. Considering the interpatient variability in the response to drugs, there are surely cases in which one of the newer drugs will produce better therapeutic effects than aspirin with

TABLE 15–4 Common Gastrointestinal Side Effects Associated
with the Nonaspirin NSAIDS*

Drug	Mild-to-Moderate Stomach Cramps, Pain, or Discomfort	Bloated Feeling or Gas	Heartburn or Indigestion	Nausea	Vomiting	Diarrhea	Constipation
Diclofenac	M	L	M	M	R	M	M
Diflunisal	M	L	M	M	L	M	L
Fenoprofen	L	L	M	M	M	L	M
Flurbiprofen	M	L	M	M	L	M	L
Ibuprofen	M	L	M	M	L	L	L
Indomethacin	M	R	M	M	L	L	L
Ketoprofen	M	M	H	M	L	M	M
Meclofenamate	M	M	M	H	U	H	L
Mefenamic acid	M	L	M	M	U	M	L
Naproxen	M	U	M	M	R	L	M
Phenylbutazone	M	R	L	M	R	R	R
Piroxicam	M	L	M	M	R	L	L
Sulindac	H	L	M	M	L	M	M
Tolmetin	M	M	M	H	M	M	L

*Incidence of side effects: H = high incidence (10% or greater); M = more frequent (3–9%); L = less frequent (1–3%); R = rare (<1%); U = unknown.
Source: Copied from *USP DI®, 14th Edition* Copyright 1994. The USP Convention, Inc. Permission granted. The USP is not responsible for any inaccuracy of quotation nor for any false or misleading implication that may arise due to the text used or due to the quotation of information subsequently changed in later editions.

206

fewer side effects.[12,105] If a patient responds equally well to a variety of NSAIDs, however, efforts should be made to use the NSAID that will produce adequate therapeutic effects at a minimal cost.[39]

ACETAMINOPHEN

Acetaminophen has several distinct differences from aspirin and the other NSAIDs. Acetaminophen does appear to be equal to aspirin and the other NSAIDs in terms of analgesic and antipyretic effects, but it does not have any appreciable anti-inflammatory or anticoagulant effects.[2,66,79] One major advantage of acetaminophen is that this drug is not associated with upper gastrointestinal tract irritation.[51] Consequently, acetaminophen has been used widely in the treatment of noninflammatory conditions associated with mild-to-moderate pain and in patients who have a history of gastric damage (such as ulcers). In addition, Reye's syndrome has not been implicated with acetaminophen use, so this drug is now preferentially used in treating fever in children and teenagers.[95] Acetaminophen is not a totally innocuous drug devoid of any adverse effects, however. High doses of acetaminophen (e.g., 15 g) can be especially toxic to the liver and may be fatal because of hepatic necrosis.[2] Consequently, therapeutic doses of acetaminophen are considered to be better tolerated than aspirin, but acetaminophen overdose is a serious problem.

The mechanism of action of acetaminophen is not fully understood. Acetaminophen does inhibit the cyclooxygenase enzyme, and its analgesic and antipyretic effects are probably mediated through prostaglandin inhibition. Why acetaminophen fails to exert anti-inflammatory and anticoagulant effects, however, is unclear. One explanation is that acetaminophen preferentially inhibits CNS prostaglandin production but has little effect on peripheral cyclooxygenase activity.[2,36] Thus, analgesia and antipyresis are produced by specifically limiting prostaglandin production in central pain interpretation and thermoregulatory centers, respectively. Tissue inflammation and platelet aggregation are peripheral events that would be unaffected by acetaminophen according to this theory.

PHARMACOKINETICS OF NSAIDS AND ACETAMINOPHEN

Aspirin is administered orally and is absorbed readily from the stomach and small intestine. Approximately 80 to 90 percent of aspirin remains bound to plasma proteins such as albumin. The remaining 10 to 20 percent is widely distributed throughout the body. The unbound or free drug exerts the therapeutic effects. Aspirin itself (acetylsalicylic acid) is hydrolyzed to an active metabolite, salicylic acid. This biotransformation occurs primarily in the bloodstream, and the salicylic acid is further metabolized by oxidation or conjugation in the liver. Excretion of salicylic acid and its metabolites occurs through the kidney. Although there is some pharmacokinetic variability within the nonaspirin NSAIDs, these drugs generally follow a pattern of absorption, protein binding, and metabolism/excretion similar to that of aspirin.

Acetaminophen is also absorbed rapidly and completely from the upper gastrointestinal tract. Plasma protein binding with acetaminophen is highly variable (20 to 50 percent) but is considerably less than with aspirin. Metabolism of acetaminophen occurs in the liver via conjugation with endogenous substrates, and the conjugated metabolites are excreted through the kidney. When high doses are ingested, a considerable amount of acetaminophen is converted in the liver to a highly reactive intermediate by-product known as N-acetyl-benzoquinoneimine. When present in sufficient amounts, this metabolite induces hepatic necrosis by binding to and inactivating certain liver proteins.

SPECIAL CONCERNS IN REHABILITATION PATIENTS

Aspirin and the other NSAIDs are among the most frequently used drugs in the rehabilitation population. Aside from the possibility of stomach discomfort, these drugs have a remarkable lack of adverse effects that will directly interfere with physical therapy. When used for various types of musculoskeletal pain and inflammation, these drugs can often provide analgesia without the sedation and euphoria associated with narcotic analgesics. Thus, the therapy session can be conducted with the benefit of pain relief but without the loss of patient attentiveness and concentration. In inflammatory conditions, NSAIDs can be used for prolonged periods without the serious side effects associated with the steroidal drugs (see Chapters 16 and 29). Of course, the limitation of NSAIDs is that they may not be as effective in moderate-to-severe pain or in severe, progressive inflammation. Still, these agents are a beneficial adjunct in many painful conditions and can usually help facilitate physical rehabilitation by relieving pain. The other clinical uses of these drugs (antipyresis, anticoagulation) may also be encountered in some patients, and these effects are also usually achieved with a minimum of adverse effects.

Acetaminophen is also frequently employed for pain relief in many physical therapy patients. Remember that this drug is equal to NSAIDs in analgesic properties but lacks anti-inflammatory effects. Since both aspirin and acetaminophen are available without prescription, the patient may inquire about the differences between these two drugs. The physical therapist should be able to provide an adequate explanation of the differential effects of aspirin and acetaminophen but should also remember that the suggested use of these agents should ultimately come from the physician.

CASE STUDY

NONSTEROIDAL ANTI-INFLAMMATORY DRUGS

Brief History. D.B., a 38-year-old man, began to develop pain in his right shoulder. He was employed as a carpenter and had recently been working rather long hours building a new house. The increasing pain required medical attention. The patient was evaluated by a physician, and a diagnosis of subacromial bursitis was made. The patient was also referred to physical therapy, and a program of heat, ultrasound, and exercise was initiated to help resolve this condition.

Problem/Influence of Medication. During the initial physical therapy evaluation, the therapist asked if the patient was taking any medication for the bursitis. The patient responded that he had been advised by the physician to take aspirin as needed to help relieve the pain. When asked if he had done this, the patient said that he had taken some aspirin once or twice, especially when his shoulder pain kept him awake at night. When he was asked specifically what type of aspirin he had taken, he named a commercial acetaminophen preparation. Evidently the patient was unaware of the difference between acetaminophen and aspirin (acetylsalicylate).

Decision/Solution. The therapist explained the difference between aspirin and acetaminophen to the patient, pointing out that acetaminophen lacks any significant anti-inflammatory effects. After consulting with the physician to confirm that aspirin was recommended for this patient, the therapist suggested that the patient should take the recommended dosage at regular intervals to help decrease the inflammation in the bursa, as well as to provide analgesia. The patient had taken aspirin in the past without any problem, but the therapist cautioned the patient to contact his physician if any adverse effects were noted (e.g., gastrointestinal distress or tinnitus).

SUMMARY

Aspirin and similarly acting drugs comprise a group of therapeutic agents that are usually referred to as NSAIDs. In addition to their anti-inflammatory effects, these drugs are also known for their ability to decrease mild-to-moderate pain (analgesia), alleviate fever (antipyresis), and inhibit platelet aggregation (anticoagulation). These drugs seem to exert all of their therapeutic effects by inhibiting the function of the cellular cyclooxygenase enzyme, which results in decreased prostaglandin and thromboxane synthesis. Aspirin is the prototypical NSAID, and the newer prescription and nonprescription drugs appear to be similar to aspirin in terms of pharmacologic effect and therapeutic efficacy. Acetaminophen also seems to be similar to aspirin in analgesic and antipyretic effects, but acetaminophen lacks anti-inflammatory and anticoagulant properties. These drugs are seen frequently in patients requiring physical therapy, and they usually provide beneficial effects (analgesia, decreased inflammation, etc.) without interfering with the rehabilitation program.

REFERENCES

1. Allison, MC, et al: Gastrointestinal damage associated with the use of nonsteroidal anti-inflammatory drugs. N Engl J Med 327:749, 1992.
2. Ameer, B and Greenblatt, DJ: Acetaminophen. Ann Intern Med 87:202, 1977.
3. Antiplatelet Trialists' Collaboration: Secondary prevention of vascular disease by prolonged antiplatelet treatment. Br Med J 296:320, 1988.
4. Asad, SI, et al: Effect of aspirin in "aspirin sensitive" patients. Br Med J 288:745, 1984.
5. Austen, KF: The role of arachadonic acid metabolites in local and systemic inflammatory processes. Drug 33(suppl 1):10, 1987.
6. Bakhle, YS: Synthesis and catabolism of cyclo-oxygenase products. Br Med Bull 39:214, 1983.
7. Bassleer, C, Henrotin, Y, and Franchimnot, P: Effects of sodium naproxen on differentiated human chondrocytes cultivated in clusters. Clin Rheumatol 11:60, 1992.
8. Benson, GD: Hepatotoxicity following the therapeutic use of antipyretic analgesics. Am J Med 75(suppl 5A):85, 1983.
9. Bland, JH: The reversibility of osteoarthritis: A review. Am J Med 74(suppl 6A):16, 1983.
10. Born, GVR, Gorog, P, and Begent, NA: The biologic background to some therapeutic uses of aspirin. Am J Med 74(suppl 6A):2, 1983.
11. Bray, ME: The pharmacology and pathophysiology of leukotriene B_4. Br Med Bull 39:249, 1983.

12. Brooks, PM and Day, RO: Drug therapy: Nonsteroidal anti-inflammatory drugs—differences and similarities. N Engl J Med 324:1716, 1991.
13. Brooks, PM and Yeomans, ND: Nonsteroidal anti-inflammatory drug gastropathy: Is it preventable? Australian New Zealand J Med 22:685, 1992.
14. Campbell, WB: Lipid-derived autacoids: Eicosanoids and platelet-activating factors. In Gilman, AG, et al (eds): The Pharmacological Basis of Therapeutics, ed 8. Pergamon Press, New York, 1990.
15. Cashman, JN: Non-steroidal anti-inflammatory drugs versus postoperative pain. J Royal Soc Med 86:464, 1993.
16. Cataldo, PA, Senagore, AJ, and Kilbride, MJ: Ketorolac and patient controlled analgesia in the treatment of postoperative pain. Surg Gynecol Obstet 176:435, 1993.
17. Chan, PS and Cervoni, P: Prostaglandins, prostacyclin, and thromboxane in cardiovascular disease. Drug Dev Res 7:341, 1986.
18. Chan, WY: Prostaglandins and nonsteroidal anti-inflammatory drugs in dysmenorrhea. Annu Rev Pharmacol Toxicol 23:131, 1983.
19. Ciabattoni, G, et al: Effects of sulindac on renal and extrarenal eicosanoid synthesis. Clin Pharmacol Ther 41:380, 1987.
20. Ciccone, CD and Zambraski, EJ: Effects of prostaglandin inhibition on renal function in deoxycorticosterone-acetate hypertensive yucatan miniature swine. Prostaglandins Med 7:395, 1981.
21. Clissold, SP: Aspirin and related derivatives of salicylic acid. Drugs 32(suppl 4):8, 1986.
22. Clive, DM and Stoff, JS: Renal syndromes associated with nonsteroidal antiinflammatory drugs. N Engl J Med 310:563, 1984.
23. Collier, S and Ghosh, P: Comparison of the effects of NSAIDs on proteoglycan synthesis by articular cartilage explant and chondrocyte monolayer cultures. Biochem Pharmacol 41:1375, 1991.
24. Committee on Infectious Diseases: Aspirin and Reye's syndrome. Pediatrics 69:810, 1982.
25. David, MJ, et al: Effects of NSAIDs on glycosyltransferase activity from human osteoarthritic cartilage. Br J Rheumatol 31(suppl 1):13, 1992.
26. Day, RO, et al: Non-steroidal anti-inflammatory drug induced upper gastrointestinal haemorrhage and bleeding. Med J Aust 157:810, 1992.
27. Deandrade, JR, et al: The use of ketorolac in the management of postoperative pain. Orthopedics 17:157, 1994.
28. Done, AK: Treatment of fever in 1982: A review. Am J Med 74(suppl 6A):27, 1983.
29. Dunn, M: The role of arachadonic acid metabolites in renal hemostasis. Drugs 33(suppl 1):56, 1987.
30. Dunn, MJ: Nonsteroidal antiinflammatory drugs and renal function. Annu Rev Med 35:411, 1984.
31. Dusting, GJ, Moncada, S, and Vane, JR: Prostaglandins, their intermediates and precursors, their cardiovascular actions and regulatory roles in normal and abnormal circulatory systems. Prog Cardiovasc Dis 21:405, 1979.
32. Dutch TIA Trial Study Group: A comparison of two doses of aspirin (30 mg vs. 283 mg a day) in patients after a transient ischemic attack or minor ischemic stroke. N Engl J Med 325:1261, 1991.
33. Emkey, RD: Aspirin and renal disease. Am J Med 74(suppl 6A):97, 1983.
34. Eriksson, L-O, Beerman, B, and Kallner, M: Renal function and tubular transport effects of sulindac and naproxen in congestive heart failure. Clin Pharmacol Ther 42:646, 1987.
35. Fields, WS: Aspirin for prevention of stroke: A review. Am J Med 74(suppl 6A):61, 1983.
36. Flower, RJ and Vane, JR: Inhibition of prostaglandin synthetase in brain explains the anti-pyretic action of paracetamol (4-acetamidophenol). Nature 240:410, 1972.
37. Freeland, GR, et al: Hepatic safety of two analgesics used over the counter: Ibuprofen and aspirin. Clin Pharmacol Ther 43:473, 1988.
38. Fretland, DJ: Review: Potential role of prostaglandins and leukotrienes in multiple sclerosis and experimental allergic encephalomyelitis. Prostaglandins Leukotrienes Essential Fatty Acids 45:249, 1992.
39. Greene, JM and Winickoff, RN: Cost-conscious prescribing of nonsteroidal anti-inflammatory drugs for adults with arthritis: A review and suggestions. Arch Intern Med 152:1995, 1992.
40. Hart, FD and Huskisson, EC: Non-steroidal anti-inflammatory drugs: Current status and rational therapeutic use. Drugs 27:232, 1984.
41. Hecker, M, Foegh, ML, and Ramwell, PW: The eicosanoids: Prostaglandins, thromboxanes, leukotrienes, and related compounds. In Katzung, BG (ed): Basic and Clinical Pharmacology, ed 5. Appleton & Lange, Norwalk, CT, 1992.
42. Henrotin, Y, Bassleer, C, and Franchimont, P: In vitro effects of etodolac and acetylsalicylic acid on human chondrocyte metabolism. Agents Actions 36:317, 1992.
43. Higgs, GA, et al: The effect of non-steroid anti-inflammatory drugs on leukocyte migration in carrageenin-induced inflammation. Eur J Pharmacol 66:81, 1980.
44. Higgs, GA and Vane, JR: Inhibition of cyclo-oxygenase and lipoxygenase. Br Med Bull 39:265, 1983.
45. Hochberg, MC: Association of nonsteroidal anti-inflammatory drugs with upper gastrointestinal disease: Epidemiologic and economic considerations. J Rheumatol 19(suppl 36):63, 1992.
46. Hollingworth, P: Paediatric rheumatology review: The use of nonsteroidal anti-inflammatory drugs in paediatric rheumatic diseases. Br J Rheumatology 32:73, 1993.
47. Hugenberg, ST, Brandt, KD, and Cole, CA. Effects of sodium salicylate, aspirin, and ibuprofen on enzymes required by the chondrocyte for synthesis of chondrotin sulfate. J Rheumatol 29:2128, 1993.

48. Insel, P: Analgesic-antipyretics and anti-inflammatory agents; drugs employed in the treatment of rheumatoid arthritis and gout. In Gilman, AG, et al (eds): The Pharmacologic Basis of Therapeutics, ed 8. Pergamon Press, New York, 1990.

49. Israel, E, Dermarkarian, R, and Rosenberg, M: The effect of a 5-lipoxygenase inhibitor on asthma induced by cold, dry air. N Engl J Med 323:1740, 1990.

50. Ivey, KJ: Gastrointestinal intolerance and bleeding with non-narcotic analgesics. Drugs 32(suppl 4): 71, 1986.

51. Ivey, KJ: Gastrointestinal effects of antipyretic analgesics. Am J Med 75(suppl 5A):53, 1983.

52. Kantor, TG: Summary: Ibuprofen—past, present and future. Am J Med 77(suppl 1A):121, 1984.

53. Kimmey, MB: NSAID, ulcers, and prostaglandins. J Rheumatol 19(suppl 36):68, 1992.

54. Kincaid-Smith, P: Effects of non-narcotic analgesics on the kidney. Drugs 32(suppl 4):109, 1986.

55. Knapp, HR: Reduced allergen-induced nasal congestion and leukotriene synthesis with an orally active 5-lipoxygenase inhibitor. N Engl J Med 323:1745, 1990.

56. Larsen, GL and Henson, PM: Mediators of inflammation. Annu Rev Immunol 1:335, 1983.

57. Lasagna, L and McMahon, FG: Introduction: Aspirin's infinite variety. Am J Med 74(suppl 6A):1, 1983.

58. Lewis, HD, et al: Protective effects of aspirin against acute myocardial infarction and death in men with unstable angina. N Engl J Med 309:396, 1983.

59. Lewis, RA, Austen, KF, and Soberman, RJ: Mechanisms of disease: Leukotrienes and other products of the 5-lipoxygenase pathway—biochemistry and relation to pathophysiology in human diseases. N Engl J Med 323:645, 1990.

60. Logan, RFA, et al: Effect of aspirin and non-steroidal anti-inflammatory drugs on colorectal adenomas: Case-control study of subjects participating in the Nottingham faecal occult blood screening programme. Br Med J 307:285, 1993.

61. Lysak, SZ, et al: Postoperative effects of fentanyl, ketorolac, and piroxicam as analgesics for outpatient laparoscopic procedures. Obstetr Gynecol 83:270, 1994.

62. Malmsten, CL: Prostaglandins, thromboxanes and leukotrienes in inflammation. Am J Med 80(suppl 4B):11, 1986.

63. Manning, PJ, et al: Inhibition of exercise-induced bronchoconstriction by MK-571, a potent leukotriene D_4-receptor antagonist. N Engl J Med 323:1736, 1990.

64. Marcus, AJ: Aspirin as an anti-thrombotic medication. N Engl J Med 309:1515, 1983.

65. McGuire, DA, Sanders, K, and Hendricks, SD: Comparison of ketorolac and opioid analgesics in postoperative ACL reconstruction outpatient pain control. Arthroscopy 9:653, 1993.

66. Mehlisch, DR: Review of the comparative analgesic efficacy of salicylates, acetaminophen and pyrazolones. Am J Med 75(suppl 5A):47, 1983.

67. Mense, S: Basic neurobiologic mechanisms of pain and analgesia. Am J Med 75(suppl 5A):4, 1983.

68. Mielke, CH: Influence of aspirin on platelets and the bleeding time. Am J Med 74(suppl 6A):72, 1983.

69. Milton, AS: Prostaglandins in fever and the mode of action of antipyretic drugs. In Milton, AS (ed): Handbook of Experimental Pharmacology, Vol 60, Pyretics and Antipyretics. Springer-Verlag, Berlin, 1982.

70. Moncada, S and Vane, JR: Pharmacology and endogenous roles of prostaglandin endoperoxides, thromboxane A_2 and prostacyclin. Pharmacol Rev 30:293, 1979.

71. Mustard, JF, Kinlough-Rathbone, RL, and Packham, MA: Aspirin in the treatment of cardiovascular disease: A review. Am J Med 74(suppl 6A):43, 1983.

72. Nissen, I, Jensen, KA, and Ohrstrom, JK: Indomethacin in the management of postoperative pain. Br J Anaesth 69:304, 1992.

73. O'Hara, DA, et al: Ketorolac tromethamine as compared with morphine sulfate for treatment of postoperative pain. Clin Pharmacol Ther 41:556, 1987.

74. Owen, PR: Prostaglandin synthetase inhibitors in the treatment of primary dysmenorrhea. Am J Obstet Gynecol 148:96, 1984.

75. Pace-Asciak, C, and Granstrom, E (eds): New Comprehensive Biochemistry, Vol 5, Prostaglandins and Related Substances. Elsevier, New York, 1983.

76. Payan, DG: Nonsteroidal anti-inflammatory drugs; nonopioid analgesics; drugs used in gout. In Katzung, BG (ed): Basic and Clinical Pharmacology, ed 5. Appleton & Lange, Norwalk, CT, 1992.

77. Pedersen, P, Nielsen, KD, and Jensen, PE: The efficacy of Na^+-naproxen after diagnostic and therapeutic arthroscopy of the knee joint. Arthroscopy 9:170, 1993.

78. Perazella, MA and Buller, GK: NSAID nephrotoxicity revisited: Acute renal failure due to parenteral ketorolac. South Med J 86:1421, 1993.

79. Peters, BH, Fraim, CJ, and Masel, BE: Comparison of 650 mg aspirin and 1000 mg acetaminophen with each other, and with placebo in moderately severe headache. Am J Med 74(suppl 6A):36, 1983.

80. Pincus, T, et al: Longterm drug therapy for rheumatoid arthritis in seven rheumatology private practices. 1. Nonsteroidal anti-inflammatory drugs. J Rheumatol 19:1874, 1992.

81. Piper, PJ: Pharmacology of leukotrienes. Br Med Bull 39:255, 1983.

82. Prescott, LF: Effects of non-narcotic analgesics on the liver. Drugs 32(suppl 4):129, 1986.

83. Rasmussen, S, et al: The clinical effect of naproxen sodium after arthroscopy of the knee: A randomized, double-blind, prospective study. Arthroscopy 9:375, 1993.

84. Redden, RJ: Ketorolac tromethamine: An oral injectable nonsteroidal anti-inflammatory for postoperative pain control. J Oral Maxillofac Surgery 50:1310, 1992.

85. Robinson, DR: Prostaglandins and the mechanism of action of anti-inflammatory drugs. Am J Med 75(suppl 4B):26, 1983.
86. Samuelsson, B: An elucidation of the arachadonic acid cascade. Discovery of prostaglandins, thromboxane and leukotrienes. Drugs 33(suppl 1):2, 1987.
87. Samuelsson, B: Leukotrienes: Mediators of immediate hypersensitivity reactions and inflammation. Science 220:568, 1983.
88. Samuelsson, B, et al: Prostaglandins and thromboxanes. Annu Rev Biochem 47:997, 1978.
89. Savage, RL, et al: Variations in the risk of peptic ulcer complications with nonsteroidal antiinflammatory drug therapy. Arthritis Rheum 36:84, 1993.
90. Settipane, GA: Aspirin and allergic diseases: A review. Am J Med 74(suppl 6A):102, 1983.
91. Stalnikowicz, R and Rachmilewitz, D: NSAID-induced gastroduodenal damage: Is prevention needed. A review and meta-analysis. J Clin Gastroenterol 17:238, 1993.
92. Steering Committee of the Physicians' Health Study Research Group: Final report on the aspirin component of the ongoing physicians' health study. N Engl J Med 321:129, 1989.
93. Suh, O, Mettlin, C, and Petrelli, NJ: Aspirin use, cancer, and polyps of the large bowel. Cancer 72:1171, 1993.
94. Szczeklik, A: Antipyretic analgesics and the allergic patient. Am J Med 75(suppl 5A):82, 1983.
95. Temple, AR: Review of comparative antipyretic activity in children. Am J Med 75(suppl 5A):38, 1983.
96. Thun, MJ, et al: Aspirin use and risk of fatal cancer. Cancer Res 53:1322, 1993.
97. Thun, MJ, Namboodiri, M, and Heath, C: Aspirin use and reduced risk of fatal colon cancer. N Engl J Med 325:1593, 1991.
98. Turner, D and Berkel, HJ: Nonsteroidal anti-inflammatory drugs for the prevention of colon cancer. Can Med Assoc J 149:595, 1993.
99. Vane, J: The evolution of non-steroidal anti-inflammatory drugs and their mechanisms of action. Drugs 33(suppl 1):18, 1987.
100. Vane, JR: Inhibition of prostaglandin synthetase as a mechanism of action for aspirin-like drugs. Nature 231:232, 1971.
101. Walt, RP: Drug therapy: Misoprostol for the treatment of peptic ulcer and antiinflammatory drug-induced gastroduodenal ulceration. N Engl J Med 327:1575, 1992.
102. Weller, JM: Medical modifiers of sports injury: The use of nonsteroidal anti-inflammatory drugs (NSAIDs) in sports soft-tissue injury. Clin Sports Med 11:625, 1992.
103. Whittle, BJR and Moncada, S: Pharmacological interactions between prostacyclin and thromboxanes. Br Med Bull 39:232, 1983.
104. Willard, JE, Lange, RA, and Hillis, LD: Current concepts: The use of aspirin in ischemic heart disease. N Engl J Med 327:175, 1992.
105. Willkens, RF: The selection of a nonsteroidal antiinflammatory drug: Is there a difference? J Rheumatol 19(suppl 36):9, 1992.
106. Yee, JT, et al. Analgesia from intramuscular ketorolac tromethamine compared to morphine in severe pain following major surgery. Pharmacotherapy 6:253, 1986.

CHAPTER 16

Pharmacologic Management of Rheumatoid Arthritis and Osteoarthritis

Rheumatoid arthritis and osteoarthritis represent the two primary pathologic conditions that affect joints and periarticular structures. Although the causes underlying these conditions are quite different from one another, both conditions can cause severe pain and deformity in various joints in the body. Likewise, pharmacologic management plays an important role in the treatment of each disorder. Since physical therapists and other rehabilitation specialists often work with patients who have rheumatoid arthritis or osteoarthritis, an understanding of the types of drugs used to treat these diseases is important.

This chapter will begin by describing the etiology of rheumatoid joint disease and the pharmacologic treatment of rheumatoid arthritis. An analogous discussion of osteoarthritis will follow. These descriptions will hopefully provide rehabilitation specialists with an understanding of the role of drug therapy in arthritis and how drug therapy can impact on physical therapy and occupational therapy.

RHEUMATOID ARTHRITIS

Rheumatoid arthritis is a chronic, systemic disorder that affects many different tissues in the body but is characterized primarily by synovitis and the destruction of articular tissue.[53,82,100] This disease is associated with pain, stiffness, and inflammation in the small synovial joints of the hands and feet, as well as in larger joints such as the knee. Although marked by periods of exacerbation and remission, rheumatoid arthritis is often progressive in nature, with advanced stages leading to severe joint destruction and bone erosion.

Specific criteria for the diagnosis of rheumatoid arthritis in adults are listed in Table 16–1. In addition to the adult form of this disease, there is also a form of arthritis that occurs in children (i.e., juvenile rheumatoid arthritis). Juvenile rheumatoid arthri-

TABLE 16–1 Criteria for the Classification of Rheumatoid Arthritis*

Criterion	Definition
1. Morning stiffness	Morning stiffness in and around the joints, lasting at least 1 hr before maximal improvement.
2. Arthritis of 3 or more joint areas	At least 3 joint areas simultaneously have had soft tissue swelling or fluid (not bony overgrowth alone) observed by a physician. The 14 possible areas are right or left PIP, MCP, wrist, elbow, knee, ankle, and MTP joints.†
3. Arthritis of hand joints	At least 1 area swollen (as defined above) in a wrist, MCP, or PIP joint.
4. Symmetric arthritis	Simultaneous involvement of the same joint areas (as defined in 2) on both sides of the body (bilateral involvement of PIPs, MCPs, or MTPs is acceptable without absolute symmetry).
5. Rheumatoid nodules	Subcutaneous nodules over bony prominences or extensor surfaces, or in juxtaarticular regions, observed by a physician.
6. Serum rheumatoid factor	Demonstration of abnormal amounts of serum rheumatoid factor by any method for which the result has been positive in <5% of normal control subjects.
7. Radiographic changes	Radiographic changes typical of rheumatoid arthritis on posteroanterior hand and wrist radiographs, which must include erosions or unequivocal bony decalcification localized in or most marked adjacent to the involved joints (osteoarthritis changes alone do not qualify).

*For classification purposes, a patient shall be said to have rheumatoid arthritis if he or she has satisfied at least 4 of these 7 criteria. Criteria 1 through 4 must have been present for at least 6 weeks.
†PIP = proximal interphalangeal; MCP = metacarpophalangeal; MTP = metatarsophalangeal.
Source: Arnett, et al: The American Rheumatism Association 1987 Revised Criteria for the Classification of Rheumatoid Arthritis. Arthritis and Rheumatism 31:315–324, 1988. Reprinted from ARTHRITIS AND RHEUMATISM Journal, copyright 1988. Used by permission of the American College of Rheumatology.

tis differs from the adult form of this disease, with the age of onset (younger than 16 years) and other criteria helping to differentiate these two types of rheumatoid joint disease. The drug treatment of adult and juvenile rheumatoid arthritis is fairly similar, however, with the exception that some drugs (e.g., corticosteroids) are used more cautiously in children.[91] Consequently, in this chapter most of the discussion of the management of rheumatoid arthritis is directed toward the adult form of this disease.

Rheumatoid arthritis affects about 1.0 percent of the population worldwide.[61] This disease occurs three times more often in women than in men, with women between the ages of 20 and 40 being especially susceptible to the onset of rheumatoid joint disease.[30,53,82] Rheumatoid arthritis often causes severe pain and suffering, frequently devastating the patient's family and social life as well as his or her job situation.[61,63] The economic impact of this disease is also staggering, with the medical costs and loss of productivity exceeding $1 billion annually in the United States.[63] Consequently, rheumatoid arthritis is a formidable and serious problem in contemporary health care.

Immune Basis for Rheumatoid Arthritis

The initiating factors in rheumatoid arthritis are not known. It is apparent, however, that the underlying basis of this disease consists of some type of autoimmune response in genetically susceptible individuals.[38,39,70,82,100] Some precipitating factor (possibly a virus or other infectious agent) appears to initiate the formation of antibodies that are later recognized by the host as antigens.[82] Subsequent formation of new antibodies to these antigens then initiates a complex chain of events involving a variety of immune system components such as mononuclear phagocytes, T lymphocytes, and B lymphocytes.[28,53] These cells basically interact with each other to produce a number of arthritogenic mediators including cytokines (interleukins, growth factors), eicosanoids (prostaglandins, leukotrienes), and destructive enzymes (proteases, collagenases).[26,27,38,56] These substances act either directly or through other cellular components of the immune system to induce synovial cell proliferation and destruction of articular cartilage and bone.[53,82] Thus, the joint destruction in rheumatoid arthritis is the culmination of a series of events that result from an inherent defect in the immune response in patients with this disease.[38,53,100]

Overview of Drug Therapy in Rheumatoid Arthritis

The drug treatment of rheumatoid arthritis has two goals: (1) to decrease joint inflammation and (2) to arrest the progression of this disease. Three general categories of drugs are available to accomplish these goals: (1) nonsteroidal anti-inflammatory drugs (NSAIDs), (2) corticosteroids, and (3) a diverse group of agents known as *disease-modifying antirheumatic drugs* (DMARDs) (Table 16–2). The NSAIDs and corticosteroids are used primarily to decrease joint inflammation, but these agents do not halt the active progression of rheumatoid arthritis. The DMARDs attempt to slow or halt

TABLE 16–2 Drug Categories Used in Rheumatoid Arthritis

I. Nonsteroidal Anti-Inflammatory Drugs

Aspirin (many trade names)	Meclofenamate (Meclofen, Meclomen)
Diclofenac (Voltaren)	Nabumetone (Relafen)
Diflunisal (Dolobid)	Naproxen (Anaprox, Naprosyn)
Etodolac (Lodine)	Oxaprozin (Daypro)
Fenoprofen (Nalfon)	Phenylbutazone (Butazolidin)
Flurbiprofen (Ansaid)	Piroxicam (Feldene)
Ibuprofen (many trade names)	Sulindac (Clinoril)
Indomethacin (Indameth, Indocin)	Tolmetin (Tolectin)
Ketoprofen (Orudis)	

II. Corticosteroids

Betamethasone (Celestone)	Paramethasone (Haldrone)
Cortisone (Cortone acetate)	Prednisolone (Hydeltrasol, others)
Dexamethasone (Decadron)	Prednisone (Deltasone, others)
Hydrocortisone (Cortef, others)	Triamcinolone (Aristocort)
Methylprednisolone (Medrol, others)	

III. Disease-Modifying Antirheumatic Drugs

Auranofin (Ridaura)	Gold sodium thiomalate (Myochrysine)
Aurothioglucose (Solganal)	Hydroxychloroquine (Plaquenil)
Azathioprine (Imuran)	Methotrexate (Rheumatrex)
Chloroquine (Aralen)	Penicillamine (Cuprimine, Depen)

the advancement of this disease, usually by interfering with the immune response that seems to be the primary underlying factor in rheumatoid arthritis. Each of these major drug categories as well as specific disease-modifying drugs is discussed in the following sections of this chapter.

Nonsteroidal Anti-Inflammatory Drugs

Aspirin and the other NSAIDs are usually considered the first line of defense in treating rheumatoid arthritis.[2,4,68,77,84] Although NSAIDs are not as powerful in reducing inflammation as corticosteroids, they are associated with fewer serious side effects, and they offer the added advantage of analgesia. Consequently, NSAIDs such as aspirin are often the first drugs employed in treating rheumatoid arthritis; in fact, this disease can often be controlled adequately for extended periods in some patients solely by the use of an NSAID.[75] In patients who continue to experience progressive joint destruction despite NSAID therapy, these drugs are often combined with one of the disease-modifying agents discussed in their respective sections of this chapter. Usually, it is not advisable to use two different NSAIDs simultaneously because there is an increased risk of side effects without any appreciable increase in therapeutic efficacy. Some amount of trial and error may be involved in selecting the best NSAID, and several agents may have to be given in succession before an optimal drug is found for that patient. As discussed in Chapter 15, aspirin appears to approximately equal the newer, more expensive NSAIDs in terms of anti-inflammatory and analgesic effects, but some of the newer drugs may produce less gastrointestinal discomfort.[40,68] The choice of a specific NSAID ultimately depends on each individual patient's response to the therapeutic effects and side effects of any given agent.[15,99]

MECHANISM OF ACTION

The pharmacology of the NSAIDs was discussed in Chapter 15. Basically, aspirin and the other NSAIDs appear to exert most or all of their anti-inflammatory and analgesic effects by inhibiting the synthesis of prostaglandins.[49,78,89] Certain prostaglandins (i.e., prostaglandin E_2 [PGE_2]) are believed to participate in the inflammatory response by increasing local blood flow and vascular permeability, and exerting a chemotactic effect on leukocytes.[15,67] Prostaglandins are also believed to sensitize pain receptors to the nociceptive effects of other pain mediators such as bradykinin.[66] NSAIDs prevent the production of all types of prostaglandins by inhibiting the cyclooxygenase enzyme that initiates their synthesis. The effect of NSAIDs on prostaglandin biosynthesis is discussed in more detail in Chapter 15.

ADVERSE SIDE EFFECTS

The problems and adverse effects of aspirin and other NSAIDs are discussed in Chapter 15. The most common problem with chronic use of NSAIDs is stomach irritation, which can lead to gastric ulceration and hemorrhage. This can be resolved to some extent by taking aspirin in an enteric-coated form so that release of the aspirin is delayed until the drug reaches the small intestine. Other pharmacologic interventions such as prostaglandin analogs and specific histamine receptor (H_2) blockers can also be used if gastropathy continues to be a limiting factor during NSAID use (see Chapter

15). Chronic NSAID use can also produce other problems such as liver toxicity and impaired renal function, especially in the elderly or debilitated patient. Still, aspirin and the other NSAIDs remain one of the mainstays in treating rheumatoid arthritis and are often used for extended periods without major adverse effects.

Corticosteroids

Corticosteroids such as prednisone are extremely effective anti-inflammatory agents, but they are associated with a number of serious side effects (see "Adverse Side Effects"). Likewise, corticosteroids are similar to NSAIDs in that they may decrease the inflammatory symptoms of rheumatoid arthritis, but they do not halt the progression of this disease. Their current use in rheumatoid arthritis is typically reserved for patients whose disease is uncontrolled by NSAIDs and who need relief from the symptoms associated with an acute exacerbation of this disease. In particular, the judicious short-term use of systemic (oral) corticosteroids can serve as a bridge between an acute flare-up of rheumatoid joint disease and successful management by other drugs such as the disease-modifying agents.[19] Corticosteroids can also be injected directly into the arthritic joint, a technique that can be invaluable in the management of acute exacerbations. There is, of course, considerable controversy about whether intra-articular corticosteroids will produce harmful catabolic effects in joints that are already weakened by arthritic changes. At the very least, the number of injections into an arthritic joint should be limited, and a common rule of thumb is to not exceed more than four injections into one joint within 1 year.[77] Consequently, corticosteroids play an important but limited role in managing rheumatoid arthritis. The extended or excessive use of these agents is not advisable, and attempts are usually made to substitute NSAIDs and disease-modifying agents as soon as possible.

MECHANISM OF ACTION

The details of the cellular effects of steroids are discussed in Chapter 29. These drugs exert some of their anti-inflammatory effects by bringing about a decrease in the synthesis of prostaglandins and leukotrienes. **Glucocorticoids** appear to promote the synthesis of a protein that inhibits the function of the phospholipase A_2 enzyme.[10,45,89] This enzyme liberates fatty acid precursors for prostaglandin and leukotriene biosynthesis, and inhibition of its function results in decreased formation of these pro-inflammatory compounds.[12] NSAIDs only inhibit prostaglandin production, whereas corticosteroids inhibit leukotriene synthesis as well. This may help explain the superior efficacy of corticosteroids in treating inflammation.[44] Corticosteroids also have immunosuppressive properties and have been shown to inhibit the migration of monocytes and neutrophils toward a site of injury.[42] This undoubtedly contributes to their anti-inflammatory effect and subsequently to their ability to treat rheumatoid arthritis.

ADVERSE SIDE EFFECTS

The side effects of corticosteroids are numerous (see Chapter 29). These drugs exert a general catabolic effect on all types of supportive tissue (i.e., muscle, tendon, bone). Osteoporosis is a particularly important problem in the arthritic patient, since many of these patients have significant bone loss before even beginning steroid therapy. Corticosteroids have been known to increase bone loss in patients with arthritis, even when these drugs are used in fairly low doses.[19,77] Corticosteroids may also cause muscle wasting and weakness, as well as hypertension, aggravation of diabetes mellitus, glaucoma, and cataracts.[19] These side effects emphasize the need to limit corticosteroid therapy as much as possible when dealing with the patient with arthritis.

Disease-Modifying Antirheumatic Drugs

The fact that NSAIDs and glucocorticoids do not slow the progression of rheumatoid arthritis has generated a great deal of interest in finding drugs that can alter the progressive nature of this disease. An eclectic group of agents has been identified as being able to arrest, or even reverse, the pathologic changes in some patients with rheumatoid arthritis. These drugs, commonly referred to as DMARDs, are also referred to as slow-acting antirheumatic drugs (SAARDs) to emphasize that a delay of several weeks to several months often occurs between the onset of drug therapy and the onset of clinical benefits.[14] The disease-modifying terminology seems to be somewhat more common, so the DMARD acronym will be used here.

Disease-modifying agents currently used in treating rheumatoid arthritis are listed in Table 16–3. As the name implies, DMARDs attempt to induce remission by modifying the pathologic process inherent to rheumatoid arthritis. In general, DMARDs inhibit the immune response thought to be underlying rheumatoid disease. Most of these drugs inhibit the function of monocytes and T and B lymphocytes that are responsible for perpetuating joint inflammation and destruction.[41] However, the exact mechanism of action of these drugs in controlling rheumatoid arthritis is often poorly understood (see later in this chapter).

Hence, disease-modifying drugs are typically used to control synovitis and erosive changes during the active stages of rheumatoid joint disease.[77,84] There is still considerable concern, however, over the safety and efficacy of DMARDs. These drugs are often ineffective in halting disease progression in some patients, and many DMARDs can produce serious side effects.[18,48,84] Despite these limitations, there has been a definite trend both to use DMARDs more frequently and to use these drugs earlier in the course of rheumatoid arthritis before excessive joint destruction has occurred.[64] The pharmacology of specific DMARDs is discussed here.

ANTIMALARIAL DRUGS

Originally used in the treatment of malaria, the drugs chloroquine (Aralen) and hydroxychloroquine (Plaquenil) have also been found to be effective in treating rheumatoid arthritis. In the past, these drugs have been used reluctantly because of the fear of retinal toxicity (see "Adverse Side Effects").[80] There is now evidence, however, that these agents can be used safely and effectively, and some clinicians feel that these drugs should be considered as a reasonable first choice when selecting a disease-modifying drug.[1,7,32,59,79]

Mechanism of Action. Antimalarials exert a number of effects, although it is unclear exactly which of these contribute to their ability to halt the progression in rheumatoid disease. These drugs are known to increase pH within certain intracellular vacuoles in macrophages and other immune-system cells.[31] This effect is believed to disrupt the ability of these cells to process antigenic proteins and present these anti-

TABLE 16–3 Disease-Modifying Antirheumatic Drugs

Drug	Trade Name	Usual Dosage	Special Considerations
Antimalarials Chloroquine	Aralen	Oral: Up to 4 mg/kg of lean body weight per day.	Periodic ophthalmic exams recommended to check for retinal toxicity.
Hydroxychloroquine	Plaquenil	Oral: Up to 6.5 mg/kg of lean body weight per day.	Similar to chloroquine.
Azathioprine	Imuran	Oral: 1 mg/kg body weight per day; can be increased after 6–8 wk up to maximum dose of 2.5 mg/kg body weight.	Relatively high toxicity; should be used cautiously in debilitated patients or patients with renal disease.
Gold compounds Auranofin	Ridaura	Oral: 6 mg one each day or 3 mg BID.*	May have a long latency (6–9 mo) before onset of benefits.
Aurothioglucose	Solganal	Intramuscular: 10 mg the 1st wk, 25 mg the 2nd and 3rd wk, then 25–50 mg each wk until total dose of 1 g. Maintenance doses of 25–50 mg every 2–4 wk can follow.	Effects occur somewhat sooner than oral gold, but still has long delay (4 mo).
Gold sodium thiomalate	Myochrysine	Similar to aurothioglucose.	Similar to aurothioglucose.
Methotrexate	Rheumatrex	Oral: 2.5–5 mg every 12 hr for total of 3 doses/wk or 10 mg once each week. Can be increased up to a maximum of 20–25 mg/wk.	Often effective in halting joint destruction, but long-term use limited by toxicity.
Penicillamine	Cuprimine, Depen	Oral: 125 or 250 mg one each day; can be increased to a maximum of 1.5 g/day.	Relatively high incidence of toxicity with long-term use.

gens to T cells.[81] Decreased T-cell stimulation results in immunosuppression and attenuation of the arthritic response.[31] Antimalarials have also been shown to stabilize lysosomal membranes and impair DNA and RNA synthesis, although the significance of these effects in their role as antiarthritics remains unclear.[58,59]

Adverse Side Effects. Chloroquine and hydroxychloroquine are usually considered the safest DMARDs.[32] The major concern with antimalarial use is that high doses of these drugs can produce irreversible retinal damage. Retinal toxicity is rare, however, when daily dosages are maintained below the levels typically used to treat rheumatoid arthritis (i.e., less than 3.5 to 4.0 mg/kg per day for chloroquine, less than 6.0 to 6.5 mg/kg per day for hydroxychloroquine).[60] Frequent ocular exams should be scheduled, however, to ensure the safe and effective use of these drugs during prolonged administration.[8] Other side effects such as headache and gastrointestinal distress can occur, but these are relatively infrequent and usually transient.

AZATHIOPRINE

Azathioprine (Imuran) is an immunosuppressant drug that is often used to prevent tissue rejection following organ transplants. Because of its immunosuppressant properties, this drug has been employed in treating cases of severe, active rheumatoid arthritis that have not responded to other agents.

Mechanism of Action. The mechanism of action of azathioprine is not known. This drug has been shown to impair the synthesis of DNA and RNA precursors, but it is unclear exactly how (or if) this is related to its immunosuppressant effects. Azathioprine can inhibit immune responses mediated by T cells and other immunocompetent cells, but the pharmacologic mechanism of these effects is not know.[84]

Adverse Side Effects. Azathioprine is relatively toxic compared to other DMARDs.[14,32] The primary side effects include fever, chills, sore throat, fatigue, loss of appetite, and nausea or vomiting; these effects often limit the use of this drug as an antiarthritic.

GOLD THERAPY

Compounds containing elemental gold were among the first drugs identified as DMARDs (Fig. 16–1). Specific compounds such as aurothioglucose (Solganal) and gold sodium thiomalate (Myochrysine) have been used in the past and are usually administered by intramuscular injection. An orally active gold compound, auranofin (Ridaura), has also been developed and offers the advantage of oral administration.[20] Auranofin is also somewhat better tolerated than parenteral gold compounds in terms of severe adverse side effects.[11,14,62,69] Gold therapy can arrest further progression of rheumatoid joint disease in many patients, but these drugs do not reverse damage that has already occurred. Hence, these drugs are now used fairly early in the course of rheumatoid arthritis, before excessive joint destruction takes place.

Mechanism of Action. Although the exact mechanism is not fully understood, gold compounds probably induce remission in patients with rheumatoid arthritis by inhibiting the maturation and function of mononuclear phagocytes.[22,57,69,88] These drugs accumulate in the lysosomes of macrophages and other synovial cells and thereby suppress the action of key components in the cellular immune reaction inherent to this disease.[20,57,90] A number of additional cellular effects have been noted (decreased lysosomal enzyme release, decreased responsiveness to prostaglandins), and

CH_2OH

H

H

O

H

HO

OH

H

H

SAu

OH

H

OH

Aurothioglucose

CH_2COONa

|

$AuSCHCOONa$

Gold Sodium Thiomalate

O

CH_2OCCH_3

O

SAuP(C_2

O

$OCCH_3$

CH_3CO

O

O

$OCCH_3$

O

FIGURE 16–1. Gold compounds used to treat rheumatoid arthritis.

Auranofin

these effects may also contribute to the effectiveness of gold compounds in treating rheumatoid arthritis.[11,41,84]

Adverse Side Effects. Adverse effects are relatively common with gold therapy, with approximately one third of patients experiencing some form of toxic effect.[71] The primary side effects caused by gold compounds are gastrointestinal distress (diarrhea, indigestion), irritation of the oral mucosa, and rashes/itching of the skin.[71,98] Other side effects include proteinuria, conjunctivitis, and blood dyscrasias (e.g., thrombocytopenia, leukopenia). As mentioned earlier, auranofin may be safer than parenteral gold compounds because it produces fewer cutaneous and potentially serious hematologic side effects, but auranofin tends to produce more gastrointestinal irritation than injected forms of gold.[49] Certain patients with rheumatoid arthritis may be genetically predisposed to the toxic side effects of gold compounds.[37,85] This is interesting in that it may be possible to predict via genetic screening which patients will not tolerate these drugs, thus sparing the patient from an unpleasant and possibly harmful toxic episode. Screening for genetic susceptibility has not been instituted on a routine basis, however, and drug therapy with gold compounds continues to be done by trial and error.

METHOTREXATE

Methotrexate (Folex, Mexate, Rheumatrex) is an antimetabolite used frequently in the treatment of cancer (see Chapter 36). There is considerable evidence that this drug is also one of the most effective DMARDs.[52,94,95] Methotrexate has been shown to slow the effects of rheumatoid arthritis as evidenced by decreased synovitis, decreased bony erosion, and less narrowing of the joint space in patients treated with this drug.[92–94] The therapeutic effects of methotrexate have also been reported as being equal to, or better than, other DMARDs such as oral gold or azathioprine, and methotrexate may offer somewhat of an advantage in terms of a more rapid onset compared to other DMARDs.[3,46,93] Hence, methotrexate's popularity as a DMARD has increased during the past few years, and this drug continues to be used on an increasing basis to treat rheumatoid arthritis in both adults and children.[35,77]

Mechanism of Action. The ability of methotrexate and similar anticancer drugs to impair DNA and RNA synthesis is well known (see Chapter 36). Methotrexate inhibits the synthesis of folic acid and thus inhibits the formation of nucleoproteins that serve as DNA precursors.[33] This inhibits cellular replication by impairing the cell's ability to produce new genetic material. Hence, the effects of methotrexate as an antirheumatic appear to mimic this drug's action as an anticancer agent. Methotrexate probably inhibits the proliferation of the rapidly replicating cells (monocytes, lymphocytes) that constitute the immune response of rheumatic joint disease much in the same way that this drug attenuates tumor cell replication in cancer.[51] Hence, methotrexate's anti-inflammatory and immunosuppressive actions seem to be mediated through its ability to slow the proliferation of key cellular components involved in rheumatoid arthritis.

Adverse Side Effects. Methotrexate is a relatively toxic drug, and a number of adverse side effects can occur.[32] The primary problems involve the gastrointestinal tract and include loss of appetite, nausea, and other forms of gastrointestinal distress (including intragastrointestinal hemorrhage).[83] Long-term methotrexate use in patients with rheumatoid arthritis has also been associated with pulmonary problems, hematologic disorders, liver dysfunction, and hair loss.[83] These side effects often limit the use of methotrexate in patients with rheumatoid arthritis, and most patients who must stop using this drug do so because of an adverse side effect rather than a loss of the drug's effectiveness.[17,65] Methotrexate does, however, offer a favorable benefit-to-risk ratio in many patients and continues to gain popularity as a DMARD.

PENICILLAMINE

Penicillamine (Cuprimine), a derivative of penicillin, is officially classified as a chelating agent that is often used in the treatment of heavy metal intoxication (e.g., lead poisoning). In addition, this drug has been used in patients with severe rheumatoid arthritis who have not responded to other measures such as gold therapy.[71]

Mechanism of Action. The basis for the antiarthritic effects of penicillamine is unknown. Reductions in serum immunoglobulin M rheumatoid factor have been observed with penicillamine, and this drug has been shown to depress T-cell function.[57,84,96] These and similar findings suggest that penicillamine works by suppressing the immune response in rheumatoid arthritis, but the exact mechanisms remain to be determined.

Adverse Side Effects. Penicillamine is considered to be moderately toxic when compared to other DMARDs.[32] Side effects that have been reported as occurring more frequently include fever, joint pain, skin rashes/itching, and swelling of lymph glands. Other adverse effects that may occur less frequently are bloody or cloudy urine, swelling of feet and legs, unusual weight gain, sore throat, and excessive fatigue.

DMARD Combinations Used in Rheumatoid Arthritis

There has been a great deal of interest in using several DMARDs simultaneously to achieve optimal effects in treating rheumatoid arthritis. The strategy of combination therapy is to attack the underlying disease process from several pharmacologic vantage points, in much the same way that combination therapies are commonly used in other disorders such as hypertension (Chapter 21) and cancer (Chapter 36). The use of DMARD combinations in treating rheumatoid arthritis, however, remains somewhat unclear. There is some evidence that increased benefits can be achieved by combining certain DMARDs such as gold and penicillamine or gold and hydroxychloroquine.[16] Other reports, however, have failed to document a significant benefit from these and other DMARD combinations.[76,77] Likewise, some combinations have been noted to be less effective because of the increased incidence of adverse side effects.[14,36] This fact is certainly understandable considering that many DMARDs have a relatively high risk of side effects when used alone, and combining these drugs will certainly increase the risk of adverse drug reactions.

Hence, there has not been an overwhelming body of evidence to support the use of combination therapy in rheumatoid arthritis. Considerable efforts are still being made, however, to find optimal combinations that can increase the effectiveness of these drugs without a substantial increase in side effects.[87,97] This is a formidable task, considering that these drugs are typically very slow acting, and the clinical trials needed to test these combinations may take months or years to complete.[74] Perhaps meticulous research will someday provide several standard DMARD combinations that can be used safely and effectively in patients with rheumatoid arthritis.

Newer and Nontraditional Therapies for Rheumatoid Arthritis

There is an ongoing search for other pharmacologic and nonpharmacologic interventions that can help arrest the progression of rheumatoid joint disease. Other drugs that can affect the immune response are currently being used on a limited basis to treat this disease. For instance, cyclosporine (Sandimmune), an immunosuppressant agent that is used to prevent rejection of organ transplants (see Chapter 37), is sometimes used to treat patients with rheumatoid arthritis who have not responded to other measures.[86] Sulfasalazine (Azulfidine), a drug that is typically used to treat inflammatory bowel disease, may also be helpful in treating rheumatoid arthritis because of its immunosuppressant effects.[84] In addition to these alternative drug therapies, there has been some evidence that dietary manipulation can help alleviate the symptoms of rheumatoid arthritis. Diets that are high in fish oil and certain fatty acids (e.g., gamma-linolenic acid) have been advocated for patients with rheumatoid arthritis because these diets may supply precursors that enhance the biosynthesis of certain endogenous anti-inflammatory and immunosuppressant compounds.[23,55] Hence, new strategies continue to be developed to add to the armamentarium of drugs that are currently available to treat rheumatoid arthritis.

OSTEOARTHRITIS

Osteoarthritis far exceeds rheumatoid arthritis as the most common form of joint disease. Osteoarthritis occurs in approximately 75 percent of 75-year-olds, with the incidence increasing to more than 90 percent in those who are 80 years of age.[53] In contrast to rheumatoid joint disease, osteoarthritis does not seem to be caused by an immune response, but rather seems to be associated with an intrinsic defect in the joint cartilage. This defect causes a slow, progressive deterioration of articular cartilage that is accompanied by degenerative bony changes including thickening of the subchondral bone, creation of subchondral bone cysts, and formation of large bony protrusions (osteophytes) at the joint margins.[82] Osteoarthritis typically occurs in large weight-bearing joints such as the knees and hips as well as some of the smaller joints in the hands and feet.[53] Patients are described as having primary osteoarthritis when there is no apparent reason for the onset of joint destruction and secondary osteoarthritis when a factor such as previous joint trauma, infection, or metabolic disease is responsible for triggering the articular changes associated with this disease. Obesity and genetic susceptibility have also been implicated as predisposing factors in osteoarthritis.[29,53] Clearly, osteoarthritis is a different form of joint disease than rheumatoid arthritis. Hence, treatment of these conditions also differs somewhat. As discussed previously, rheumatoid arthritis is characterized by a severe inflammatory response that is perpetuated by a cellular immune reaction. Thus, drug therapy in rheumatoid disease consists of agents that are focused on directly relieving these inflammatory symptoms (i.e., NSAIDs or glucocorticoids) or drugs that attempt to arrest the cellular immune response that causes this inflammation (DMARDs). Treatment of joint inflammation is not a major focus of drug therapy in osteoarthritis, however. A mild inflammatory synovitis does occur in osteoarthritis, but this is secondary to the articular damage inherent to this disease.[53] Also, drug therapy represents one of the primary interventions in rheumatoid arthritis, whereas treatment of osteoarthritis is dominated by nonpharmacologic measures such as physical therapy, weight loss, and joint replacement in the advanced stages of this disease.[82]

Hence, drug therapy is often not initiated during the early stages of osteoarthritis.[25] When joint pain begins to be a problem, simple analgesics such as the NSAIDs and acetaminophen have been the major form of drug therapy. A second pharmacologic strategy known as **viscosupplementation** has emerged recently. This technique is directed at changing the consistency and properties of synovial fluid in osteoarthritic joints. The roles of these two primary pharmacologic interventions in osteoarthritis are discussed here.

NSAIDs and Acetaminophen

NSAIDs are typically the first drugs used for the symptomatic treatment of pain in osteoarthritis.[25] These drugs are used primarily for their analgesic properties, although the anti-inflammatory effects of the NSAIDs are also helpful in controlling the mild synovitis that typically occurs secondary to joint destruction.[13,25] As discussed in Chapter 15, there are no clear differences in the therapeutic effects of different NSAIDs when these drugs are used orally to treat pain. Selection of a specific NSAID depends primarily on each patient's ability to tolerate each drug's side effects, especially in terms of NSAID-induced gastropathy.

Acetaminophen can also be used to control pain in osteoarthritis, especially in patients who are at a higher risk for gastric ulcer or other NSAID-induced side effects.[25] Acetaminophen will not, however, contribute any anti-inflammatory effects. This is of less concern when acetaminophen is used in osteoarthritis versus rheumatoid arthritis because the inflammatory symptoms are much milder in osteoarthritis. Hence, acetaminophen provides a relatively safe and effective form of analgesia for patients with osteoarthritis who do not need anti-inflammatory effects.[13,25]

There is no doubt that the analgesia produced by NSAIDs or acetaminophen plays an extremely valuable role in the management of osteoarthritis. These drugs can allow the patient to maintain a more active lifestyle and participate in various activities including exercise programs and other forms of physical and occupational therapy.[9,40] One must recall, however, that these drugs do not alter the progressive course of joint destruction and osteoarthritic changes. There is preliminary evidence, in fact, that some of the NSAIDs may actually impair cartilage formation by inhibiting the synthesis of proteoglycans and other key cartilaginous components (see Chapter 15).[6,21,24,43,47] At the present time, however, NSAIDs and acetaminophen remain the cornerstone of the pharmacologic treatment of joint pain in osteoarthritis.

Viscosupplementation

Viscosupplementation is a clinical procedure that is being used increasingly in the treatment of osteoarthritis. This technique uses a substance known as hyaluronan to restore the lubricating properties of synovial fluid in osteoarthritic joints.[72] Hyaluronan is a polysaccharide that can be injected into an arthritic joint to help restore the normal viscosity of the synovial fluid.[50] This helps reduce joint stresses and thus limits the progression of articular destruction seen in osteoarthritis.[34] This technique can provide substantial benefits in 65 to 80 percent of the patients receiving treatment.[73]

When used to treat osteoarthritis, viscosupplementation typically consists of 2 to 10 weekly injections of hyaluronan. Patients often experience a decrease in pain within a few days after injection, and pain continues to diminish within the first few weeks after beginning treatment. Duration of relief is variable, but most patients who respond to viscosupplementation experience beneficial effects for 6 months to 1 year after a series of injections.[5,73]

Hence, viscosupplementation may actually attenuate the progressive changes in joint structure and function typically seen in osteoarthritis. This fact suggests that viscosupplementation may represent one of the first disease-modifying pharmacologic techniques available for treating osteoarthritic joints.[25] Future clinical studies will be needed to determine if viscosupplementation provides long-term benefits without excessive adverse effects in patients with osteoarthritis.

Special Concerns for Antiarthritic Drug Therapy in Rehabilitation Patients

Drugs used to treat rheumatoid arthritis and osteoarthritis often play a vital role in permitting optimal rehabilitation of patients with joint disease. By decreasing pain and inflammation, these drugs help facilitate a more active and vigorous program of exercise and functional activity. Some drugs, such as the disease-modifying drugs used in rheumatoid arthritis and viscosupplementation in osteoarthritis, appear to be able to impair or even halt the progression of joint destruction. This may enable the therapist to help restore muscle strength and joint function rather than to simply employ a program of maintenance therapy during a steady downward progression in patients with arthritis.

The influence of antiarthritic drugs on the rehabilitative process depends primarily on the type of drugs being used. Beginning with the NSAIDs, there is little concern for adverse effects on physical therapy procedures. These drugs are relatively safe and are not usually associated with the type of side effects that will directly influence the physical therapy of patients with rheumatoid arthritis or osteoarthritis. If the corticosteroids are used, the therapist must be aware of the many adverse side effects of these drugs. In particular, the catabolic effects of these agents on supporting tissues (muscle, tendon, bone, skin) must be considered. Range-of-motion and strengthening programs must be used judiciously to avoid fractures and soft-tissue injuries. Care must also be taken to prevent skin breakdown, especially when splints and other protective orthotic devices are employed.

The disease-modifying agents used in rheumatoid arthritis are each associated with a number of side effects that could influence rehabilitation. Some of these drugs such as the gold compounds and methotrexate may cause headache and nausea, which may be bothersome during the therapy session. Joint pain and swelling may also occur with drugs like methotrexate and penicillamine, and this may also become a problem during rehabilitation. A variety of other side effects can occur, depending on the particular DMARD being used and the sensitivity of the individual patient. Therapists should be aware of any change in patient response, not only when a new drug is being started but also during the prolonged use of DMARDs.

Finally, the use of viscosupplementation to restore synovial fluid function in osteoarthritic joints is fairly new, and it is not yet clear if this technique will have any side effects that will have a direct impact on physical rehabilitation. Likewise, it remains to be seen if there are any rehabilitation techniques (exercise, physical agents) that could enhance the effectiveness of viscosupplementation. It is hoped that this technique will work synergistically with physical therapy to improve function in patients with osteoarthritic joints.

CASE STUDY

RHEUMATOID ARTHRITIS

Brief History. A.T., a 75-year-old woman, was diagnosed several years ago with rheumatoid joint disease. Currently she is being seen three times each week in physical therapy as an outpatient for a program of paraffin and active exercise to her wrists and hands. Resting splints were also fabricated for both hands, and these are worn at night to prevent joint deformity. The patient was also instructed in a home exercise program to maintain joint mobility in both upper extremities. Pharmacologic management in this patient originally consisted of NSAIDs, beginning with aspirin and later switching to ibuprofen. Six months ago, she was also placed on auranofin (Ridaura), which was instituted in an attempt to halt the progressive arthritic changes. This orally administered gold compound was given at a dosage of 3 mg twice each day.

Problem/Influence of Medication. The combination of an NSAID and a disease-modifying drug along with the physical therapy program seemed to be helping to decrease the patient's pain and joint stiffness. However, she began to develop skin rashes and itching on her arms and legs. The therapist noticed this while preparing the patient for her paraffin treatment. It seemed that these rashes might be occurring as a side effect of the auranofin. The therapist brought this to the attention of the physician, and he concurred that this was probably a side effect of the gold therapy.

Decision/Solution. The patient was temporarily removed from auranofin therapy to see if this skin reaction would subside. In the interim, the therapist discontinued paraffin so that the rashes and itching on the distal forearm would not be exacerbated. To continue to provide gentle heat, a warm whirlpool (100°F) was substituted for the paraffin bath. Also, the night splints were temporarily discontinued to prevent irritation to the affected areas. After 2 weeks, the skin rashes had virtually disappeared, and the original physical therapy program was resumed. After another week, the physician restarted auranofin administration. No other adverse effects were noted, and the patient continued to notice improvements in her arthritic condition.

SUMMARY

Rheumatoid arthritis and osteoarthritis represent two distinct forms of joint disease that can produce devastating effects on the structure and function of synovial joints. Fortunately, management of these conditions has improved substantially through advancements in drug therapy. Rheumatoid arthritis can be treated pharmacologically with NSAIDs, glucocorticoids, and various DMARDs. NSAIDs, including aspirin, represent the primary form of drug therapy in the early stages of this disease, and these drugs are often used in conjunction with other drugs as the arthritic condition increases in severity. Glucocorticoids are often effective in decreasing the joint inflammation typically found in rheumatoid arthritis, but long-term use of these agents is limited because of their many toxic effects. Disease-modifying drugs can slow or halt the progressive nature of rheumatoid arthritis by suppressing the immune response inherent to this disease. Although there is some concern about the efficacy and safety of these drugs, DMARDs have been a welcome addition to the rather limited arsenal of drugs used to treat rheumatoid arthritis.

Drug treatment of osteoarthritis differs somewhat from rheumatoid arthritis, with management of pain using NSAIDs and acetaminophen constituting the major form of drug therapy. A newer technique known as viscosupplementation has also been used to help restore the lubricating properties of the synovial fluid in osteoarthritic joints. It remains to be seen, however, if this technique will become widely accepted as a safe and effective treatment for osteoarthritis. In any event, drug therapy along with nonpharmacologic measures such as physical therapy can provide an effective way of dealing with the potentially devastating effects of rheumatoid arthritis and osteoarthritis.

REFERENCES

1. Adams, EM, Yocum, DE, and Bell, CL: Hydroxychloroquine in the treatment of rheumatoid arthritis. Am J Med 75:321, 1983.
2. Agambar, L and Flower, R: Anti-inflammatory drugs. Physiotherapy 76:198, 1990.
3. Alarcon, GS, et al: Radiographic evidence of disease progression in methotrexate treated and non-methotrexate disease modifying antirheumatic drug treated rheumatoid arthritis patients: A meta-analysis. J Rheumatol 19:1868, 1992.
4. Baker, DG and Rabinowitz, JL: Current concepts in the treatment of rheumatoid arthritis. J Clin Pharmacol 26:2, 1986.
5. Balazs, EA and Denlinger, JL: Viscosupplementation: A new concept in the treatment for osteoarthritis. J Rheumatol 20(suppl 39):3, 1993.
6. Bassleer, C, Henrotin, Y, and Franchimont, P: Effects of sodium naproxen on differentiated human chondrocytes cultivated in clusters. Clin Rheumatol 11:60, 1992.
7. Bell, CL: Hydroxychloroquine sulfate in rheumatoid arthritis: Long term response rate and predictive parameters. Am J Med 75(suppl 1A):46, 1983.
8. Bernstein, HN: Ophthalmologic considerations and testing in patients receiving long-term antimalarial therapy. Am J Med 75(suppl 1A):25, 1983.
9. Blackwell, GJ, et al: Macrocortin: A polypeptide causing the anti-phospholipase effect of glucocorticoids. Nature 287:147, 1980.
10. Bland, JH: The reversibility of osteoarthritis: A review. Am J Med 74:16, 1983.
11. Blodgett, RC: Auranofin: Experience to date. Am J Med 75(suppl 6A):86, 1983.
12. Bomalaski, JS and Clark, MA: Review: Phospholipase A_2 and arthritis. Arthritis Rheum 36:190, 1993.
13. Bradley, JD, et al: Treatment of knee osteoarthritis: Relationship of clinical features of joint inflammation to the response to a nonsteroidal antiinflammatory drug or pure analgesic. J Rheumatol 19:1950, 1992.
14. Brooks, PM: The use of suppressive agents for the treatment of rheumatoid arthritis. Aust NZ J Med 23:193, 1993.
15. Brooks, PM and Day, RO: Drug therapy: Nonsteroidal anti-inflammatory drugs—differences and similarities. N Engl J Med 324:1716, 1991.
16. Brooks, PM and Schwarzer, AC: Combination chemotherapy in rheumatoid arthritis. Ann Rheum Dis 50:507, 1991.
17. Buchbinder, R, et al: Methotrexate therapy in rheumatoid arthritis: A life table review of 587 patients treated in community practice. J Rheumatol 20:639, 1993.
18. Butler, RC and Goddard, DH: Controversy in the treatment of rheumatoid arthritis. Lancet 2:278, 1984.
19. Caldwell, JR and Furst, DE: The efficacy and safety of low-dose corticosteroids for rheumatoid arthritis. Semin Arthritis Rheum 21:1, 1991.

20. Chaffman, M, et al: Auranofin: A preliminary review of its pharmacologic properties and therapeutic use in rheumatoid arthritis. Drugs 27:378, 1984.
21. Collier, S and Ghosh, P: Comparison of the effects of NSAIDs on proteoglycan synthesis by articular cartilage explant and chondrocyte monolayer cultures. Biochem Pharmacol 41:1375, 1991.
22. Crooke, ST and Mirabelli, CK: Molecular mechanisms of action of auranofin and other gold complexes as related to their biological activities. Am J Med 75(suppl 6A):109, 1983.
23. Darlington, LG and Ramsey, NW: Review of dietary therapy for rheumatoid arthritis. Br J Rheumatol 32:507, 1993.
24. David, MJ, et al: Effects of NSAIDs on glycosyltransferase activity from human osteoarthritic cartilage. Br J Rheumatol 31(suppl 1):13, 1992.
25. Dieppe, P: Drug treatment of osteoarthritis. J Bone Joint Surg 75(B):673, 1993.
26. Dinarello, CA and Wolff, SM: The role of interleukin-1 in disease. N Engl J Med 328:106, 1993.
27. Dooley, MA, et al: The effects of nonsteroidal drug therapy in early rheumatoid arthritis on serum levels of soluble interleukin-2 receptor, CD4, and CD8. J Rheumatol 20:1857, 1993.
28. Fathman, CG: What a rheumatologist needs to know about T cell receptor structure and function. J Rheumatol 19(suppl 32):12, 1992.
29. Felson, DT, et al: Obesity and knee osteoarthritis. Ann Intern Med 109:18, 1988.
30. Ferguson, GG: Pathophysiology: Mechanisms and Expression. WB Saunders, Philadelphia, 1984.
31. Fox, RI: Mechanism of action of hydroxychloroquine as an antirheumatic drug. Semin Arthritis Rheum 23(suppl 1):82, 1993.
32. Fries, JF, et al: The relative toxicity of alternate therapies for rheumatoid arthritis: Implications for the therapeutic progression. Semin Arthritis Rheum 23(suppl 1):68, 1993.
33. Furst, DE and Kremer, JM: Methotrexate in rheumatoid arthritis. Arthritis Rheum 31:305, 1988.
34. Ghosh, P, et al: The effects of intraarticular administration of hyaluronan in a model of early osteoarthritis in sheep. II. Cartilage composition and proteoglycan metabolsim. Semin Arthritis Rheum 22(suppl 1):31, 1993.
35. Giannini, EH, et al: Comparative safety and efficacy of advanced drug therapy in children with juvenile rheumatoid arthritis. Semin Arthritis Rheum 23:34, 1993.
36. Haar, D, et al: A double-blind comparative study of hydroxychloroquine and dapsone, alone and in combination, in rheumatoid arthritis. Scand J Rheumatol 22:113, 1993.
37. Hakala, M, et al: Association of different HLA antigens with various toxic effects of gold salts in rheumatoid arthritis. Ann Rheum Dis 45:177, 1986.
38. Harris, ED: Mechanisms of disease: Rheumatoid arthritis: Pathophysiology and implications for therapy. N Engl J Med 322:1277, 1990.
39. Harris, ED: Pathogenesis of rheumatoid arthritis. Am J Med 80(suppl 4B):4, 1986.
40. Hart, FD, and Huskisson, EC: Non-steroidal anti-inflammatory drugs: Current status and rational therapeutic use. Drugs 27:232, 1984.
41. Harth, M: Mechanisms of action of disease modifying antirheumatic drugs. J Rheumatol 19(suppl 32): 100, 1993.
42. Haynes, RC: Adrenocorticotropic hormone; adrenocortical steroids and their synthetic analogs; inhibitors of the synthesis and actions of adrenocortical hormones. In Gilman, AG, et al (eds): The Pharmacological Basis of Therapeutics. Pergamon Press, New York, 1990.
43. Henrotin, Y, Bassleer, C, and Franchimont, P: In vitro effects of etodolac and acetylsalicylic acid on human chondrocyte metabolism. Agents Actions 36:317, 1992.
44. Higgs, GA and Vane, JR: Inhibition of cyclo-oxygenase and lipooxygenase. Br Med Bull 39:265, 1983.
45. Hirata, F, et al: A phospholipase A_2 inhibitory protein in rabbit neutrophils induced by glucocorticoids. Proc Natl Acad Sci 77:2533, 1980.
46. Hoffmeister, RT: Methotrexate therapy in rheumatoid arthritis: 15 years experience. Am J Med 75(suppl 6A):69, 1983.
47. Hugenberg, ST, Brandt, KD, and Cole, CA: Effect of sodium salicylate, aspirin, and ibuprofen on enzymes required by the chondrocyte for synthesis of chondroitin sulfate. J Rheumatol 20:2128, 1993.
48. Ianuzzi, L, et al: Does drug therapy slow radiographic deterioration in rheumatoid arthritis? N Engl J Med 309:1023, 1983.
49. Insel, P: Analgesic-antipyretics and antiinflammatory agents; drugs employed in the treatment of rheumatoid arthritis and gout. In Gilman, AG, et al (eds): The Pharmacologic Basis of Therapeutics. Pergamon Press, New York, 1990.
50. Iwata, H: Pharmacologic and clinical aspects of intraarticular injection of hyaluronate. Clin Orthop 289:285, 1993.
51. Jaffe, IA: New approaches to the management of rheumatoid arthritis. J Rheumatol 19(suppl 36): 2, 1992.
52. Kremer, JM: Long-term methotrexate therapy in rheumatoid arthritis: A review. J Rheumatol 12(suppl 12):25, 1985.
53. Kumar, V, Cotran, RS, and Robbins, SL: Basic Pathology, ed 5. WB Saunders, Philadelphia, 1992.
54. Larsen, GL and Henson, PM: Mediators of inflammation. Annu Rev Immunol 1:335, 1983.
55. Leventhal, LJ, Boyce, EG, and Zurier, RB: Treatment of rheumatoid arthritis with gammalinolenic acid. Ann Intern Med 119:867, 1993.

56. Lewis, RA, Austen, KF, and Soberman, RJ: Mechanisms of disease: Leukotrienes and other products of the 5-lipoxygenase pathway—biochemistry and relation to pathophysiology in human diseases. N Engl J Med 323:645, 1990.
57. Lipsky, PE: Remission-inducing therapy in rheumatoid arthritis. Am J Med 75(suppl 4B):40, 1983.
58. Mackenzie, AH: Pharmacologic actions of 4-aminoquinolone compounds. Am J Med 75(suppl 1A): 5, 1983.
59. Mackenzie, AH: Antimalarial drugs for rheumatoid arthritis. Am J Med 75(suppl 6A):49, 1983.
60. Mackenzie, AH: Dose refinements in long-term therapy of rheumatoid arthritis with antimalarials. Am J Med 75(suppl 1A):40, 1983.
61. Markenson, JA: Worldwide trends in the socioeconomic impact and long-term prognosis of rheumatoid arthritis. Semin Arthritis Rheum 21(suppl 1):4, 1991.
62. Mazanec, DJ, et al: Oral chrysotherapy in rheumatoid arthritis: Auranofin. Cleveland Clinic experience and literature review. Cleve Clin Q 52:123, 1985.
63. McDuffie, FC: Morbidity impact of rheumatoid arthritis on society. Am J Med 78(suppl 1A):1, 1985.
64. McGuire, JL and Ridgway, WM: Aggressive drug therapy for rheumatoid arthritis. Hosp Pract 28: 45, 1993.
65. McKendry, RJR and Dale, P: Adverse effects of low-dose methotrexate therapy in rheumatoid arthritis. J Rheumatol 20:1850, 1993.
66. Mense, S: Basic neurobiologic mechanisms of pain and analgesia. Am J Med 75(suppl 5A):4, 1983.
67. Moncada, S and Vane, JR: Pharmacology and endogenous roles of prostaglandin endoperoxides, thromboxane A_2, and prostacyclin. Pharmacol Rev 30:293, 1979.
68. O'Brien, WM: Pharmacology of NSAIDs: Practical review for clinicians. Am J Med 75(suppl 4B): 32, 1983.
69. O'Duffy, JD and Luthra HS: Current status of disease-modifying drugs in progressive rheumatoid arthritis. Drugs 27:373, 1984.
70. Panayi, GS: The immunopathogenesis of rheumatoid arthritis. Br J Rheumatol 32(suppl 1):4, 1993.
71. Payan, DG: Nonsteroidal anti-inflammatory drugs; nonopioid analgesics; drugs used in gout. In Katzung, BG (ed): Basic and Clinical Pharmacology, ed 5. Appleton & Lange, Norwalk, CT, 1992.
72. Pelletier, J-P and Martel-Pelletier, J: The pathophysiology of osteoarthritis and the implications of the use of hyaluronan and hylan as therapeutic agents in viscosupplementation. J Rheumatol 20(suppl 39): 19, 1993.
73. Peyron, JG: Intraarticular hyaluronan injections in the treatment of osteoarthritis: State-of-the-art review. J Rheumatol 20(suppl 39):10, 1993.
74. Pincus, T: Limitations of randomized clinical trials to recognize possible advantages of combination therapies in rheumatic disease. Semin Arthritis Rheum 23(suppl 1):2, 1993.
75. Pincus, T, et al: Long-term drug therapy for rheumatoid arthritis in seven rheumatology private practices. 1. Nonsteroidal anti-inflammatory drugs. J Rheumatol 19:1874, 1992.
76. Porter, DR, Capell, HA, and Hunter, J: Combination therapy in rheumatoid arthritis: No benefit of addition of hydroxychloroquine to patients with a suboptimal response to intramuscular gold therapy. J Rheumatol 20:645, 1993.
77. Porter, DR and Sturrock, RD: Fortnightly review: Medical management of rheumatoid arthritis. Br Med J 307:425, 1993.
78. Robinson, DR: Prostaglandins and the mechanism of action of anti-inflammatory drugs. Am J Med 75(suppl 4B):26, 1983.
79. Runge, LA: Risk/benefit analysis of hydroxychloroquine sulfate treatment in rheumatoid arthritis. Am J Med 75(suppl 1A):52, 1983.
80. Rynes, RI: Ophthalmologic safety of long-term hydroxychloroquine treatment. Am J Med 75(suppl 1A):35, 1983.
81. Salmeron, G and Lipsky, PE: Immunosuppressive potential of antimalarials. Am J Med 75(suppl 1A): 19, 1983.
82. Schiller, AL: Bones and joints. In Rubin, E and Farber, JL (eds): Pathology, ed 2. JB Lippincott, Philadelphia, 1994.
83. Scully, CJ, Anderson, CJ, and Cannon, GW: Long-term methotrexate therapy for rheumatoid arthritis. Semin Arthritis Rheum 20:317, 1991.
84. Spencer-Green, G: Drug treatment of arthritis: Update on conventional and less conventional methods. Postgrad Med 93:129, 1993.
85. Stockman, A, et al: Genetic markers in rheumatoid arthritis: Relationship to toxicity from d-penicillamine. J Rheumatol 13:269, 1986.
86. Symposium (various authors): An international consensus report: The use of cyclosporin A in rheumatoid arthritis. Br J Rheumatol 32(suppl 1):1, 1993.
87. Symposium (various authors): Combination therapy in the treatment of rheumatoid arthritis. Semin Arthritis Rheum 23(suppl 1):1, 1993.
88. Tsokos, GC: Immunomodulatory treatment in patients with rheumatic diseases: Mechanisms of actions. Semin Arthritis Rheum 17:24, 1987.
89. Vane, J: The evolution of non-steroidal anti-inflammatory drugs and their mechanisms of actions. Drugs 33(suppl 1):18, 1987.

90. Walz, DT, et al: Biologic actions and pharmacokinetic studies of auranofin. Br J Med 75(suppl 6A):90, 1983.
91. Ward, DJ and Tidswell, ME: Rheumatoid arthritis and juvenile chronic arthritis. In Downie, PA (ed): Cash's Textbook of Orthopaedics and Rheumatology for Physiotherapists. JB Lippincott, Philadelphia, 1984.
92. Weinblatt, ME, Coblyn, JS, and Fox, DA: Efficacy of low-dose methotrexate in rheumatoid arthritis. N Engl J Med 312:818, 1985.
93. Weinblatt, ME, et al: The effects of drug therapy on radiographic progression of rheumatoid arthritis. Results of a 36-week randomized trial comparing methotrexate and auranofin. Arthritis Rheum 36:613, 1993.
94. Weinstein, A, et al: Low-dose methotrexate treatment of rheumatoid arthritis: Long-term observations. Am J Med 79:331, 1985.
95. Wells, WL, et al: Studies on the effects of low-dose methotrexate on rat adjuvant arthritis. J Rheumatol 12:904, 1985.
96. Wernick, R, et al: IgG and IgM rheumatoid factors in rheumatoid arthritis. Arthritis Rheum 26:593, 1983.
97. Wilke, WS and Clough, JD: Therapy for rheumatoid arthritis: Combinations of disease-modifying drugs and new paradigms of treatment. Semin Arthritis Rheum 21(suppl 1):21, 1991.
98. Wilkinson, SM, et al: Suspected cutaneous drug toxicity in rheumatoid arthritis: An evaluation. Br J Rheumatol 32:798, 1993.
99. Willkens, RF: The selection of a nonsteroidal antiinflammatory drug: Is there a difference? J Rheumatol 19(suppl 36):9, 1992.
100. Zvaifler, NJ: Pathogenesis of the joint disease of rheumatoid arthritis. Am J Med 75(suppl 6A):3, 1983.

CHAPTER 17

Patient-Controlled Analgesia

Patient-controlled analgesia (PCA) was first introduced into clinical practice in the early 1980s as an alternative way to administer analgesic medications. The basic principle behind PCA is that the patient can self-administer small doses of the drug (usually an opioid) at relatively frequent intervals to provide optimal pain relief. These small doses are typically delivered intravenously or into the spinal canal by some type of machine (pump) that is controlled by the patient. Patient-controlled analgesia has several apparent advantages over more traditional dosing regimens. In particular, PCA systems often provide equivalent or increased analgesic effects with the use of less drug and a lower incidence of side effects. This fact has generated a great deal of interest and increased use of PCA in a variety of clinical situations. For instance, PCA systems have been used to help manage acute pain following surgery, and PCAs have also been used to treat pain in patients with cancer and other conditions associated with chronic pain.

Hence, PCA continues to gain acceptance as an optimal method for treating pain. Because PCA is used extensively to treat acute and chronic pain, rehabilitation specialists should be aware of some of the fundamental principles governing PCA. This chapter begins by discussing the basic concepts and strategies of PCA, followed by some of the practical aspects of PCA, including the types of analgesics used, the possible routes of administration, and the types of machines used to administer the drugs. An indication of why PCA is often clinically superior to more traditional methods of analgesia is then presented. Finally, potential problems associated with PCA and the specific ways that PCA can impact on patients receiving physical therapy and occupational therapy are discussed. It is hoped that this will provide the reader with a better understanding of why PCA systems are often a preferred method of managing pain in contemporary practice.

PHARMACOKINETIC BASIS FOR PCA

To provide optimal management of pain, analgesic drugs should be delivered into the bloodstream or other target tissues (epidural space, intrathecal space) in a predictable and fairly constant manner. The goal is to maintain drug levels within a fairly well defined range, or **therapeutic window**. Such a therapeutic window for analgesia is represented schematically by the shaded area in Figure 17–1. If drug levels are below this window, the analgesic is below the minimum analgesic concentration and the patient is in pain. Drug levels above the window may produce adequate analgesia but may also produce side effects such as sedation. The traditional method of administering analgesics is to give relatively large doses with relatively large time intervals between each dosage. For instance, opioid analgesics are typically injected intramuscularly every 3 to 4 hours to manage severe pain, thus creating large fluctuations in the amount of drug present in the body. These large fluctuations are illustrated by the dark, solid lines in Figure 17–1. As illustrated in Figure 17–1, this traditional method of administration is associated with long periods of time when the drug concentration falls below the therapeutic window, allowing pain to occur, or above the therapeutic window, causing sedation.

Figure 17–1 also illustrates why PCA systems are better at maintaining drug levels within the therapeutic (analgesic) window. Systems using some form of PCA deliver small doses of the analgesic on a relatively frequent basis, as indicated by the dashed lines in Figure 17–1. Drug levels are maintained within the analgesic range; there are shorter periods of time when the drug concentration falls below the therapeutic window (i.e., below the shaded area), and there is virtually no time when side effects occur because the concentration rises above the therapeutic window. Hence, analgesia can be achieved more effectively with a reduced incidence of side effects.

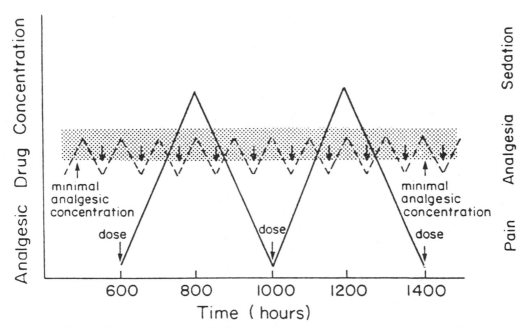

FIGURE 17–1. Pharmacokinetic model for PCA using opioid drugs. Conventional intramuscular injection is indicated by the long solid lines; PCA is indicated by the short dashed lines; and the therapeutic window for analgesia is indicated by the shaded area. (From Ferrante, et al,[7] 457–461, with permission.)

PCA DOSING STRATEGIES AND PARAMETERS

The fact that PCA enables the patient to self-deliver small doses of the analgesic at frequent intervals illustrates the need for specific dosing parameters that control the amount and frequency of analgesic administration. Several terms are used to describe these parameters and indicate each parameter's role in safeguarding against excessive drug delivery.[6] The basic terms that describe PCA dosing strategies are indicated here.

Loading Dose

A single large dose is given initially to establish analgesia. This **loading dose** is used to bring levels of the analgesic to the therapeutic window illustrated by the shaded area in Figure 17–1.

Demand Dose

The amount of drug that is self-administered by the patient each time he or she activates the PCA delivery mechanism is known as the **demand dose**. The magnitude of these doses for some commonly used opioid analgesics are listed in Table 17–1.

Lockout Interval

The minimum amount of time allowed between each demand dose is called the **lockout interval.** After the patient self-administers a dose, the PCA delivery system will not deliver the next dose until the lockout interval has expired. Typical lockout intervals for commonly used opioids are listed in Table 17–1.

1- and 4-Hour Limits

Some PCA systems can be set to limit the total amount of drug given in a 1- or 4-hour period. The use of these parameters is somewhat questionable, however, because other parameters such as the demand dose and lockout interval automatically limit the total amount of drug that can be given in a specific period of time.

Background Infusion Rate

In some patients, a small amount of the analgesic is infused continuously to maintain a low, background level of analgesia. Demand doses are superimposed on the background infusion whenever the patient feels an increase in pain (e.g., the so-called breakthrough pain that may occur when the patient coughs or changes position). The

TABLE 17–1 Parameters for PCA Using Opioid Medications

Drug (Concentration)	Demand Dose	Lockout Interval (min)
Fentanyl (10 μg/mL)	10–20 μg	5–10
Hydromorphone (0.2 mg/mL)	0.05–0.25 mg	5–10
Meperidine (10 mg/mL)	5–30 mg	5–12
Methadone (1 mg/mL)	0.5–2.5 mg	8–20
Morphine (1 mg/mL)	0.5–3.0 mg	5–12
Nalbuphine (1 mg/mL)	1–5 mg	5–10
Oxymorphone (0.25 mg/mL)	0.2–0.4 mg	8–10

Source: Ferrante,[6] p 292, with permission.

use of background infusion basically combines the technique of continuous infusion with PCA, which may provide optimal analgesia with minimal side effects.[14]

Successful Versus Total Demands

Successful demands occur when the patient activates the PCA delivery system and actually receives a demand dose of the drug. Demands made during the lockout interval would not be successful but would be added to the number of successful demands to indicate the total demands. A large number of unsuccessful demands may indicate that the PCA parameters are not effective in providing adequate analgesia. Hence, most PCA systems record the number of total demands so that the demand dose can be adjusted if a large number of unsuccessful demands are being made.

TYPES OF ANALGESICS USED FOR PCA

The primary medications used during PCA are the opioid analgesics (see Chapter 14) and the local anesthetics (see Chapter 12).[6] Opioids such as morphine, meperidine, and fentanyl are powerful analgesics that act primarily on the spinal cord and brain to inhibit the transmission and perception of nociceptive impulses. Opioids must be used cautiously because these drugs can cause serious side effects and because the potential for overdose with opioids is fairly high. As explained earlier, PCA often provides a safer and more effective way to administer these powerful drugs by preventing large fluctuations in plasma opioid levels.

Local anesthetics such as bupivacaine have also been used during PCA. These drugs, which block transmission along afferent sensory neurons, can be administered epidurally to block sensation at the spinal cord level. Local anesthetics have been used as the single anesthetic agent when PCA is used during labor and childbirth.[8,9] These drugs have also been mixed with opioids to provide optimal PCA during labor or following surgery.[11,12] Hence, local anesthetics serve as an alternative or adjunct to opioids during PCA.

ADMINISTRATION ROUTES DURING PCA

Intravenous PCA

Perhaps the simplest and most common method of PCA administration is through the peripheral IV route. When PCA will be needed for a fairly short period of time (e.g., for the first few days after surgery), typically a needle is inserted into a peripheral vein and then is connected to a catheter or IV line. Small intermittent doses of the analgesic can then be administered through the catheter and delivered directly into the systemic circulation.

When IV PCA will be needed for longer periods, a catheter can be implanted surgically in a large central vein with the tip of the catheter advanced to the right atrium of the heart. The catheter is then tunneled through subcutaneous tissues and brought out through the patient's skin to allow administration of PCA. Alternatively, the catheter can be connected to a small container known as an *access port* that is implanted subcutaneously within the patient's body (Fig. 17–2). This type of catheter-port system is used to provide a method of IV drug delivery that is located primarily

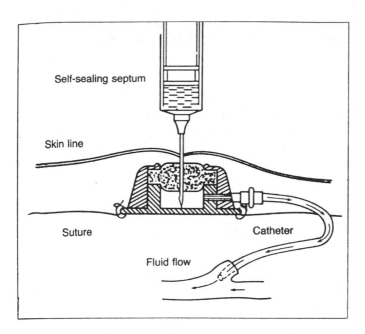

FIGURE 17-2. Schematic representation of an implantable vascular access port that can be used with PCA. The port can be connected to a PCA pump via a percutaneous needle, and a catheter leads from the port to a large central vein. (From Knox, LS: Implantable venous access devices. Crit Care Nurse 7:71, 1987, with permission.)

within the patient's body. Injections can be made through the skin and into the port through a self-sealing silicone rubber septum located on the port. When these ports are used during PCA, the external PCA source is connected to the port via a special (Huber) needle that is inserted through the skin and into the port (see Fig. 17-2). The analgesic drug is then given from the PCA pump through a catheter into the port and ultimately into the systemic circulation. This provides an effective way of getting small frequent doses of the drug into the bloodstream with less risk of infection or displacement of the intravenous catheter. This type of PCA-port delivery also enables the patient to be disconnected from the PCA delivery system for short periods of time by removing the needle from the port. This allows the patient to bathe or get dressed without risking damage to the indwelling port-IV system.[4]

Epidural and Intrathecal PCA

PCA can also be achieved by administering drugs directly into the spaces surrounding the spinal cord. This is typically done by inserting a small catheter so that the tip of the catheter lies in either the epidural space or the subarachnoid space at a specific level of the spinal cord (Fig. 17-3). Delivery of the drug into the subarachnoid space is usually referred to as **intrathecal administration** because the catheter is placed within the sheath of membranes that surrounds the spinal cord (intrathecal means "within a sheath"; see Chapter 2). If this type of PCA is intended for fairly short-term use, the catheter can be externalized through the skin on the midline of the patient's back and held in place by surgical tape. For longer-term use, the catheter is often tunneled through the subcutaneous tissues in the patient's abdominal wall, after which the catheter can either be brought out through the skin on the patient's side (see Fig. 17-3) or connected to some type of implanted access port or drug reservoir. In either case, PCA is then achieved by delivering the drug through the catheter and into the area directly surrounding the spinal cord.

Administration of drugs into the epidural or intrathecal space is obviously more difficult than simple intravenous delivery using a peripheral vein. Spinal delivery does, however, offer advantages in terms of providing effective analgesia with less drug. For instance, it is estimated that epidural morphine is 5 to 10 times more potent than IV morphine, indicating that much more drug must be administered by the IV route to achieve adequate analgesia.[4] Likewise, a study involving women who had undergone caesarean delivery showed that the amount of opioid (hydromorphone) required to provide analgesia during the first and second postoperative day was three to four times higher when administered via the IV route as compared to the epidural route.[16] In addition, intrathecal administration often requires even less drug than with the epidural route because the analgesic is being delivered within the spinal membranes and into the CSF. Analgesic requirements can be as much as 10 times lower when hydrophilic drugs like morphine are administered intrathecally versus epidurally because these drugs do not pass easily through the dura mater.[4]

Hence, the route of administration used during PCA can have dramatic effects on the amount of drug needed to provide adequate analgesia. Therefore, selection of the desired route will depend on several factors, including how long PCA will be required and whether or not the more complex methods (i.e., spinal delivery, surgically implanted catheters and ports) will offer substantial benefits over simpler techniques that use a peripheral IV route.

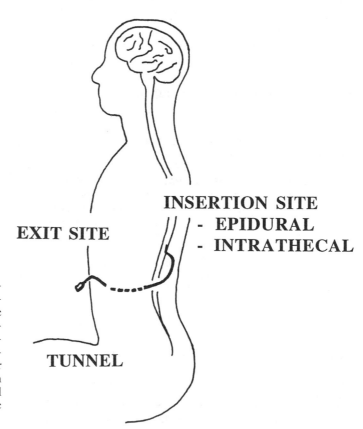

FIGURE 17–3. Schematic illustration of PCA spinal delivery. The catheter delivers the analgesic into either the epidural or intrathecal (subarachnoid space. Catheters for long-term use are tunneled under the skin *(dashed line)* and can exit on the anterior-lateral flank for connection to the PCA pump.

EXIT SITE

INSERTION SITE
- EPIDURAL
- INTRATHECAL

TUNNEL

PCA Pumps

The increase in popularity and use of PCA has been largely because of the development of infusion devices that can administer the analgesic in a safe and accurate manner. These devices, or *pumps*, vary in technologic sophistication and cost, but they all share some common features.[17] These features are summarized in Table 17–2. PCA pumps essentially allow the practitioner to set specific parameters of drug delivery (demand dose, lockout interval, etc.). The pump must then provide features to safeguard the patient against pump malfunction and warn the patient or caregiver if drug delivery is interrupted.

Pumps used for PCA fall into two basic categories: external and internal (implantable) pumps.[17] The most basic type of external pump is a simple syringe driver (Fig. 17–4). A syringe containing the medication is placed in a viselike machine that advances the syringe a small amount when the patient activates the pump. A second type of pump uses some sort of peristaltic action that sequentially compresses a piece of tubing to milk the medication through the tubing toward the patient. A third type of pump known as a cassette system works by drawing the medication into a fluid container within the pump and then expelling the selected amount of medication out of the chamber into tubing that leads to the patient. In most cases, these external pumps are activated when the patient pushes a button located on the end of a pendant that is connected to the pump (see Fig. 17–4).

Internal, or implantable, pumps are placed surgically beneath the patient's skin and connected to a catheter that leads to the patient's bloodstream or perispinal spaces (epidural or intrathecal). This basically creates a closed system within the patient's body. These pumps typically contain a reservoir that is filled with the medication. The reservoir can be refilled by inserting a Huber needle through the skin and into the pump via a resealable septum located on the outside of the pump (Fig. 17–5). Some implantable pumps use a rotatory peristaltic mechanism to milk the medication out of the pump. Other pumps use a bellows system to compress a chamber within the pump, thus expelling a given quantity of the drug from the pump. Implantable pumps are often programmed through the skin using some sort of electronic control device.

TABLE 17–2 Basic Features of Some Common PCA Pumps

Feature	Abbott PMP	Bard Ambulatory PCA Infuser	Pharmacia/Deltec Infuser
Size	$6.75 \times 4.0 \times 23$	$4.75 \times 3.4 \times 1.2$ (100-mL container) $4.75 \times 3.4 \times 2.75$ (250-mL container)	$1.1 \times 3.5 \times 6.3$ (50-mL cassette) $1.1 \times 3.5 \times 7.8$ (100-mL cassette)
Power source	Wall plug in AC 2×9 alkaline battery; attachable battery pack	Lithium 3×3 V battery	Alkaline 9 V
Drive mechanism	Rotary peristaltic	Linear peristaltic	Linear peristaltic
Bolus dose	0.1–25 mL (or mg/hr)	0.1–20 mL (or mg/hr)	0.1–6 mL (or mg/mL)
Reservoir	0.1–1000 mL (or mg or μg)	Maximum of 240 mL	50–100 mL
Lockout	5–99 min	3 min–10 hr	5–999 min
Hourly limit	Maximum 25 mL	1–30 mL	0–6 mL

Source: Adapted from Shaw,[17] p 3422, with permission.

FIGURE 17–4. An example of a syringe driver pump that is commonly used with PCA.

The type of pump selected for a given patient depends primarily on which method (external or implantable) will best serve the patient's needs as well as other factors including cost and availability of a given type of pump. Advances in pump technology will continue to improve the devices that are available, and future developments will undoubtedly provide devices that are even more efficient in providing PCA.

COMPARISON OF PCA TO TRADITIONAL METHODS OF ANALGESIC ADMINISTRATION

From the pharmacokinetic perspective discussed previously, it is apparent that giving small, frequent doses of analgesic through PCA should be superior to administering large doses given at infrequent intervals. Many clinical studies have attempted

FIGURE 17–5. An example of an implantable, electronically controlled PCA pump. This pump is implanted surgically in the patient's abdomen and can be refilled periodically through a self-sealing septum.

to verify this by comparing IV PCA using opioid drugs with traditional IM opioid injection. Although some studies have not shown any clear advantages or disadvantages of PCA,[5,7,15] most controlled trials indicate that PCA offers distinct advantages in terms of using less drug to provide improved analgesia without an increase in side effects.[1,3,10,18,19] Patients also reported a much higher level of satisfaction with PCA versus traditional IM dosing, which seems to be related to the increased feeling of control over their pain offered to patients receiving PCA.[3,18] Hence, PCA systems afford some obvious advantages when compared to more traditional methods such as periodic IM injection.

One must then consider how PCA-like administration would compare to continuous infusion of an analgesic drug. As discussed in Chapter 14, it is sometimes feasible to administer opioid analgesics by slow, continuous infusion into the bloodstream or into some other area such as the epidural or intrathecal space. Continuous infusion would obviously provide the best way of maintaining drug concentration within a given therapeutic range. Studies have indeed shown that continuous infusion of opioids into the epidural space may produce somewhat better pain relief than with IV PCA.[2,12] This is understandable considering that epidural delivery places the drug much closer to the spinal cord than does IV delivery. It would be more helpful to compare continuous epidural infusion with analogous PCA delivery into the epidural space. Studies that have made the comparison of continuous epidural infusion with epidural PCA have failed to show any clear advantage of continuous infusion.[9,11,13] In fact, continuous epidural infusion was often associated with the need for more drug to provide an equivalent level of analgesia compared to epidural PCA.[4,9,13] Hence, epidural PCA seems to be superior to continuous delivery of analgesics into the epidural space.

Thus, PCA has been shown to have certain advantages over more traditional methods such as intermittent IM injection or continuous epidural infusion. One must also consider that PCA decreases the need for other health professionals (physicians, nurses, pharmacists) to be directly involved in administering analgesics or adjusting the rate of analgesic delivery. IM injection, for instance, requires that the nurse be available at the proper time to inject the proper amount of the correct drug into the correct patient. This clearly takes the locus of control out of the patient's hands and makes the patient feel more dependent on an outside person to provide pain relief. When PCA systems are used appropriately, pain control is literally in the patient's hands. Likewise, continuous infusion often requires frequent adjustments by a qualified person who must attempt to match the dose of analgesic to the patient's pain level. This is especially difficult if pain levels are changing, such as in the patient recovering from surgery. With PCA, the patient is able to automatically titrate the amount of analgesia according to his or her pain. Again, this underscores a key advantage of PCA: this technique is superior to more traditional methods of analgesia because the person most qualified to judge his or her pain is empowered to self-administer the analgesic according to his or her own needs.

PROBLEMS AND SIDE EFFECTS OF PCA

Pharmacologic Side Effects

Side effects typically seen when opioids are used for PCA include sedation, pruritus, and gastrointestinal problems (nausea, vomiting). The incidence of these side effects, however, is not significantly increased during PCA versus more traditional methods of opioid administration such as intermittent intramuscular dosing.[3] Respiratory depression is another common side effect of opioid use, but again, there is no increased incidence of this problem when opioids are given via PCA.[3] In fact, the risk of respiratory depression is believed to be negligible when opioids are administered through spinal routes (epidural and intrathecal).[4] Hence, there does not seem to be an increase in the side effects commonly seen when PCA techniques are used to administer opioids, and the side effects commonly associated with these drugs may even be reduced during certain types of PCA application.

The incidence of side effects during PCA with local anesthetics is not well defined. Local anesthetics could conceivably cause sensory loss and motor weakness below the level of spinal administration. The possibility of these effects is directly dependent on the dose and site of administration, with the likelihood being greater when higher doses of local anesthetic are administered into the subarachnoid space.[21] Also, administration of local anesthetics with a vasoconstrictor (epinephrine) has been shown to cause excessive inhibition of motor function (dense motor block) because the anesthetic is not dispersed as easily by the local circulation.[11] Hence, transient sensory and motor loss must always be considered as a potential side effect when local anesthetics are used during PCA.

Problems with PCA Delivery

Other problems that can occur with PCA systems include errors on the part of the operator (nurse, physician, etc.) or the patient, or mechanical problems with the pump-delivery system.[20] These problems are summarized in Table 17–3. Operator er-

TABLE 17–3 Summary of Problems That Can Occur During PCA Therapy

Operator errors	Patient errors	Mechanical problems
Misprogramming PCA device	Failure to understand PCA therapy	Failure to deliver on demand
Failure to clamp or unclamp tubing	Misunderstanding PCA pump device	Cracked drug vials or syringes
Improperly loading syringe or cartridge	Intentional analgesic abuse	Defective one-way valve at Y connector
Inability to respond to safety alarms		Faulty alarm system
Misplacing PCA pump key		Malfunctions (e.g., lock)

Source: White,[20] p 81, 1987, with permission.

rors typically occur because the pump is not programmed correctly, or some other error occurs in loading the analgesic into the pump. Errors on the part of the patient can occur if the patient is not properly educated in PCA use or if the patient lacks adequate cognitive skills to use the PCA correctly. Finally, mechanical problems, including pump malfunction and clogging or displacement of the delivery tubing, may preclude delivery of the analgesic. Members of the health-care team should be alert for signs that the drug is being overdelivered during PCA, as evidenced by an increase in analgesic side effects, or that the analgesic is being underdelivered, as indicated by inadequate pain control.

SPECIAL CONCERNS FOR PCA IN REHABILITATION PATIENTS

When used appropriately, PCA offers several advantages to patients receiving physical therapy and occupational therapy. As discussed previously, PCA often provides analgesia with a lower chance of certain side effects such as sedation. Patients will be more alert and have a clearer sensorium while still receiving optimal pain control. Likewise, PCA prevents large fluctuations in plasma analgesic concentration and helps maintain analgesic concentration within a more finite range (see Fig. 17–1). This decreases the need to schedule rehabilitation at the time when analgesic concentrations are at optimal levels because concentrations should always be within the appropriate range. Patients may also be more mobile using various PCA systems as compared to more traditional analgesic methods. The use of PCA may allow patients to begin ambulation sooner following surgery, and PCA systems can help decrease the need for the patient to be bed-bound for long periods because of severe pain or the side effects from high, intermittent doses of analgesics.[17,19] Hence, rehabilitation specialists should acknowledge the advantages of PCA and capitalize on these advantages whenever possible in patients receiving PCA.

Rehabilitation specialists should also be aware of potential problems that can occur in patients receiving PCA. In particular, by monitoring the patient's signs and symptoms, therapists can help detect problems in PCA delivery. Therapists should use visual analog scales or some other valid measurement tool to routinely assess pain in patients receiving PCA. Patients exhibiting inadequate pain management or an unexplained increase in pain may be using a PCA system that is underdelivering the analgesic drug. The medical and nursing staff should be notified so that the delivery problem can be identified and rectified. Conversely, signs of respiratory depression or excessive sedation may indicate that the patient is being overdosed by the PCA system. This can obviously be a life-threatening situation that requires immediate attention. Hence, it is the responsibility of all health-care workers including rehabilitation specialists to look for signs of PCA malfunction every time they interact with the patient.

CASE STUDY

PATIENT-CONTROLLED ANALGESIA

Brief History. S.G., a 61-year-old man, was being treated for severe osteoarthritis in the right knee. Following an unsuccessful course of conservative therapy, S.G. was admitted to the hospital for a total knee replacement. The surgery was performed successfully, and PCA was instituted for postoperative pain management. PCA consisted of an external syringe pump connected to an IV catheter. The analgesic used was meperidine at a concentration of 10 mg/mL. Parameters for PCA were set by the physician to allow a demand dose of 1 mL (10 mg) with a lockout interval of 10 minutes. An initial or loading dose of 10 mg was also provided at the conclusion of the surgery. Physical therapy was initiated at the patient's bedside on the afternoon following surgery. The therapist found the patient groggy from the surgery, but the patient was coherent and able to understand simple commands. Pain, as assessed using a visual analog scale (VAS), was rated in the 4- to 5-cm range of a 10-cm scale (10 cm being equivalent to "worst pain imaginable"). The patient was observed using his PCA during the therapy session, and he seemed to understand how to use this device properly.

Problem/Influence of Drug Therapy. When seen at the bedside on the day following surgery, the patient was in obvious discomfort. Pain was rated in the 8- to 9-cm range of the VAS. The patient stated that he had been using the PCA as instructed and that the device had been recording his successful attempts with an audible signal. Upon closer inspection, however, the therapist noticed that the syringe was not properly engaged in the pump mechanism. Hence, the syringe was not being propelled forward, and the demand dose was not being administered.

Decision/Solution. The PCA malfunction was brought to the attention of the nursing staff, and the problem was quickly rectified. The syringe containing the opioid had apparently been refilled earlier in the day and had not been installed properly into the pump's syringe driver. The patient was given an initial 10-mg infusion, and PCA was then resumed according to the original dosing parameters. The remainder of the patient's recovery was uneventful, and he was able to participate actively and enthusiastically in the rehabilitation sessions.

SUMMARY

PCA allows the patient to self-administer a small amount of analgesic medication on a relatively frequent basis. This technique has been used to administer drugs such as opioids and local anesthetics. PCA can often provide better pain control using smaller quantities of the drug and with a lower incidence of side effects. The patient is allowed to self-administer a small dose of the drug by pressing a button that is connected to some type of pump. These PCA pumps vary in their cost, level of sophistication, and location (external versus surgically implanted), but all pumps are capable of being programmed to prevent the patient from exceeding certain dosing parameters. PCA systems continue to increase in popularity and are now used in a variety of clinical situations to manage acute and chronic pain. Rehabilitation specialists should be aware that PCA can provide improved pain control and enhance the patient's recovery. Human error or mechanical malfunction during PCA, however, may cause excessive or inadequate drug delivery, so therapists should also be alert for any signs that patients are receiving too much or too little analgesic during PCA.

REFERENCES

1. Albert, JM and Talbott, TM: Patient-controlled analgesia versus conventional intramuscular analgesia following colon surgery. Dis Colon Rectum 31:83, 1988.
2. Allaire, PH, et al: A prospective randomized comparison of epidural infusion of fentanyl and intravenous administration of morphine by patient-controlled analgesia after radical retropubic prostatectomy. Mayo Clin Proc 67:1031, 1992.
3. Ballantyne, JC, et al: Postoperative patient-controlled analgesia: Meta-analysis of initial randomized controlled trails. J Clin Anesth 5:182, 1993.
4. Chrubasik, J, Chrubasik, S, and Martin, E: Patient-controlled spinal opiate analgesia in terminal cancer. Drugs 43:799, 1992.
5. Dahl, JB, et al: Patient-controlled analgesia: A controlled trial. Acta Anaesthesiol Scand 31:744, 1987.
6. Ferrante, FM: Patient-controlled analgesia. Anesthesiol Clin North Am 10:287, 1992.
7. Ferrante, FM, et al: A statistical model for pain in patient-controlled analgesia and conventional intramuscular opioid regimens. Anesth Analg 67:457, 1988.
8. Gambling, DR, et al: Comparison of patient-controlled epidural analgesia and conventional intermittent "top-up" injections during labor. Anesth Analg 70:256, 1990.
9. Gambling, DR, et al: A comparative study of patient-controlled epidural analgesia (PCEA) and continuous infusion epidural analgesia (CIEA) during labour. Can J Anaesth 35:249, 1988.
10. Hecker, BR and Albert, L: Patient-controlled analgesia: A randomized, prospective comparison between two commercially available PCA pumps and conventional analgesic therapy for postoperative pain. Pain 35:115, 1988.
11. Lysak, SZ, Eisenach, JC, and Dobson, CE: Patient-controlled epidural analgesia during labor: A comparison of three solutions with a continuous infusion control. Anesthesiology 72:44, 1990.
12. Madej, TH, et al: Hypoxaemia and pain relief after lower abdominal surgery: Comparison of extradural and patient-controlled analgesia. Br J Anaesth 69:554, 1992.
13. Marlowe, S, Englstrom, R, and White, PF: Epidural patient-controlled analgesia (PCA): An alternative to continous epidural infusions. Pain 37:97, 1989.
14. McCoy, EP, Furness, G, and Wright, PMC: Patient-controlled analgesia with and without background infusion: Analgesia assessed using the demand-delivery ratio. Anaesthesia 48:256, 1993.
15. McGrath, D, et al: Comparison of one technique of patient-controlled postoperative analgesia with intramuscular meperidine. Pain 37:265, 1989.
16. Parker, RK, and White, PF: Epidural patient-controlled analgesia: An alternative to intravenous patient-controlled analgesia for pain relief after cesarean delivery. Anesth Analg 75:245, 1992.
17. Shaw, HL: Treatment of intractable cancer pain by electronically controlled parenteral infusion of analgesic drugs. Cancer 72(suppl):3416, 1993.
18. Spetzler, B and Anderson, L: Patient-controlled analgesia in the total joint arthroplasty patient. Clin Orthop 215:122, 1987.
19. Wasylak, TJ, et al: Reduction of postoperative morbidity following patient-controlled morphine. Can J Anaesth 37:726, 1990.
20. White, PF: Mishaps with patient-controlled analgesia. Anesthesiology 66:81, 1987.
21. Wild, L and Coyne, C: Epidural analgesia. Am J Nursing 4:26, 1992.

Autonomic and Cardiovascular Pharmacology

CHAPTER 18

Introduction to Autonomic Pharmacology

The human nervous system can be divided into two major functional areas: the somatic nervous system and the autonomic nervous system (ANS). The somatic division is concerned primarily with voluntary function—that is, control of the skeletal musculature. The ANS is responsible for controlling bodily functions that are largely involuntary, or automatic, in nature. For instance, the control of BP and other aspects of cardiovascular function is under the influence of the ANS. Other involuntary, or vegetative, functions such as digestion, elimination, and thermoregulation are also controlled by this system.

Considering the potential problems that can occur in various systems, such as the cardiovascular and digestive systems, the use of therapeutic drugs to alter autonomic function is one of the major areas of pharmacology. Drugs affecting autonomic function are prescribed routinely to many patients, including those individuals seen for physical and occupational therapy. The purpose of this chapter is to review some of the primary anatomic and physiologic aspects of the ANS. This review is intended to provide rehabilitation specialists with a basis for understanding the pharmacologic effects and clinical applications of the autonomic drugs, which are discussed in subsequent chapters.

ANATOMY OF THE AUTONOMIC NERVOUS SYSTEM: SYMPATHETIC AND PARASYMPATHETIC DIVISIONS

The ANS can be roughly divided into two areas: the sympathetic and parasympathetic nervous systems. The *sympathetic*, or thoracolumbar, division arises primarily from neurons located in the thoracic and upper lumbar regions of the spinal cord. The *parasympathetic*, or craniosacral, division is composed of neurons originating in the midbrain, brainstem, and sacral region of the spinal cord. There are many other anatomic and functional characteristics differentiating these two divisions, and these are briefly discussed later in this chapter. For a more detailed discussion of the

247

anatomic and functional organization of the ANS, the reader is referred to several excellent sources listed at the end of this chapter.[1,10,12,14,22]

Preganglionic and Postganglionic Neurons

The somatic nervous system uses one neuron to reach from the CNS to the periphery. In the somatic motor system, for instance, the alpha motor neuron begins in the spinal cord and extends all the way to the skeletal muscle; that is, it does not synapse until it reaches the muscle cell. In both the sympathetic and parasympathetic divisions, however, two neurons are used in sequence to reach from the CNS (i.e., brain or spinal cord) to the peripheral organ or tissue that is being supplied. The first neuron begins somewhere in the CNS and extends a certain distance toward the periphery before synapsing with a second neuron, which completes the journey to the final destination. The synapse of these two neurons is usually in one of the autonomic ganglia (see "Sympathetic Organization" and "Parasympathetic Organization"). Hence, the first neuron in sequence is termed the *preganglionic neuron*, and the second is referred to as the *postganglionic neuron*.

In both the sympathetic and parasympathetic divisions, preganglionic fibers are myelinated type B fibers, and postganglionic fibers are the small, unmyelinated type C fibers. In the sympathetic division, preganglionic neurons tend to be relatively short, while the sympathetic postganglionic neurons are relatively long. The opposite is true for the parasympathetic division, with the preganglionic neurons being relatively long and the postganglionic neurons short. The location of preganglionic and postganglionic fibers in each autonomic division is presented here.

Sympathetic Organization

The cell bodies for the sympathetic preganglionic fibers arise from the intermediolateral gray columns of the thoracic and upper lumbar spinal cord. The preganglionic fibers leave the spinal cord via the ventral root of the spinal nerve and end in a sympathetic ganglion. The sympathetic ganglia are located in three areas: (1) the paired paravertebral, or chain, ganglia, which lie bilaterally on either side of the vertebral column; (2) a group of unpaired prevertebral ganglia, which lie anterior to the aorta (e.g., the celiac plexus, the superior and inferior mesenteric ganglia); and (3) a small number of terminal ganglia, which lie directly in the tissue that is innervated (e.g., the bladder and rectum).

When the preganglionic fiber reaches one of the sympathetic ganglia, it synapses with a postganglionic fiber. Actually, one sympathetic preganglionic neuron may synapse with many postganglionic fibers. (The ratio of preganglionic to postganglionic fibers in the sympathetic chain ganglia is usually 1:15 to 20.) The postganglionic fiber then leaves the ganglion to travel to the effector tissue that it supplies (i.e., the heart, peripheral arteriole, sweat gland, etc.).

Parasympathetic Organization

Parasympathetic preganglionic neurons originate in the midbrain and brainstem (cranial portion) or the sacral region of the spinal cord. Neurons comprising the cranial portion of the parasympathetics exit the CNS via cranial nerves III, VII, IX, and X. Cranial nerve X (vagus nerve) is particularly significant because it contains approximately 75 percent of the efferent component of the entire parasympathetic division. Neurons composing the preganglionic fibers of the sacral portion exit the spinal cord via the pelvic splanchnic nerves.

As in the sympathetic division, parasympathetic preganglionic neurons synapse in the periphery with a postganglionic fiber. This synapse usually takes place in a terminal ganglion that is located directly in the organ or tissue supplied by the postganglionic neuron. Consequently, the parasympathetic ganglia are usually embedded directly in the organ or tissue that is innervated.

FUNCTIONAL ASPECTS OF THE SYMPATHETIC AND PARASYMPATHETIC DIVISIONS

Except for skeletal muscle, virtually all tissues in the body are innervated in some way by the ANS. Table 18-1 summarizes the innervation and effects of the sympathetic and parasympathetic divisions on some of the major organs and tissues in the body. As indicated in Table 18-1, some organs, such as the heart, are innervated by both sympathetic and parasympathetic neurons. Other tissues, however, may only be

TABLE 18-1 Response of Effector Organs to Autonomic Stimulation

Organ	Sympathetic*	Parasympathetic†
Heart	Increased contractility (beta-1)	Decreased heart rate (musc)
	Increased heart rate (beta-1)	Slight decrease in contractility (musc)
Arterioles	Vasoconstriction of skin and viscera (alpha-1)	No parasympathetic innervation
	Vasodilation of skeletal muscle and liver (beta-2)	
Lung	Bronchodilation (beta-2)	Bronchoconstriction (musc)
Eye		
Radial muscle	Contraction (alpha-1)	Relaxation (musc)
Ciliary muscle	Relaxation (beta-2)	Contraction (musc)
Gastrointestinal function	Decreased motility (alpha-1,-2; beta-1,-2)	Increased motility and secretion (musc)
Kidney	Increased renin secretion (alpha-1, beta-1)	No parasympathetic innervation
Urinary bladder		
Detrusor	Relaxation (beta-2)	Contraction (musc)
Trigone and sphincter	Contraction (alpha-1)	Relaxation (musc)
Sweat glands	Increased secretion (musc‡)	No parasympathetic innervation
Liver	Glycogenolysis and gluconeogenesis (alpha, beta-2)	Glycogen synthesis (musc)
Fat cells	Lipolysis (alpha, beta-1)	No parasympathetic innervation

*The primary receptor subtypes that mediate each response are listed in parentheses (e.g, alpha-1, beta-2). If no subtype is designated, it is because the particular alpha or beta subtype has not been conclusively determined.

†Note that all organ responses to parasympathetic stimulation are mediated via muscarinic (musc) receptors.

‡Represents response due to sympathetic postganglionic cholinergic fibers.

supplied by the sympathetic division. The peripheral arterioles, for instance, are innervated by the sympathetic division but receive no parasympathetic innervation.

If an organ *is* innervated by both the sympathetic and parasympathetic divisions, a physiologic antagonism typically exists between these divisions.[10] That is, if both divisions innervate the tissue, one division usually increases function, whereas the other decreases activity. For instance, the sympathetics increase heart rate and stimulate cardiac output, whereas the parasympathetics cause bradycardia. However, it is incorrect to state that the sympathetics are always excitatory in nature and that the parasympathetics are always inhibitory. In tissues such as the gastrointestinal tract, the parasympathetics tend to increase intestinal motility and secretion, whereas the sympathetics slow down intestinal motility. The effect of each division on any tissue must be considered according to the particular organ or gland in question.

One generalization that can be made regarding sympathetic and parasympathetic function is that the sympathetic division tends to mobilize body energy, whereas the parasympathetic division tends to conserve and store body energy. Typically, sympathetic discharge is increased when the individual is faced with some stressful situation. This situation initiates the classic fight-or-flight scenario in which the person must either flee or defend himself or herself. Sympathetic discharge causes increased cardiac output, decreased visceral blood flow (thus leaving more blood available for skeletal muscle), increased cellular metabolism, and several other physiologic changes that facilitate vigorous activity. In contrast, the parasympathetic division tends to have the opposite effect. Parasympathetic discharge slows down the heart and generally brings about changes that encourage inactivity. Parasympathetic discharge tends to increase intestinal digestion and absorption, an activity that stores energy for future needs.

Finally, activation of the sympathetic division tends to result in a more massive and diffuse reaction than does parasympathetic activation. Parasympathetic reactions tend to be fairly discrete and to affect only one organ or tissue. For instance, the parasympathetic fibers to the myocardium can be activated to slow down the heart without a concomitant emptying of the bowel through an excitatory effect on the lower gastrointestinal tract. When the sympathetic division is activated, effects are commonly observed on many tissues throughout the body. The more diffuse sympathetic reactions routinely produce a simultaneous effect on the heart, total peripheral vasculature, general cellular metabolism, and so on.

FUNCTION OF THE ADRENAL MEDULLA

The adrenal medulla synthesizes and secretes norepinephrine and epinephrine directly into the bloodstream. Typically, the secretion from the adrenal medulla contains about 20 percent norepinephrine and 80 percent epinephrine.[10] These two hormones are fairly similar in action, except that **epinephrine** increases cardiac function and cellular metabolism to a greater extent than **norepinephrine** because epinephrine has a higher affinity for certain receptors than norepinephrine (i.e., epinephrine binds more readily to the beta subtype of adrenergic receptors; see "Autonomic Receptors").[10]

The adrenal medulla is innervated by sympathetic neurons. During normal, resting conditions, the adrenal medulla secretes small amounts of epinephrine and norepinephrine. During periods of stress, however, a general increase in sympathetic discharge causes an increased release of epinephrine and norepinephrine from the adrenal medulla. Since these hormones are released directly into the bloodstream, they tend to circulate extensively throughout the body. Circulating epinephrine and norepinephrine can reach tissues that are not directly innervated by the sympathetic neurons, thus augmenting the general sympathetic effect. Also, the circulating epinephrine and norepinephrine are removed from the body more slowly than norepinephrine that is produced locally at the sympathetic postganglionic nerve terminals. As a result, adrenal release of epinephrine and norepinephrine tends to prolong the effect of the sympathetic reaction.

Consequently, the adrenal medulla serves to augment the sympathetic division of the ANS. In situations where a sudden increase in sympathetic function is required (i.e., the fight-or-flight scenario), the adrenal medulla works with the sympathetics to produce a more extensive and lasting response.

AUTONOMIC INTEGRATION AND CONTROL

Most of the autonomic control over various physiologic functions is manifested through autonomic reflexes; that is, homeostatic control of BP, thermoregulation, and gastrointestinal function depend on the automatic reflex adjustment in these systems through the sympathetic and/or parasympathetic divisions. Autonomic reflexes are based on the following strategy: some peripheral sensor monitors a change in the particular system. This information is relayed to a certain level of the CNS, where it is integrated. An adjustment is made in the autonomic discharge to the specific organ or tissue, which will alter its activity to return physiologic function back to the appropriate level.

A practical example of this type of autonomic reflex control is the so-called baroreceptor reflex, which is important in the control of BP. In this particular example, pressure sensors (i.e., baroreceptors) located in the large arteries of the thorax and neck monitor changes in BP and heart rate. A sudden drop in BP is sensed by these baroreceptors, and this information is relayed to the brainstem. In the brainstem, this information is integrated, and a compensatory increase occurs in sympathetic discharge to the heart and peripheral vasculature, and parasympathetic outflow to the heart is decreased. The result is an increase in cardiac output and an increase in peripheral vascular resistance, which effectively brings BP back to the appropriate level. The baroreceptor reflex works in the opposite fashion if BP were to suddenly increase, with the ultimate result being a return to normal pressure levels because of a decrease in sympathetic outflow and an increase in cardiac parasympathetic discharge.

The baroreceptor response is just one example of the type of reflex activity employed by the ANS. The control of other involuntary functions usually follows a similar pattern of peripheral monitoring, central integration, and altered autonomic discharge. Body temperature, for instance, is monitored by thermoreceptors located in the skin, viscera, and hypothalamus. When a change in body temperature is monitored by these sensors, this information is relayed to the hypothalamus and appropriate adjustments are made in autonomic discharge in order to maintain thermal homeostasis (e.g., sweating is increased or decreased and blood flow is redistributed). Many other autonomic reflexes that control other visceral and involuntary functions operate in a similar manner.

Integration of autonomic responses is often fairly complex and may occur at several levels of the CNS. Some reflexes, such as emptying of the bowel and bladder, are integrated primarily at the level of the sacral spinal cord. Other reflexes, such as the baroreceptor reflex previously discussed, are integrated at higher levels in the so-called vasomotor center located in the brainstem. Also, the hypothalamus is important in regulating the ANS, and many functions including body temperature, water balance, and energy metabolism are controlled and integrated at the hypothalamus. To add to the complexity, higher levels of the brain such as the cortex and limbic system may also influence autonomic function through their interaction with the hypothalamus, brainstem, and spinal cord. This information is important pharmacologically because drugs that act on the CNS have the potential to alter autonomic function by influencing the central integration of autonomic responses. Drugs that affect the cortex, limbic system, and brainstem may indirectly alter the response of some of the autonomic reflexes by altering the relationship between afferent input and efferent sympathetic and parasympathetic outflow.

AUTONOMIC NEUROTRANSMITTERS

Acetylcholine and Norepinephrine

There are four sites of synaptic transmission in the efferent limb of the ANS: (1) the synapse between preganglionic and postganglionic neurons in the sympathetic division, (2) the analogous preganglionic-postganglionic synapse in the parasympathetic division, (3) the synapse between the sympathetic postganglionic neuron and the effector cell, and (4) the parasympathetic postganglionic–effector cell synapse. Figure 18–1 summarizes the chemical neurotransmitter that is present at each synapse.

As indicated in Figure 18–1, the transmitter at the preganglionic-postganglionic synapse in both divisions is acetylcholine. The transmitter at the parasympathetic

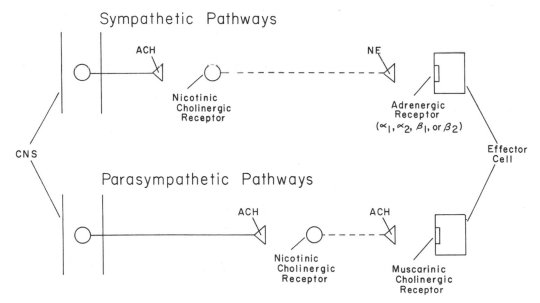

FIGURE 18–1. Autonomic neurotransmitters and receptors. Preganglionic neurons *(solid lines)* release acetylcholine (ACh). Postganglionic neurons *(dashed lines)* release ACh in the parasympathetic pathways and norepinephrine (NE) in the sympathetic pathways.

postganglionic–effector cell synapse is also acetylcholine. The transmitter at the sympathetic postganglionic–effector cell synapse is usually norepinephrine. A small number of sympathetic postganglionic fibers, however, also use acetylcholine as their neurotransmitter.

Consequently, all preganglionic neurons and parasympathetic postganglionic neurons are said to be cholinergic in nature because of the presence of acetylcholine at their respective synapses. Most sympathetic postganglionic neurons use norepinephrine and are referred to as **adrenergic**. (Norepinephrine is sometimes referred to as noradrenaline; hence the term "adrenergic.") An exception to this scheme is the presence of certain sympathetic postganglionic fibers that use acetylcholine as their neurotransmitter. These sympathetic cholinergic neurons innervate sweat glands and certain blood vessels in the face, neck, and lower extremities.

Other Autonomic Neurotransmitters

In recent years, it has become apparent that several nonadrenergic, noncholinergic neurotransmitters may also be present in the ANS. Purinergic substances such as adenosine and adenosine triphosphate have been implicated as possible transmitters in the gastrointestinal tract.[4,17,19] Several peptides such as substance P and vasoactive intestinal polypeptide have been identified as possibly participating in the autonomic control of intestinal and respiratory function.[2,3]

Whether these nonadrenergic, noncholinergic substances are true neurotransmitters is still uncertain. They may act as cotransmitters that are released from the synaptic terminal along with the classic autonomic transmitters (i.e., acetylcholine and norepinephrine). These other substances, however, may simply be produced locally and serve to modulate synaptic activity without actually being released from the presynaptic terminal. Additional information will be necessary to fully identify the role of these and other nonadrenergic, noncholinergic substances as autonomic neurotransmitters.

AUTONOMIC RECEPTORS

Since there are two primary neurotransmitters involved in autonomic discharge, there are two primary classifications of postsynaptic receptors. **Cholinergic** receptors are located at acetylcholine synapses, and adrenergic receptors are located at norepinephrine synapses. As indicated in Figure 18–2, each type of receptor has several subclassifications. The location and functional significance of these classifications and subclassifications are presented here.

Cholinergic Receptors

Cholinergic receptors are subdivided into two categories: **nicotinic** and **muscarinic**. Although acetylcholine will bind to all cholinergic receptors, certain receptors bind preferentially with the drug nicotine. Other receptors have a specific affinity for muscarine, a naturally occurring compound found in certain poisonous mushrooms. Thus the terms "nicotinic" and "muscarinic" were derived.

Nicotinic cholinergic receptors are located at the junction between preganglionic

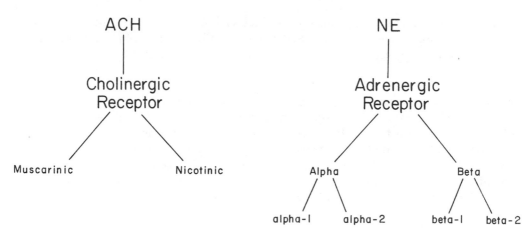

FIGURE 18–2. Receptor classifications and subclassifications for acetylcholine (ACh) and norepinephrine (NE), the two primary neurotransmitters used in the autonomic nervous system.

and postganglionic neurons in both the sympathetic and parasympathetic pathways (see Fig. 18–1). This fact is significant pharmacologically because any drug that affects these nicotinic receptors will affect activity in both divisions of the ANS. The cholinergic nicotinic receptor located in the ANS is sometimes referred to as a type I (or N_N) nicotinic receptor to differentiate it from the type II (or N_M) nicotinic receptors, which are located at the skeletal neuromuscular junction.

Muscarinic cholinergic receptors are located at all the synapses between cholinergic postganglionic neurons and the terminal effector cell, including all the parasympathetic terminal synapses, as well as the sympathetic postganglionic cholinergic fibers, which supply sweat glands and some specialized blood vessels. Current research suggests that there are probably several different types of muscarinic receptors; that is, M_1, M_2, and M_3 muscarinic subtypes may exist.[5,8,12,16,18,20] At present, however, these muscarinic receptors can be regarded as being functionally similar.

Thus, cholinergic muscarinic receptors ultimately mediate the effect on the tissue itself. Table 18–2 summarizes the primary physiologic responses when muscarinic receptors are stimulated on various tissues in the body. Note that the specific response to stimulation of a muscarinic cholinergic receptor depends on the tissue in question. Stimulation of muscarinic receptors on the myocardium, for instance, causes a decrease in heart rate, whereas stimulation of muscarinic receptors in the intestinal wall leads to increases in smooth muscle contraction and glandular secretion.

Adrenergic Receptors

As shown in Figure 18–2, the adrenergic receptors are subdivided into two primary categories: alpha- and beta-adrenergic receptors. **Alpha receptors** are further subdivided into alpha-1 and alpha-2 receptors, and **beta receptors** are subdivided into beta-1 and beta-2 receptors.[11] These divisions are based on a different sensitivity of each receptor subcategory to different endogenous and exogenous agents. Alpha-1 receptors, for instance, bind more readily with certain agonists and antagonists, whereas alpha-2 receptors bind preferentially with other agents. Specific agents that bind to each adrenergic receptor subcategory are identified in Chapter 20.

In the ANS, the various types of adrenergic receptors are found on the effector cell in the innervated tissue. In other words, these receptors are located at the terminal synapse between sympathetic postganglionic adrenergic neurons and the tissue they supply. The basic characteristics of each adrenergic receptor subtype are briefly outlined here.

Alpha-1 Receptors. A primary location of these receptors is the smooth muscle located in various tissues throughout the body. Alpha-1 receptors are located on the smooth muscle located in the peripheral vasculature, intestinal wall, radial muscle of the iris, ureters, urinary sphincter, and spleen capsule. The response of each tissue when the alpha-1 receptor is stimulated depends on each respective tissue (see Table 18–2).

Alpha-2 Receptors. The alpha-2 receptors were originally identified by their presence on the presynaptic terminal of certain adrenergic synapses.[6] These presynaptic alpha-2 receptors appear to modulate norepinephrine release from the presynaptic terminal; that is, they seem to decrease norepinephrine release, thus serving as a form of

TABLE 18–2 Autonomic Receptor Locations and Responses

Receptor	Primary Location(s)	Response
Cholinergic		
Nicotinic	Autonomic ganglia	Mediate transmission to postganglionic neuron
Muscarinic	All parasympathetic effector cells:	
	Visceral and bronchiole smooth muscle	Contraction (generally)
	Cardiac muscle	Decreased heart rate
	Exocrine glands (salivary, intestinal, lacrimal)	Increased secretion
	Sweat glands	Increased secretion
Adrenergic		
Alpha-1	Vascular smooth muscle	Contraction
	Intestinal smooth muscle	Relaxation
	Radial muscle iris	Contraction (mydriasis)
	Ureters	Increased motility
	Urinary sphincter	Contraction
	Spleen capsule	Contraction
Alpha-2	CNS inhibitory synapses	Decreased sympathetic discharge from CNS
	Presynaptic terminal at peripheral adrenergic synapses	Decreased norepinephrine release
	Gastrointestinal tract	Decreased motility and secretion
	Pancreatic islet cells	Decreased insulin secretion
Beta-1	Cardiac muscle	Increased heart rate and contractility
	Kidney	Increased renin secretion
	Fat cells	Increased lipolysis
Beta-2	Bronchiole smooth muscle	Relaxation (bronchodilation)
	Some arterioles (skeletal muscle, liver)	Vasodilation
	Gastrointestinal smooth muscle	Decreased motility
	Skeletal muscle and liver cells	Increased cellular metabolism
	Uterus	Relaxation
	Gallbladder	Relaxation

negative feedback that limits the amount of neurotransmitter released from the pre-synaptic terminal.[7,15,21] Also, alpha-2 receptors have been found postsynaptically on certain CNS adrenergic synapses involved in the control of sympathetic discharge.[13] Stimulation of these centrally located alpha-2 receptors is believed to inhibit sympa-thetic discharge from the brainstem. The importance of central alpha-2 receptors in controlling cardiovascular function and the possible use of alpha-2 agonists to control BP are discussed in Chapter 21. Alpha-2 receptors are also located in the gastrointesti-nal tract and pancreas, and stimulation of these receptors at these sites causes de-creased intestinal motility and decreased insulin secretion, respectively.

Beta-1 Receptors. These receptors predominate in the heart and kidneys (see Table 18–2).[9] The cardiac beta-1 receptors have received a tremendous amount of at-tention with regard to pharmacologic antagonism of their function through the use of the so-called beta blockers. Beta-1 receptors are also located on fat cells, and stimula-tion of these receptors increases lipolysis.

Beta-2 Receptors. Beta-2 receptors are found primarily on the smooth muscle of certain vasculature, the bronchioles, the gallbladder, and the uterus.[9] Their presence in bronchiole smooth muscle is especially important in the pharmacologic management of respiratory conditions such as asthma (see Chapter 26). These receptors are also re-sponsible for mediating changes in the metabolism of skeletal muscle and liver cells.

Table 18–2 summarizes receptor subtypes that are located on the primary organs and tissues in the body, and the associated response when the receptor is stimulated. Exactly which receptor subtype is located on any given tissue depends on the tissue in question. Note that some tissues may have two or more different subtypes of adrener-gic receptor (e.g., skeletal muscle arterioles appear to have alpha-1 and beta-2 recep-tors). Also, the response of a tissue when the receptor is stimulated is dependent on the specific receptor-cell interaction. Stimulation of the vascular alpha-1 receptor, for instance, results in smooth-muscle contraction and vasoconstriction, whereas stimula-tion of the intestinal alpha-1 receptor results in relaxation and decreased intestinal motility. This difference is caused by the way the receptor is coupled to the cell's inter-nal biochemistry at each location. As discussed in Chapter 4, the surface receptor at one cell may be coupled to the internal enzymatic machinery of the cell so that it stim-ulates cell function. The same receptor subtype at a different tissue will be linked to in-hibitory enzymes that slow down cell function. Refer to Chapter 4 for a more detailed description of how surface receptors are coupled to cell function.

PHARMACOLOGIC SIGNIFICANCE OF AUTONOMIC RECEPTORS

Perhaps no area of research has contributed more to pharmacology than the iden-tification, classification, and subclassification of autonomic receptors. The realization that various tissues have distinct subtypes of receptors has enabled the use of drugs that affect certain tissues and organs while causing minimal effects on other tissues. For instance, a beta-1 antagonist (i.e., a drug that specifically blocks the beta-1 adrener-gic receptor) will slow down heart rate and decrease myocardial contractility without causing any major changes in the physiologic functions that are mediated by the other autonomic receptors.

However, several limitations of autonomic drugs must be realized. First, a drug that binds preferentially to one receptor subtype will bind to that receptor at all of its locations. For example, a muscarinic antagonist that decreases activity in the gastrointestinal tract will also decrease bronchial secretions in the lungs and cause urinary retention because of relaxation of the detrusor muscle of the bladder. Also, no drug is entirely specific for only one receptor subtype. For instance, the so-called beta-1–specific antagonists atenolol and metoprolol have a 10- to 20-fold greater affinity for beta-1 receptors than for beta-2 receptors.[9] At high enough concentrations, however, these drugs will affect beta-2 receptors as well. Finally, organs and tissues in the body do not contain only one subtype of receptor. For example, the predominant receptor in the bronchioles is the beta-2 subtype, but some beta-1 receptors are also present. Thus, a patient using a beta-1–specific drug such as metoprolol may experience some respiratory effects as well.[9]

Consequently, many side effects as well as beneficial effects of autonomic drugs can be attributed to the interaction of various agents with different receptors. The significance to autonomic receptor subtypes as well as the use of specific cholinergic and adrenergic drugs in treating various problems are covered in more detail in Chapters 19 and 20.

SUMMARY

The ANS is primarily responsible for controlling involuntary, or vegetative, functions in the body. The sympathetic and parasympathetic divisions of the ANS often function as physiologic antagonists to maintain homeostasis of various activities, including BP control, thermoregulation, digestion, and elimination. The primary neurotransmitters used in synaptic transmission within the ANS are acetylcholine and norepinephrine. These chemicals are found at specific locations in each autonomic division, as are their respective cholinergic and adrenergic receptors. The two primary types of autonomic receptors (cholinergic and adrenergic) are subdivided according to differences in drug affinity. Receptor subtypes are located in specific tissues throughout the body and are responsible for mediating the appropriate tissue response. Most autonomic drugs exert their effects by interacting in some way with autonomic synaptic transmission so that a fairly selective and isolated effect is achieved.

REFERENCES

1. Appenzeller, O: The Autonomic Nervous System: An Introduction to Basic and Clinical Concepts. Elsevier, New York, 1982.
2. Barnes, PJ: Non-adrenergic non-cholinergic neural control of human airways. Arch Int Pharmacodyn Ther 280:208, 1986.
3. Bauer, V and Matusak, O: The non-adrenergic non-cholinergic innervation and transmission in the small intestine. Arch Int Pharmacodyn Ther 280(suppl):137, 1986.
4. Burnstock, G: Neurotransmitters and trophic factors in the autonomic nervous system. J Physiol 313: 1, 1981.
5. Cortes, R, et al: Muscarinic cholinergic receptor subtypes in the human brain. II. Quantitative autoradiographic studies. Brain Res 362:239, 1986.
6. Davey, MJ: Alpha adrenoceptors: An overview. J Mol Cell Cardiol 18(suppl 5):1, 1986.
7. Dixon, WR, Mosimann, WF, and Weiner, N: The role of presynaptic feedback mechanisms in regulation of norepinephrine release by nerve stimulation. J Pharmacol Exp Ther 209:196, 1979.
8. Evans, RA, et al: Differential ontogeny of putative M1 and M2 muscarinic receptor binding sites in the murine cerebral cortex and heart. J Pharmacol Exp Ther 235:612, 1985.
9. Gerber, JG and Nies, AS: Beta-adrenergic blocking drugs. Annu Rev Med 36:145, 1985.
10. Guyton, AC: Basic Neuroscience: Anatomy and Physiology. WB Saunders, Philadelphia, 1987.

11. Heinsimer, JA and Lefkowitz, RJ: Adrenergic receptors: Biochemistry, regulation, molecular mechanism, and clinical implications. J Lab Clin Med 100:641, 1982.
12. Katzung, BG: Introduction to autonomic pharmacology. In Katzung, BG (ed): Basic and Clinical Pharmacology, ed 5. Appleton & Lange, Norwalk, CT, 1992.
13. Koss, MC: Review article: Pupillary dilation as an index of central nervous system alpha-2 adrenoceptor activation. J Pharmacol Methods 15:1, 1986.
14. Lefkowitz, RJ, Hoffman, BB, and Taylor, P: Neurohumoral transmission: The autonomic and somatic motor nervous systems. In Gilman, AG, et al (eds): The Pharmacological Basis of Therapeutics, ed 8. Pergamon Press, New York, 1990.
15. Levitt, B and Hieble, JP: Prejunctional alpha-2 adrenoceptors modulate stimulation-evoked norepinephrine release in rabbit lateral saphenous vein. Eur J Pharmacol 132:197, 1986.
16. Magous, R, Baudiere, B, and Bali, J-P: Muscarinic receptors in isolated gastric fundic mucosal cells. Binding-activity relationships. Biochem Pharmacol 34:2269, 1985.
17. Manzini, S, Maggi, CA, and Meli, A: Pharmacological evidence that at least 2 different non-adrenergic non-cholinergic inhibitory systems are present in the rat small intestine. Eur J Pharmacol 123:229, 1986.
18. Potter, LT, Flynn, DD, and Hanchett, HE: Independent M_1 and M_2 receptors: Ligands, autoradiography and functions. Trends Pharmacol Sci (suppl):22, 1984.
19. Su, C: Purinergic neurotransmission and neuromodulation. Annu Rev Pharmacol Toxicol 23:397, 1983.
20. Vickroy, TW, et al: Agonist binding to multiple muscarinic receptors. Fed Proc 43:2785, 1984.
21. Westfall, TC: Evidence that noradrenergic neurotransmitter release is regulated by presynaptic receptors. Fed Proc 43:1352, 1984.
22. Williams, PL, et al (eds): Gray's Anatomy, ed 37. Churchill Livingstone, New York, 1989.

CHAPTER 19

Cholinergic Drugs

This chapter discusses drugs that affect the activity at **cholinergic** synapses—that is, synapses using acetylcholine as a neurotransmitter. These cholinergic synapses are very important in a number of different physiologic systems. As discussed in Chapter 18, acetylcholine is one of the primary neurotransmitters in the autonomic nervous system (ANS), especially the parasympathetic autonomic division. Consequently, many of the drugs discussed in this chapter are administered to alter the response of various tissues to autonomic parasympathetic control. Acetylcholine is also the neurotransmitter at the skeletal neuromuscular junction. Certain cholinergic stimulants are used to treat a specific problem at the skeletal neuromuscular junction (i.e., myasthenia gravis). Cholinergic synapses are also found in specific areas of the brain, and some anticholinergic drugs are used to decrease the symptoms of such diverse problems as parkinsonism and motion sickness. Consequently, these drugs are used in a variety of clinical situations.

The purpose of this chapter is to present an overview of these drugs in the context that they share a common mode of action; that is, they influence cholinergic activity. Considering the diverse clinical applications of cholinergic and anticholinergic agents, physical therapists and occupational therapists will likely encounter patients taking these agents. Some knowledge of the pharmacodynamics of these medications will enable the rehabilitation specialist to understand the therapeutic rationale behind drug administration as well as the patient's response to the drug.

Autonomic cholinergic drugs can be divided into two general categories: cholinergic stimulants and anticholinergic drugs. Cholinergic stimulants effectively increase activity at acetylcholine synapses, whereas anticholinergic drugs decrease synaptic activity. Cholinergic stimulants and anticholinergic agents can be further characterized according to functional or pharmacodynamic criteria, and these criteria will be discussed in more detail in this chapter.

CHOLINERGIC RECEPTORS

Many autonomic cholinergic drugs affect synaptic activity by interacting with the acetylcholine receptor located on the postsynaptic membrane. At each cholinergic

259

synapse, postsynaptic receptors are responsible for recognizing the acetylcholine molecule and transducing the chemical signal into a postsynaptic response. As discussed in Chapter 18, cholinergic receptors can be subdivided into muscarinic and nicotinic receptors according to their affinity for certain drugs.

Muscarinic cholinergic receptors are generally found on the peripheral tissues supplied by parasympathetic postganglionic neurons—that is, on effector organs such as the gastrointestinal tract, urinary bladder, heart, eye, and so on. Acetylcholine synapses found in specific areas of the CNS also use the muscarinic subtype of cholinergic receptor. Nicotinic cholinergic receptors are located in the autonomic ganglia (nicotinic type I or N_N) and at the skeletal neuromuscular junction (nicotinic type II or N_M). Refer to Chapter 18 for a more detailed discussion of cholinergic receptor subclassification.

The existence of different varieties of cholinergic receptors is important pharmacologically. Some drugs are relatively specific for a certain cholinergic receptor subtype, whereas others tend to bind rather indiscriminately to all cholinergic receptors. Obviously the more specific drugs are preferable because they tend to produce a more precise response with fewer side effects. As this chapter will point out, however, specificity is only a relative term, and drugs that bind preferentially to one receptor subtype may produce a variety of responses.

CHOLINERGIC STIMULANTS

Cholinergic stimulants increase activity at acetylcholine synapses. Chemically, many agents are capable of potently and effectively stimulating cholinergic activity. However, only a few drugs exhibit sufficient safety and relative specificity to be used in clinical situations. These clinically relevant drugs can be subdivided into two categories depending on their mechanism of action. Direct-acting cholinergic stimulants exert their effects by binding directly with the cholinergic receptor (Fig. 19–1). Indirect-acting cholinergic stimulants increase synaptic activity by inhibiting the acetylcholinesterase enzyme located at the cholinergic synapse (see Fig. 19–1). Table 19–1 lists specific direct-acting and indirect-acting cholinergic stimulants, and the rationale for their use is presented here.

Direct-Acting Cholinergic Stimulants

Direct-acting stimulants bind directly to the cholinergic receptor and activate the receptor, which in turn initiates a cellular response. These stimulants may be considered true cholinergic agonists, and they function in a manner similar to the acetylcholine molecule. By definition, acetylcholine itself is a direct-acting cholinergic stimulant. Exogenously administered acetylcholine is not used therapeutically, however, because it is degraded rapidly and extensively by the acetylcholinesterase enzyme, which is found ubiquitously throughout the body.

As mentioned previously, there are many pharmacologic agents that can directly stimulate cholinergic receptors. A certain degree of drug specificity is desirable, however, when considering these agents for therapeutic purposes. For instance, drugs that have a greater specificity for the muscarinic cholinergic receptor are more beneficial. These muscarinic cholinergic stimulants will primarily affect the peripheral tissues

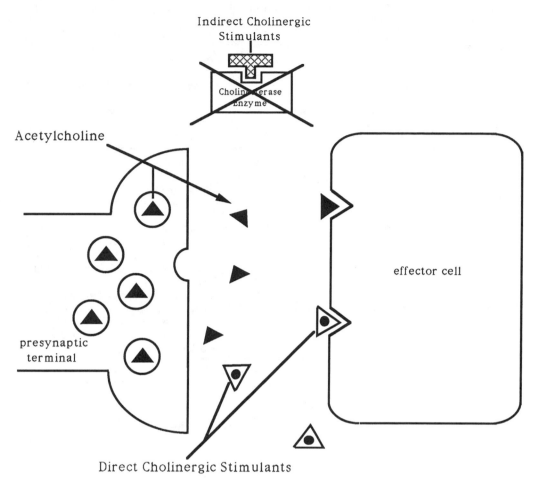

FIGURE 19–1. Mechanism of action of cholinergic stimulants. Direct-acting stimulants bind directly to the postsynaptic cholinergic receptor. Indirect-acting stimulants inhibit the cholinesterase enzyme, thus allowing acetylcholine to remain in the synaptic cleft.

while exerting a minimal effect on the cholinergic receptors located in the autonomic ganglia and the neuromuscular junction. (Recall that the cholinergic receptors found in the autonomic ganglia and at the skeletal neuromuscular junction are the nicotinic type I and nicotinic type II, respectively.)

Consequently, only a few agents are suitable for clinical use as direct-acting cholinergic stimulants. For systemic administration, bethanechol (Duvoid, Urecholine) is the primary direct-acting cholinergic stimulant used clinically (see Table 19–1). Bethanechol appears to preferentially stimulate muscarinic cholinergic receptors, although some amount of stimulation of the ganglionic nicotinic receptor may also occur.[14] Other direct-acting cholinergic stimulants such as carbachol and pilocarpine are limited to topical use in ophthalmologic conditions (glaucoma). These antiglaucoma drugs would produce too many side effects if administered systemically but are relatively specific when administered directly to the eye. Likewise, methacholine is a direct-acting cholinergic stimulant that can be administered locally to the lungs via in-

TABLE 19–1 Cholinergic Stimulants

Generic Name	Trade Name(s)	Primary Clinical Use(s)*
Direct-Acting (Cholinergic Agonists)		
Bethanechol	Duvoid, Urecholine, others	Postoperative gastrointestinal and urinary atony
Carbachol	Isopto Carbachol, Miostat	Glaucoma
Methacholine	Provocholine	Diagnosis of asthma
Pilocarpine	Pilocar, Adsorbocarpine, many others	Glaucoma
Indirect-Acting (Cholinesterase Inhibitors)		
Ambenonium	Mytelase	Myasthenia gravis
Demecarium	Humorsol	Glaucoma
Echothiophate	Phospholine Iodide	Glaucoma
Edrophonium	Reversol, Tensilon	Myasthenia gravis, reversal of neuromuscular blocking drugs
Isoflurophate	Floropryl	Glaucoma
Neostigmine	Prostigmin	Postoperative gastrointestinal and urinary atony, myasthenia gravis, reversal of neuromuscular blocking drugs
Physostigmine	Isopto Eserine, Antilirium	Glaucoma, reversal of CNS toxicity caused by anticholinergic drugs
Pyridostigmine	Mestinon, Regonol	Myasthenia gravis, reversal of neuromuscular blocking drugs

*Agents used to treat glaucoma are administered topically, that is, directly to the eye. Agents used for other problems are given systemically by oral administration or injection.

halation to test for airway hyperresponsiveness when diagnosing patients for asthma. Clinical applications of direct-acting cholinergic stimulants are summarized in Table 19–1.

Indirect-Acting Cholinergic Stimulants

Indirect-acting stimulants increase activity at cholinergic synapses by inhibiting the acetylcholinesterase enzyme. This enzyme is normally responsible for destroying acetylcholine after this neurotransmitter is released from the presynaptic terminal. Indirect-acting stimulants inhibit the acetylcholinesterase, thus allowing more acetylcholine to remain at the synapse. The result is an increase in cholinergic synaptic transmission.

Because of their effect on the acetylcholinesterase enzyme, indirect-acting stimulants are also referred to as *cholinesterase inhibitors* or *anticholinesterase agents*. The exact way in which these drugs inhibit the acetylcholinesterase enzyme varies depending on each individual agent. The net effect is similar, however, in that the enzyme's ability to degrade acetylcholine is diminished by these drugs.

Unlike the systemic direct-acting cholinergic stimulants (bethanechol), cholinesterase inhibitors display a relative lack of specificity regarding which cholinergic synapses they stimulate. These drugs tend to inhibit the acetylcholinesterase found at all cholinergic synapses. Thus, they may exert a stimulatory effect on the peripheral muscarinic cholinergic synapses, as well as the cholinergic synapses found at the autonomic ganglia, at the skeletal neuromuscular junction, and within certain aspects of the CNS. In appropriate doses, however, these indirect-acting stimulants tend to predominantly affect the skeletal neuromuscular junction and peripheral tissues containing muscarinic receptors. This specificity may be because the drug has better access to the peripheral cholinergic synapses than to synapses located in the CNS and autonomic ganglia. Still, some adverse side effects of the indirect-acting cholinergic stimulants may be caused by their relatively nonspecific activity.

The primary indirect-acting cholinergic stimulants currently in use are neostigmine and pyridostigmine. Several other agents are also used therapeutically to treat systemic conditions such as myasthenia gravis and ophthalmologic disorders such as glaucoma. These indirect-acting agents are summarized in Table 19–1.

Clinical Applications of Cholinergic Stimulants

Direct-acting and indirect-acting cholinergic stimulants are used to treat the decrease in smooth-muscle tone that sometimes occurs in the gastrointestinal tract and urinary bladder following abdominal surgery or trauma. Indirect-acting stimulants are also used in the treatment of glaucoma and myasthenia gravis, and to reverse the effects from an overdose of other drugs such as neuromuscular blocking agents and anticholinergic drugs. Each of these applications is briefly discussed here.

Gastrointestinal and Urinary Bladder Atony. After surgical manipulation or other trauma to the viscera, there is often a period of atony (i.e., lack of tone) in the smooth muscle of these organs. As a result, intestinal peristalsis is diminished or absent, and the urinary bladder becomes distended, leading to urinary retention. Under normal circumstances, acetylcholine released from parasympathetic postganglionic neurons would stimulate smooth-muscle contraction in these tissues. Consequently, cholinergic agonists (i.e., drugs that mimic or enhance the effects of acetylcholine) are administered to treat this problem. Bethanechol and neostigmine, a direct-acting and an indirect-acting cholinergic stimulant, respectively, are the drugs most frequently used to treat this condition until normal gastrointestinal and urinary function is resumed.

Glaucoma. Glaucoma is an increase in intraocular pressure brought on by an accumulation of aqueous humor within the eye.[19] If untreated, this increased pressure leads to impaired vision and blindness. Cholinergic stimulation via the parasympathetic supply to the eye increases the outflow of aqueous humor, thus preventing excessive accumulation. If evidence of increased intraocular pressure exists, cholinergic stimulants are among the drugs that may be used to treat this problem.[12] Direct-acting and indirect-acting cholinergic drugs (see Table 19–1) are usually applied topically to the eye by placing the drug directly within the conjunctival sac to treat glaucoma. This application concentrates the action of the drug on the eye, thus limiting the side effects that might occur if these agents were given systemically.

Myasthenia Gravis. Myasthenia gravis is a disease affecting the skeletal neuromuscular junction and is characterized by skeletal muscle weakness and profound fatigability.[2,5] As the disease progresses, the fatigue increases in severity and in the number of muscles involved. In advanced stages, the patient requires respiratory support because of a virtual paralysis of the respiratory musculature. In myasthenia gravis, the number of cholinergic receptors located postsynaptically at the neuromuscular junction is diminished.[2,4] As a result, acetylcholine released from the presynaptic terminal cannot sufficiently excite the muscle cell to reach threshold. Thus, the decreased receptivity of the muscle cell accounts for the clinical symptoms of weakness and fatigue.

Myasthenia gravis appears to be caused by an autoimmune response whereby an antibody to the neuromuscular cholinergic receptor is produced.[13] Although no cure is available, cholinesterase inhibitors such as neostigmine and pyridostigmine may help alleviate the muscular fatigue associated with this disease. These indirect-acting cholinergic agonists inhibit the acetylcholinesterase enzyme at the neuromuscular junction, allowing the endogenous acetylcholine released from the presynaptic terminal to remain at the myoneural junction for a longer period of time. The endogenously released acetylcholine is able to provide adequate excitation of the skeletal muscle cell and thus allow a more sustained muscular contraction.

Reversal of Neuromuscular Blockage. Drugs that block transmission at the skeletal neuromuscular junction are often used during general anesthesia to maintain skeletal muscle paralysis during surgical procedures (see Chapter 11). These skeletal muscle paralytic agents include curarelike drugs (e.g., tubocurarine, gallamine, pancuronium). Occasionally, the neuromuscular blockage caused by these drugs must be reversed. For instance, an accelerated recovery from the paralytic effects of these neuromuscular blockers may be desired at the end of the surgical procedure. Consequently, indirect-acting cholinergic stimulants are sometimes used to inhibit the acetylcholinesterase enzyme at the neuromuscular junction, thus allowing endogenously released acetylcholine to remain active at the synaptic site and effectively overcome the neuromuscular blockade until the curarelike agents have been metabolized.

Reversal of Anticholinergic-Induced CNS Toxicity. Indirect-acting cholinergic stimulants (e.g., physostigmine) are sometimes used to reverse the toxic effects of anticholinergic drugs on the CNS. An overdose of anticholinergic drugs may produce toxic CNS effects such as delirium, hallucinations, and coma. By inhibiting acetylcholine breakdown, indirect-acting stimulants enable endogenously released acetylcholine to overcome the anticholinergic drug effects.

Adverse Effects of Cholinergic Stimulants

Cholinergic stimulants are frequently associated with a number of adverse side effects caused by the relative nonspecificity of these drugs. Even a drug like bethanechol, which is relatively specific for muscarinic receptors, may stimulate muscarinic receptors on many different tissues. For example, administering bethanechol to increase gastrointestinal motility may also result in bronchoconstriction if this drug reaches muscarinic receptors in the upper respiratory tract. Indirect-acting stimulants (i.e., the cholinesterase inhibitors) show even less specificity and will increase synaptic activity at all synapses that they reach, including nicotinic cholinergic synapses.

The adverse effects associated with both the direct-acting and indirect-acting cholinergic stimulants mimic the effects that would occur during exaggerated parasympathetic activity. This notion is logical considering that the parasympathetic autonomic division exerts its effects on peripheral tissues by releasing acetylcholine from postganglionic neurons. Consequently, the primary adverse effects of cholinergic stimulants include gastrointestinal distress (nausea, vomiting, diarrhea, abdominal cramping), increased salivation, bronchoconstriction, bradycardia, and difficulty in visual accommodation. Increased sweating and vasodilation of facial cutaneous blood vessels (flushing) may also occur because of an effect on the respective tissues supplied by special sympathetic postganglionic neurons that release acetylcholine. The incidence of these side effects varies from patient to patient, but the onset and severity of these adverse effects increase as higher drug doses are administered.

ANTICHOLINERGIC DRUGS

In contrast to drugs that stimulate cholinergic activity, anticholinergic drugs attempt to diminish the response of tissues to cholinergic stimulation. In general, these drugs are competitive antagonists of the postsynaptic cholinergic receptors; that is, they bind reversibly to the cholinergic receptor but do not activate it. This binding blocks the receptor from the effects of endogenously released acetylcholine, thus diminishing the cellular response to cholinergic stimulation. (See Chapter 4 for a more detailed description of the mechanism by which drugs function as competitive antagonists.)

Anticholinergic drugs can be classified as antimuscarinic or antinicotinic agents, depending on their specificity for the two primary subtypes of cholinergic receptors. This chapter focuses on the antimuscarinic agents, with the antinicotinic drugs being discussed elsewhere in this text. Mecamylamine and trimethaphan, for example, are drugs that are relatively specific for the nicotinic type I receptor located in the autonomic ganglia. These nicotinic type I antagonists are sometimes used to treat extremely high blood pressure. The use of antinicotinic drugs in treating hypertensive emergencies is discussed in Chapter 21. Antinicotinic drugs that block the skeletal neuromuscular junction (i.e., the nicotinic type II drugs) are sometimes used as an adjunct in general anesthesia and are used to produce skeletal muscle paralysis during surgery. These so-called neuromuscular blockers are discussed in Chapter 11.

Source and Mechanism of Action of Antimuscarinic Anticholinergic Drugs

The prototypical antimuscarinic anticholinergic drug is atropine (Fig. 19–2). *Atropine* is a naturally occurring substance that can be obtained from the extract of plants such as belladonna and jimsonweed. Other natural, semisynthetic, and synthetic antimuscarinic anticholinergic agents have been developed that are similar in structure or function to atropine.

As mentioned previously, antimuscarinic anticholinergic drugs all share the same basic mechanism of action: they block the postsynaptic cholinergic muscarinic receptor. However, certain antimuscarinic agents seem to preferentially affect some tissues more than others. For instance, certain antimuscarinics seem to preferentially antagonize gastrointestinal muscarinic receptors, whereas others have a predominant effect on CNS cholinergic synapses. This fact suggests some degree of specificity of these drugs, which may be because of differences in the muscarinic receptor at gastrointestinal versus central synapses. Indeed, there is evidence that as many as three muscarinic receptor subtypes may exist at different locations in the body; these subtypes are designated M_1, M_2, and M_3 receptors.[3,7,8,11,16] Some drugs may be more selective for a certain receptor subtype than for others. This drug-receptor specificity is far from complete, however, and virtually every antimuscarinic drug will antagonize cholinergic receptors on a number of different tissues, leading to a number of side effects with

$$H_3C-\overset{\overset{O}{\|}}{C}-O-CH_2-CH_2-\overset{\overset{CH_3}{|}}{\underset{\underset{CH_3}{|}}{N^+}}-CH_3$$

acetylcholine

atropine

FIGURE 19–2. Structures of acetylcholine and atropine. Atropine and similar agents antagonize the effects of acetylcholine by blocking muscarinic cholinergic receptors.

these drugs (see "Side Effects of Anticholinergic Drugs"). Perhaps as more is learned about muscarinic receptor subtypes, more selective anticholinergic drugs may be developed.

Clinical Applications of Antimuscarinic Drugs

The primary clinical applications of antimuscarinic anticholinergic drugs include the treatment of certain gastrointestinal disorders. These drugs may also be helpful in managing Parkinson's disease. In addition, they have been used to treat a variety of other clinical disorders involving many other physiologic systems. The clinical applications of antimuscarinic agents are discussed here, and specific drugs used in various clinical situations are outlined in Table 19–2.

Gastrointestinal System. Stimulation of the gastrointestinal tract via parasympathetic cholinergic neurons generally produces an increase in gastric secretions and an increase in gastrointestinal motility. Consequently, certain antimuscarinic anticholinergics tend to reverse this stimulation by blocking the effects of endogenously released acetylcholine. Clinically, these drugs are used as an adjunct in peptic ulcer. The rationale is that they will limit secretion of gastric acid, thus reducing irritation of the stomach mucosa. Also, antimuscarinic anticholinergic drugs have been approved for treat-

TABLE 19–2 Common Anticholinergic Drugs*

Generic Name	Trade Name(s)	Primary Clinical Use(s)*
Anisotropine	Valpin	Peptic ulcer
Atropine	Dey-Dose, others	Peptic ulcer, irritable bowel syndrome, neurogenic bladder, bronchospasm, preoperative antisecretory agent, cardiac arrhythmias (e.g., symptomatic bradycardia, postmyocardial infarction, asystole)
Belladonna	Generic	Peptic ulcer, irritable bowel syndrome, dysmenorrhea, nocturnal enuresis
Clidinium	Quarzan	Peptic ulcer, irritable bowel syndrome
Cyclopentolate	Pentolate, Cyclogyl, others	Induces mydriasis for ophthalmologic procedures
Dicyclomine	Bentyl, others	Irritable bowel syndrome
Glycopyrrolate	Robinul	Peptic ulcer, preoperative antisecretory agent
Homatropine	Homapin	Peptic ulcer, irritable bowel syndrome
Hyoscyamine	Cystospaz, Levsin, others	Peptic ulcer, irritable bowel syndrome, urinary bladder hypermotility, preoperative antisecretory agent
Ipratropium	Atrovent	Antiasthmatic
Isopropamide	Darbid	Peptic ulcer, irritable bowel syndrome
Mepenzolate	Cantil	Peptic ulcer
Methantheline	Banthine	Peptic ulcer, neurogenic bladder
Methscopolamine	Pamine	Peptic ulcer
Oxybutynin	Ditropan	Neurogenic bladder
Oxyphencyclimine	Daricon	Peptic ulcer
Propantheline	Pro-Banthine, Norpanth, others	Peptic ulcer, irritable bowel syndrome
Scopolamine	Transderm-Scop	Motion sickness, preoperative antisecretory agent
Tridihexethyl	Pathilon	Peptic ulcer, irritable bowel syndrome

*Anticholinergic drugs used specifically to treat Parkinson's disease are listed in Table 10–2, Chapter 10.

ment of irritable bowel syndrome. This condition is characterized by hyperactivity of gastrointestinal smooth muscle and includes problems such as irritable colon and spastic colon. These antimuscarinic agents are sometimes referred to as *antispasmodics* because of their reported ability to decrease gastrointestinal smooth-muscle tone or spasms.

Drugs used to treat peptic ulcer and irritable bowel syndrome are listed in Table 19–2. Although these agents are approved for use in these conditions, considerable doubt exists as to how effective they are in actually resolving these gastrointestinal disorders. Their use in treating peptic ulcer has essentially been replaced by other agents such as the H_2 histamine receptor blockers (see Chapter 27), but antimuscarinic anticholinergics may still be used if other drugs are ineffective or poorly tolerated. These drugs will not cure peptic ulcer or prevent its recurrence when the medication is discontinued.[9,14,18] In essence, they only treat a symptom of the problem (increased gastric secretion), without really addressing the cause of the increased secretion (e.g., emotional stress). Likewise, the efficacy of these drugs in treating irritable bowel syndrome has also been questioned. There is little evidence that these drugs are actually effective in treating this problem.[10,14]

Finally, antimuscarinic anticholinergic drugs used to treat gastrointestinal problems are often combined with other agents such as antianxiety drugs. Librax, for instance, is the trade name for a combination of chlordiazepoxide and clidinium (an antianxiety agent and an anticholinergic agent, respectively). These combination products are supposedly better at relieving gastrointestinal problems where emotional factors are also present.

Parkinson's Disease. The pharmacologic management of Parkinson's disease is discussed in detail in Chapter 10. Consequently, the use of anticholinergic drugs in this disorder will only be mentioned briefly at this time. Parkinsonism is a movement disorder caused by a deficiency of the neurotransmitter dopamine in the basal ganglia. This deficiency leads to an overactivity of central cholinergic synapses. Hence, anticholinergic drugs should be beneficial in helping resolve this increase in central cholinergic influence.

Certain anticholinergic drugs such as benztropine, biperiden, and trihexyphenidyl are approved for use in treating Parkinson's disease (see Chapter 10, Table 10–2 for a more complete list). As mentioned, these drugs seem to preferentially block the central muscarinic cholinergic synapses involved in parkinsonism. This does not mean that these drugs do not affect other peripheral muscarinic receptors. Indeed, these antiparkinsonian drugs are associated with a number of side effects such as dry mouth, constipation, and urinary retention, which are caused by their antagonistic effect on muscarinic receptors located outside of the brain. Their primary effect, however, is to decrease the influence of central cholinergic synapses in parkinsonism.

Cardiovascular System. Atropine is sometimes used to block the effects of the vagus nerve (cranial nerve X) on the myocardium. Release of acetylcholine from vagal efferent fibers slows heart rate and the conduction of the cardiac action potential throughout the myocardium. Atropine reverses the effects of excessive vagal discharge and is used to treat the symptomatic bradycardia that may accompany myocardial infarction.[1,15] Atropine may also be useful in treating other cardiac arrhythmias such as atrioventricular nodal block and ventricular asystole.[15]

Motion Sickness. Antimuscarinics (scopolamine in particular) are used frequently in the treatment of motion sickness. Scopolamine appears to block cholinergic transmission from areas of the brain and brainstem that mediate motion-related nausea and vomiting (i.e., the vestibular system and reticular formation). These drugs are often administered transdermally via small patches that adhere to the skin.[17]

Preoperative Medication. Atropine and related antimuscarinics are occasionally used preoperatively to decrease respiratory secretions during general anesthesia. Their use in this capacity has declined considerably, however, because the newer inhalation forms of general anesthesia do not stimulate bronchial secretions to the same extent as earlier general anesthetics (see Chapter 11). Antimuscarinics may also be administered to prevent bradycardia during surgery, especially in children.

Urinary Tract. Atropine and several synthetic antimuscarinics have been used to alleviate urinary frequency and incontinence caused by hypertonicity of the urinary bladder. Increased bladder tone results if the normal reflex control of bladder function is disrupted (i.e., the so-called neurogenic bladder syndrome) or a urinary tract infection irritates the bladder. Antimuscarinics inhibit contraction of the bladder detrusor muscle, thus allowing the bladder to fill more normally with a decreased frequency of urination and less chance of incontinence.

Respiratory Tract. Stimulation of the upper respiratory tract via the vagus causes bronchoconstriction. Anticholinergic drugs that block the effects of vagal-released acetylcholine will relax bronchial smooth muscle. Consequently, atropine and some synthetic derivatives have been used to treat the bronchospasm that occurs in patients with asthma. Although anticholinergics are not usually the initial drugs used in treating asthma, they have been used successfully in patients who are unable to tolerate more conventional forms of antiasthmatic drug therapy such as the adrenergic agonists.[6,20] The use of anticholinergics in treating respiratory disorders is discussed in more detail in Chapter 26.

Eye. Atropine and similar antimuscarinics block the acetylcholine-mediated contraction of the pupillary sphincter muscle, thus causing dilation of the pupil (mydriasis). During an ophthalmologic exam, these drugs may be applied topically in order to dilate the pupil, thus allowing a more detailed inspection of internal eye structures such as the retina.

Cholinergic Poisoning. Cholinergic poisoning can occur in several situations such as eating wild mushrooms, being exposed to certain insecticides, or being exposed to certain types of chemical warfare.[11] These potentially life-threatening occurrences typically require emergency treatment with atropine or an analogous anticholinergic agent. In cases of severe poisoning, fairly high doses of these drugs must often be administered for several days.

Side Effects of Anticholinergic Drugs

Considering the diverse uses of the anticholinergic drugs named previously, these drugs can obviously affect a number of different tissues. A systemically administered anticholinergic agent cannot be targeted for one specific organ without also achieving a response in other tissues as well. For instance, an antimuscarinic drug administered to decrease motility in the gastrointestinal tract may also affect other tissues containing muscarinic receptors (e.g., the bladder, bronchial smooth muscle, eye, heart). As higher doses are administered for any given problem, the chance of additional effects in tissues other than the target organ is also increased.

Consequently, antimuscarinic anticholinergic drugs are associated with a number of side effects. Exactly which symptoms (if any) will be encountered depends on a number of factors such as the specific anticholinergic agent, the dosage of the drug, and the individual response of each patient. The most common side effects include dryness of the mouth, blurred vision, urinary retention, constipation, and tachycardia. Each of these side effects is caused by blockade of muscarinic receptors on the tissue or organ related to the side effect. Some patients also report symptoms such as confusion, dizziness, nervousness, and drowsiness, presumably because of an interaction of antimuscarinic drugs with CNS cholinergic receptors. These CNS-related symptoms occur more frequently with anticholinergic drugs that readily cross the blood-brain barrier.

SUMMARY

Drugs affecting acetylcholine-mediated responses are classified as cholinergic stimulants and anticholinergic drugs. Cholinergic stimulants increase cholinergic activity by binding to the acetylcholine receptor and activating the receptor (direct-acting stimulants) or by inhibiting the acetylcholinesterase enzyme, thus allowing more acetylcholine to remain active at the cholinergic synapse (indirect-acting stimulants). Anticholinergic drugs inhibit cholinergic activity by acting as competitive antagonists; that is, they bind to the cholinergic receptor but do not activate it.

Cholinergic stimulants and anticholinergic drugs affect many tissues in the body and are used to treat a variety of clinical problems. Cholinergic stimulants are often administered to increase gastrointestinal and urinary bladder tone, to treat glaucoma and myasthenia gravis, and to reverse the neuromuscular blockade produced by curarelike drugs. Anticholinergic drugs are used principally to decrease gastrointestinal motility and secretions and to decrease the symptoms of Parkinson's disease, but they may also be used to treat problems in several other physiologic systems. Because of the ability of cholinergic stimulants and anticholinergic drugs to affect many different tissues, these drugs may be associated with a number of side effects. Considering the diverse clinical applications of cholinergic stimulants and anticholinergic drugs, physical and occupational therapists may frequently encounter patients taking these drugs. Rehabilitation specialists should be aware of the rationale for drug administration as well as possible adverse side effects of cholinergic stimulants and anticholinergic agents.

REFERENCES

1. Adgey, AAJ, et al: Incidence, significance, and management of early bradyarrhythmia complicating acute myocardial infarction. Lancet 2(7578):1097, 1968.
2. Drachman, DH: Myasthenia gravis. N Engl J Med 298:136, 1978.
3. Evans, RA, et al: Differential ontogeny of putative M_1 and M_2 muscarinic receptor binding sites in the murin cerebral cortex and heart. J Pharmacol Exp Ther 235:612, 1985.
4. Fambrough, DM, Drachman, DB, and Satyamurti, S: Neuromuscular junction in myasthenia gravis: Decreased acetylcholine receptors. Science 182:293, 1973.
5. Grob, D (ed): Myasthenia gravis: Pathophysiology and management. Ann NY Acad Sci 377:1, 1981.
6. Gross, NJ and Skorodin, MS: Anticholinergic, antimuscarinic bronchodilators. Am Rev Respir Dis 129: 856, 1984.
7. Hammer, R and Giachetti, A: Muscarinic receptor subtypes: Biochemical and functional characterization. Life Sci 31:2991, 1982.
8. Hirschowitz, BI, et al (eds): Symposium: Subtypes of muscarinic receptors. Trends Pharmacol Sci (suppl): 1, 1984
9. Ivey, KJ: Anticholinergics: Do they work in peptic ulcer? Gastroenterology 68:154, 1975.
10. Ivey, KJ: Are anticholinergics of use in the irritable colon syndrome? Gastroenterology 68:1300, 1974.
11. Katzung, BG: Cholinoceptor-blocking drugs. In Katzung, BG (ed): Basic and Clinical Pharmacology, ed 5. Appleton & Lange, Norwalk, CT, 1992.
12. Leopold, IH and Duzman, E: Observations on the pharmacology of glaucoma. Annu Rev Pharmacol Toxicol 26:401, 1986.
13. Lindstorm, J: Immunobiology of myasthenia gravis, experimental autoimmune myasthenia gravis, and Lambert-Eaton syndrome. Annu Rev Immunol 3:109, 1985.
14. McEvoy, GK (ed): American Hospital Formulary Service-Drug Information. American Society of Hospital Pharmacists, Bethesda, MD, 1987.
15. National Conference on Cardiopulmonary Resuscitation (CPR) and Emergency Cardiac Care (ECC): Standards and Guidelines for Cardiopulmonary Resuscitation (CPR) and Emergency Cardiac Care (ECC). JAMA 255:2841, 1986.
16. Potter, LT, et al: Independent M_1 and M_2 receptors: Ligands, autoradiography and functions. Trends Pharmacol Sci (suppl):22, 1984.
17. Price, NM, et al: Transdermal scopolamine in the prevention of motion sickness at sea. Clin Pharmacol Ther 29:414, 1981.
18. Saco, LS, et al: Double-blind controlled trial of bethanechol and antacid versus placebo and antacid in the treatment of erosive esophagitis. Gastroenterology 82:1369, 1982.
19. Scwartz, B: The glaucomas. N Engl J Med 299:182, 1978.
20. Skorodin, MS, et al: Oxitropium bromide: A new anticholinergic bronchodilator. Ann Allerg 56:229, 1986.

CHAPTER 20

Adrenergic Drugs

The purpose of this chapter is to describe drugs that either stimulate activity at norepinephrine synapses (adrenergic agonists) or inhibit norepinephrine influence (adrenergic antagonists). To be more specific, this chapter will focus on drugs that primarily influence activity in the sympathetic nervous system through their effect on adrenergic synapses. Norepinephrine is usually the neurotransmitter at the junction between sympathetic postganglionic neurons and peripheral tissues. Consequently, most of the adrenergic agonists discussed in this chapter will be used to augment sympathetic responses, while the adrenergic antagonists will be used to attenuate sympathetic-induced activity. In fact, adrenergic agonists are sometimes referred to as **sympathomimetic,** and antagonists are referred to as **sympatholytic,** because of their ability to increase and decrease sympathetic activity, respectively.

As in Chapter 19, the drugs discussed here are categorized according to a common mode of action rather than according to common clinical applications. Most of the drugs introduced in this chapter will again appear throughout this text when they are classified according to their use in treating specific problems. For instance, the beta-selective adrenergic antagonists (i.e., beta blockers, see "Beta Antagonists") are collectively introduced in this chapter. Individual beta blockers, however, are also discussed in subsequent chapters with regard to their use in specific problems such as hypertension (see Chapter 21), angina pectoris (see Chapter 22), and cardiac arrhythmias (see Chapter 23).

The drugs described in this chapter are used to treat a variety of disorders, which range from severe cardiovascular and respiratory problems to the symptoms of the common cold. Because of the widespread use of these drugs in cardiovascular disease and other disorders, many patients seen in physical and occupational therapy will be taking adrenergic agonists or antagonists. In this chapter, the basic pharmacodynamic mechanisms, clinical applications, and adverse effects of these drugs are introduced. The relevance of specific adrenergic drugs to physical rehabilitation is addressed in more detail in subsequent chapters that categorize their use according to specific disorders (hypertension, angina, asthma, etc.).

Many adrenergic agonists and antagonists exert their effects by binding directly to the appropriate postsynaptic receptor. Since a great deal of the specificity (or lack of specificity) of these drugs depends on the drug-receptor interaction, adrenergic receptor classes and subclasses are briefly reviewed here.

ADRENERGIC RECEPTOR SUBCLASSIFICATIONS

As discussed in Chapter 18, adrenergic receptors can be divided into two primary categories: alpha and beta receptors. Each category can then be subdivided, so that there are ultimately four receptor subtypes: alpha-1, alpha-2, beta-1, and beta-2.[24,26] Adrenergic receptor subtypes are located on specific tissues throughout the body, and the response mediated by each receptor depends on the interaction between that receptor and the respective tissue. Refer to Chapter 18 for a more detailed description of adrenergic receptor locations and responses.

The primary uses of adrenergic agonists and antagonists according to their selectivity for individual receptor subtypes are summarized in Table 20–1. In general, a specific agonist is used to mimic or increase the response mediated by that receptor, whereas the antagonist is used to decrease the receptor-mediated response.

Clinically useful adrenergic agonists and antagonists display variable amounts of specificity for each receptor subtype. Some drugs are fairly specific and bind to only one receptor subtype (e.g., a specific alpha-1 agonist like phenylephrine preferentially stimulates the alpha-1 subtype). Other drugs show a moderate amount of specificity and perhaps affect one major receptor category. An example is the nonselective beta antagonist propranolol, which blocks beta-1 and beta-2 receptors but has little or no effect on alpha receptors. Finally, other drugs such as ephedrine are rather nonspecific and affect alpha and beta receptors fairly equally. In some clinical situations, adminis-

TABLE 20–1 Summary of Adrenergic Agonist/Antagonist Use According to Receptor Specificity

Primary Receptor Location: Response When Stimulated	Agonist Use(s)*	Antagonist Use(s)*
Alpha-1 receptor Vascular smooth muscle: vasoconstriction	Hypotension Nasal congestion Paroxysmal supra-ventricular tachycardia	Hypertension
Alpha-2 receptor CNS synapses (inhibitory): decreased sympathetic discharge from brainstem	Hypertension	No significant clinical use
Beta-1 receptor Heart: increased heart rate and force of contraction	Cardiac decompensation	Hypertension Arrhythmia Angina pectoris Prevention of reinfarction
Beta-2 receptor Bronchioles: bronchodilation Uterus: relaxation	Prevent bronchospasm Prevent premature labor	No significant clinical use

*Primary clinical condition(s) that the agonists or antagonists are used to treat. See text for specific drugs in each category and a discussion of treatment rationale.

tering a fairly selective drug may be desirable, whereas other problems may benefit from a drug that interacts with more than one receptor subtype. Use of selective versus nonselective adrenergic drugs is considered in the sections that describe "Adrenergic Agonists" and "Adrenergic Antagonists" in this chapter.

"Receptor selectivity," however, is a relative term. Even though an adrenergic drug is reported to be selective for only one receptor subtype, a certain affinity for other receptor subtypes may also occur to a lesser degree. A beta-1–specific drug, for instance, binds preferentially to beta-1 receptors but may also show some slight affinity for beta-2 receptors. Selectivity is also dose-related, with the relative degree of receptor selectivity decreasing as higher doses are administered. Consequently, some side effects of the so-called selective drugs may be caused by stimulation of other receptor subtypes, especially at higher drug doses.

ADRENERGIC AGONISTS

Drugs that stimulate the adrenergic receptors are presented here according to their relative specificity for each receptor subtype. The drugs that primarily activate alpha receptors are discussed first, followed by beta-selective drugs, and finally drugs that have mixed alpha and beta agonist activity.

Alpha Agonists

ALPHA-1–SELECTIVE AGONISTS

General Indications

Alpha-1 agonists bind directly to and activate the alpha-1 receptor that is located primarily on vascular smooth muscle, thus leading to smooth-muscle contraction and vasoconstriction. Because of their vasoconstrictive properties, these drugs are able to increase blood pressure by increasing peripheral vascular resistance. Consequently, certain alpha-1 agonists are administered systemically to treat acute hypotension that may occur in emergencies such as shock or during general anesthesia. A second primary clinical application of these drugs is the treatment of nasal congestion (i.e., the runny nose, stuffy head feelings often associated with the common cold). In appropriate doses, alpha-1 agonists preferentially constrict the vasculature in the nasal and upper respiratory mucosa, thus decreasing the congestion and mucosal discharge. A third application of alpha-1 agonists is to decrease heart rate during attacks of paroxysmal supraventricular tachycardia. By increasing peripheral vascular resistance, these drugs bring about a reflex decrease in heart rate through the cardiac baroreceptor reflex.

Specific Agents

Methoxamine (Vasoxyl):   This drug is used to increase blood pressure in severe, acute hypotension and to normalize heart rate in paroxysmal supraventricular tachycardia. It is usually administered by injection (intramuscularly or intravenously) to allow a rapid onset.

Oxymetazoline (Afrin, Nafrine, many others):   This drug is used in nose drops and nasal sprays to decrease nasal congestion through alpha-1–mediated vasoconstriction. Higher or systemic doses may also cause hypotension, presumably because of stimulation of CNS alpha-2 receptors in a manner similar to clonidine (see "Alpha-2–Selective Agonists").

Phenylephrine (Neo-Synephrine, Sinex, many others):   Like methoxamine, phenylephrine can be administered systemically to treat hypotension and tachycardia. In addition, phenylephrine is administered topically to treat nasal congestion and is found in many over-the-counter spray decongestants.

Pseudoephedrine (Novafed, Sudafed, many others):   Pseudoephedrine is administered orally for its decongestant effects, is found in many over-the-counter preparations, and is commonly used to help relieve cold symptoms.

Xylometazoline (Otrivin, Neo-Synephrine Long-Acting, others):   This drug is similar to oxymetazoline.

Adverse Effects

The primary side effects associated with alpha-1–specific agonists are caused by excessive stimulation of alpha-adrenergic responses. Some of the more frequent side effects include increased blood pressure, headache, and an abnormally slow heart rate (because of reflex bradycardia). Some patients also report feelings of chest pain, difficulty breathing, and feelings of nervousness. These side effects are quite variable from patient to patient and are usually dose-related (i.e., they occur more frequently at higher doses).

ALPHA-2–SELECTIVE AGONISTS

General Indications

Alpha-2–selective drugs are used in the treatment of hypertension for a rather unique reason. Alpha-2 receptors have been identified in the brain and brainstem. When stimulated, these central alpha-2 receptors exert an *inhibitory* effect on sympathetic discharge from the vasomotor center in the brainstem.[32,34] Diminished sympathetic discharge results in a decrease in blood pressure.

Consequently, alpha-2 agonists appear to exert their antihypertensive effects by preferentially stimulating central alpha-2 receptors that, in turn, inhibit sympathetic discharge. Whether alpha-2 agonists exert their primary effects on central presynaptic or postsynaptic receptors is unclear. Stimulation of presynaptic alpha-2 receptors located at peripheral adrenergic synapses results in a decrease in norepinephrine release from the presynaptic terminal.[11,33,36,48] Decreased norepinephrine release at central synapses might account for the general decrease in sympathetic discharge seen with alpha-2 agonists. Similarly, alpha-2 receptors have also been identified postsynaptically at specific central synapses, and these postsynaptic receptors are believed to directly inhibit sympathetic discharge.[21,32] Thus, alpha-2 agonists may exert their antihypertensive effects by stimulating either central presynaptic or postsynaptic receptors, or by acting on inhibitory presynaptic and postsynaptic receptors simultaneously. The use of alpha-2 agonists in lowering blood pressure is discussed in more detail in Chapter 21.

Specific Agents

Clonidine (Catapres):   Clonidine is used in treating mild-to-moderate hypertension and is especially useful in patients who are unable to tolerate alpha-1 antagonists such as prazosin (see "Alpha Antagonists"). Clonidine, however, is not usually successful when used alone in the long-term treatment of essential hypertension and is usually used only for short-term management or in combination with other antihypertensive drugs. Clonidine also has sedative properties and has been used as an analgesic, an antianxiety drug, and an adjunct in general anesthesia.

Guanabenz (Wytensin): Guanabenz appears to be similar to clonidine in efficacy and clinical use.

Methyldopa (Aldomet): Methyldopa has been used as an antihypertensive drug for some time, but its mechanism of action is poorly understood. Currently, methyldopa is believed to exert its effects by being converted to alpha-methylnorepinephrine in the body.[19] Alpha-methylnorepinephrine is a potent alpha-2 agonist that lowers blood pressure by stimulating inhibitory central adrenergic receptors in a manner similar to clonidine and guanabenz.

Adverse Effects

Use of alpha-2–specific drugs may be associated with some relatively minor side effects such as dizziness, drowsiness, and dry mouth. More pronounced adverse effects such as difficulty in breathing, an unusually slow heart rate, and persistent fainting may indicate a toxic accumulation or overdose of these drugs.

Beta Agonists

BETA-1–SELECTIVE AGONISTS

General Indications

The beta-1 receptor is located primarily on the myocardium, and stimulation of the receptor results in increased heart rate and increased force of myocardial contraction (i.e., increased cardiac output). Consequently, beta-1 agonists are used primarily to increase cardiac output in emergency situations such as cardiovascular shock or if complications develop during cardiac surgery. Beta-1 agonists may also be used to increase cardiac function in the short-term treatment of certain types of heart disease.

Specific Agents

Dobutamine (Dobutrex): Dobutamine is used for short-term management of cardiac decompensation that sometimes occurs during exacerbations of heart disease or following cardiac surgery. This drug is often administered via intravenous pump infusion to allow relatively stable plasma levels.

Dopamine (Dopastat, Intropin): In addition to its ability to stimulate dopamine receptors, this drug directly stimulates beta-1–adrenergic receptors. At higher doses, dopamine may also indirectly stimulate adrenergic activity by increasing the release of norepinephrine from presynaptic storage sites. Clinically, this drug is used to treat cardiac decompensation in a manner similar to dobutamine. Dopamine is also used to increase cardiac output in acute or severe hypotension. Dopamine is especially useful in the management of hypotension with decreased renal blood flow. Dopamine is able to increase cardiac output by stimulating beta-1 adrenoceptors while vasodilating the renal vasculature through an effect on renal dopamine receptors. This effectively increases blood pressure and renal perfusion, thus facilitating normal kidney function.

Adverse Effects

Because of their cardiostimulatory effects, beta-1–selective drugs may induce side effects such as chest pain and cardiac arrhythmias in some patients. Shortness of breath and difficulty in breathing (i.e., feelings of chest constriction) have also been reported.

BETA-2–SELECTIVE AGONISTS

General Indications

One important location of beta-2 receptors is on bronchiole smooth muscle. When stimulated, the receptor mediates relaxation of the bronchioles. Consequently, most beta-2 agonists are administered to treat the bronchospasm associated with respiratory ailments such as asthma, bronchitis, and emphysema.[6,13] Since a nonselective beta agonist will also stimulate the myocardium (beta-1 effect), beta-2–selective agonists are often used preferentially in treating asthma, especially if the patient also has some cardiac abnormality such as ischemia or arrhythmias.[13,55] Another clinically important location of beta-2 receptors is on uterine muscle. When stimulated, these receptors cause inhibition or relaxation of the uterus. As a result, drugs such as ritodrine and terbutaline are used to inhibit premature uterine contractions during pregnancy, thus preventing premature labor and delivery.[4,5]

Specific Agents

Beta-2–selective bronchodilators: This group of drugs includes albuterol (Proventil, Ventolin), bitolterol (Tornalate), fenoterol (Berotec), isoetharine (Bronkometer, Bronkosol, others), metaproterenol (Alupent, Metaprel), and pirbuterol (Maxair). These agents are similar pharmacologically and are used for their ability to stimulate beta-2 receptors located on pulmonary smooth muscle, thus causing bronchodilation in patients with asthma and similar conditions. Ethylnorepinephrine (Bronkephrine) and isoproterenol (Isuprel) can also be included with this group, but these are somewhat less beta-2–selective and affect beta-1 receptors as well. Beta-2 bronchodilators are often administered by oral inhalation so that the drug is applied directly to bronchial membranes. Albuterol and similar agents, for example, are packaged in small aerosol inhalers so that the patient can self-administer the drug at the onset of a bronchospastic attack. The use of these drugs in treating respiratory conditions is addressed in more detail in Chapter 26.

Ritodrine (Yutopar):   The primary clinical application of this drug is to inhibit premature labor.[4] Ritodrine activates uterine beta-2 receptors, which mediate relaxation of uterine muscle. This drug is usually administered initially via intravenous pump infusion, and maintenance therapy is accomplished through oral administration.

Terbutaline (Brethine, Bricanyl):   Terbutaline is usually administered by oral inhalation for the treatment of bronchospasm (i.e., similar to albuterol). Terbutaline has also been administered systemically to inhibit premature labor and thus prolong pregnancy (i.e., similar to ritodrine).

Adverse Effects

The primary side effects associated with beta-2–specific drugs include nervousness, restlessness, and trembling. These adverse symptoms may be caused by stimulation of central beta-adrenergic receptors. There is also some suggestion that excessive use of beta-2 agonists may cause increased airway hyperresponsiveness that could lead to severe and possibly fatal asthmatic attacks.[6,47] This fact has generated debate about the safe and effective use of these drugs in treating asthma, and the contemporary use of beta-2 agonists along with other antiasthmatic drugs is described in Chapter 26. When used to prevent premature labor, drugs such as ritodrine have also been associated with increases in maternal heart rate and systolic blood pressure, as well as maternal pulmonary edema. These changes in maternal cardiopulmonary function can be quite severe and may be fatal to the mother.

Drugs with Mixed Alpha and Beta Agonist Activity

GENERAL INDICATIONS

Several drugs are available that display a rather mixed agonistic activity with regard to adrenergic receptor subtypes. Some drugs like epinephrine and ephedrine appear to be able to stimulate all four adrenergic receptor subtypes. Other drugs such as norepinephrine bind to both types of alpha receptors, bind to beta-1 receptors to a lesser extent, and show little or no affinity for beta-2 receptors. Another group of indirect adrenergic agonists appear to act as nonselective agonists because of their ability to increase the release of norepinephrine from presynaptic storage sites. Because of the ability of many of these multiple-receptor drugs to affect a number of adrenoceptor subtypes, their clinical uses are quite varied. Specific agents with mixed agonistic activity and their respective applications are presented here.

SPECIFIC AGENTS

Amphetamines: Drugs such as amphetamine (Biphetamine), dextroamphetamine (Dexedrine, others), and methamphetamine (Desoxyn) are known for their powerful sympathomimetic effects. These drugs appear to increase norepinephrine release and decrease norepinephrine reuptake and breakdown at adrenergic synapses, thus increasing activity at synapses with norepinephrine-sensitive receptors (i.e., alpha-1, alpha-2, and beta-1 receptors). These drugs may also exert similar effects on certain dopaminergic synapses. Amphetamines are used on a limited basis to treat attention-deficit disorder in children and to increase mental alertness in adults with narcolepsy. Use of these drugs to suppress appetite or to combat normal sleepiness is discouraged because of their high potential for abuse, and these drugs are classified in the United States as schedule II controlled substances (see Chapter 1 for a description of controlled substance classification).

Ephedrine (Efedron Nasal, Ectasule Minus): Ephedrine displays agonistic activity at all four adrenoceptor subtypes. This drug is sometimes administered for its alpha-1 effects and can be used to treat severe, acute hypotension or nasal congestion. When treating hypotension in emergency situations (e.g., shock), ephedrine is administered by injection (intravenously, intramuscularly, or subcutaneously). As a nasal decongestant, ephedrine is administered orally and the dosage is adjusted appropriately. Ephedrine is also sometimes administered for its beta-2 agonistic activity and can be taken via oral inhalation or oral tablets to treat asthma-related bronchospasm. Finally, ephedrine has been administered to produce a general excitatory effect on central adrenergic receptors and has been used to treat conditions associated with a decrease in CNS arousal (e.g., narcolepsy).

Epinephrine (Adrenalin, Bronkaid Mist, Primatene Mist, others):   Like ephedrine, epinephrine appears to stimulate all adrenergic receptor subtypes and is administered for a variety of reasons. Epinephrine is found in many antiasthmatic inhalation products because of its ability to stimulate beta-2 receptors on the bronchi. Because it stimulates vascular alpha-1 receptors, epinephrine may be applied topically to produce local vasoconstriction and control bleeding during minor surgical procedures (e.g., suturing superficial wounds). Likewise, epinephrine may be mixed with a local anesthetic when the anesthetic is injected during minor surgical and dental procedures. The vasoconstriction produced by the epinephrine prevents the anesthetic from being washed away by the local blood flow, thus prolonging the effects of the anesthetic. Because of a potent ability to stimulate the heart (beta-1 effect), epinephrine is frequently administered during cardiac arrest to reestablish normal cardiac rhythm. Finally, epinephrine is often the drug of choice in treating anaphylactic shock. Anaphylactic shock is a hypersensitive allergic reaction marked by cardiovascular collapse (decreased cardiac output, hypotension) and severe bronchoconstriction. Epinephrine is ideally suited to treat this problem because of its ability to stimulate the heart (beta-1 effect), vasoconstrict the periphery (alpha-1 effect), and dilate the bronchi (beta-2 effect).

Mephentermine (Wyamine):   The mechanism by which mephentermine works is somewhat unclear. Although this drug has some direct beta-agonist activity, some alpha stimulation may also occur because of the release of presynaptic norepinephrine. This drug is used primarily for its antihypotensive effects and is administered by injection to treat the sudden, severe decrease in blood pressure sometimes seen during general anesthesia.

Metaraminol (Aramine):   Metaraminol appears to exert a direct stimulatory effect on both alpha- and beta-adrenergic receptors, and may also act as an indirect agonist by increasing the release of presynaptic norepinephrine. This drug is usually administered by injection (intramuscularly, intravenously, or subcutaneously) to treat hypotension occurring in shock or general anesthesia.

Norepinephrine (Levophed):   Norepinephrine stimulates both types of alpha receptors as well as beta-1 receptors but displays very little agonistic activity toward beta-2 receptors. It is usually administered intravenously to treat hypotension during shock or general anesthesia.

Phenylpropanolamine (Acutrim, Dexatrim, Rhindecon, others):   The exact mechanism of this drug is unclear. Although it may directly stimulate alpha and beta receptors, this drug probably exerts its effects by increasing the release of presynaptic norepinephrine; thus, phenylpropanolamine is an indirect-acting, nonselective agonist. Phenylpropanolamine has two primary uses: as a nasal decongestant and as an appetite suppressant or "diet" drug. Nasal decongestant properties derive from its alpha-1–agonistic activity. Phenylpropanolamine appears to act as an appetite suppressant by increasing the release of norepinephrine within the hypothalamus. In this regard, it is similar to amphetamine-like compounds, which may also suppress feeding behavior by increasing adrenergic influence in the brain. Phenylpropanolamine is taken orally for both nasal decongestion and appetite suppression.

ADVERSE EFFECTS

Because of the general ability of many of the drugs described previously to produce CNS excitation, some of the primary side effects are nervousness, restlessness, and anxiety. Because these agents also tend to stimulate the cardiovascular system, prolonged or excessive use may also lead to complications such as hypertension, arrhythmias, and even cardiac arrest. When used to treat bronchospasm, prolonged administration via inhalation may also cause some degree of bronchial irritation with some agents.

ADRENERGIC ANTAGONISTS

Adrenergic antagonists or blockers bind to adrenergic receptors but do not activate the receptor. These agents are often referred to as sympatholytic drugs because of their ability to block the receptors that typically mediate sympathetic responses (i.e., alpha and beta receptors). Clinically useful adrenergic antagonists usually show a fairly high degree of specificity for one of the major receptor classifications. They tend to bind preferentially to either alpha- or beta-adrenergic receptors. Specific drugs may show an additional degree of specificity within the receptor class. For instance, a beta blocker may bind rather selectively to only beta-1 receptors, or it may bind fairly equally to both beta-1 and beta-2 receptors.

The general clinical applications of alpha antagonists and beta antagonists are presented here. Specific agents within each major group are also discussed.

Alpha Antagonists

GENERAL INDICATIONS

Alpha antagonists are administered primarily to reduce peripheral vascular tone by blocking the alpha-1 receptors located on vascular smooth muscle. When stimulated by endogenous catecholamines (norepinephrine, epinephrine), the alpha-1 receptor initiates vasoconstriction.

Consequently, alpha antagonists are used in conditions where peripheral vasodilation would be beneficial. A principal application of these agents, for instance, is in treating hypertension.[10,50] These drugs seem to attenuate the peripheral vasoconstriction mediated by excessive adrenergic influence, thus decreasing blood pressure through a decrease in peripheral vascular resistance. These agents may also be used in patients with a pheochromocytoma, which is a tumor that produces large quantities of epinephrine and norepinephrine. Alpha antagonists are often administered prior to and during the removal of such a tumor, thus preventing the hypertensive crisis that may occur from excessive alpha-1 stimulation from catecholamines released from the tumor. Similarly, alpha antagonists have been used to successfully prevent and treat the sudden increase in blood pressure that often occurs during an autonomic crisis.[45] These drugs have been used to promote vasodilation in conditions of vascular insufficiency, including peripheral vascular disease and Raynaud's phenomenon. However, the success of these drugs in treating vascular insufficiency has been somewhat limited.

A group of drugs known collectively as *ergot alkaloids* display some alpha-blocking ability as well as other unique properties. Ergot alkaloids, which include the ergoloid mesylates and ergotamine, are used clinically for diverse problems including treatment of vascular headache and improvement of mental function in presenile dementia.

Because the primary uses of alpha antagonists involve their ability to decrease vascular tone, the clinically useful alpha antagonists tend to be somewhat alpha-1 selective. Alpha-2 receptors should not be selectively antagonized because this event may ultimately lead to an increase in peripheral vascular tone through an increase in sympathetic discharge. Certain alpha-2 receptors are located in the brainstem, and stimulation of these receptors appears to decrease sympathetic outflow from the vasomotor center. Thus, blocking these centrally located alpha-2 receptors is counterproductive when a decrease in vascular tone is desired.

SPECIFIC AGENTS

Ergoloid mesylates (Gerimal, Hydergine, others): These compounds, also known as dihydrogenated ergot alkaloids, exhibit some ability to produce peripheral vasodilation by blocking peripheral alpha-1 receptors. The primary clinical application of ergoloid mesylates is to increase mental acuity and alertness in geriatric patients with dementia related to Alzheimer's disease. These drugs supposedly increase mental function by increasing cerebral blood flow or by increasing oxygen utilization in the brain. The mechanism of action of these drugs is probably a moot point, however, because there is no evidence that they produce any significant clinical benefits in treating dementia of the Alzheimer's type.[52] These drugs are usually administered orally or sublingually.

Ergotamine (Ergomar, Ergostat): Ergotamine and similar drugs such as dihydroergotamine exert a number of complex effects. At higher doses, these drugs act as competitive alpha antagonists, hence their inclusion here. However, these drugs appear to produce vasoconstriction in blood vessels that have low vascular tone and vasodilation in vessels that have high vascular tone. Exactly how they accomplish these rather contradictory effects is unclear, but these drugs essentially function as partial agonists because they display agonistic (stimulatory) activity in vessels with low tone and antagonistic (inhibitory) activity in vessels with high tone. Clinically, these drugs are used for their ability to prevent or abort vascular headaches (migraine, cluster headaches) by vasoconstricting cerebral vessels.[40] That is, their alpha-agonistic ability in dilated cerebral vessels may explain their primary clinical usefulness. These drugs can also stimulate 5-hydroxytryptamine (serotonin) receptors, and some, if not all, of their antimigraine effects have been attributed to an agonistic effect on vascular serotonin receptors.[41,42] When used in headache suppression, these drugs are administered by a number of routes, including oral, oral inhalation, sublingual, rectal, and even injection.

Phenoxybenzamine (Dibenzyline): Phenoxybenzamine is a noncompetitive alpha-1 blocker, which essentially means that it binds irreversibly to the alpha-1 receptor. This drug tends to have a slow onset, but its effects last much longer than those of the competitive blockers (e.g., phentolamine and prazosin). Phenoxybenzamine is used primarily to control blood pressure prior to the removal of a pheochromocytoma. The drug has also been used for other purposes such as management of essential hypertension and treatment of vasospastic disease (Raynaud's phenomenon). Phenoxybenzamine is usually administered orally.

Phentolamine (Regitine):   Phentolamine is a competitive alpha antagonist used primarily to control blood pressure during management of pheochromocytoma. The drug is usually administered via intravenous or intramuscular injection. Phentolamine is not usually used to treat essential hypertension because with prolonged use, effectiveness tends to decrease and patients begin to develop adverse side effects.

Prazosin (Minipress):   Prazosin is a competitive alpha-1 antagonist that is used primarily in the long-term management of hypertension,[22,51] is administered orally, and tends to produce vasodilation in both arteries and veins.

Other alpha-1 receptor antagonists: Several new alpha-1 selective antagonists have been developed, and some of the more promising agents include doxazosin (Cardura)[49,51] and terazosin (Hytrin).[28,50] These drugs are gaining favor in treating hypertension because they lower blood pressure while producing beneficial effects on serum lipid profiles (decreased total cholesterol, decreased triglycerides) as well as producing favorable effects on glucose metabolism.[28,49–51] These drugs are typically administered orally, and their role in treating hypertension will be discussed in more detail in Chapter 21.

ADVERSE EFFECTS OF ALPHA-1 ANTAGONISTS

One of the primary adverse effects associated with alpha antagonists is reflex tachycardia. By blocking alpha-1 receptors, these drugs tend to decrease blood pressure by decreasing peripheral vascular resistance. As blood pressure falls, a compensatory increase in cardiac output is initiated via the baroreceptor reflex. The increased cardiac output is mediated in part by an increase in heart rate, hence the reflex tachycardia. A second major problem with these drugs is orthostatic hypotension. Dizziness and syncope following changes in posture are quite common due to the decrease in peripheral vascular tone. With alpha antagonists, orthostatic hypotension may be a particular problem just after drug therapy is initiated, in geriatric patients, or following exercise.

Beta Antagonists

GENERAL INDICATIONS

Beta antagonists are generally administered for their effect on the beta-1 receptors that are located on the heart.[20,23] When stimulated, these receptors mediate an increase in cardiac contractility and rate of contraction. By blocking these receptors, beta antagonists reduce the rate and force of myocardial contractions. Consequently, beta antagonists are frequently used to decrease cardiac workload in conditions such as hypertension and certain types of angina pectoris. Beta blockers may also be used to normalize heart rate in certain forms of cardiac arrhythmias. Specific clinical applications of individual beta blockers are summarized in Table 20–2.

Another important function of beta blockers is their ability to limit the extent of myocardial damage following a heart attack and to reduce the risk of fatality following myocardial infarction.[8,17,25,29,37,39,46,54] Apparently, these drugs help reduce the workload of the damaged heart, thus allowing the heart to recover more completely following infarction. Likewise, there is increasing evidence that some beta blockers can help im-

TABLE 20–2 Summary of Common Beta Blockers

Generic Name	Trade Name(s)	Selectivity	Primary Indications
Acebutolol	Sectral	Beta-1	Hypertension
Atenolol	Tenormin	Beta-1	Angina pectoris, hypertension, prevent reinfarction
Betaxolol	Kerlone	Beta-1	Hypertension
Bisoprolol	Zebeta	Beta-1	Hypertension
Carteolol	Cartrol	Nonselective	Hypertension
Esmolol	Brevibloc	Beta-1	Arrhythmias
Labetalol	Normodyne, Trandate	Nonselective	Hypertension
Metoprolol	Lopressor	Beta-1	Angina pectoris, hypertension, prevent reinfarction
Nadolol	Corgard	Nonselective	Angina pectoris, hypertension
Penbutolol	Levatol	Nonselective	Hypertension
Pindolol	Visken	Nonselective	Hypertension
Propranolol	Inderal	Nonselective	Angina pectoris, arrhythmias, hypertension, prevent reinfarction, prevent vascular headache
Sotalol	Betapace	Nonselective	Arrhythmias
Timolol	Blocadren	Nonselective	Hypertension, prevent reinfarction, prevent vascular headache

*Only indications listed in the United States product labeling are included in this table. All drugs are fairly similar pharmacologically, and some may be used for appropriate cardiovascular conditions not specifically listed in product labeling.

prove cardiac function in certain types of heart failure,[3,35,38] and this idea is addressed in more detail in Chapter 24.

Clinically useful beta antagonists are classified as beta-1–selective if they predominantly affect the beta-1 subtype, or beta-nonselective if they have a fairly equal affinity for beta-1 and beta-2 receptors (see Table 20–2). Beta-1–selective drugs are also referred to as *cardioselective* because of their preferential effect on the myocardium. Even if a beta antagonist is nonselective (i.e., blocks both beta-1 and beta-2 receptors), the beta-1 blockade is clinically beneficial. When stimulated, beta-2 receptors, which are found primarily on bronchial smooth muscle, cause bronchodilation. Blockade of these beta-2 receptors may lead to smooth-muscle contraction and bronchoconstriction. Thus, drugs that selectively block beta-2 receptors have no real clinical significance because they promote bronchoconstriction.[44]

Currently, a number of beta blockers are used clinically; selection of a specific agent depends on factors such as cardioselectivity, duration of action (half-life), and several other ancillary properties of each drug. Certain beta blockers, for instance, produce added effects such as mild peripheral vasodilation or stabilization of cardiac membranes that can be beneficial in treating certain cardiovascular conditions.[18,44,53] Clinical applications of specific beta blockers are discussed in more detail in Chapters 21 through 24.

SPECIFIC AGENTS

Acebutolol (Sectral): Acebutolol is described as a relatively cardioselective beta blocker[12] that tends to bind preferentially to beta-1 receptors at lower doses but binds to both types of beta receptors as dosages increase. Primary clinical applications are for treatment of hypertension and prevention and treatment of cardiac arrhythmias. The drug is usually administered orally.

Atenolol (Tenormin): Like acebutolol, atenolol is regarded as beta-1 selective but tends to be less beta-specific at higher doses. The drug is administered orally for the long-term treatment of both hypertension and chronic, stable angina.

Labetalol (Normodyne, Trandate): Labetalol is a nonselective beta blocker. This drug also appears to have some alpha-1–selective blocking effects.[7] Labetalol is used primarily in the management of hypertension and, while usually given orally, may be injected intravenously in emergency hypertensive situations.

Metoprolol (Lopressor): Metoprolol is considered a cardioselective beta blocker[30] and has been approved for use in the long-term management of hypertension, as well as in the prevention of myocardial reinfarction. As an antihypertensive, metoprolol is usually administered orally. In the prevention of reinfarction, metoprolol is initiated by intravenous injection and then followed up by oral administration.

Nadolol (Corgard): Nadolol is a nonselective beta blocker that is administered orally as an antihypertensive and antianginal agent. This drug has somewhat of an advantage over other nonselective beta blockers (propranolol) in that nadolol often needs to be taken only once each day.[16]

Pindolol (Visken): Pindolol is a nonselective beta blocker that also exhibits some intrinsic sympathomimetic activity,[14,43] which means that pindolol not only blocks the beta receptor from the effects of endogenous catecholamines but also stimulates the receptor to some extent (i.e., it acts as a partial beta agonist). This advantage protects the beta receptor from excessive endogenous stimulation while still preserving a low level of background sympathetic activity. Pindolol is used primarily in the long-term management of hypertension.

Propranolol (Inderal): Propranolol, the classic nonselective beta blocker,[27] is approved for use in hypertension, angina pectoris, cardiac arrhythmias, and prevention of myocardial reinfarction. In addition, propranolol has been used in the prevention of vascular headache and as an adjunct to alpha blockers in treating pheochromocytoma. Propranolol is usually administered orally for the long-term management of the conditions listed previously, but it may be administered via intravenous injection for the immediate control of arrhythmias.

Timolol (Blocadren): This nonselective beta blocker is administered orally for treatment of hypertension and prevention of myocardial reinfarction.[15]

Other beta antagonists: Several newer beta blockers are currently available including betaxolol (Kerlone), bisoprolol (Zebeta), carteolol (Cartrol), esmolol (Brevibloc), penbutolol (Levatol), and sotalol (Betapace). These agents have various ancillary properties and clinical applications, but they are all used primarily for their ability to block cardiac beta receptors. Clinical applications and relative selectivity of these drugs are summarized in Table 20–2.

ADVERSE EFFECTS

When nonselective beta blockers are used, some antagonism of beta-2 receptors also occurs.[2] The antagonism of beta-2 receptors on bronchiole smooth muscle often leads to some degree of bronchoconstriction and an increase in airway resistance. Although this event is usually not a problem in individuals with normal pulmonary function, patients with respiratory problems such as asthma, bronchitis, and emphysema may be adversely affected by nonselective beta antagonists.[9,20] In these patients, one of the beta-1–selective drugs should be administered.

Selective and nonselective beta blockers are also associated with several other adverse effects. The most serious of these effects results from excessive depression of cardiac function. By slowing down the heart too much, these agents can lead to cardiac failure, especially if there is some pre-existing cardiac disease. Because of their antihypertensive properties, beta blockers may produce orthostatic hypotension, and dizziness and syncope may occur following abrupt changes in posture. Patients taking beta blockers for prolonged periods have also been reported to have an increase in centrally related side effects such as depression, lethargy, and sleep disorders.[1,31] These behavioral side effects may be because of interaction of the beta blockers with CNS receptors.

Various other relatively minor side effects have also been reported, including gastrointestinal disturbances (nausea, vomiting) and allergic responses (fever, rash). However, these are fairly uncommon and tend to be resolved by adjusting the dosage or the specific type of medication.

Other Drugs That Inhibit Adrenergic Neurons

GENERAL INDICATIONS

Several agents are available that inhibit activity at adrenergic synapses by interfering with the release of norepinephrine. Rather than directly blocking the postsynaptic receptor, these drugs typically inhibit or deplete the presynaptic terminal of stored norepinephrine. These drugs are used primarily to decrease peripheral adrenergic influence and to treat problems such as hypertension and cardiac arrhythmias.

SPECIFIC AGENTS

Bretylium (Bretylol):   Bretylium appears to directly inhibit the release of norepinephrine from adrenergic nerve terminals. With prolonged use, this drug may also replace presynaptic norepinephrine in a manner similar to guanadrel and guanethidine (see the next two agent listings in this section). Bretylium is used primarily in the treatment of cardiac arrhythmias (see Chapter 23). While usually given orally for the long-term management of ventricular arrhythmias, bretylium is injected intravenously for the emergency treatment of ventricular tachycardia and ventricular fibrillation.

Guanadrel (Hylorel):   Guanadrel is taken up by the presynaptic terminal and appears to directly inhibit the release of norepinephrine. With prolonged use, guanadrel slowly replaces norepinephrine in the presynaptic vesicles. This substitution of guanadrel for norepinephrine further inhibits activity at postsynaptic adrenergic synapses by creating a false neurotransmitter. Guanadrel also replaces stored norepinephrine in the adrenal medulla, thus decreasing adrenal influence on cardiovascular function. Guanadrel is administered orally for management of hypertension.

Guanethidine (Ismelin):   Similar in action and effects to guanadrel, this drug is actively transported into the presynaptic terminal by the norepinephrine pump, where it inhibits norepinephrine release and later replaces stored norepinephrine. Unlike guanadrel, guanethidine selectively affects postganglionic sympathetic adrenergic nerve terminals and does not affect release of norepinephrine from the adrenal medulla. Guanethidine is usually administered orally for the management of moderate-to-severe hypertension.

Metyrosine (Demser):   Metyrosine inhibits the enzyme that initiates catecholamine synthesis (epinephrine, norepinephrine), and this drug is used to diminish catecholamine stores prior to removal of a catecholamine-producing tumor (pheochromocytoma).

Reserpine (Serpalan, Serpasil, others):   Reserpine inhibits the presynaptic synthesis of catecholamines (norepinephrine, epinephrine) as well as 5-hydroxytryptamine (serotonin). This inhibition eventually causes a depletion of presynaptic neurotransmitter stores in several tissues including postganglionic nerve terminals, adrenal medulla, and brain. Unlike guanethidine and guanadrel, reserpine does not appear to actually replace the presynaptic neurotransmitter, but simply prevents more transmitter from being resynthesized. Reserpine is used primarily in the treatment of mild-to-moderate hypertension and is administered orally. The antihypertensive effects of this drug are caused, in part, by the inhibition of peripheral adrenergic nerve terminals, although some of its antihypertensive effects may also be because of the inhibition of CNS catecholamine activity.

ADVERSE EFFECTS

Orthostatic hypotension is occasionally a problem with the aforementioned drugs, and dizziness and syncope sometimes occur after a sudden change in posture. Some patients also experience gastrointestinal disturbances including nausea, vomiting, and diarrhea. Peripheral edema as evidenced by swelling in the feet and legs has also been reported.

SUMMARY

This chapter classifies and describes a variety of drugs according to their stimulatory (agonistic) or inhibitory (antagonistic) effect on adrenergic function. In general, adrenergic agonists are administered according to their ability to evoke specific tissue responses via specific adrenergic receptors. Alpha-1–adrenergic agonists are used as antihypotensive agents because of their ability to increase peripheral vascular resistance; they may also be used as nasal decongestants because of their ability to vasoconstrict the nasal mucosa. Agonists selective for alpha-2 receptors are administered to treat hypertension because of their ability to inhibit sympathetic discharge from the CNS. Cardioselective beta-1 agonists are used primarily for their ability to stimulate the heart, and beta-2 agonists are used in the treatment of asthma and premature labor because of their ability to relax bronchiole and uterine smooth muscle, respectively.

Alpha-adrenergic antagonists are used primarily as antihypertensive drugs because of their ability to block vascular alpha-1 receptors. Beta-adrenergic antagonists (beta blockers) are administered primarily for their inhibitory effects on myocardial function and are used in the prevention and treatment of hypertension, angina pectoris, arrhythmias, and myocardial reinfarction. Many of the drugs introduced in this chapter are discussed further in later chapters that deal with specific clinical conditions (e.g., hypertension, asthma, and other disorders).

REFERENCES

1. Avorn, J, Everitt, DE, and Weiss, S: Increased antidepressant use in patients prescribed beta-blockers. JAMA 255:357, 1986.
2. Bauer, K, Rakusen, S, and Kaik, G: Pulmonary effects of long-term beta-2 blockade in healthy subjects: Comparative study of oral metaprolol OROS. Am Heart J 120(suppl):473, 1990.
3. Bristow, MR: Pathophysiologic and pharmacologic rationales for clinical management of chronic heart failure with beta-blocking agents. Am J Cardiol 71:C12, 1993.
4. Canadian Preterm Labor Investigators Group: Treatment of preterm labor with the beta-adrenergic agonist ritodrine. N Engl J Med 327:308, 1992.
5. Caritis, SN: Treatment of preterm labour. A review of therapeutic options. Drugs 26:243, 1983.
6. Chung, KF: The current debate concerning beta-agonists in asthma. A review. J Royal Soc Med 86:96, 1993.
7. Cressman, MD and Gifford, RW: Labetalol: The first combined alpha and beta blocker. J Cardiovasc Med 9:593, 1984.
8. Cruickshank, JM: Beta-blockers: Primary and secondary prevention. J Cardiovasc Pharmacol 20(suppl 11):S55, 1992.
9. Cruickshank, JM: The clinical importance of cardioselectivity and lipophilicity in beta blockers. Am Heart J 100:160, 1980.
10. Davey, MJ: The pharmacological basis for the use of alpha-1 adrenoceptor antagonists in the treatment of essential hypertension. Br J Clin Pharmacol 21(suppl 1):5S, 1986.
11. Davey, MJ: Alpha adrenoceptors: An overview. J Mol Cell Cardiol 18(suppl 5):1, 1986.
12. DeBono, G, et al: Acebutolol: 10 years of experience. Am Heart J 109:1211, 1985.
13. Executive Committee, American Academy of Allergy and Immunology: Inhaled beta-2 adrenergic agonists in asthma. J Allergy Clin Immunol 91;1234, 1993.
14. Frishman, WH: Pindolol: A new beta-adrenoceptor antagonist with partial agonist activity. N Engl J Med 308:940, 1983.
15. Frishman, WH: Drug therapy: Atenolol and timolol, two new systemic beta-adrenoceptor antagonists. N Engl J Med 306:1456, 1982.
16. Frishman, WH: Nadolol: A new beta-adrenoceptor antagonist. N Engl J Med 305:678, 1981.
17. Frishman, WH, Furberg, CD, and Friedewald, WT: Beta-adrenergic blockade for survivors of acute myocardial infarction. N Engl J Med 310:830, 1984.
18. Frolich, ED: Vasodilating beta-blockers: Systemic and regional hemodynamic effects. Am Heart J 121:1012, 1991.
19. Gerber, JG and Nies, AS: Antihypertensive agents and the drug therapy of hypertension. In Gilman, AG, et al (eds): The Pharmacological Basis of Therapeutics, ed 8. Pergamon Press, New York, 1990.
20. Gerber, JG and Nies, AS: Beta-adrenergic blocking drugs. Annu Rev Med 36:145, 1985.
21. Gillis, RA, Gatti, PJ, and Quest, JA: Mechanism of the anti-hypertensive effect of alpha-2 agonists. J Cardiovasc Pharmacol 7(suppl 8):S38, 1985.
22. Graham, RM and Pettinger, WA: Drug therapy: Prazocin. N Engl J Med 300:232, 1979.
23. Hansson, L: Review of state-of-the-art beta-blocker therapy. Am J Cardiol 67:43B, 1991.
24. Heinsimer, JA and Lefkowitz, R: Adrenergic receptors: Biochemistry, regulation, molecular mechanisms and clinical implications. J Lab Clin Med 100:641, 1982.
25. Held, P: Effects of beta-blockers on ventricular dysfunction after myocardial infarction: Tolerability and survival effects. Am J Cardiol 71:39C, 1993.
26. Hoffman, BB: Adrenoceptor-activating drugs. In Katzung, BG (ed): Basic and Clinical Pharmacology, ed 5. Appleton & Lange, Norwalk, CT, 1992.
27. Holland, OG and Kaplan, NM: Propranolol in the treatment of hypertension. N Engl J Med 294:930, 1976.
28. Horky, K: Alpha-1 blockade in the management of hypertension. J Clin Pharmacol 33:874, 1993.
29. International Collaborative Study Group: Reduction of infarct size with the early use of timolol in acute myocardial infarction. N Engl J Med 310:9, 1984.
30. Koch-Weser, J: Metoprolol. N Engl J Med 301:698, 1979.
31. Koella, WP: CNS-related effects of beta-blockers with special reference to mechanisms of action. Eur J Clin Pharmacol 28(suppl 1):55, 1985.
32. Koss, MC: Review article: Pupillary dilation as an index of central nervous system alpha-2 adrenoceptor activation. J Pharmacol Methods 15:1, 1986.
33. Langer, SZ: Presynaptic receptors and their role in the regulation of transmitter release. Br J Pharmacol 60:481, 1977.
34. Langer, SZ, Cavero, I, and Massingham, R: Recent developments in noradrenergic neurotransmission and its relevance to the mechanism of action of certain antihypertensive agents. Hypertension 2:372, 1980.
35. Leung, W-H, et al: Improvement in exercise performance and hemodynamics by labetolol in patients with idiopathic dilated cardiomyopathy. Am Heart J 119:884, 1990.

36. Levitt, B and Hieble, JP: Prejunctional alpha-2 adrenoceptors modulate stimulation-evoked norepinephrine release in rabbit lateral saphenous vein. Eur J Pharmacol 132:197, 1986.
37. Levy, S: Secondary prevention after myocardial infarction: In favor of beta-blockers. J Cardiovasc Pharmacol 16(suppl 6):S50, 1990.
38. Nemanich, JW, et al: Effects of metoprolol on rest and exercise cardiac function and plasma catecholamines in chronic congestive heart failure secondary to ischemic or idiopathic cardiomyopathy. Am J Cardiol 66:843, 1990.
39. Pearle, DL: Pharmacologic management of ischemic heart disease with beta-blockers and calcium channel blockers. Am Heart J 120(suppl):739, 1990.
40. Peatfield, R: Migraine. Current concepts of pathogenesis and treatment. Drugs 26:364, 1983.
41. Peroutka, SJ: 5-hydroxytryptamine receptor subtypes and the pharmacology of migraine. Neurology 43(suppl 3):34, 1993.
42. Raskin, NJ: Acute and prophylactic treatment of migraine: Practical approaches and pharmacologic rationale. Neurology 43(suppl 3):39, 1993.
43. Schirger, A, et al: Pindolol, a new beta-adrenergic blocking agent with intrinsic sympathomimetic activity in the management of mild and moderate hypertension. Mayo Clin Proc 58:315, 1983.
44. Shanks, RG: Clinical pharmacology of vasodilating beta-blocking drugs. Am Heart J 121:1006, 1991.
45. Sizemore, GW and Winternitz, WW: Autonomic hyper-reflexia: Suppression with alpha-adrenergic blocking agents. N Engl J Med 282:795, 1970.
46. Sleight, P: Use of beta adrenoceptor blockade during and after acute myocardial infarction. Annu Rev Med 37:415, 1986.
47. Spitzer, WO, et al: The use of beta-agonists and the risk of death and near death from asthma. N Engl J Med 326:501, 1992.
48. Starke, K and Altmann, KP: Inhibition of adrenergic neurotransmission by clonidine: An action on prejunctional alpha-receptors. Neuropharmacology 12:339, 1973.
49. Symposium (various authors): Management of coronary heart disease risk factors in hypertensive patients: Clinical experience with doxazosin. Am Heart J 121:245, 1991.
50. Symposium (various authors): Clinical application of alpha$_1$-receptor blockade: Terazosin in the management of hypertension. J Clin Pharmacol 33:866, 1993.
51. Taylor, SH and Grimm, RH: New developments in the role of alpha$_1$-adrenergic receptors in cardiovascular disease. Am Heart J 119:655, 1990.
52. Thompson, TL, et al: Lack of efficacy of hydergine in patients with Alzheimer's disease. N Engl J Med 323:445, 1990.
53. Turner, P: Which ancillary properties of beta-adrenoceptor blocking drugs influence their therapeutic or adverse effects: A review. J Royal Soc Med 84:672, 1991.
54. Vedin, JA and Wilhelmsson, CE: Beta receptor blocking agents in the secondary prevention of coronary heart disease. Annu Rev Pharmacol Toxicol 23:29, 1983.
55. Webb-Johnson, DC and Andrews, JL: Bronchodilator therapy. N Engl J Med 297:476, 1977.

CHAPTER 21

Antihypertensive Drugs

Hypertension is defined as a sustained, reproducible increase in blood pressure. Hypertension is one of the most common diseases affecting adults living in industrialized nations; approximately 15 to 20 percent of adult Americans are believed to be hypertensive.[2,29] If left untreated, the sustained increase in blood pressure associated with hypertension can lead to cardiovascular problems (stroke, heart failure), renal disease, and blindness.[27,50,78] These and other medical problems ultimately lead to an increased mortality rate in hypertensive individuals.

Although there is a general consensus regarding the adverse effects of hypertension, some debate exists as to exactly how much of an increase in blood pressure constitutes hypertension. Generally, diastolic values greater than 90 mm Hg and/or systolic values greater than 140 mm Hg warrant a diagnosis of hypertension. A more detailed classification scheme is shown in Table 21–1. Patients are usually classified as having mild, moderate, or severe hypertension depending on the extent of their elevated blood pressure. As might be expected, the incidence of morbidity and mortality increases as the hypertension becomes more severe. Hence, pharmacologic and nonpharmacologic methods are implemented to decrease blood pressure in most patients to a diastolic value of less than 85 mm Hg and a systolic value of less than 125 mm Hg.[32]

Hypertension is often described as a silent killer because of the lack of symptoms throughout most of the course of this disease. Patients may feel perfectly well into the advanced stages of hypertension. Rehabilitation specialists dealing with hypertensive patients are usually treating some problem other than the increased blood pressure (i.e., hypertension is not the reason the patient is referred to physical therapy and occupational therapy). Considering the prevalence of hypertension, however, many patients receiving therapy for various other problems will also be taking antihypertensive drugs, so some knowledge of the pharmacology of these agents is essential.

The pharmacologic management of hypertension has evolved to where blood pressure can be controlled for extended periods in most patients. There are currently several major categories of antihypertensive agents, and new drugs are continually being added to the antihypertensive arsenal. Each group of antihypertensive drugs is discussed under the appropriate section in this chapter, as well as how several different drugs can be used together when treating hypertension. To better understand how

TABLE 21-1 Classification of BP*

Category	Range (mm Hg)
Normal BP	Systolic < 140; diastolic < 85
High-normal BP	Diastolic 85–89
Mild hypertension	Diastolic 90–104
Moderate hypertension	Diastolic 105–114
Severe hypertension	Diastolic ≥ 115
Borderline isolated systolic hypertension	Systolic 140–159; diastolic < 90
Isolated systolic hypertension	Systolic ≥ 160; diastolic < 90

*The diastolic pressure is the primary value used to make a diagnosis of mild, moderate, or severe hypertension. "Isolated" hypertension indicates an increase in only the systolic value, with the diastolic pressure remaining relatively normal.
Source: From Joint National Committee on Detection, Evaluation, and Treatment of High Blood Pressure,[55] p 1047, with permission.

these drugs work in decreasing blood pressure, the normal control of blood pressure and the possible mechanisms that generate a hypertensive state are briefly discussed here.

NORMAL CONTROL OF BLOOD PRESSURE

Blood pressure is normally maintained by the complex interaction of several physiologic systems.[11,28] Short-term control of blood pressure is accomplished primarily by the baroreceptor reflex (see Chapter 18). The baroreflex monitors and corrects changes in blood pressure within a matter of seconds by altering cardiac output and peripheral vascular resistance. The more long-term management of blood pressure is accomplished primarily by the kidneys through their control of fluid balance. Changes in blood pressure through the renal handling of fluid and electrolytes usually take place over a period of several hours to several days. Together these two systems interact to maintain blood pressure within a fairly narrow range.

Although the control of blood pressure is a fairly complex subject, the actual factors that determine blood pressure can be simplified somewhat. At any given time, blood pressure is the product of cardiac output and the total resistance in the peripheral vasculature. This relationship is illustrated by the following equation:

$$BP = (CO) \times (TPR)$$

where BP = blood pressure, CO = cardiac output, and TPR = total peripheral resistance in the systemic vasculature. As indicated by this equation, BP can be maintained at a relatively constant level by changes in either CO or TPR. A decrease in CO, for instance, can potentially be offset by an increase in TPR so that BP does not appreciably change. Conversely, a sudden fall in TPR will necessitate an increase in CO if BP is to be maintained.

The relevance of this simple equation to antihypertensive therapy will become apparent as different drugs are discussed. Some antihypertensive drugs exert their effects by primarily acting on CO, others primarily affect TPR, and some agents decrease both factors in an attempt to lower blood pressure.

PATHOGENESIS OF HYPERTENSION

Essential Versus Secondary Hypertension

Hypertension can be divided into two major categories: secondary hypertension and primary, or essential, hypertension. In secondary hypertension, the elevated blood pressure can be attributed to some specific abnormality such as renal artery stenosis, catecholamine-producing tumors, endocrine disorders, or cerebral damage. The treatment of secondary hypertension is rather straightforward, with efforts focused on correcting the underlying pathology (e.g., the cause of the problem can be dealt with directly by surgery). Secondary hypertension, however, accounts for only about 5 percent of the patients diagnosed with hypertension.[29] The remaining 95 percent of hypertensive individuals are classified as having primary, or essential, hypertension. In essential hypertension, there is no clear, readily discernible cause of the elevated blood pressure.

Consequently, the exact cause of hypertension in the majority of patients is unknown. Many theories have been proposed to explain how blood pressure increases and eventually becomes sustained in essential hypertension. Some of the major factors that may account for the increased blood pressure in essential hypertension are presented here.

Possible Mechanisms in Essential Hypertension

The voluminous literature dealing with potential causes and mechanisms of essential hypertension cannot be fully reviewed here. As stated previously, the exact cause of hypertension in most patients is not known. There appears to be a rather complex interaction of genetic and environmental factors that ultimately leads to adaptive changes in the cardiovascular system of the patient with essential hypertension.[7,8,33,36] Diet, stress, and other external factors, for example, are associated with increased blood pressure. These factors seem to be more influential in certain patients, suggesting a possible genetic predisposition to hypertension. Other risk factors such as cigarette smoking and alcohol abuse clearly play a role in potentiating the onset and maintenance of hypertension. The point is that essential hypertension is probably not caused by only one factor, but may be caused by a subtle, complex interaction of many factors. The exact way in which these factors interact probably varies from person to person, so that the cause of this disease really must be regarded individually rather than being based on one common etiology.

Despite the fact that the actual cause of hypertension is unknown, studies in humans and in animal models that mimic essential hypertension have suggested that the sympathetic nervous system may be a final common pathway in mediating and perpetuating the hypertensive state. That is, the factors described earlier may interact in such a way as to cause a general increase in sympathetic activity, which then becomes the common denominator underlying the elevated blood pressure in essential hypertension.[1,19,26,56,95,102,104] Increased sympathetic activity should produce a hypertensive effect because of the excitatory effect of sympathetic neurons on the heart and peripheral vasculature. Increased sympathetic drive may initially increase blood pressure by increasing cardiac output. In later stages, cardiac output often returns to normal levels, with the increased blood pressure being due to an increase in vascular resistance. The reasons for this shift from elevated cardiac output to elevated peripheral vascular resistance are somewhat unclear. A sustained increase in sympathetic activity, however, may be the initiating factor that begins a sequence of events ultimately resulting in essential hypertension.

Once blood pressure does become elevated, hypertension seems to become self-perpetuating to some extent. The increased blood pressure may invoke adaptive changes in the peripheral vasculature so that peripheral vessels become less compliant and vascular resistance increases.[9,33,82] The peripheral vasculature also appears to be more reactive to pressor substances such as norepinephrine and angiotensin II,[12,20] and relaxation of the vasculature by vasodilating substances such as nitrous oxide seems to be impaired in patients with essential hypertension.[77] Reflex mechanisms that control blood pressure (the baroreceptor reflex) may decrease in sensitivity, thus blunting the normal response to elevated pressure.[95,100] Increased sympathetic discharge to the kidneys and altered renal hemodynamics may also cause changes in renal function that contribute to the increase in blood pressure.[19,59]

The possible factors involved in initiating and maintaining essential hypertension are summarized in Figure 21–1. Ultimately, certain environmental factors may turn on the sympathetic division of the autonomic nervous system in susceptible individuals. Increased sympathetic discharge then creates a vicious cycle whereby increased sympathetic effects in conjunction with the increased blood pressure itself help perpetuate the hypertension. Exactly how various factors initiate the increased sympathetic discharge is not fully understood and may in fact vary from patient to patient. It is hoped that future studies will elaborate on the exact role of such factors in causing essential hypertension and that treatment can then be focused on preventing the changes that initially increase blood pressure.

DRUG THERAPY

Several major categories of drugs exist for the treatment of essential hypertension. These categories include diuretics, sympatholytic drugs, vasodilators, angiotensin-converting enzyme inhibitors, and calcium channel blockers. The primary sites of action and effects of each category are summarized in Table 21–2. The mechanism of action, rationale for use, specific agents, and adverse effects of drugs in each category are discussed in the next few sections of this chapter.

DIURETICS

Mechanism of Action and Rationale for Use

Diuretics increase the formation and excretion of urine. These drugs are used as antihypertensive agents because of their ability to increase the renal excretion of water and sodium, thus decreasing the volume of fluid within the vascular system. This situation is somewhat analogous to the decrease in pressure that would occur inside a balloon if some of the air inside the balloon were allowed to leak out. Consequently, diuretics appear to have a rather direct effect on blood pressure through their ability to simply decrease the amount of fluid in the vascular system.

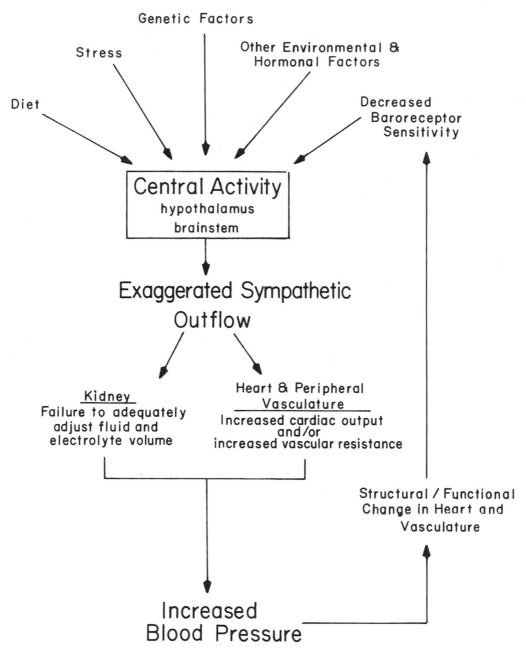

FIGURE 21–1. Schematic diagram of the possible mechanisms in essential hypertension. Various factors interact to turn on sympathetic outflow to the kidneys, heart, and peripheral vasculature, resulting in elevated blood pressure. Hypertension also causes structural and functional changes in the vasculature that help maintain the elevated pressure.

Diuretics are often the first type of drugs used to treat hypertension.[76] They are relatively inexpensive and seem to work well in a large percentage of patients with mild-to-moderate hypertension.[44] The use of diuretics alone and in conjunction with other antihypertensives is discussed in more detail in "Stepped-Care Approach to Hypertension."

TABLE 21–2 Antihypertensive Drug Categories

Category	Primary Site(s) of Action	Primary Antihypertensive Effect(s)
Diuretics	Kidneys	Decrease plasma fluid volume
Sympatholytics	Various sites within the sympathetic division of the autonomic nervous system	Decrease sympathetic influence on the heart and/or peripheral vasculature
Vasodilators	Peripheral vasculature	Lower vascular resistance by directly vasodilating peripheral vessels
Angiotensin-converting enzyme inhibitors	Angiotensin-converting enzyme located in the lungs and other tissues	Prevent the conversion of angiotensin I to angiotensin II (angiotensin II is a potent vasoconstrictor)
Calcium channel blockers	Limit calcium entry into vascular smooth muscle and cardiac muscle	Decrease vascular smooth-muscle contraction; decrease myocardial force and rate of contraction

Although they differ chemically, all diuretics exert their beneficial effects by directly acting on the kidneys to increase water and sodium excretion.[6,63] Diuretic drugs can be subclassified according to their chemical structure or the manner in which they affect kidney function. The primary subclassifications of diuretics are listed here.

Classification of Diuretics

Thiazide Diuretics. Thiazide drugs share a common chemical nucleus as well as a common mode of action. These drugs act primarily on the early portion of the distal tubule of the nephron, where they inhibit sodium reabsorption. By inhibiting sodium reabsorption, more sodium is retained within the nephron, creating an osmotic force that also retains more water in the nephron. Since more sodium and water are passed through the nephron, from which they will ultimately be excreted from the body, a diuretic effect is produced. Thiazides are the most frequently used type of diuretic for hypertension. Specific types of thiazide drugs are listed in Table 21–3.

Loop Diuretics. These drugs act primarily on the ascending limb of the loop of Henle (hence the term "loop diuretic"). They exert their diuretic effect by inhibiting the reabsorption of sodium and chloride from the nephron, thereby also preventing the reabsorption of water that follows these electrolytes. Specific types of loop diuretics are listed in Table 21–3.

Potassium-Sparing Diuretics. Several different drugs with diuretic properties are classified as potassium-sparing because of their ability to prevent potassium secretion into the distal tubule. Normally, a sodium-potassium exchange occurs in the distal tubule, whereby sodium is reabsorbed and potassium is secreted. Potassium-sparing agents interfere with this exchange in various ways (depending on the specific drug) so that potassium is spared from excretion and sodium remains in the tubule, from which it is excreted. Although these agents do not produce a diuretic effect to the same extent as the loop and thiazide drugs, potassium-sparing drugs have the advantage of reducing potassium loss and thus preventing hypokalemia. Specific potassium-sparing drugs are listed in Table 21–3.

TABLE 21-3 Diuretic Drugs Used to Treat Hypertension

Thiazide diuretics

Bendroflumethiazide (Naturetin)	Hydroflumethiazide (Diucardin, Saluron)
Benzthiazide (Exna, Hydrex)	Methyclothiazide (Enduron, others)
Chlorothiazide (Diuril)	Metolazone (Diulo, Zaroxolyn)
Chlorthalidone (Hygroton, others)	Polythiazide (Renese)
Cyclothiazide (Anhydron)	Quinethazone (Hydromox)
Hydrochlorothiazide (Esidrix, others)	Trichlormethiazide (Metahydrin, Naqua)

Loop diuretics	**Potassium-sparing diuretics**
Bumetanide (Bumex)	Amiloride (Midamor)
Ethacrynic acid (Edecrin)	Spironolactone (Aldactone)
Furosemide (Lasix, Furoside, others)	Triamterene (Dyrenium)

Adverse Effects of Diuretics

The most serious side effects of diuretics are fluid depletion and electrolyte imbalance.[34,87] By the very nature of their action, diuretics decrease extracellular fluid volume as well as produce sodium depletion (**hyponatremia**) and potassium depletion (**hypokalemia**). Hypokalemia is a particular problem with the thiazide and loop diuretics but occurs less frequently when the potassium-sparing agents are used. Hypokalemia and other disturbances in fluid and electrolyte balance can produce serious metabolic and cardiac problems and may even prove fatal in some individuals. Consequently, patients must be monitored closely, and the drug dosage should be maintained at the lowest effective dose. Also, potassium supplements are used in some patients to prevent hypokalemia.

Fluid depletion may also be a serious problem during diuretic therapy. A decrease in blood volume may cause a reflex increase in cardiac output and peripheral vascular resistance because of activation of the baroreflex (see Chapter 18). This occurrence may produce an excessive demand on the myocardium, especially in patients with cardiac disease. Decreased blood volume may also activate the renin-angiotensin system, thereby causing further peripheral vasoconstriction and increased cardiac workload. Again, these effects of fluid depletion may be especially serious in patients with certain types of heart failure.

Other, less serious, but bothersome, side effects of diuretic therapy include gastrointestinal disturbances and weakness-fatigue. **Orthostatic hypotension** may occur because of the relative fluid depletion produced by these drugs. Changes in mood and confusion may also occur in some patients.

SYMPATHOLYTIC DRUGS

As discussed previously, the preponderance of evidence indicates that an increase in sympathetic activity may be an underlying factor in essential hypertension. Consequently, drugs that interfere with sympathetic discharge (i.e., sympatholytic agents) should be valuable as antihypertensive agents. These sympatholytic drugs can be classified according to where and how they interrupt sympathetic activity.[101] Sympatholytic drugs used to treat hypertension include beta-adrenergic blockers, alpha-adrenergic blockers, presynaptic adrenergic neurotransmitter depletors, centrally acting drugs, and ganglionic blockers (Table 21–4). Each of these categories is discussed here.

Beta Blockers

MECHANISM OF ACTION AND RATIONALE FOR USE

Beta-adrenergic blockers have been used extensively to decrease blood pressure and are a mainstay of antihypertensive therapy in many patients.[38,49,79,85] Beta blockers exert their primary effect on the heart, where they decrease heart rate and force of myocardial contraction. In hypertensive patients, these drugs lower blood pressure by slowing down the heart and reducing cardiac output. This statement, however, is probably an oversimplification of how beta blockers produce an antihypertensive effect. In addition to their direct effect on the myocardium, beta blockers also produce a general decrease in sympathetic tone.[85] Exactly how this decrease in sympathetic activity occurs remains to be determined. Some theories suggest (1) that beta blockers may have a central inhibitory effect on sympathetic activity, (2) that they influence renin release from the kidneys and within the CNS, (3) that they impair sympathetic activity in the ganglia or at the presynaptic adrenergic terminals, or (4) that they act by a combination of these and other factors.[85] Regardless of the exact mechanism of their action, beta blockers remain one of the most effective and well-tolerated types of antihypertensive drugs.[22,43]

SPECIFIC AGENTS

Beta-adrenergic blockers that are approved for use in hypertension are listed in Table 21–4. These drugs are all effective in decreasing blood pressure, but certain beta blockers have additional properties that make them more suitable in specific pa-

TABLE 21–4 Sympatholytic Drugs Used to Treat Hypertension

Beta blockers
  Acebutolol (Sectral)
  Atenolol (Tenormin)
  Betaxolol (Kerlone)
  Bisoprolol (Zebeta)
  Carteolol (Cartrol)
  Labetalol (Normodyne; Trandate)
  Metoprolol (Lopressor)
  Nadolol (Corgard)
  Oxprenolol (Trasicor)
  Penbutolol (Levatol)
  Pindolol (Visken)
  Propranolol (Inderal)
  Sotalol (Betapace)
  Timolol (Blocadren)
Alpha blockers
  Doxazosin (Cardura)
  Phenoxybenzamine (Dibenzyline)
  Prazosin (Minipress)
  Terazosin (Hytrin)

Presynaptic adrenergic inhibitors
  Guanadrel (Hylorel)
  Guanethidine (Ismelin)
  Reserpine (Serpalan, others)

Centrally acting agents
  Clonidine (Catapres)
  Guanabenz (Wytensin)
  Guanfacine (Tenex)
  Methyldopa (Aldomet)

Ganglionic blockers
  Mecamylamine (Inversine)
  Trimethaphan (Arfonad)

tients.[22,98,103] As discussed in Chapter 20, some beta blockers are relatively selective for beta-1 receptors (cardioselective) and tend to affect the heart more than lungs and other tissues (see Table 20–2). Certain beta blockers such as pindolol and acebutolol function as partial agonists and are said to have *intrinsic sympathomimetic activity* because they block the effects of excessive endogenous catecholamines while still producing a normal background level of sympathetic stimulation to the heart.[25,37,83] Some agents such as labetalol and propranolol are able to normalize the excitability of the cardiac cell membrane; these drugs are said to have *membrane-stabilizing activity*.[25,98] Finally, labetalol and some of the newer beta blockers produce peripheral vasodilation as well as cardiac beta blockade, making these drugs especially useful in decreasing blood pressure.[21,40,86,90] Hence, selection of a specific beta blocker is based on these additional properties along with consideration for the individual needs of each patient.

ADVERSE EFFECTS

Nonselective beta blockers (i.e., those with a fairly equal affinity for beta-1 and beta-2 receptors) may produce bronchoconstriction in patients with asthma and similar respiratory disorders. Cardiovascular side effects include excessive depression of heart rate and myocardial contractility as well as orthostatic hypotension. Other side effects include depression, fatigue, gastrointestinal disturbances, and allergic reactions. Beta blockers are generally well tolerated by most patients, however, and the incidence of side effects is relatively low.

Alpha Blockers

MECHANISM OF ACTION AND RATIONALE FOR USE

Drugs that block the alpha-1–adrenergic receptor on vascular smooth muscle will promote a decrease in vascular resistance.[24,46] Since total peripheral vascular resistance often increases in essential hypertension, blocking vascular adrenergic receptors should be an effective course of action. In a sense, alpha blockers act directly on the tissues that ultimately mediate the increased blood pressure—that is, the peripheral vasculature. In the past, the use of alpha blockers in mild-to-moderate essential hypertension was somewhat limited because these drugs are sometimes *too* effective and tend to cause problems with hypotension. It is now recognized that alpha-1 antagonists may offer specific advantages in treating hypertension, including an ability to improve blood lipid profiles (decreased triglycerides and total cholesterol, increased high-density lipoprotein–cholesterol ratio) and produce a favorable effect on glucose metabolism and insulin resistance.[53,89,94,97] Hence, alpha blockers are gaining acceptance in the treatment of mild-to-moderate hypertension as well as being included in the antihypertensive regimen of patients having more severe cases of high blood pressure.

SPECIFIC AGENTS

The characteristics of individual alpha blockers are discussed in Chapter 20. Basically, these drugs can be differentiated according to their relative alpha-1 selectivity, duration of action, and other pharmacokinetic properties. Prazosin has been the primary alpha blocker used in the past, but newer agents such as doxazosin and terazosin are gaining acceptance in treating hypertension. Prazosin and other alpha blockers approved as antihypertensives are listed in Table 21–4.

ADVERSE EFFECTS

One of the primary problems with alpha blockers is reflex tachycardia. When peripheral vascular resistance falls because of the effect of these drugs, the baroreceptor reflex often responds by generating a compensatory increase in heart rate. This tachycardia may be a significant problem, especially if there is any history of cardiac disease. To prevent reflex tachycardia, a beta blocker may be administered with the alpha blocker. The beta blocker will negate the increase in heart rate that is normally mediated through the sympathetic innervation to the heart.

The other major adverse effect with alpha blockers is orthostatic hypotension. Blockade of alpha-1 receptors in peripheral arteries and veins often promotes pooling of blood in the lower extremities when a patient stands up. Therapists should be alert for the symptoms of orthostatic hypotension (i.e., dizziness and syncope), especially for the first few days during which an alpha blocker is being administered.

Presynaptic Adrenergic Inhibitors

MECHANISM OF ACTION AND RATIONALE FOR USE

Drugs that inhibit the release of norepinephrine from the presynaptic terminals of peripheral adrenergic neurons may be used effectively in some individuals with hypertension. Some agents, such as reserpine, act primarily by inhibiting the presynaptic synthesis of norepinephrine. Other agents (guanadrel, guanethidine) replace norepinephrine in the presynaptic terminal, thus creating a false neurotransmitter. In either case, loss of norepinephrine from the presynaptic terminal decreases the excitation of the heart and peripheral vasculature, resulting in decreased blood pressure.

SPECIFIC AGENTS

Drugs that inhibit the presynaptic synthesis and storage of norepinephrine are discussed in Chapter 20. The drugs in this category used to treat hypertension are listed in Table 21–4. These drugs are often used in conjunction with other agents in the stepped-care approach to hypertension (see "Stepped-Care Approach to Hypertension").

ADVERSE EFFECTS

Orthostatic hypotension is sometimes a problem with these agents. Other bothersome side effects include gastrointestinal disturbances such as nausea, vomiting, and diarrhea.

Centrally Acting Agents

MECHANISM OF ACTION AND RATIONALE FOR USE

Several drugs currently available seem to inhibit sympathetic discharge from the brainstem. These agents act like alpha-2 agonists; that is, they appear to directly stimulate alpha-2 receptors located in the CNS. As discussed in Chapter 20, activation of these central alpha-2 receptors results in a decrease in sympathetic outflow.[64,65,80,101] Consequently, centrally acting drugs offer a rather unique approach to hypertension because these drugs limit sympathetic activity at the source (brainstem vasomotor center) rather than at the periphery (cardiovascular neuroeffector junction).

SPECIFIC AGENTS

The primary drugs in this category are clonidine, guanabenz, guanfacine, and methyldopa (see Table 21–4). The first three drugs act directly on the alpha-2 receptor, whereas methyldopa acts as an alpha-2 agonist after being converted in vivo to alpha-methylnorepinephrine.

ADVERSE EFFECTS

At therapeutic doses, these drugs are associated with some troublesome but relatively minor side effects including dry mouth, dizziness, and drowsiness.

Ganglionic Blockers

MECHANISM OF ACTION AND RATIONALE FOR USE

Drugs that block synaptic transmission at autonomic ganglia will dramatically and effectively reduce blood pressure by decreasing systemic sympathetic activity.[96] These agents are essentially nicotinic cholinergic antagonists (see Chapter 18), which block transmission at the junction between presynaptic and postsynaptic neurons in sympathetic and parasympathetic pathways. Because of the effect of these agents on both divisions of the autonomic nervous system, ganglionic blockers are used very sparingly in treating hypertension. Currently, these drugs are used primarily to reduce blood pressure in emergency situations, such as a hypertensive crisis.[13]

SPECIFIC AGENTS

Ganglionic blockers currently used to decrease blood pressure in a hypertensive crisis are listed in Table 21–4.

ADVERSE EFFECTS

As might be expected, ganglionic blockers produce a multitude of side effects because of the inhibition of both sympathetic and parasympathetic responses. Some adverse effects include gastrointestinal discomfort (nausea, constipation), urinary retention, visual disturbances, and orthostatic hypotension. At higher doses, they may even exhibit some neuromuscular blocking activity. These and other side effects may be quite severe in some patients. Fortunately, ganglionic blockers are usually not used for extended periods of time, because the patient is placed on other antihypertensive drugs when the hypertensive crisis is resolved.

·

VASODILATORS

Mechanism of Action and Rationale for Use

Drugs that directly vasodilate the peripheral vasculature will produce an antihypertensive effect by decreasing peripheral vascular resistance.[14,105] Although other drugs such as the alpha blockers may ultimately produce vasodilation by interrupting adrenergic supply to the vasculature, the vasodilators exert an inhibitory effect directly on vascular smooth-muscle cells. Vasodilators are believed to inhibit smooth-muscle contraction by increasing the intracellular production of second messengers such as cyclic guanosine monophosphate (cyclic GMP) (see Chapter 4). Increased amounts of cyclic GMP inhibit the function of the contractile process in the vascular smooth-muscle cell, thus leading to vasodilation.

Specific Agents

The primary vasodilators used in hypertension are hydralazine (Apresoline) and minoxidil (Loniten) (Table 21–5). These drugs are not usually the first medications used in patients with hypertension but tend to be added to the drug regimen if other agents (diuretics, beta blockers) prove inadequate. Other vasodilators include diazoxide (Hyperstat) and nitroprusside (Nipride, Nitropress), but these drugs are usually only given in emergency situations to treat a patient in hypertensive crisis.

TABLE 21–5 Antihypertensive Vasodilators, ACE Inhibitors, and Calcium Channel Blockers

Vasodilators	
Diazoxide (Hyperstat)	Minoxidil (Loniten)
Hydralazine (Apresoline)	Nitroprusside (Nipride, Nitropress)

ACE Inhibitors	
Benazepril (Lotensin)	Lisinopril (Prinivil, Zestril)
Captopril (Capoten)	Quinapril (Accupril)
Enalapril (Vasotec)	Ramipril (Altace)
Fosinopril (Monopril)	

Calcium Channel Blockers	
Diltiazem (Cardizem)	Nicardipine (Cardene)
Felodipine (Plendil)	Nifedipine (Adalat, Procardia)
Isradipine (DynaCirc)	Verapamil (Calan, Isoptin)

Adverse Effects

Although vasodilators are effective in lowering blood pressure, these drugs are associated with a number of adverse effects. Reflex tachycardia often occurs because of baroreflex responses attempting to compensate for the fall in vascular resistance produced by these drugs. This side effect is analogous to the increased heart rate that often occurs when alpha blockers are used to decrease peripheral vascular resistance. Other common reactions include dizziness, postural hypotension, weakness, nausea, fluid retention, and headaches. Minoxidil also increases hair growth on the face, ears, forehead, and other hairy body surfaces. This increased hair growth is often a cause for discontinued use of this drug in women. Some men, however, have applied minoxidil cutaneously to treat baldness, and a topical preparation of this drug (Rogaine) is marketed as a potential hair-growth stimulant.

ANGIOTENSIN-CONVERTING ENZYME INHIBITORS

Mechanism of Action and Rationale for Use

Captopril (Capoten) and several similar drugs work by inhibiting the enzyme that converts angiotensin I to angiotensin II.[5,18,54,68,93] Hence, these drugs are commonly referred to as angiotensin-converting enzyme (ACE) inhibitors. Angiotensin II is part of the renin-angiotensin system that exists in the body. In the systemic circulation, the renin-angiotensin system acts by a sequence of events that are summarized in Figure 21–2. Renin is an enzyme produced primarily in the kidneys. When blood pressure falls, renin is released from the kidneys into the systemic circulation. Angiotensinogen is a peptide that is produced by the liver and circulates continually in the bloodstream. When renin contacts angiotensinogen, angiotensinogen is transformed into angiotensin I. The circulating angiotensin I is then transformed by angiotensin-converting enzyme into angiotensin II. The converting enzyme is located in the vasculature of many tissues, especially the lung. Angiotensin II is an extremely potent vasoconstrictor. Consequently, the fall in blood pressure that activated the renin-angiotensin system is rectified by the increase in vascular resistance caused by angiotensin II.

The sequence of events just described illustrates the role of the renin-angiotensin system in normal blood pressure regulation. Exactly what goes wrong with this system in patients with essential hypertension is not fully understood. Some of these patients display increased levels of circulating renin, hence their classification as having high-renin hypertension. Why renin production is elevated in these patients, however, is often unclear. ACE inhibitors may also help decrease blood pressure in patients who do not have a substantial increase in circulating renin, suggesting that the renin-angiotensin system may affect blood pressure in more ways than just through angiotensin II–mediated vasoconstriction. For instance, a complete, functioning renin-angiotensin system has been identified within the brain[31,42] and in the heart and vascular walls.[99] This suggests that some of the hypertensive effects of this system may be mediated through CNS mechanisms or by changes directly in the vascular tissues.

Regardless of where ACE inhibitors ultimately exert their effect, these drugs are gaining acceptance as antihypertensive agents either when used alone or in conjunction with other drugs.[41,51] In fact, ACE inhibitors appear to have several advantages

FIGURE 21–2. The renin-angiotensin system and the pressor effect of angiotensin II.

over other antihypertensives, such as having a lower incidence of cardiovascular side effects. ACE inhibitors, for example, are not associated with reflex tachycardia or orthostatic hypotension.[54,81] Studies on animals have also suggested that ACE inhibitors may be especially successful in preventing the adverse structural changes (hypertrophy) seen in the heart and vasculature during prolonged hypertension.[15,69,99] Hence, these drugs continue to gain acceptance and popularity in the treatment of various stages of hypertension.

Specific Agents

ACE inhibitors used to treat hypertension are listed in Table 21–5. These drugs have been shown to be effective in many cases of mild-to-moderate essential hypertension, and they may be used alone or in combination with beta blockers or diuretics.

Adverse Effects

ACE inhibitors are generally well tolerated in most patients. Some individuals may experience an allergic reaction as evidenced by skin rash. This reaction usually disappears when the dosage is reduced or when administration is discontinued. Other problems (gastrointestinal discomfort, dizziness, chest pain, persistent dry cough) may occur in some patients, but major adverse effects are relatively rare.

CALCIUM CHANNEL BLOCKERS

Drugs that selectively block calcium entry into vascular smooth-muscle cells were originally developed to treat certain forms of angina pectoris and cardiac arrhythmias (Chapters 22 and 23, respectively). Calcium channel blockers are now recognized as being beneficial in the treatment of essential hypertension.[16,52,71,73,74] Calcium appears to play a role in activating the contractile element in smooth muscle much in the same way that calcium initiates actin-myosin interaction in skeletal muscle cells. Drugs that block calcium entry into vascular smooth muscle will inhibit the contractile process, leading to vasodilation and decreased vascular resistance.[39,48,62] Calcium channel blockers also tend to decrease heart rate and myocardial contraction force, and some of their antihypertensive properties may derive from their inhibitory effect on the heart.[48,60,61] Consequently, calcium channel blockers are another useful addition to the antihypertensive arsenal.[73,91]

Specific Agents

The primary calcium channel blockers used to treat hypertension are listed in Table 21–5. These agents have all been shown to be effective in treating hypertension, but whether one of these drugs has any distinct clinical advantages over the others is uncertain. The pharmacology of these drugs is discussed in more detail in Chapter 22.

Adverse Effects

These drugs may cause excessive vasodilation as evidenced by swelling in the feet and ankles, and some patients may also experience orthostatic hypotension. Abnormalities in heart rate (too fast, too slow, irregular) may also occur, and reflex tachycardia, caused by excessive peripheral vasodilation, has been noted with nifedipine. Other bothersome side effects include dizziness, headache, and nausea.

STEPPED-CARE APPROACH TO HYPERTENSION

In many hypertensive patients, more than one type of drug must be given to successfully control blood pressure. In general, the more severe the hypertension, the greater the need for a combination of several agents. To provide some type of rationale for effective drug use, a stepped-care approach is often implemented. The object of a stepped-care approach is to begin drug therapy with certain types of drugs and then, if additional drugs are needed, to follow a logical progression in each patient. One type of stepped-care system is outlined in Table 21–6. Typically, drug therapy is initiated with either a thiazide diuretic, a beta blocker, an ACE inhibitor, or a calcium channel blocker (step 1). If blood pressure is not adequately controlled, other types of antihypertensive drugs are instituted as outlined in steps 2 through 4 (see Table 21–6).

A stepped-care approach is generally regarded as the most effective way to use different types of antihypertensive drugs.[72] The stepped-care approach is not a set protocol, however, but only acts as a guideline for drug administration. Specific programs

TABLE 21–6 Stepped-Care Approach to Hypertension

STEP 1: In patients with mild hypertension, drug therapy is usually initiated with a single agent (monotherapy) from one of the following classes: a diuretic, a beta blocker, an ACE inhibitor, or a calcium channel blocker.

STEP 2: If a single drug is unsuccessful in reducing blood pressure, a second agent is added. The second drug can be from one of the initial classes not used in step 1, or it can be from a second group that includes the centrally acting agents (clonidine, guanabenz), presynaptic adrenergic inhibitors (reserpine, guanethidine), alpha-1 blockers (prazosin, doxazosin), and vasodilators (hydralazine, minoxidil).

STEP 3: A third agent is added, usually from one of the classes listed in step 2 that has not already been used. Three different agents from three different classes are often administered concurrently in this step.

STEP 4: A fourth drug is added from still another class.

can (and should) be tailored to individual patients by substituting various drugs at each step.[51,67,88]

NONPHARMACOLOGIC TREATMENT OF HYPERTENSION

Although several effective and relatively safe drugs exist for treating hypertension, the use of nondrug methods in decreasing blood pressure should not be overlooked,[3,55,58,70,92] especially in cases of mild or borderline hypertension.[47,58] Certain dietary modifications such as sodium restriction, low-fat diets, and diets high in certain fish oils have been helpful in some patients.[10,75] Decreasing the use of alcohol and tobacco may also help lower blood pressure. Generally, a decrease in body weight will produce an antihypertensive effect.[23,66,84] Regular exercise may help decrease blood pressure by decreasing body weight or by mechanisms unrelated to weight loss.[4] Many forms of behavior modification and stress management techniques have also been suggested as nonpharmacologic methods of blood pressure control.

Considerable debate exists as to whether or not mild hypertension should be treated initially with drugs, or if a trial with one or more nonpharmacologic techniques should be employed first.[3,17,35,45,58] This decision must be made on an individual basis with consideration given to the patient's lifestyle and chance of compliance with a nondrug approach. There is ample evidence, however, that optimal results are obtained when lifestyle changes are combined with antihypertensive drug therapy.[30,66,75] Hence, changes in lifestyle and behavior should be encouraged in all hypertensive patients, regardless of whether drug therapy is initiated. Patients should be encouraged to quit smoking, lose weight, manage stress, and modify their diet, even if blood pressure is reduced pharmacologically.

SPECIAL CONCERNS IN REHABILITATION PATIENTS

Considering the prevalence of hypertension, therapists will undoubtedly work with many patients taking blood pressure medications. These drugs produce a diverse array of side effects that can influence the rehabilitation session. Primary among these are hypotension and orthostatic hypotension. Since the major action of these drugs is to lower blood pressure, physical therapists and occupational therapists should be cautious when their patients change posture suddenly or engage in other activities that may lower blood pressure.

Activities that produce widespread vasodilation must be avoided or used very cautiously, especially if vasodilating drugs are used. Systemically applied heat (whirlpool, Hubbard tank), for instance, may cause blood pressure to fall precipitously if alpha blockers, calcium channel blockers, or direct-acting vasodilators are being administered. Similarly, exercise may cause vasodilation in skeletal musculature, which may potentiate the peripheral vasodilation induced by these antihypertensive drugs. Also, if beta blockers are given, exercise tolerance may also be impaired somewhat since the myocardial response to sympathetic stimulation will be blunted.

Aside from being aware of the side effects of antihypertensive drugs, therapists may also play an important role in encouraging patient compliance in dealing with high blood pressure. Although drug therapy can control blood pressure in many individuals, patients are often forgetful or hesitant about taking their medications, largely because hypertension is usually asymptomatic until the late stages of this disease. The patient will probably feel fine even when the drug is not taken, or the patient may actually avoid taking the drug because of some bothersome side effect (i.e., the patient may actually feel better without the drug). The idea that hypertension is a silent killer must be continually reinforced in some patients. Through their close contact with the patient, rehabilitation specialists are often in a good position to remind the patient of the consequences of noncompliance. Also, therapists can help suggest and supervise nonpharmacologic methods of lowering blood pressure (e.g., stress management, relaxation techniques, exercise programs). Physical therapists and occupational therapists can play a valuable role in helping patients realize the importance of long-term pharmacologic and nonpharmacologic management of hypertension.

CASE STUDY

HYPERTENSION

Brief History. H.C. is a 55-year-old man who works as an attorney for a large corporation. He is consistently faced with a rather demanding work schedule, often working 12- to 14-hour days, 6 days each week. In addition, he is 25 to 30 pounds overweight and is a habitual cigarette smoker. He has a long history of high blood pressure, which has been managed fairly successfully over the past 15 years through the use of different drugs. Currently, H.C. is in step 3 of the stepped-care approach to hypertensive therapy, and three drugs are being administered to control his blood pressure. He is receiving a diuretic (furosemide, 100 mg/day), a cardioselective beta blocker (metoprolol, 200 mg/day), and a vasodilator (minoxidil, 20 mg/day).

While rushing to a business luncheon, H.C. was hit by an automobile as he was crossing the street. He was admitted to the hospital, where radiologic examination revealed a fracture of the right pelvis. Further examination did not reveal any other significant internal injuries. The pelvic fracture appeared stable at the time of admission, and internal fixation was not required. H.C. remained in the hospital and was placed on bed rest. Two days after admission, a physical therapist was called in to consult on this case. The physical therapist suggested a progressive ambulation program using the facility's therapeutic pool. The buoyancy provided by the pool would allow a gradual increase in weight bearing while protecting the fracture site.

Problem/Influence of Medication. To guard against patient hypothermia, the water temperature in the therapeutic pool was routinely maintained at 95°F. The therapist was concerned that immersing the patient in the pool would cause excessive peripheral vasodilation. Because the patient was taking a vasodilating drug (minoxidil), the additive effect of the warm pool and vasodilating agent might cause profound hypotension because of a dramatic decrease in total peripheral resistance. Also, because this patient was taking a cardioselective beta blocker (metoprolol), his heart would not be able to sufficiently increase cardiac output to offset the decreased peripheral resistance.

Decision/Solution. When the patient was in the pool, the therapist monitored heart rate and blood pressure at frequent, regular intervals. Blood pressure did decrease when the patient was ambulating in the pool, but not to a point of concern because the patient's active leg muscle contractions facilitated venous return, and the buoyancy of the water decreased the effects of gravity on venous pooling in the lower extremities. In fact, only at the end of the rehabilitation session, when the patient came out of the pool, did hypotension became a potential problem. The patient was still experiencing peripheral vasodilation because of the residual effects of the warm water, but he no longer had the advantage of active muscle contractions and water buoyancy to help maintain his blood pressure. To prevent a hypotensive episode at the end of the session, the therapist placed the patient supine on a stretcher as soon as he came out of the water. Also, the patient's legs were quickly toweled dry, and vascular support stockings were placed on the patient's legs as soon as possible. These precautions allowed the patient to progress rapidly through his rehabilitation without any adverse incidents. When he was eventually discharged from the hospital, he was ambulating with crutches, with partial weight bearing on the side of the pelvic fracture.

SUMMARY

Hypertension is a common disease marked by a sustained increase in blood pressure. If untreated, hypertension leads to serious problems such as stroke, renal failure, and problems in several other physiologic systems. Although the cause of hypertension is discernible in a small percentage of patients, the majority of hypertensive individuals are classified as having essential hypertension, which means that the cause of their elevated blood pressure is unknown. Fortunately, several types of drugs are currently available to adequately control blood pressure in essential hypertension. Drugs such as diuretics, sympatholytics (alpha blockers, beta blockers, etc.), vasodilators, angiotensin-converting enzyme inhibitors, and calcium channel blockers have all been used in treating hypertension. These agents are usually prescribed according to a stepped-care protocol, where therapy is initiated with one drug, and subsequent agents are added as required. Rehabilitation specialists should be aware of the potential side effects of these drugs. Physical and occupational therapists assume an important role in making patients aware of the sequelae of hypertension, and therapists should actively encourage patients to comply with pharmacologic and nonpharmacologic methods of lowering blood pressure.

REFERENCES

1. Abboud, FM: The sympathetic nervous system in hypertension: State of the art review. Hypertension 4(suppl II):208, 1982.
2. Alderman, MH: Mild hypertension: New light on an old controversy. Am J Med 69:653, 1980.
3. Andrews, G, et al: Hypertension: Comparison of drug and non-drug treatments. Br Med J 284:1523, 1982.
4. Arroll, B and Beaglehole, R: Does physical activity lower blood pressure: A critical review of the clinical trials. J Clin Epidemiol 45:439, 1992.
5. Bauer, JH: Role of angiotensin converting enzyme inhibitors in essential and renal hypertension. Am J Med 77(suppl 2a):43, 1984.
6. Bennet, WM, et al: Do diuretics have antihypertensive properties independent of natriuresis? Clin Pharmacol Ther 22:499, 1977.
7. Beyer, KH and Peuler, J: Hypertension: Perspectives. Pharmacol Rev 34:287, 1982.
8. Bohr, DF: What makes the pressure go up? A hypothesis. Hypertension 3(suppl II):160, 1981.
9. Bohr, DF and Webb, RC: Vascular smooth muscle function and its changes in hypertension. Am J Med 77(suppl 4a):3, 1984.
10. Bonaa, KH, et al: Effect of eicosapentaenoic and docosahexaenoic acids on blood pressure in hypertension. N Engl J Med 322:795, 1990.
11. Brody, MJ: New developments in our knowledge of blood pressure regulation. Fed Proc 40:2257, 1981.
12. Buhler, FR, et al: Elevated adrenaline and increased alpha-adrenoceptor mediated vasoconstriction in essential hypertension. J Cardiovasc Pharm 4(suppl I):S134, 1982.
13. Calhoun, DA and Oparil, S: Current concepts: Treatment of hypertensive crisis. N Engl J Med 323:1177, 1990.
14. Campese, VM: Minoxidil: A review of its pharmacological properties and therapeutic use. Drugs 22:257, 1981.
15. Chevalier, B, et al: Molecular basis for regression of cardiac hypertrophy. Am J Cardiol 73:10c, 1994.
16. Chobanian, AV (ed): Symposium: Role of calcium channel blockers in the management of hypertension. Am J Med 81(suppl 6a):1, 1986.
17. Chobanian, AV: Treatment of mild hypertension: The debate intensifies. J Cardiovasc Med 8:883, 1983.
18. Chobanian, AV and Warren, JV (eds): Symposium: Update on the clinical utility of converting enzyme inhibitors in cardiovascular disease. Am J Med 81(suppl 4c):1, 1986.
19. Ciccone, CD and Zambraski, EJ: Effects of acute renal denervation on kidney function in deoxycorticosterone acetate-hypertensive swine. Hypertension 8:925, 1986.
20. Ciccone, CD and Zambraski, EJ: Effects of phenoxybenzamine, metoprolol, captopril, and meclofenamate on cardiovascular function in deoxycorticosterone acetate hypertensive Yucatan miniature swine. Can J Physiol Pharmacol 61:149, 1983.
21. Cressman, MD and Gifford, RW: Labetalol: The first combined alpha and beta blocker. J Cardiovasc Med 9:593, 1984.
22. Cruickshank, JM: The clinical importance of cardioselectivity and lipophilicity in beta blockers. Am Heart J 100:160, 1980.
23. Cutler, J: The effects of nonpharmacologic interventions on blood pressure of persons with high normal levels: Results of the trials of hypertension prevention, phase I. JAMA 267:1213, 1992.
24. Davey, MJ: The pharmacological basis for the use of alpha$_1$-adrenoceptor antagonists in the treatment of essential hypertension. Br J Clin Pharmacol 21(suppl 1):5S, 1986.
25. DeBono, G, et al: Acebutolol: 10 years of experience. Am Heart J 109:1211, 1985.
26. Dickinson, CJ: Neurogenic hypertension revisited. Clin Sci 60:471, 1981.
27. Doyle, AE and Donnan, GA: Stroke as a clinical problem in hypertension. J Cardiovasc Pharmacol 15(suppl 1):S34, 1990.
28. Dustan, HP: Physiologic regulation of arterial pressure: An overview. Hypertension 4:62, 1982.
29. Epstein, M and Oster, JR: Hypertension: A Practical Approach. WB Saunders, Philadelphia, 1984.
30. Fagerberg, B, et al: Cardiovascular effects of weight reduction versus antihypertensive drug treatment: A comparative, randomized, 1-year study of obese men with mild hypertension. J Hypertension 9:431, 1991.
31. Ferrario, CM: The renin-angiotensin system: Importance in physiology and pathology. J Cardiovasc Pharmacol 15(suppl 3):S1, 1990.
32. Fletcher, AE and Bulpitt, CJ: Current concepts: How far should blood pressure be lowered? N Engl J Med 326:251, 1992.

33. Folkow, B: Physiologic aspects of primary hypertension. Physiol Rev 62:347, 1982.
34. Freis, ED: The cardiovascular risks of thiazide diuretics. Clin Pharmacol Ther 39:239, 1986.
35. Freis, ED: Should mild hypertension be treated? N Engl J Med 307:306, 1982.
36. Friedman, GD, et al: Precursors of essential hypertension: Body weight, alcohol and salt use, and parental history of hypertension. Prev Med 17:387, 1988.
37. Frishman, WH: Pindolol: A new beta-adrenoceptor antagonist with partial agonist activity. N Engl J Med 308:940, 1983.
38. Frishman, WH: Beta-adrenoceptor antagonists: New drugs and new indications. N Engl J Med 305:500, 1981.
39. Frishman, WH, Landau, A, and Cretkovic, A: Combination drug therapy with calcium-channel blockers in the treatment of systemic hypertension. J Clin Pharmacol 33:752, 1993.
40. Frohlich, ED: Vasodilating beta-blockers: Systemic and regional hemodynamic effects. Am Heart J 121:1012, 1991.
41. Frohlich, ED, Cooper, RA, and Lewis, EJ: Review of the overall experience of captopril in hypertension. Arch Intern Med 144:1441, 1984.
42. Ganong, WF: The brain renin-angiotensin system. Annu Rev Physiol 46:17, 1984.
43. Gerber, JG and Nies, AS: Beta-adrenergic blocking drugs. Annu Rev Med 36:145, 1985.
44. Gifford, RW: The role of diuretics in the treatment of hypertension. Am J Med 77(suppl 4a):102, 1984.
45. Gifford, RW, et al: The dilemma of "mild" hypertension: Another viewpoint of treatment. JAMA 250:3171, 1983.
46. Gillis, RA, Gatti, PJ, and Quest, JA: Mechanism of the antihypertensive effect of alpha$_2$-antagonists. J Cardiovasc Pharmacol 7(suppl 8):S38, 1985.
47. Gillum, RF, et al: Nonpharmacologic therapy of hypertension: The independent effects of weight reduction and sodium restriction in overweight borderline hypertensive patients. Am Heart J 105:128, 1983.
48. Hansson, L: Calcium antagonists: An overview. Am Heart J 122:308, 1991.
49. Hansson, L: Review of state-of-the-art beta-blocker therapy. Am J Cardiol 67:43B, 1991.
50. Hebert, PR, et al: Recent evidence on drug therapy of mild to moderate hypertension and decreased risk of coronary heart disease. Arch Intern Med 153:578, 1993.
51. Hollenberg, NK: Treatment of hypertension: The place of angiotensin converting enzyme inhibitors in the nineties. J Cardiovasc Pharmacol 20(suppl 10):S29, 1992.
52. Hollenberg, NK (ed): Symposium: Calcium channel blockers: New insights into their role in the management of hypertension. Am J Med 82(suppl 3b):1, 1987.
53. Horky, K: Alpha$_1$-blockade in the management of hypertension. J Clin Pharmacol 33:874, 1993.
54. Johnston, CI, Arnolda, L, and Hiwatari, M: Angiotensin-converting enzyme inhibitors in the treatment of hypertension. Drugs 27:271, 1984.
55. Joint National Committee on Detection, Evaluation, and Treatment of High Blood Pressure: The 1984 report. Arch Intern Med 144:1045, 1984.
56. Julius, S: Autonomic nervous system dysregulation in human hypertension. Am J Cardiol 67:3B, 1991.
57. Kaplan, NM: Use of non-drug therapy in treating hypertension. Am J Med 77(suppl 4a):96, 1984.
58. Kaplan, NM: New choices for the initial drug therapy of hypertension. Am J Cardiol 51:1786, 1983.
59. Katholi, RE: Renal nerves in the pathogenesis of hypertension in experimental animals and humans. Am J Physiol 245:F1, 1983.
60. Katz, AM, et al: Cellular actions and pharmacology of the calcium channel blocking drugs. Am J Med 79(suppl 4a):2, 1985.
61. Kenny, J: Calcium channel blocking agents and the heart. Br Med J 291:1150, 1985.
62. Klaus, D: The role of calcium antagonists in the treatment of hypertension. J Cardiovasc Pharmacol 20(suppl 6):S5, 1992.
63. Kokko, JP: Site and mechanism of action of diuretics. Am J Med 77(suppl 4a):11, 1984.
64. Koss, MC: Review article: Pupillary dilation as an index of central nervous system alpha-2 adrenoceptor activation. J Pharmacol Methods 15:1, 1986.
65. Langer, SZ, Cavero, I, and Massingham, R: Recent developments in noradrenergic neurotransmission and its relevance to the mechanism of action of certain antihypertensive agents. Hypertension 2:372, 1980.
66. Langford, HG, et al: Effect of drug and diet treatment of mild hypertension on diastolic blood pressure. Hypertension 17:210, 1991.
67. Laragh, JH: Modification of stepped care approach to antihypertensive therapy. Am J Med 77(suppl 2a):78, 1984.
68. Laragh, JH (ed): Symposium: Converting enzyme inhibition for understanding and management of hypertensive disorders and congestive heart failure. Am J Med 77(suppl 2a):1, 1984.
69. Levy, BI, et al: Long-term effects of angiotensin-converting enzyme inhibitors on the arterial wall of adult spontaneous hypertensive rats. Am J Cardiol 71:8E, 1993.
70. Marley, J, Davis, N, and Joy, M: Is the non-pharmacological treatment of hypertension neglected? J Royal Soc Med 84:540, 1991.
71. Massie, BM, et al: Calcium channel blockers as antihypertensive agents. Am J Med 77(suppl 4a):135, 1984.

72. Moser, M: Initial treatment of adult patients with essential hypertension: I. Why conventional stepped-care therapy of hypertension is still indicated. Pharmacotherapy 5:189, 1985.
73. Muller, FB, et al: Use of calcium antagonists as monotherapy in the management of hypertension. Am J Med 77(suppl 2b):11, 1984.
74. Murphy, MB, Scriven, AJI, and Dollery, CT: Role of nifedipine in treatment of hypertension. Br Med J 287:257, 1983.
75. Neaton, JD, et al: Treatment of mild hypertension study: Final results. JAMA 270:713, 1993.
76. Oglivie, RI, et al: Report of the Canadian hypertension society consensus conference: Pharmacologic treatment of essential hypertension. Can Med Assoc J 149:575, 1993.
77. Panza, JA, et al: Abnormal endothelium-dependent vascular relaxation in patients with essential hypertension. N Engl J Med 323:22, 1990.
78. Reaven, GM: Treatment of hypertension: Focus on prevention of coronary artery disease. J Clin Endocrinol Metab 76:537, 1993.
79. Robertson, JIS, et al (eds): Symposium: Beta-blockade in the 1980's: Focus on atenolol. Drugs 25(suppl 2):1, 1983.
80. Sambhi, MP and Villarreal, H: Central alpha-adrenoceptors: Basic mechanisms and clinical applications in cardiovascular disease. Chest 83(suppl):293, 1983.
81. Sassano, P, et al: Antihypertensive effect of enalapril as first-step treatment of mild and moderate uncomplicated essential hypertension. Am J Med 77(suppl 2a):18, 1984.
82. Schachter, M: Drug-induced modification of vascular structure: Effects of antihypertensive drugs. Am Heart J 122:316, 1991.
83. Schirger, A, et al: Pindolol, a new beta-adrenergic blocking agent with intrinsic sympathomimetic activity in the management of mild and moderate hypertension. Mayo Clin Proc 58:315, 1983.
84. Schotte, DE and Stunkard, AJ: The effects of weight reduction on blood pressure in 301 obese patients. Arch Intern Med 150:1701, 1990.
85. Scriabine, A: Beta-adrenoceptor blocking drugs in hypertension. Annu Rev Pharmacol Toxicol 19:269, 1979.
86. Shanks, RG: Clinical pharmacology of vasodilating beta-blocking drugs. Am Heart J 121:1006, 1991.
87. Sonnenblick, M, Friedlander Y, and Rosin, AJ: Diuretic-induced severe hyponatremia: A review and analysis of 129 reported patients. Chest 103:601, 1993.
88. Stokes, GS: Optimal drug treatment in hypertension. J Cardiovasc Pharmacol 16(suppl 7):S105, 1990.
89. Symposium (various authors): Management of coronary heart disease risk factors in hypertensive patients: Clinical experience with doxazosin. Am Heart J 121:245, 1991.
90. Symposium (various authors): Clinical challenges in hypertension: Therapeutic applications of new vasodilating beta-blockers. J Cardiovasc Pharmacol 18(suppl 4):S1, 1991.
91. Symposium (various authors): Expanding the role of calcium antagonists in hypertension. J Cardiovasc Pharmacol 17(suppl 4):S1, 1991.
92. Symposium (various authors): New vistas on nonpharmacological approaches to hypertension. J Cardiovasc Pharmacol 16(suppl 8):S1, 1990.
93. Symposium (various authors): The renin-angiotensin system as a therapeutic target. J Cardiovasc Pharmacol 16(suppl 4):S1, 1990.
94. Symposium (various authors): Clinical applications of alpha$_1$-receptor blockade: Terazosin in the management of hypertension. J Clin Pharmacol 33:866, 1993.
95. Tarazi, RC: Pathophysiology of essential hypertension: Role of the autonomic nervous system. Am J Med 75(suppl 4a):2, 1983.
96. Taylor, P: Agents acting at the neuromuscular junction and autonomic ganglia. In Gilman, AG, et al (eds): The Pharmacological Basis of Therapeutics, ed 8. Pergamon Press, New York, 1990.
97. Taylor, SH and Grimm, RH: New developments in the role of alpha$_1$-adrenergic receptors in cardiovascular disease. Am Heart J 119:655, 1990.
98. Turner, P: Which ancillary properties of beta-adrenoceptor blocking drugs influence their therapeutic and adverse effects: A review. J Royal Soc Med 84:672, 1991.
99. Unger, TU and Gohlke, P: Tissue renin-angiotensin systems in the heart and vasculature: Possible involvement in the cardiovascular actions of converting enzyme inhibitors. Am J Cardiol 65:31, 1990.
100. Wallin, BG, Delius, W, and Hagbarth, KE: Comparison of sympathetic activity in normo- and hypertensive subjects. Circ Res 33:9, 1973.
101. Weber, MA and Drayer, JIM: Central and peripheral blockade of the sympathetic nervous system. Am J Med 77(suppl 4a):110, 1984.
102. Westfall, TC and Meldrum, MJ: Alterations in the release of norepinephrine at the vascular neuroeffector junction in hypertension. Annu Rev Pharmacol Toxicol 25:621, 1985.
103. Wood, AJ: Pharmacologic differences between beta blockers. Am Heart J 108:1070, 1984.
104. Zambraski, EJ, Ciccone, CD, and Izzo, JL: The role of the sympathetic nervous system in 2-kidney DOCA-hypertensive Yucatan miniature swine. Clin Exp Hypertens [A] 8:411, 1986.
105. Zsoter, TT: Vasodilators. Can Med Assoc J 129:424, 1983.

CHAPTER 22

Treatment of Angina Pectoris

Angina pectoris is pain in the chest region resulting from myocardial ischemia. Attacks of angina pectoris begin suddenly and are often described as a sensation of intense compression and tightness in the retrosternal region, with pain sometimes radiating to the jaw or left arm. In many patients, episodes of angina pectoris are precipitated by physical exertion. Some forms of angina, however, may occur spontaneously even when the patient is at rest or asleep.

The basic problem in angina pectoris is that the supply of oxygen to the heart is insufficient to meet myocardial demands at a given point in time, which results in an imbalance between myocardial oxygen supply and demand (Fig. 22-1).[11] This imbalance leads to myocardial ischemia, which results in several metabolic, electrophysiologic, and contractile changes in the heart. The painful symptoms inherent to angina pectoris seem to result from the accumulation of metabolic by-products such as lactic acid. Presumably, these metabolic by-products act as nociceptive substances and trigger the painful compressive sensations characteristic of angina pectoris.

Although angina pectoris is believed to be caused by the buildup of lactic acid and other metabolites, the exact mechanisms responsible for mediating anginal pain remain unknown. During an anginal attack, whether metabolites mediate painful sensations via specific nociceptors, mechanoreceptors, or chemoreceptors is unclear.[33] Also, the emotional state of the patient and other factors that influence central pain perception play an obvious role in angina pectoris. In fact, the majority of anginal attacks may be silent in many patients, and myocardial ischemia may frequently occur without producing any symptoms.[12,17,41,46] Clearly, there is much information regarding the nature of angina pectoris still remaining to be clarified.

Considering the prevalence of ischemic heart disease in the United States, many patients receiving physical therapy and occupational therapy may suffer from angina pectoris. These patients may be undergoing rehabilitation for a variety of clinical disorders, including, but not limited to, coronary artery disease. This chapter describes the three primary drug groups used to treat angina pectoris, as well as the pharmacologic management of specific forms of angina. Physical therapists and occupational therapists should be aware of the manner in which these drugs work and the ways in which antianginal drugs can influence patient performance in rehabilitation sessions.

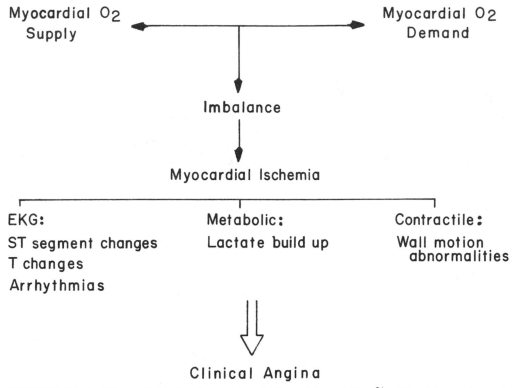

FIGURE 22–1. Myocardial ischemia equation. (Adapted from Miller,[36] p 26, with permission.)

DRUGS USED TO TREAT ANGINA PECTORIS

Drugs used to treat angina pectoris attempt to restore or maintain the balance between myocardial oxygen supply and myocardial oxygen demand. Two drug groups (organic nitrates and beta blockers) exert their effects primarily by decreasing myocardial oxygen demand. A third group (calcium channel blockers) works mainly by increasing myocardial oxygen supply. The primary drug categories used to treat angina and specific agents within each category are presented here.

ORGANIC NITRATES

Mechanism of Action and Rationale for Use

Organic nitrates consist of drugs such as nitroglycerin and isosorbide dinitrate (Table 22–1). The ability of these agents to dilate vascular smooth muscle is well established. Nitrates are actually drug precursors (prodrugs) that become activated when they are converted to nitrous oxide within vascular smooth muscle.[10,20,43] Nitrous oxide causes vasodilation by increasing the production of cyclic guanosine monophosphate (cyclic GMP) within the muscle cell. Cyclic GMP acts as a second messenger that inhibits smooth-muscle contraction, probably by initiating the phosphorylation of specific contractile proteins.[28,65]

TABLE 22–1 Organic Nitrates

Dosage Form	Onset of Action	Duration of Action
Nitroglycerin		
Oral	20–45 min	4–6 hr
Buccal (extended release)	2–3 min	3–5 hr
Sublingual	1–3 min	30–60 min
Ointment	30 min	4–8 hr
Transdermal patches	Within 30 min	8–24 hr
Isosorbide dinitrate		
Oral	15–40 min	4–6 hr
Oral (extended release)	30 min	12 hr
Chewable	2–5 min	1–2 hr
Sublingual	2–5 min	1–2 hr
Erythrityl tetranitrate		
Oral	30 min	Up to 6 hr
Chewable	Within 5 min	2 hr
Buccal	Within 5 min	2 hr
Sublingual	Within 5 min	2–3 hr
Pentaerythritol tetranitrate		
Oral	20–60 min	4–5 hr
Amyl nitrite		
Inhaled	30 sec	3–5 min

For years nitrates were believed to relieve angina attacks by dilating the coronary arteries; that is, they supposedly increased blood flow to the myocardium. We now know, however, that these drugs exert their primary antianginal effects by producing a general vasodilation in the vasculature throughout the body, not just the coronary vessels.[2,44] By producing dilation in the systemic venous system, nitrates decrease the amount of blood returning to the heart (*cardiac preload*). By dilating systemic peripheral arterioles, these drugs decrease the pressure against which the heart must pump (*cardiac afterload*). A decrease in cardiac preload and afterload decreases the amount of work the heart must perform; hence, myocardial oxygen demand decreases.

Consequently, nitroglycerin and other organic nitrates seem to primarily decrease myocardial oxygen demand rather than directly increase oxygen supply. Nitrates can also dilate the coronary arteries to some extent because an increase in coronary artery flow has been documented with these drugs.[9,34] The *primary* way that these drugs relieve angina pectoris, however, is through their ability to decrease cardiac work, thus decreasing myocardial oxygen demand.

Specific Agents

Nitroglycerin (Nitro-Bid, Nitrostat, Nitro-Dur, Many Others). In addition to being used as a powerful explosive, nitroglycerin is perhaps the most well known of the antianginal drugs. The explosive nature of this agent is rendered inactive by diluting it with lactose, alcohol, or propylene glycol. Nitroglycerin is administered for both the prevention and the treatment of anginal attacks and is available in oral, buccal, sublingual, and transdermal forms (see Table 22–1).

Sublingual administration of nitroglycerin is the best method to treat an acute attack of angina. Placed under the tongue, the drug is rapidly absorbed through the oral mucosa into the systemic circulation. Therapeutic effects usually begin within 2 minutes when nitroglycerin is administered sublingually. Sublingual administration also spares the nitroglycerin from the first-pass effect. The drug is able to reach the systemic circulation before first passing through the liver, where it is inactivated (see Chapter 2).

For the prevention of angina, extended-release versions of this drug, which can be taken buccally, that is, between the cheek and gum, have been developed. Oral preparations have also been developed,[18] but this method of administration is limited since nitroglycerin undergoes extensive first-pass degradation in the liver when absorbed directly from the intestines.

For prophylaxis of angina, nitroglycerin can also be administered transdermally via ointment or medicated patches placed on the skin (see Table 22–1). Nitroglycerin-impregnated patches or disks are applied cutaneously like a small bandage, with the drug slowly and continuously absorbed through the skin and into the systemic circulation.[22,48,54] Transdermal administration of nitroglycerin using these patches has been regarded favorably because of the ease and convenience of administration. Evidence exists, however, that the length of the effect of the nitroglycerin from a single patch may be somewhat limited and that patches may have to be changed more than once every 24 hours.[7,48]

Continuous administration of nitroglycerin through transdermal patches can also cause drug tolerance, thus reducing the antianginal effectiveness of this medication.[5,15,40] Tolerance to nitrate drugs is rather short-lived, however, and normal responses to nitrate drugs can be restored within only a few hours after withdrawing these agents.[29] Consequently, patients may benefit from having intervals during each day when they do not wear their patches. Daily administration, for example, might be optimized by wearing the patch for 12 to 14 hours followed by a 10- to 12-hour nitrate-free interval.[53] This method of intermittent nitroglycerin administration may provide beneficial effects with less chance of developing drug tolerance.[1,42]

Nitroglycerin ointment is another way to provide continuous transdermal administration of this drug.[49] The ointment is applied directly to the skin on the patient's chest or back, in much the same way as any topical ointment or skin cream. Although somewhat messy and inconvenient, administration of nitroglycerin via an ointment probably results in higher plasma levels of the drug as well as more prolonged effects than with medicated patches.[14] This method is not as popular as transdermal patches, however, because patches are much more convenient and easier to apply. Likewise, tolerance may occur if nitroglycerin is applied continually through topical ointments.

Isosorbide Dinitrate. Like nitroglycerin, isosorbide dinitrate is used for the treatment of acute episodes of angina as well as for the prevention of the onset of anginal attacks. The antianginal and hemodynamic effects last longer with isosorbide, however, so this drug is often classified as a long-acting nitrate. For acute attacks, isosorbide is administered sublingually, buccally, or by chewable tablets (see Table 22–1). For prevention of angina, this drug is usually given by oral tablets.

Erythrityl Tetranitrate. Erythrityl tetranitrate is also classified as a long-acting nitrate. When administered sublingually, this drug requires somewhat longer to take action, but the effects tend to last longer than with sublingually administered nitroglycerin. Consequently, erythrityl tetranitrate is used primarily for the prevention rather than the acute treatment of anginal attacks. This drug can be administered orally, sublingually, buccally, or by chewable tablets (see Table 22–1).

Pentaerythritol Tetranitrate (Peritrate). Pentaerythritol tetranitrate is a long-acting nitrate similar in function to erythrityl tetranitrate, is used primarily in the prevention of anginal attacks, and is administered orally.

Amyl Nitrite. This drug is supplied in small ampules that can be broken open so that the drug is inhaled during acute anginal attacks. Absorption of the drug through the nasal membranes causes peripheral vasodilation and decreased cardiac preload and afterload. Clinical use of inhaled amyl nitrite is very limited, however, and this type of antianginal treatment has generally been replaced by safer and more convenient methods of nitrate administration (e.g., nitroglycerin patches).

Adverse Side Effects of Nitrates

The primary adverse effects associated with the organic nitrates are headache, dizziness, and orthostatic hypotension.[2] These effects are related to the ability of these drugs to dilate peripheral blood vessels and decrease peripheral resistance. Nausea may also be a problem in some patients. As indicated earlier, tolerance to the beneficial effects of nitrates can occur during the continuous administration of these drugs, but providing daily nitrate-free intervals should prevent this problem.

BETA-ADRENERGIC BLOCKERS

Mechanism of Action and Rationale for Use

By antagonizing beta-1 receptors on the myocardium, beta blockers tend to decrease heart rate and the force of myocardial contraction,[19,55] thus producing an obvious decrease in the work the heart must perform and decreasing myocardial oxygen demand. Beta blockers help maintain an appropriate balance between myocardial oxygen supply and demand by preventing an increase in myocardial oxygen demand.

Consequently, beta blockers are given to certain patients with angina to limit the oxygen demands of the heart.[19,24,45] This prophylactic administration prevents the onset of an anginal attack. The use of beta blockers in specific forms of angina is reviewed later in this chapter when the various types of angina are discussed.

Specific Agents

Individual beta blockers were discussed in Chapter 20. Beta blockers effective in treating angina pectoris are listed in Table 22–2. Various beta blockers seem to display a fairly equal effect in treating angina pectoris.[61] The choice of which beta blocker will provide optimal results in any particular individual depends primarily on the chemical characteristics and side effects of the drug relative to the particular needs of each patient.[62]

TABLE 22-2 Beta Blockers Used to Treat Angina Pectoris

Generic Name	Trade Name	Usual Oral Dose
Acebutolol	Sectral	200–600 mg 2 times a day
Atenolol	Tenormin	50–100 mg once a day
Carteolol	Cartrol	2.5–10.0 mg once a day
Labetalol	Normodyne, Trandate	200–400 mg 2 times a day
Metoprolol	Lopressor	50–200 mg 2 times a day
Nadolol	Corgard	40–240 mg once a day
Penbutolol	Levatol	20 mg once a day
Pindolol	Visken	5–20 mg 2 times a day
Propranolol	Inderal	10–120 mg 2–4 times a day
Sotalol	Betapace	80–160 mg 2 times a day
Timolol	Blocadren	10–30 mg 2 times a day

Adverse Side Effects

Beta blockers that bind to both beta-1 and beta-2 receptors (nonselective agents, see Table 20–2) may induce bronchoconstriction in patients with asthma or similar respiratory problems. These patients should be given one of the more cardioselective beta antagonists such as atenolol or metoprolol. Beta blockers may also produce excessive cardiac depression in individuals with certain types of cardiac disease. The beta blockers are generally well tolerated in most patients, however, with major problems being fairly infrequent.

CALCIUM CHANNEL BLOCKERS

Mechanism of Action and Rationale for Use

These drugs block the entry of calcium into vascular smooth muscle.[8,23,56] In vascular smooth muscle, calcium ions facilitate contraction by initiating actin-myosin interaction.[4] Calcium channel blockers decrease the entry of calcium into vascular smooth-muscle cells, thus causing relaxation and vasodilation. By blocking calcium entry into coronary artery smooth muscle, these drugs mediate coronary vasodilation, with a subsequent increase in the supply of oxygen to the myocardium. Consequently, a primary role of calcium channel blockers in angina pectoris is to directly increase coronary blood flow, thus increasing myocardial oxygen supply.[56,58,59]

Calcium channel blockers also cause some degree of systemic vasodilation, and some of their antianginal effects may be related to a decrease in myocardial oxygen demand caused by a decrease in cardiac preload and afterload; that is, they may exert some of their beneficial effects in a manner similar to that of organic nitrates.[23] Also, calcium channel blockers limit the entry of calcium into cardiac striated cells, thus decreasing myocardial contractility and oxygen demand. The *primary* beneficial effects of these drugs in angina pectoris, however, are related to their ability to dilate the coronary arteries and peripheral vasculature. Calcium channel blockers can also affect myocardial excitability by altering the conduction of electrical activity throughout the myocardium.[4,58] This effect seems to be more important when these drugs are used to treat cardiac arrhythmias (see Chapter 23).

The calcium channel blockers currently used to treat angina pectoris are listed in Table 22–3. Although the chemistry and exact mechanism of action of each drug are somewhat distinct, all of these agents exert their effects by limiting calcium entry into specific cardiovascular tissues. Individual agents are discussed here.

Specific Agents

Bepridil (Bepadin, Vascor). Bepridil is a nonselective calcium channel blocker that inhibits calcium influx into vascular smooth muscle and cardiac striated muscle. It can vasodilate coronary and peripheral vessels, hence its use in angina pectoris. Bepridil also decreases heart rate (negative chronotropic effect) and cardiac contractility (negative inotropic effect) through an inhibitory effect on the myocardium.

Diltiazem (Cardizem). Like the other calcium channel blockers, diltiazem is able to vasodilate the coronary arteries and the peripheral vasculature. Diltiazem also produces some depression of electrical conduction in the sinoatrial and artrioventricular nodes, an effect that may cause slight bradycardia. Adverse side effects appear to occur somewhat less frequently with diltiazem as compared to other antianginal calcium channel blockers.[47]

Nifedipine (Procardia) and Other Dihydropyridines. Nifedipine and similar drugs are members of the dihydropyridine class of calcium channel blockers. This class is distinguished by drugs with an *-ipine* suffix, including felodipine (Plendil), isradipine (DynaCirc), and nicardipine (Cardene). These drugs are relatively selective for vascular smooth muscle as compared to cardiac striated muscle, and they vasodilate the coronary arteries and peripheral vasculature without exerting any major effects on cardiac excitability or contractility.[59]

Verapamil (Calan, Isoptin). Verapamil has been used to treat angina because of its ability to vasodilate the coronary vessels. Verapamil, however, seems to be only moderately effective compared to the other antianginal drugs.[25] Verapamil exerts considerable effects on myocardial excitability and is probably more valuable in its ability to control cardiac arrhythmias (see Chapter 23).[56]

Adverse Side Effects

The primary problems associated with the calcium channel blockers are related to the peripheral vasodilation produced by these agents. Headache, flushing or feelings

TABLE 22–3 Calcium Channel Blockers

Generic Name	Trade Name	Usual Oral Dose
Bepridil	Bepadin, Vascor	200–300 mg once a day
Diltiazem	Cardizem	60–90 mg 3 or 4 times a day
Felodipine	Plendil	5–10 mg once a day
Isradipine	DynaCirc	2.5–10 mg 2 times a day
Nicardipine	Cardene	20 mg 3 times a day
Nifedipine	Procardia	10–30 mg 3 or 4 times a day
Verapamil	Calan, Isoptin	80–160 mg 3 times a day

of warmth, and dizziness may occur in some patients. Peripheral edema, as evidenced by swelling in the feet and legs, may also occur, and nausea may be fairly common. Nonselective calcium channel blockers that affect the myocardium (e.g., bepridil, verapamil) can cause disturbances in cardiac rhythm. Finally, animal studies suggest that long-term use of calcium channel blockers may lead to significant levels of skeletal muscle fatigue and weakness.[21]

TREATMENT OF SPECIFIC TYPES OF ANGINA PECTORIS

All forms of angina pectoris are not the same. Traditionally, angina has been subclassified according to the factors that precipitate the angina and the pathophysiologic mechanisms responsible for producing myocardial ischemia.[11] Table 22–4 summarizes the different types of angina and the drugs used in each type. The major forms of angina and the primary drugs used to treat each type are also discussed here.

Stable Angina

Stable angina is the most common form of ischemic heart disease.[50] The primary problem in stable angina is that myocardial oxygen demand greatly exceeds oxygen supply. Stable angina is also frequently referred to as effort or exertional angina since attacks are usually precipitated by a certain level of physical exertion. If the patient exercises beyond a certain level of his or her capacity, the coronary arteries are unable to deliver the oxygen needed to sustain that level of myocardial function, and an anginal episode occurs. The inability of the coronary arteries to adequately deliver oxygen in stable angina is usually caused by some degree of permanent coronary artery occlusion (e.g., coronary artery atherosclerosis or stenosis).

Because stable angina is caused primarily by an increase in myocardial oxygen demand, treatment of this form of angina has consisted mainly of beta blockers and organic nitrates. Beta blockers are administered prophylactically to decrease the workload of the heart, thus limiting myocardial oxygen requirements.[55] Nitrates can also be given as a preventive measure to blunt myocardial oxygen needs, and nitroglycerin can be administered transdermally through patches or ointments, or long-acting ni-

TABLE 22–4 Types of Angina Pectoris

Classification	Cause	Drug Therapy
Stable angina	Myocardial oxygen demand exceeds oxygen supply; usually brought on by physical exertion	Usually treated with either a beta blocker or long-acting nitrate
Variant angina	Myocardial oxygen supply decreases due to coronary vasospasm; may occur with patient at rest	Treated primarily with a calcium channel blocker
Unstable angina	Myocardial oxygen supply decreases at the same time that oxygen demand increases; may occur at any time	May require a combination of drugs, that is, a calcium channel blocker plus a beta blocker

trates (isosorbide dinitrate, erythrityl tetranitrate) can be administered orally. Nitroglycerin can also be taken sublingually at the onset of an attack or just before activities that routinely precipitate an attack.

Calcium channel blockers can also be given to treat stable angina.[35,39,51,52,63] These drugs decrease cardiac workload directly by limiting calcium entry into myocardial cells and indirectly by producing peripheral vasodilation and thus decreasing cardiac preload and afterload. Hence, calcium channel blockers are administered in stable angina for their effect on the myocardium and peripheral vasculature rather than for their ability to dilate the coronary arteries.

Finally, a combination of various antianginal drugs is often used in patients with stable angina. A beta blocker and long-acting nitrate may be administered together, for instance, or a beta blocker and calcium channel blocker may be used in combination.[38] Likewise, a combination of all three types of drugs (nitrate, beta blocker, and calcium channel blocker) may be used in patients with severe stable angina.[35]

Variant Angina (Prinzmetal's Ischemia)

In variant angina, the primary problem is that oxygen supply to the myocardium *decreases* because of coronary artery vasospasm.[11] Vasospasm causes oxygen supply to decrease even though oxygen demand has not changed, and this phenomenon can occur even when the patient is at rest. In some patients with variant angina, the coronary arteries appear to be supersensitive to endogenous vasoconstrictive agents, and a variety of emotional or environmental stimuli may trigger coronary vasospasm.[30,60] In many patients, however, the reason for this spontaneous coronary vasoconstriction is unknown.

Calcium channel blockers are usually the drugs of choice in treating the variant form of angina.[3] These drugs limit the entry of calcium into the coronary vessels, thus attenuating or preventing the vasospasm underlying variant angina.[31] If calcium channel blockers are not tolerated, long-acting nitrates may be used instead. Calcium channel blockers are especially effective in treating variant angina, however, and most patients with this form of angina respond well to these agents. If patients do not respond to singular use of calcium channel blockers, long-acting nitrates may be added to calcium channel blockers for management of severe variant angina.[64]

Unstable Angina

"Unstable" angina is a rather ambiguous term used to identify several serious and potentially life-threatening forms of myocardial ischemia. In unstable angina, oxygen demand often increases at the same time that oxygen supply decreases; that is, coronary vasoconstriction is superimposed on an increase in myocardial oxygen requirements.[11,36] Hence, unstable angina is somewhat of a combination of stable and variant angina. As a result, anginal attacks may begin with minimal levels of exertion, or spontaneously even when the patient is at rest. Unstable angina is also associated with episodes of increased platelet aggregation and thrombosis in the affected coronary arteries that can lead to myocardial infarction.[11] Hence, unstable angina is generally regarded as the most serious and potentially dangerous form of this disease.

Various combinations of antianginal drugs are often used to treat unstable angina.[52] For instance, combining a calcium channel blocker with a long-acting nitrate is often effective because unstable angina is caused by both coronary artery vasospasm, which is resolved primarily by the calcium channel blocker, and increased myocardial oxygen demand, which is resolved primarily by the nitrate.[13] Likewise, beta blockers have also been used alone or in various combinations with calcium channel blockers and nitrates to treat unstable angina.[26,52] The optimal combination of antianginal drugs must typically be determined on a patient-by-patient basis. Other drugs such as aspirin, heparin, and thrombolytic agents may also be administered to decrease the risk of coronary thrombosis in patients with stable angina; the use of these agents is described in more detail in Chapter 25.

NONPHARMACOLOGIC MANAGEMENT OF ANGINA PECTORIS

The drugs used to treat angina are effective and relatively safe for long-term use. These agents, however, really only treat a symptom of heart disease, namely, the pain associated with myocardial ischemia. Antianginal drugs do not cure any cardiac conditions, nor do they exert any beneficial long-term effects on cardiac function. Consequently, efforts are made in many patients with angina to resolve the underlying disorder responsible for causing an imbalance in myocardial oxygen supply and demand.

Nonpharmacologic treatment usually begins by identifying any potentiating factors that might initiate or exacerbate anginal attacks. For instance, hypertension, congestive heart failure, anemia, and thyrotoxicosis may all contribute to the onset of aging.[55] In some cases, treatment of one of these potentiating factors may effectively resolve the angina, thus making subsequent drug therapy unnecessary. Lifestyle changes including exercise, weight control, giving up smoking, and stress management may also be helpful in decreasing or even eliminating the need for antianginal drugs. Finally, a number of surgical techniques that try to increase coronary blood flow may be attempted. Revascularization procedures such as coronary artery bypass and coronary artery angioplasty may be successful in increasing myocardial oxygen supply, thus attenuating anginal attacks in some patients. Regardless of what strategy is pursued, a permanent solution to the factors that precipitate myocardial ischemia should be explored in all patients with angina pectoris.

SPECIAL CONCERNS IN REHABILITATION PATIENTS

Physical therapists and occupational therapists must be aware of patients who are taking medications for angina pectoris and of whether the medications are taken prophylactically or during an attack. For the patient with stable angina who takes nitroglycerin at the onset of an anginal episode, therapists must make sure the drug is always near at hand during therapy sessions. Since many activities in rehabilitation (exercise, functional training, etc.) increase myocardial oxygen demand, anginal attacks may occur during the therapy session. If the nitroglycerin tablets are in the patient's hospital room (inpatients) or were left at home (outpatients), the anginal attack will be prolonged and possibly quite severe. A little precaution in making sure patients bring their nitroglycerin to therapy can prevent some tense movements while waiting to see if an anginal attack will subside.

For patients taking antianginal drugs prophylactically (i.e., at regular intervals), having the drug actually present during the rehabilitation session is not as crucial, providing that the patient has been taking the medication as prescribed. Therapists must still be aware, however, that many rehabilitation activities may disturb the balance between myocardial oxygen supply and demand, particularly by increasing oxygen demand beyond the ability of the coronary arteries to increase oxygen supply to the heart. Consequently, therapists must be aware of the cardiac limitations in their patients with angina and use caution in not overtaxing the heart to the extent that the antianginal drugs are ineffective.

Another important consideration in rehabilitation is the effect of antianginal drugs on the response to an exercise bout. Some patients taking these drugs may experience an *increase* in exercise tolerance because the patient is not as limited by symptoms of angina.[7,32] Certain drugs, however, may blunt the ability of the heart to respond to an acute exercise bout. Beta blockers and certain calcium channel blockers, for instance, slow down heart rate and decrease myocardial contractility during exercise.[6,16,27,37,57] At any absolute exercise workload, the myocardial response (e.g., heart rate) of the patient taking these drugs will be lower than if the drug was not taken. Consequently, the heart may not be able to handle some workloads. This blunted exercise response must be taken into account when patients engage in cardiac conditioning activities, and exercise workloads should be adjusted accordingly.

Finally, therapists should be aware of how the side effects of the antianginal drugs may impact on the therapy session. The nitrates and calcium channel blockers both produce peripheral vasodilation and can lead to hypotension. This decrease in blood pressure may be exaggerated when the patient suddenly sits up or stands up (orthostatic hypotension). Also, conditions that produce peripheral vasodilation, such as heat or exercise, may produce an additive effect on the drug-induced hypotension, thus leading to dizziness and syncope. Therapists should be aware that patients taking nitrates and calcium channel blockers may experience hypotension when systemic heat is applied or when their patients perform exercises that use large muscle groups.

CASE STUDY

ANTIANGINAL DRUGS

Brief History. T.M. is a 73-year-old man who is retired from his job as an accountant. He has a long history of diabetes mellitus, which has progressively worsened over the past decade despite insulin treatments. He also has a history of stable (classic) angina, which has been managed by nitroglycerin. The patient self-administers a nitroglycerin tablet sublingually (0.4 mg per tablet) at the onset of an anginal attack. Recently, this patient was admitted to the hospital for treatment of a gangrenous lesion on his left foot. When this lesion failed to respond to conservative treatment, a left below-knee amputation was performed. Following the amputation, the patient was referred to physical therapy for strengthening and a preprosthetic evaluation.

 Problem/Influence of Medication. A program of general conditioning and strengthening was initiated at the patient's bedside the day following surgery. The third day following the amputation, the therapist decided to bring the patient to the physical therapy department for a more intensive program, including standing activities with the parallel bars. The patient arrived in the department via wheelchair and began complaining immediately of chest pains. The patient had not brought his nitroglycerin tablets with him to the therapy session. The therapist immediately phoned the nursing floor, and the patient's medication was rushed to the physical therapy department. While waiting for the nitroglycerin to arrive, the patient's vital signs were monitored and he was placed in a supine position on a mat table. The drug was administered sublingually while the patient remained supine, and his chest pain subsided.

Decision/Solution. Evidently the exertion and apprehension of merely being transported to the physical therapy department was sufficient to trigger an attack of angina in this patient. The fact that his medication was not readily available created a rather anxious situation, which, fortunately, was resolved without any serious incident. To prevent a repeat of this predicament, the therapist contacted the nursing staff and requested that the patient always bring his medication with him to physical therapy. On subsequent occasions when the patient did experience the onset of angina, he was immediately placed in a supine position and the drug was administered sublingually. The patient was placed supine to prevent any orthostatic hypotension that may occur with nitroglycerin. The patient was eventually fitted with a temporary prosthesis and transferred to an extended-care facility to continue his rehabilitation.

SUMMARY

Pain in the chest region, or angina pectoris, is a common symptom of ischemic heart disease. Anginal pain usually occurs because of an imbalance between myocardial oxygen supply and myocardial oxygen demand. Organic nitrates, beta blockers, and calcium channel blockers are the primary drugs used to treat angina pectoris. Organic nitrates and beta blockers exert their effects primarily by decreasing myocardial oxygen demand, whereas calcium channel blockers primarily increase myocardial oxygen supply. Several forms of angina pectoris can be identified, and specific types of antianginal drugs are used alone or in combination with each other to treat or prevent various forms of angina.

Rehabilitation specialists must be aware of any patients who suffer from angina pectoris and the possibility of patients having an anginal attack during a therapy session. Therapists should also be cognizant of what drugs are being taken to control the patient's angina, as well as the possibility that side effects of antianginal drugs may influence certain rehabilitation procedures.

REFERENCES

1. Abrams, J: Management of myocardial ischemia: Role of intermittent nitrate therapy. Am Heart J 120(suppl):762, 1990.
2. Abrams, J: Nitroglycerin and long-acting nitrates in clinical practice. Am J Med 74(suppl 6b):85, 1983.
3. Antman, E, et al: Nifedipine therapy for coronary-artery spasm: Experience in 127 patients. N Engl J Med 302:1269, 1980.
4. Antman, EM, et al: Calcium channel blocking agents in the treatment of cardiovascular disorders. Part I: Basic and clinical electrophysiologic events. Ann Intern Med 93:875, 1980.

5. Armstrong, PW and Moffat, JA: Tolerance to organic nitrates: Clinical and experimental perspectives. Am J Med 74(suppl 6b):72, 1983.
6. Bailey, DG and Carruthers, SG: Interaction between oral verapamil and beta blockers during submaximal exercise: Relevance of ancillary properties. Clin Pharmacol Ther 49:370, 1991.
7. Bassan, M: The day-long antianginal effectiveness of nitroglycerin patches. A double-blind study using dose-titration. Chest 99:1120, 1991.
8. Braunwald, E: Mechanism of action of calcium-channel blocking agents. N Engl J Med 307:1618, 1982.
9. Brown, BG, et al: The mechanism of nitroglycerin action: Stenosis vasodilation as a major component of the drug response. Circulation 64:1089, 1981.
10. Cohn, JN: Pharmacologic mechanisms of nitrates in myocardial ischemia. Am J Cardiol 70:G38, 1992.
11. Cohn, PF: Mechanisms of myocardial ischemia. Am J Cardiol 70:14G, 1992.
12. Cohn, PF: Silent myocardial ischemia: Classification, prevalence and prognosis. Am J Med 79(suppl 3a):2, 1985.
13. Conti, CR, et al: Nitrates for treatment of unstable angina pectoris and coronary vasospasm. Am J Med 74(suppl 6b):40, 1983.
14. Curry, SH, et al: Plasma nitroglycerin concentrations and hemodynamics: Effects of sublingual, ointment and controlled-release forms of nitroglycerin. Clin Pharmacol Ther 36:765, 1984.
15. Dalal, JJ and Parker, JO: Nitrate cross-tolerance: Effect of sublingual isosorbide nitrate and nitroglycerin during sustained nitrate therapy. Am J Cardiol 54:286, 1984.
16. Dargie, HJ, Grant, S, and McLenachan, J: Angina, ischemia, and effort tolerance with vasodilating beta-blockers. Am Heart J 121:1017, 1991.
17. Deanfield, JE and Selwyn, AP: Character and causes of transient myocardial ischemia during daily life. Am J Med 80(suppl 4c):19, 1986.
18. Degre, SG, et al: Effect of oral sustained-release nitroglycerin on exercise capacity in angina pectoris: Dose-response relation and duration of action during double-blind crossover randomized acute therapy. Am J Cardiol 51:1595, 1983.
19. deMuinck, ED and Lie, KI: Safety and efficacy of beta-blockers in the treatment of stable angina pectoris. J Cardiovasc Pharmacol 16(suppl 5):S123, 1990.
20. Fung, HL: Clinical pharmacology of organic nitrates. Am J Cardiol 72:C9, 1993.
21. Gallant, EM and Goettl, VM: Effects of calcium antagonists on mechanical responses of mammalian skeletal muscle. Eur J Pharmacol 117:259, 1985.
22. Greco, R, et al: Long-term efficacy of nitroglycerin patch in stable angina pectoris. Am J Cardiol 65:9J, 1990.
23. Hansson, L: Calcium antagonists: An overview. Am Heart J 122:308, 1991.
24. Hansson, L: Review of state-of-the-art beta-blocker therapy. Am J Cardiol 67:43B, 1991.
25. Henry, PD: Comparatitive pharmacology of calcium antagonists: Nifedipine, verapamil and diltiazem. Am J Cardiol 46:1047, 1980.
26. Hugenholtz, PG, et al: Nifedipine in the treatment of unstable angina, coronary spasm and myocardial ischemia. Am J Cardiol 47:163, 1981.
27. Hughson, RL and Kowalchuk, JM: Beta-blockade and oxygen delivery to muscle during exercise. Can J Physiol Pharmacol 69:285, 1991.
28. Ignarro, LJ and Kadowitz, PJ: The pharmacological and physiological role of cyclic GMP in vascular smooth muscle relaxation. Annu Rev Pharmacol Toxicol 25:171, 1985.
29. Jordan, RA, et al: Rapidly developing tolerance to transdermal nitroglycerin in congestive heart failure. Ann Intern Med 104:295, 1985.
30. Kaski, JC, et al: Local coronary supersensitivity to diverse vasoconstrictive stimuli in patients with variant angina. Circulation 74:1255, 1986.
31. Kimura, E and Kishida, H: Treatment of variant angina with drugs: A survey of 11 cardiology institutes in Japan. Circulation 63:844, 1981.
32. Lai, C, et al: Effect of calcium antagonists on exercise tests. J Cardiovasc Pharmacol 20(suppl 5):S55, 1992.
33. Maseri, A, et al: Mechanisms of ischemic cardiac pain and silent myocardial ischemia. Am J Med 79(suppl 3a):7, 1985.
34. McGregor, M: Pathogenesis of angina pectoris and role of nitrates in relief of myocardial ischemia. Am J Med 74(suppl 6b):21, 1983.
35. Meluzin, J, et al: Effects of nifedipine and diltiazem on myocardial ischemia in patients with severe stable angina pectoris treated with nitrates and beta-blockers. J Cardiovasc Pharmacol 20:864, 1992.
36. Miller, AB: Mixed ischemic subsets. Comparison of the mechanism of silent ischemia and mixed angina. Am J Med 79(suppl 3a):25, 1985.
37. Mooy, J, et al: The effects of verapamil and propranolol on exercise tolerance in hypertensive patients. Clin Pharmacol Ther 41:490, 1987.
38. Morse, JR and Neston, RW: Double-blind crossover comparison of the antianginal effects of nifedipine and isosorbide dinitrate in patients with exertional angina receiving propranolol. J Am Coll Cardiol 6:1395, 1985.
39. Moskowitz, RM, et al: Nifedipine therapy for stable angina pectoris: Preliminary results of effects on angina frequency and treadmill exercise response. Am J Cardiol 44:811, 1979.

40. Nabel, EG, et al: Effects of dosing intervals on the development of tolerance to high dose transdermal nitroglycerin. Am J Cardiol 63:663, 1989.
41. Nesto, RW and Phillips, RT: Silent myocardial ischemia: Clinical characteristics underlying mechanisms and indications for treatment. Am J Med 81(suppl 4a):12, 1986.
42. Paciaroni, E and Luca, C: Discontinuous transdermal nitroglycerin as treatment for stable angina in the elderly: A double-blind multicentre study. Eur Heart J 12:1076, 1991.
43. Parker, JO: Nitrates and angina pectoris. Am J Cardiol 72:3C, 1993.
44. Parratt, JR: Nitroglycerin—the first one hundred years: New facts about an old drug. J Pharm Pharmacol 31:801, 1979.
45. Pearle, DL: Pharmacologic management of ischemic heart disease with beta-blockers and calcium channel blockers. Am Heart J 120(suppl):739, 1990.
46. Pepine, CJ: Clinical aspects of silent myocardial ischemia in patients with angina and other forms of coronary heart disease. Am J Med 80(suppl 4c):25, 1986.
47. Pepine, CJ, et al: Clinical outcome after treatment of rest angina with calcium channel blockers: Comparative experience during the initial year of therapy with diltiazem, nifedipine and verapamil. Am Heart J 106:1341, 1983.
48. Reichek, N: Long-acting nitrates: Relative utility of nitroglycerin patches. Am J Med 76(suppl 6A):63, 1984.
49. Reichek, N, Goldstein, RE, and Redwood, DR: Sustained effects of nitroglycerin ointment in patients with angina pectoris. Circulation 50:348, 1974.
50. Roberts, R: Stable angina as a manifestation of ischemic heart disease: Medical management. Circulation 72(suppl V):V145, 1985.
51. Rouleau, J-L, et al: Mechanism of relief of pacing-induced angina with oral verapamil: Reduced oxygen demand. Circulation 67:94, 1983.
52. Rutherford, JD, et al: Pharmacologic management of angina and acute myocardial infarction. Am J Cardiol 72:C16, 1993.
53. Scheidt, S: Angina: Evolution of the role of nitrates. Am Heart J 120(suppl):757, 1990.
54. Scheidt, S: Update on transdermal nitroglycerin: An overview. Am J Cardiol 56:31, 1985.
55. Scheidt, S: Beta-blockade for angina and arrhythmias: An overview. Drugs 25(suppl 2):153, 1983.
56. Schwartz, A and Triggle, DJ: Cellular action of calcium channel blocking drugs. Annu Rev Med 35:325, 1984.
57. Stewart, JK, et al: Effects of diltiazem or propranolol during exercise training of hypertensive men. Med Sci Sports Exerc 22:171, 1990.
58. Stone, PH, et al: Calcium channel blocking agents in the treatment of cardiovascular disorders. Part II: Hemodynamic effects and clinical applications. Ann Intern Med 93:886, 1980.
59. Struyker-Boudier, HAJ, Smits, JFM, and DeMey, JGR: The pharmacology of calcium antagonists: A review. J Cardiovasc Pharmacol 15(suppl 4):S1, 1990.
60. Symposium (various authors): Triggering and circadian variation of onset of acute cardiovascular disease. Am J Cardiol 66:1G, 1990.
61. Thadani, U, et al: Comparison of five beta-adrenoreceptor antagonists with different ancillary properties during sustained twice daily therapy in angina pectoris. Am J Med 68:243, 1980.
62. Turner, P: Which ancillary properties of beta-adrenoceptor blocking drugs influence their therapeutic and adverse effects: A review. J Royal Soc Med 84:672, 1991.
63. Wagniart, P, et al: Increased exercise tolerance and reduced electrocardiographic ischemia with diltiazem in patients with stable angina pectoris. Circulation 66:23, 1982.
64. Winniford, MD, et al: Concomitant calcium antagonist plus isosorbide dinitrate therapy for markedly active variant angina. Am Heart J 108:1269, 1984.
65. Zelis, R: Mechanisms of vasodilation. Am J Med 74(suppl 6b):3, 1983.

CHAPTER 23

Treatment of Cardiac Arrhythmias

An *arrhythmia* can be broadly defined as any significant deviation from normal cardiac rhythm.[4,37] Various problems in the origination and conduction of electrical activity in the heart can lead to distinct types of arrhythmias. If untreated, disturbances in normal cardiac rhythm result in impaired cardiac pumping ability, and certain arrhythmias are associated with cerebrovascular accidents, cardiac failure, and other sequelae that can be fatal.[23,32] Fortunately, a variety of drugs are available to help establish and maintain normal cardiac rhythm.

This chapter presents the primary antiarrhythmic drugs and the therapeutic rationale for their use. Many patients seen in rehabilitation are given these drugs to help control and prevent the onset of arrhythmias. Physical therapists and occupational therapists often work directly with cardiac patients in cardiac rehabilitation and fitness programs. Likewise, cardiac patients taking antiarrhythmic drugs may be seen in rehabilitation for any number of other neuromuscular or musculoskeletal disorders. Consequently, therapists should have some knowledge of the clinical use of these drugs.

To understand how antiarrhythmic drugs exert their effects, we first review the origin and spread of electrical activity throughout the heart. This chapter begins with a brief discussion of cardiac electrophysiology, followed by a presentation of the basic mechanisms responsible for producing disturbances in cardiac rhythm and the common types of arrhythmias seen clinically. Finally, antiarrhythmic drugs are presented according to their mechanism of action and clinical use.

CARDIAC ELECTROPHYSIOLOGY

Cardiac Action Potentials

The action potential recorded from a cardiac Purkinje's fiber is shown in Figure 23–1. At rest, the interior of the cell is negative relative to the cell's exterior. As in other excitable tissues (neurons, skeletal muscle), an action potential occurs when the cell in-

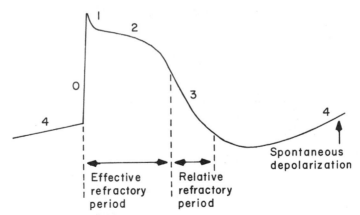

FIGURE 23–1. The cardiac action potential recorded from a Purkinje's cell. The effective refractory period is the time during which the cell cannot be depolarized, and the relative refractory period is the time in which a supranormal stimulus is required to depolarize the cell. Action potential phases (0–4) and the ionic basis for each phase are discussed in the text. (From Keefe, Kates, and Harrison,[22] p 364, with permission.)

terior suddenly becomes positive (*depolarizes*), primarily because of the influx of sodium ions. The cell interior then returns to a negative potential (*repolarizes*), primarily because of the efflux of potassium ions. The cardiac action potential, however, has several features that distinguish it from action potentials recorded in other nerves and muscles.[4,15] The cardiac action potential is typically divided into several phases (see Fig. 23–1). The ionic movement that occurs in each phase is outlined here.

Phase 0: Rapid depolarization occurs because of the sudden influx of sodium ions into the cell. At some threshold level, the cell membrane suddenly becomes permeable to sodium ions because of the opening of sodium channels or gates, similar to the spike seen in skeletal muscle depolarization.

Phase 1: An early, brief period of repolarization occurs because of potassium leaving the cell. Specific potassium channels in the cell membrane open to allow potassium to leave the cell.

Phase 2: The action potential undergoes a plateau phase, primarily because of the opening of calcium channels and a slow, prolonged influx of calcium ions into the cell. Because the efflux of positively charged potassium ions that occurred in phase 1 is balanced by the influx of positively charged calcium ions, there is no net change in the charge within the cell. Thus, the cell's potential remains relatively constant for a brief period of time, creating the distinctive plateau seen in Figure 23–1. This phase 2 plateau is important in cardiac cells because it prolongs the cell's effective refractory period (i.e., the time interval between successive action potentials). The plateau basically enables the heart to enter a period of rest (*diastole*) so that the cardiac chambers can fill with blood before the next contraction (*systole*).

Phase 3: At the end of the plateau, repolarization is completed. This is primarily because of the closing (*inactivation*) of the calcium channels, thus terminating the entry of calcium into the cell. Repolarization is completed by the unopposed exit of potassium ions.

Phase 4: In certain cardiac cells (such as the one shown in Fig. 23–1), phase 4 consists of a slow, spontaneous depolarization. This spontaneous depolarization was originally thought to be caused by a gradual accumulation of positively charged potassium ions within the cell. The cell probably depolarizes spontaneously, however, because of the influx of positive ions such as sodium.[6,15] The cell may automatically start to increase its permeability to sodium, thus allowing positively charged ions to leak into the cell. When enough positive charges enter the cell, threshold is reached and phase 0 is initiated.

Action potentials recorded from various cardiac cells may vary somewhat from the action potential described previously. Some cells, for instance, may totally lack phase 1 and have a much slower phase 0. Such cells are said to have a slow response as opposed to the fast response just described. Also, action potentials from the nodal cells (see the next section,"Normal Cardiac Rhythm") differ somewhat from the fast response cells. The fundamental ionic fluxes that occur during cardiac action potentials are similar in all cardiac cells, however. This ionic activity is pharmacologically significant because various antiarrhythmic drugs will affect the movement of sodium and other ions in an attempt to establish and maintain normal cardiac rhythm.

Normal Cardiac Rhythm

Certain cardiac cells are able to initiate and maintain a spontaneous automatic rhythm. Even in the absence of any neural or hormonal input, these cells will automatically generate an action potential. They are usually referred to as *pacemaker cells* in the myocardium. Pacemaker cells have the ability to depolarize spontaneously because of a rising phase 4 in the cardiac action potential (see Fig. 23–1). As described previously, the resting cell automatically begins to depolarize during phase 4 until the cell reaches threshold and an action potential is initiated.

Pacemaker cells are found primarily in the sinoatrial (SA) node and in the atrioventricular (AV) node (Fig. 23–2). Although many other cardiac cells also have the ability to generate an automatic rhythm, the pacemaker cells in the SA node usually dominate and control cardiac rhythm in the normal heart.

Normal Conduction of the Cardiac Action Potential

The normal propagation of the cardiac action potential is illustrated in Figure 23–2. The action potential originates in the SA node and is conducted throughout both atria via the atrial muscle cells. While spreading through the atria, the action potential reaches the AV node. From the AV node, the action potential is passed on to the ventricles via a specialized conducting system known as the *bundle of His*. The bundle of His is composed primarily of specialized conducting cells known as *Purkinje's fibers*. As the bundle leaves the AV node, it divides into left and right branches, which supply the respective ventricles. The action potential is distributed to all parts of the ventricles via the bundle branches and Purkinje's fibers (see Fig. 23–2).

MECHANISMS OF CARDIAC ARRHYTHMIAS

The origin of the cardiac action potential and system of action potential propagation represents normal cardiac excitation and conduction. Any number of factors can

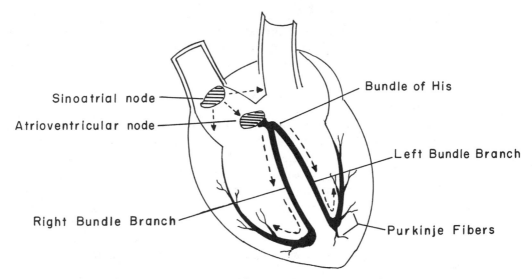

FIGURE 23–2. Schematic representation of the conduction system of the heart. Conduction normally follows the pathways indicated by the dashed lines. Impulses originate in the sinoatrial node and are transmitted to the atrioventricular node. Impulses are then conducted from the atrioventricular node to the ventricles by the bundle of His and the bundle branches.

disrupt the normal cardiac excitation process, however, thus resulting in arrhythmic contractions. Such factors include disease, metabolic and electrolyte imbalances, abnormal autonomic influence on the heart, toxicity to other drugs (e.g., digitalis), and myocardial ischemia and infarction.[37,38,45] Regardless of what the initiating factor is in producing arrhythmias, the mechanism underlying a disturbance in cardiac rhythm can be attributed to one of the three basic abnormalities listed here.[37,41]

1. *Abnormal impulse generation:* The normal automatic rhythm of the cardiac pacemaker cells has been disrupted. Injury and disease may directly render the SA and AV cells incapable of maintaining normal rhythm. Also, cells that do not normally control cardiac rhythm may begin to compete with pacemaker cells, thus creating multiple areas of automaticity.
2. *Abnormal impulse conduction:* The conduction of impulses throughout the myocardium has been interrupted. Various diseases and local damage may result in the delay or failure of an action potential to reach certain areas. These conduction impairments or heart blocks can prevent a smooth and synchronous contraction, thus creating an abnormal rhythm.
3. *Simultaneous abnormalities of impulse generation and conduction:* A combination of both factors listed previously may cause cardiac arrhythmias.

TYPES OF ARRHYTHMIAS

Cardiac arrhythmias are described by many different terms according to their site of origin, nature of the disturbed heartbeat, or impairment in cardiac conduction.[37,45] This text cannot fully describe all of the various forms of arrhythmias occurring clinically. To understand when various antiarrhythmic drugs are used, however, some basic terms describing cardiac arrhythmias must be defined. Some of the more commonly occurring arrhythmias are listed in Table 23–1. For a more detailed description of the electrophysiologic nature and diagnosis of these arrhythmias, the reader is referred to several other sources on this topic.[4,13,37,45]

CLASSIFICATION OF ANTIARRHYTHMIC DRUGS

Drugs used to treat cardiac arrhythmias are traditionally placed in one of four distinct classes according to their mechanism of action.[6,22,43] These classifications are summarized in Table 23–2. Although the accuracy of this classification system has been criticized somewhat, this method of categorizing antiarrhythmic drugs is still commonly used to describe these drugs.[27,40] The mechanism of action and specific agents within each class are described here.

CLASS I: SODIUM CHANNEL BLOCKERS

Mechanism of Action and Rationale for Use

Class I antiarrhythmic drugs have an affinity for sodium channels in nerve and muscle cell membranes. These drugs appear to interact in some way with sodium channels and to inhibit them from opening.[3,10,20] Exactly how these drugs interfere with sodium channel function is somewhat unclear. We do not know if these drugs in-

TABLE 23–1 Common Forms of Arrhythmias

Classification	Characteristic Rhythm
Sinus arrhythmias	
Sinus tachycardia	> 100 beats/min
Sinus bradycardia	< 60 beats/min
Sick sinus syndrome	Severe bradycardia (< 50 beats/min); periods of sinus arrest
Supraventricular arrhythmias	
Atrial fibrillation and flutter	Atrial rate > 300 beats/min
Atrial tachycardia	Atrial rate > 140–200 beats/min
Premature atrial contractions	Variable
Atrioventricular junctional arrhythmias	
Junctional rhythm	40–55 beats/min
Junctional tachycardia	100–200 beats/min
Conduction disturbances	
Atrioventricular block	Variable
Bundle branch block	Variable
Fascicular block	Variable
Ventricular arrhythmias	
Premature ventricular contractions	Variable
Ventricular tachycardia	140–200 beats/min
Ventricular fibrillation	Irregular, totally uncoordinated rhythm

TABLE 23–2 Classification of Antiarrhythmic Drugs

Generic Names	Trade Names
Class I: Sodium channel blockers	
Subclass A	
Disopyramide	Norpace
Procainamide	Promine, Pronestyl
Quinidine	Cardioquin, Duraquin, others
Subclass B	
Lidocaine	Xylocaine, Lidopen
Mexiletine	Mexitil
Moricizine*	Ethmozine
Phenytoin	Dilantin
Tocainide	Tonocard
Subclass C	
Encainide	Enkaid
Flecainide	Tambocor
Propafenone	Rythmol
Class II: Beta blockers	
Acebutolol	Sectral
Atenolol	Tenormin
Esmolol	Brevibloc
Metoprolol	Lopressor
Nadolol	Corgard
Oxprenolol	Trasicor
Propranolol	Inderal
Sotalol	Betapace
Timolol	Blocadren
Class III: Drugs that prolong repolarization	
Amiodarone†	Cordarone
Bretylium	Bretylol
Class IV: Calcium channel blockers	
Diltiazem	Cardizem
Verapamil	Calan, Isoptin

*Also has some class IC properties.
†Also has some class I properties.

hibit sodium channel function by directly binding to the channel or by a more general effect on the cardiac cell membrane.[5] Many class I agents (e.g., lidocaine) are also used as local anesthetics,[17] and the possible ways in which these drugs may interact with sodium channels are discussed in more detail in Chapter 12.

Because sodium influx plays an important role during action potential generation during phase 0 of the cardiac action potential, inhibition of sodium channels tends to decrease membrane excitability. Thus, class I drugs tend to stabilize the cardiac cell membrane and normalize the rate of firing of cardiac cells. Although all class I drugs exert their antiarrhythmic effects by inhibiting sodium channel function, various agents affect myocardial excitation and conduction in slightly different ways. Class I drugs are typically subclassified according to how they influence cardiac electrophysiology (see Table 23–2). These subclassifications and specific agents in each group are presented here.

Specific Agents

Class IA. Drugs in this group are similar in that they produce a moderate slowing of phase 0 depolarization and a moderate slowing of action potential propagation throughout the myocardium. These drugs also prolong repolarization of the cardiac cell, thus lengthening the time interval before a second action potential can occur (i.e., they increase the effective refractory period). Class IA agents include quinidine, procainamide, and disopyramide (see Table 23–2). Class IA drugs are used to treat a variety of arrhythmias that originate in the ventricles or the atria.

Class IB. These drugs display only a minimal ability to slow phase 0 depolarization, and they produce only a minimal slowing of cardiac conduction. In contrast to IA drugs, class IB agents usually shorten cardiac repolarization; that is, the effective refractory period is decreased. Class IB drugs include lidocaine, mexiletine, moricizine, phenytoin, and tocainide (see Table 23–2). These drugs are primarily used to treat ventricular arrhythmias such as ventricular tachycardia and premature ventricular contractions (PVCs). Lidocaine is especially effective in treating some patients with severe ventricular arrhythmias that occur following myocardial infarction and cardiac surgery.[34] Routine use of this drug in all patients who have had an acute myocardial infarction has been questioned, however, and administration of lidocaine and other class I drugs should be considered on a patient-by-patient basis following infarction.[1,39]

Class IC. These drugs produce both a marked decrease in the rate of phase 0 depolarization and a marked slowing of cardiac conduction. They have little effect on repolarization, however. Class IC drugs, which include encainide, flecainide, and propafenone (see Table 23–2), appear to be best suited to treat ventricular arrhythmias, such as ventricular tachycardia and PVCs.

Adverse Side Effects

Despite their use in treating arrhythmias, the most common side effect associated with all antiarrhythmic drugs is an aggravation of cardiac rhythm disturbances.[11,28–31] Since class I drugs affect sodium channel function and cardiac excitability, some paradoxic changes in cardiac rhythm may occur. Class I drugs are also associated with a variety of annoying side effects such as dizziness, visual disturbances, and nausea.[29] These symptoms are often important, however, because they may indicate the presence of arrhythmias even when the pulse or ECG is not being directly monitored.[31] Arrhythmias and other side effects vary greatly according to the exact agent used and the sensitivity of individual patients.

CLASS II: BETA BLOCKERS

Mechanisms of Action and Rationale for Use

Drugs that block beta-1 receptors on the myocardium are one of the mainstays in the treatment of arrhythmias. Beta blockers are effective because they decrease cardiac automaticity and prolong the effective refractory period, thus slowing heart rate.[16,33] Beta blockers also slow down conduction through the myocardium. These drugs are most effective in treating heart rate problems that originate in the atria (supraventricular arrhythmias), especially problems originating in the AV node.[16] Some ventricular arrhythmias may also respond to treatment with beta blockers.

Specific Agents

Individual beta blockers are presented in Chapter 20. Beta blockers shown to be effective in treating arrhythmias include acebutolol, atenolol, esmolol, metoprolol, nadolol, oxprenolol, propranolol, sotalol, and timolol (see Table 23–2). Choice of a specific beta blocker depends to a large extent on the exact type of arrhythmia present and the individual patient's response to the drug.

Adverse Side Effects

Because of the ability of beta blockers to slow down the heart, patients with poor cardiac pumping ability may experience heart failure when given these drugs. Also, beta blockers may produce excessive slowing of cardiac conduction in some individuals, resulting in an increase in arrhythmias. Both of these problems are relatively rare, however, and beta blockers are well tolerated by most patients when used to treat arrhythmias.

CLASS III: DRUGS THAT PROLONG REPOLARIZATION

Mechanism of Action and Rationale for Use

These agents delay repolarization of cardiac cells, thus prolonging the effective refractory period.[6,19,22] This delay lengthens the time interval before a subsequent action potential can be initiated, thus slowing and stabilizing the heart rate. Exactly how class III drugs exert this effect is unknown. Some evidence suggests that these agents may inhibit sympathetic adrenergic discharge onto the myocardium.[74] These agents may also directly decrease myocardial excitability and slow down cardiac conduction.[42] Class III drugs are primarily used to treat ventricular arrhythmias such as ventricular tachycardia and ventricular fibrillation.

Specific Agents

Class III drugs currently in use include bretylium and amiodarone (see Table 23–2). Both drugs prolong repolarization in cardiac cells. Amiodarone also appears to have some properties similar to class I drugs and may directly decrease myocardial excitability and conduction by inhibiting sodium channel function.[26]

Adverse Side Effects

An initial increase in cardiac arrhythmias may occur when class III drugs are instituted, but this is often transient. Amiodarone is also associated with a number of frequent and potentially serious side effects.[21,26] Most notable is pulmonary toxicity, including interstitial pneumonitis and pulmonary fibrosis, which can be fatal. Liver damage may also occur in some patients taking amiodarone. Bretylium appears to be somewhat safer than amiodarone, although orthostatic hypotension may occur when bretylium is administered.[9]

CLASS IV: CALCIUM CHANNEL BLOCKERS

Mechanism of Action and Rationale for Use

Class IV drugs have a selective ability to block calcium entry into myocardial and vascular smooth-muscle cells. These drugs inhibit calcium influx by binding to specific channels in the cell membrane.[7,35,36] As discussed previously in this chapter, calcium entry plays an important role in the generation of the cardiac action potential, especially during phase 2. By inhibiting calcium influx into myocardial cells, calcium channel blockers can alter the excitability and conduction of cardiac tissues.

Calcium channel blockers decrease the rate of discharge of the SA node, and they inhibit conduction velocity through the AV node.[2,18] These drugs are most successful in treating arrhythmias caused by atrial dysfunction, such as supraventricular tachycardia and atrial fibrillation.

Specific Agents

The pharmacology of specific calcium channel blockers is presented in Chapter 22. Of the calcium channel blockers currently in use, verapamil and diltiazem are currently approved for treating arrhythmias (Table 23–2). Of these two drugs, verapamil appears to be more effective as an antiarrhythmic,[2,8,25] and this drug has been used to treat both acute and chronic forms of supraventricular arrhythmias, as well as arrhythmias induced by digitalis.[12,14,44] Diltiazem is only moderately effective in treating arrhythmias, and other calcium channel blockers such as nifedipine and similar dihydropyridines (see Chapter 22) do not have any substantial effects on cardiac rhythm. These other calcium channel blockers are more effective in dilating vascular smooth muscle and are used more frequently to treat angina pectoris (see Chapter 22).

Adverse Side Effects

Because drugs like verapamil slow down heart rate by inhibiting calcium entry into cardiac muscle cells, excessive bradycardia (less than 50 beats per minute) may occur in some patients receiving these drugs. Calcium channel blockers also limit calcium entry into vascular smooth muscle, which may cause peripheral vasodilation and lead to dizziness and headaches in some patients.

SPECIAL CONCERNS IN REHABILITATION PATIENTS

The primary problems associated with antiarrhythmic drugs in rehabilitation patients are related to the side effects of these agents. Therapists should be aware of the potential for increased arrhythmias or changes in the nature of arrhythmias with these drugs. This concern may be especially important in patients involved in exercise and cardiac rehabilitation programs. Therapists who supervise such patients often can detect the presence of arrhythmias by monitoring ECG recordings. If an ECG recording is not available, palpation of pulses for rate and regularity may detect rhythm disturbances. Also, the presence of other side effects such as faintness or dizziness may signal the presence of cardiotoxic drug effects and increased arrhythmias.[31] Consequently, therapists treating patients for both cardiac and noncardiac disorders may help detect the cardiotoxic effects of antiarrhythmic drugs by being alert for any side effects. By playing a role in the early detection of increased arrhythmias, therapists can alert the physician to a problem and avert any potentially serious or even fatal consequences.

Other concerns related to the side effects are fairly minor. Hypotension may occur with some agents, especially with bretylium (class III) and the calcium channel blockers (class IV). Therapists should be aware that patients may become dizzy, especially after sudden changes in posture.

CASE STUDY

ANTIARRHYTHMIC DRUGS

Brief History. M.R. is a 48-year-old man with a history of coronary artery disease and cardiac rhythm disturbances. Specifically, he has experienced episodes of paroxysmal supraventricular tachycardia, with his heart rate often exceeding 180 beats per minute. He has been treated for several years with the nonspecific beta blocker propranolol (Inderal). Oral propranolol (60 mg/day) has successfully diminished his episodes of tachycardia. In an effort to improve his myocardial function and overall cardiovascular fitness, the patient recently enrolled as an outpatient in a cardiac rehabilitation program. Under the supervision of a physical therapist, he attended cardiac training sessions three times each week. A typical session consisted of warm-up calisthenics, bicycle ergometry, and cool-down stretching activities. Each session lasted approximately 45 minutes.

Problem/Influence of Medication. Propranolol and the other beta blockers are successful in reducing various supraventricular arrhythmias. These drugs, however, also attenuate the cardiac response to exercise. Heart rate and cardiac output are lower at any absolute workload, and maximal heart rate and cardiac output are attenuated by beta blockade. Consequently, the exercise response of a patient taking a beta blocker will be less than if the patient is not taking the drug. This consideration is important because the exercise prescription for any given patient must take into account the patient's maximal exercise capacity. Typically, patients exercise at some submaximal percentage of their maximal ability. If maximal exercise capacity is influenced by the beta blocker, the exercise prescription must be adjusted accordingly.

Decision/Solution. Prior to beginning the rehabilitation program, the patient underwent a graded exercise test (GXT). All patients with cardiac disorders should undergo a GXT before beginning a cardiac rehabilitation program. Patients taking beta blockers and other drugs that affect cardiac function must also be tested under the conditions in which they will eventually be exercising. The GXT accurately determined the patient's exercise workload while he was taking his normal dosage of propranolol. Consequently, the prescribed exercise workload was adjusted by the therapist for the effect of the beta blocker.

During the cardiac rehabilitation sessions, the therapist periodically monitored heart rate, blood pressure, and ECG. No significant episodes of arrhythmias were noted, and the patient progressed rapidly through the program. He was eventually discharged from the formal program with instructions of how to continue his rehabilitation exercises at home and at a local health club.

SUMMARY

Cardiac arrhythmias may arise because of disturbances in the origination and conduction of electrical activity in the heart. These changes in cardiac rhythm can be controlled to a large extent by several groups of drugs including sodium channel blockers, beta blockers, calcium channel blockers, and drugs that prolong the cardiac action potential. These agents work by different cellular mechanisms to stabilize heart rate and improve the conduction of electrical impulses throughout the myocardium. Although these drugs are often successful in preventing or resolving arrhythmias, rehabilitation specialists should be cognizant of patients who are taking these agents. Therapists should also be alert for any changes in cardiac function or other side effects that may signal toxicity of these drugs.

REFERENCES

1. Antman, EM and Berlin, JA: Declining incidence of ventricular fibrillation in myocardial infarction: Implications for the prophylactic use of lidocaine. Circulation 86:764, 1992.
2. Antman, EM, et al: Calcium channel blocking agents in the treatment of cardiovascular disorders. Part I: Basic and clinical electrophysiologic effects. Ann Intern Med 93:875, 1980.
3. Bean, BP, Cohen, CJ, and Tsien, RW: Lidocaine block of cardiac sodium channels. J Gen Physiol 81:613, 1983.
4. Berne, RM and Levy, MN: Cardiovascular Physiology, ed 6. Mosby Year Book, St Louis, 1992.
5. Bhise, SB, et al: Liquid membrane phenomena in antiarrhythmic action. Int J Pharm 28:145, 1986.
6. Bigger, JT and Hoffman, BF: Antiarrhythmic drugs. In Gilman, AG, et al (eds): The Pharmacological Basis of Therapeutics, ed 8. Pergamon Press, New York, 1990.
7. Braunwald, E: Mechanism of action of calcium-channel-blocking agents. N Engl J Med 307:1618, 1982.
8. Bush, LR, et al: Comparative effects of verapamil, diltiazem and felodipine during experimental digitalis-induced arrhythmias. Pharmacology 34:111, 1987.
9. Castle, L: Therapy of ventricular tachycardia. Am J Cardiol 54:1A, 1984.
10. Colatsky, TJ: Mechanisms of action of lidocaine and quinidine on action potential duration in rabbit cardiac Purkinje fibers. An effect on steady state sodium currents? Circ Res 50:17, 1982.
11. Dhein, S, et al: Comparative study on the proarrhythmic effects of some antiarrhythmic agents. Circulation 87:617, 1993.
12. Edwards, JD and Kishen, R: Significance and management of intractable supraventricular arrhythmias in critically ill patients. Crit Care Med 144:280, 1986.
13. Ellestad, MH: Stress Testing: Principles and Practice, ed 3. FA Davis, Philadelphia, 1986.
14. Ferraris, VA, et al: Verapamil prophylaxis for postoperative atrial dysrhythmias: A prospective, randomized, double-blind study using drug level monitoring. Ann Thorac Surg 43:530, 1987.
15. Gadsby, DC and Wit, AL: Normal and abnormal electrical activity in cardiac cells. In Mandel, WJ (ed): Cardiac Arrhythmias: Their Mechanisms, Diagnosis and Management. JB Lippincott, Philadelphia, 1987.
16. Gerber, JG and Nies, AS: Beta-adrenergic blocking drugs. Annu Rev Med 36:145, 1985.
17. Gintant, GA and Hoffman, BF: The role of local anesthetic effects in the actions of antiarrhythmic drugs. In Strichartz, GR (ed): Handbook of Experimental Pharmacology: Local Anesthetics, Vol 81. Springer-Verlag, Berlin, 1987.
18. Henry, PD: Comparative pharmacology of calcium antagonists: Nifedipine, verapamil and diltiazem. Am J Cardiol 46:1047, 1980.

19. Hondeghem, LM: Development of class III antiarrhythmic agents. J Cardiovasc Pharmacol 20(suppl 2):S17, 1992.
20. Hondeghem, LM and Katzung, BG: Antiarrhythmic agents: The modulated receptor mechanism of action of sodium and calcium channel blocking drugs. Annu Rev Pharmacol Toxicol 24:387, 1984.
21. Horowitz, LN, et al: Use of amiodarone in the treatment of persistent and paroxysmal atrial fibrillation resistant to quinidine therapy. J Am Coll Cardiol 6:1402, 1985.
22. Keefe, DLD, Kates, RE, and Harrison, DC: New antiarrhythmic drugs: Their place in therapy. Drugs 22:363, 1981.
23. Kochs, M, Eggeling, T, and Hombach, V: Pharmacological therapy in coronary heart disease: Prevention of life-threatening ventricular tachycardias and sudden cardiac death. Eur Heart J 14(suppl E):107, 1993.
24. Kopia, GA and Lucchesi, BR: Antifibrillation action of bretylium: Role of the sympathetic nervous system. Pharmacology 34:37, 1987.
25. Krikler, DM: Verapamil in arrhythmia. Br J Clin Pharmacol 21(suppl 2):183S, 1986.
26. Naccarelli, GV, et al: Amiodarone: Pharmacology and antiarrhythmic and adverse effects. Pharmacotherapy 5:298, 1985.
27. Nattel, S: Comparative mechanisms of action of antiarrhythmic drugs. Am J Cardiol 72:F13, 1993.
28. Nygaard, TW, et al: Adverse reactions to antiarrhythmic drugs during therapy for ventricular arrhythmias. JAMA 256:55, 1986.
29. Podrid, PJ: Safety and toxicity of antiarrhythmic drug therapy: Benefit versus risk. J Cardiovasc Pharmacol 17(suppl 6):S65, 1991.
30. Podrid, PJ: Aggravation of arrhythmia: A complication of antiarrhythmic drug therapy. Eur Heart J 10(suppl E):66, 1989.
31. Podrid, PJ: Can antiarrhythmic drugs cause arrhythmias? J Clin Pharmacol 24:313, 1984.
32. Pritchett, ELC: Drug therapy: Management of atrial fibrillation. N Engl J Med 326:1264, 1992.
33. Scheidt, S: Beta-blockage for angina and arrhythmias: An overview. Drugs 25(suppl 2):153, 1983.
34. Scheinman, MM: Treatment of cardiac arrhythmias in patients with acute myocardial infarction. Am J Surg 145:707, 1983.
35. Schwartz, A: Molecular and cellular aspects of calcium channel antagonism. Am J Cardiol 70:6F, 1992.
36. Schwartz, A and Triggle, DJ: Cellular action of calcium channel blocking drugs. Annu Rev Med 35:325, 1987.
37. Smith, WM: Mechanisms of cardiac arrhythmias and conduction disturbances. In Hurst, JW (ed): The Heart, Arteries and Veins, ed 7. McGraw-Hill, New York, 1990.
38. Surawicz, B: The interrelationship of electrolyte abnormalities and arrhythmias. In Mandel, WJ (ed): Cardiac Arrhythmias: Their Mechanisms, Diagnosis and Management. JB Lippincott, Philadelphia, 1987.
39. Teo, KK, Yusuf, S, and Furberg, CD: Effects of prophylactic antiarrhythmic drug therapy in acute myocardial infarction: An overview of results from randomized controlled trials. JAMA 270:1589, 1993.
40. Williams, EMV: Classifying antiarrhythmic actions: By facts or speculation. J Clin Pharmacol 32:964, 1992.
41. Wit, AL: Cellular electrophysiologic mechanisms of cardiac arrhythmias. Ann NY Acad Sci 432:1, 1984.
42. Wit, AL and Coromilas, J: Role of alterations in refractoriness and conduction in the genesis of reentrant arrhythmias. Am J Cardiol 72:3F, 1993.
43. Woosley, RL: Antiarrhythmic drugs. Annu Rev Pharmacol Toxicol 31:427, 1991.
44. Yeh, S-J, et al: Effects of oral diltiazem in paroxysmal supraventricular tachycardia. Am J Cardiol 52:271, 1983.
45. Zipes, DP and Jalife, J (eds): Cardiac Electrophysiology: From Cell to Bedside. WB Saunders, Philadelphia, 1990.

CHAPTER 24

Treatment of Congestive Heart Failure

Congestive heart failure is a chronic condition in which the heart is unable to pump a sufficient quantity of blood to meet the needs of peripheral tissues.[29] Essentially, the pumping ability of the heart has been compromised by some form of myocardial disease of dysfunction. The congestive aspect of heart failure arises from the tendency for fluid to accumulate in peripheral tissues because of the inability of the heart to maintain proper circulation. The pathophysiology of congestive heart failure is fairly complex; the possible causes and mechanisms of heart failure are addressed in more detail in "Pathophysiology of Congestive Heart Failure."

The primary symptoms associated with congestive heart failure are peripheral edema and a decreased tolerance for physical activity.[29] Dyspnea and shortness of breath are also common, especially if the left heart is failing and pulmonary congestion is present (see the next section). In severe cases, cyanosis is present because the heart cannot deliver oxygen to peripheral tissues.

Congestive heart failure represents one of the major illnesses present in industrialized nations.[23,54] In the United States, approximately 2 million physician office visits and 2 percent of all hospital admissions each year are for the treatment of congestive heart failure.[39] Also, this disease is associated with serious consequences, and the prognosis for congestive heart failure is often poor.[51] Approximately 34 to 48 percent of patients with severe congestive heart failure die within 1 year.[45]

Consequently, the effective treatment of congestive heart failure is a critical and challenging task. Pharmacotherapy represents one of the primary methods of treatment in congestive heart failure, and the drugs discussed in this chapter play a vital role in the optimal management of this disease. As with other cardiac problems, the prevalence of congestive heart failure necessitates that members of the health-care community be aware of the pharmacologic management of this disease. Rehabilitation specialists will often treat patients with heart failure, and therapists should be cognizant of the drugs used to treat this problem.

PATHOPHYSIOLOGY OF CONGESTIVE HEART FAILURE

Vicious Cycle of Heart Failure

The mechanisms underlying chronic heart failure are complex and may include biochemical disturbances in the cardiac cell, altered genetic expression of myocardial proteins, and systemic changes in hemodynamic and neurohormonal factors.[30] Heart failure also tends to be self-perpetuating because an aberration in cardiac function often initiates a vicious cycle that leads to further decrements in cardiac function.[18,55] Figure 24–1 illustrates the way in which such a vicious cycle might be generated by the interaction of cardiac and neurohumoral factors. The sequence of events depicted in Figure 24–1 is discussed briefly here.

1. *Decreased cardiac performance:* Any number of factors that affect cardiac pumping ability may be responsible for initiating a change in myocardial performance. Factors such as ischemic heart disease, myocardial infarction, valve dysfunction, and

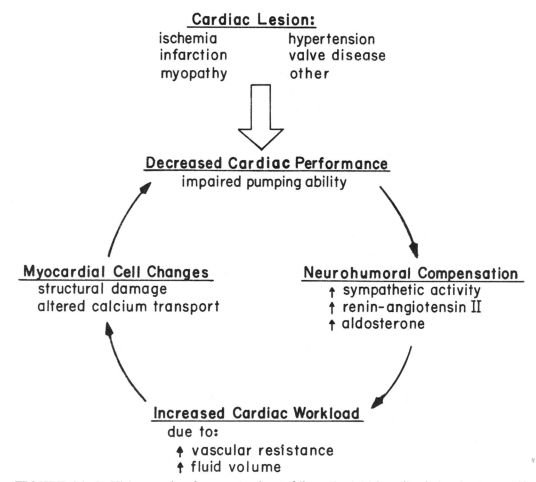

FIGURE 24–1. Vicious cycle of congestive heart failure. An initial cardiac lesion begins a self-perpetuating decrease in myocardial performance.

hypertension may all compromise the pumping ability of the heart. Also, cardiomyopathy may result from other diseases and infections.

2. *Neurohumoral compensations:* The body responds to the decreased cardiac pumping ability in a number of ways. In the early stages of failure, the heart itself often compensates by an increase in contractility and myocardial hypertrophy. As heart failure becomes more pronounced, cardiac output decreases and the peripheral tissues begin to be deprived of adequate oxygen delivery. As a result, several important compensatory changes in neural and hormonal control of cardiac function occur. A general increase in sympathetic nervous system activity often occurs. Increased sympathetic drive and increased circulating catecholamines stimulate the heart and constrict visceral and cutaneous blood vessels.[17] The renin-angiotensin system is activated, and increased secretion of aldosterone and antidiuretic hormone occurs.

3. *Increased cardiac workload:* The neurohormonal changes described previously contribute to peripheral vasoconstriction, as well as a general increase in sodium and water retention. This places additional strain on the heart by increasing cardiac preload (the volume of blood returning to the heart) and cardiac afterload (the pressure that the heart must pump against).

4. *Changes in myocardial cell function:* The increased workload on the heart leads to or exaggerates alterations in cell function. Increased cardiac workload may lead to further structural damage to the already compromised myocardial cell.[30,55] Also, studies on the molecular basis of heart failure have suggested that alterations in calcium transport, energy production/utilization, and beta receptor density may occur.[30,45] Continued stress on the heart may exacerbate these changes, leading to more cellular dysfunction. Increased dysfunction on the cellular level results in a further decrease in cardiac performance, thus completing the cycle shown in Figure 24–1.

The changes in cardiac function described previously represent a simplification of the interaction of central and peripheral factors in congestive heart failure. This description does, however, illustrate the primary problems that occur in this disease, as well as the manner in which heart failure tends to be self-perpetuating.

Congestion in Left and Right Heart Failure

The primary problem in heart failure is that the heart is unable to push blood forward through the circulatory system, thus causing pressure to build up in the veins that return blood to the heart. In effect, blood begins to back up in the venous system, increasing the pressure gradient for fluid to move out of the capillary beds. The net movement of fluid out of the capillaries causes the edema or congestion typically found in advanced stages of heart failure.

Although heart disease commonly affects the entire myocardium, congestive heart failure is sometimes divided into left and right heart failure (Fig. 24–2). In *left heart failure,* the left atrium and ventricle are unable to adequately handle the blood returning from the lungs. This causes pressure to build up in the pulmonary veins, and fluid accumulates in the lungs. Consequently, left heart failure is associated with pulmonary edema (see Fig. 24–2A). In *right heart failure,* the right atrium and ventricle are unable to handle blood returning from the systemic circulation. This causes fluid to accumulate in the peripheral tissues, and ankle edema and organ congestion (liver, spleen) are typical manifestations of right heart failure (see Fig. 24–2B). If both left and right heart failure occur simultaneously, congestion is found in the lungs as well as the periphery.

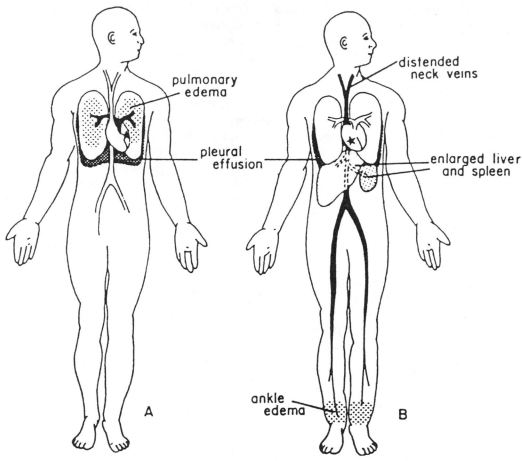

FIGURE 24–2. Effects of congestive heart failure. (*A*) Left-sided heart failure results primarily in pulmonary edema. (*B*) Right-sided heart failure results in peripheral edema (swollen ankles, enlarged organs). (From Kent, TH and Hart, MN: Introduction to Human Disease, ed 2. Appleton-Century-Crofts, Norwalk, 1987, p 141, with permission.)

PHARMACOTHERAPY

One of the basic goals in congestive heart failure is to improve the pumping ability of the heart. Drug administration should selectively increase cardiac contractile performance and produce what is referred to as a *positive inotropic effect*. "Inotropic" refers to the force of muscular contraction, and the primary drugs used to exert a positive inotropic effect are the cardiac glycosides such as digitalis. In addition to increasing cardiac contractility, drugs that decrease cardiac workload through an effect on peripheral vascular tone and fluid volume are recognized as beneficial in congestive heart failure. Included in this group are the diuretics and angiotensin-converting enzyme inhibitors. Other drugs that either directly increase myocardial performance or decrease cardiac workload have also been used to treat congestive heart failure. The primary drug groups used to treat congestive heart failure are listed in Table 24–1. The mechanism of action and specific agents within each group are presented here.

TABLE 24–1 Primary Drugs Used in Congestive Heart Failure

Drug Group	Primary Effect
Digitalis glycosides	Increase cardiac pumping ability
Deslanoside	
Digitoxin	
Digoxin	
Diuretics	Decrease vascular fluid volume
Thiazides, loop diuretics, and so on	
Angiotensin-converting enzyme inhibitors	Prevent angiotensin-induced vasoconstriction; limit aldosterone secretion
Benazepril	
Captopril	
Enalapril	
Lisinopril	
Quinapril	
Ramipril	
Others	
Amrinone, milrinone	Increase myocardial contractility
Dopamine, dobutamine	Increase myocardial contractility
Vasodilators	Decrease peripheral vascular resistance

DIGITALIS

The cardiac glycosides are a group of drugs consisting of digitalis, digoxin, digitoxin, and several other similar agents (Table 24–2). For simplicity, the term "digitalis" is often used to represent these drugs. Although the widespread use of digitalis has been questioned somewhat,[37] digitalis continues to be one of the primary drugs used to treat congestive heart failure.[13,21,33] There is little doubt that digitalis improves cardiac pumping ability in a number of patients, but the efficacy of this drug varies greatly, depending on the individual patient and underlying cardiac problem.[6,35,41,57] Also, the use of digitalis is limited to some extent by the toxic effects of this drug.[25,37,40]

The current consensus is that digitalis is a useful drug when used cautiously and specifically in certain cases of congestive heart failure, rather than as a panacea for all forms of this disease.[6,13,41,44] Also, other agents including diuretics, angiotensin-converting enzyme (ACE) inhibitors, and vasodilators (see the respective headings later in this chapter) are often used in combination with digitalis to provide better clinical effects than can be achieved using digitalis alone.

TABLE 24–2 Digitalis Glycosides

Generic Name	Trade Name	Dosage*
Deslanoside	Cedilanid-D	*Digitalization:* IV, 1.6 mg
		Maintenance: Switch to an orally active glycoside
Digitoxin	Crystodigin	*Digitalization:* Oral 0.6 mg initially, 0.4 mg after 4–6 hr, 0.2 mg after another 4–6 hr
		Maintenance: 0.05–0.3 mg once per day
Digoxin	Lanoxin	*Digitalization:* Oral, total of 0.75–1.25 mg divided into 2 or more doses with each dose given every 6–8 hr
		Maintenance: 0.125–0.5 mg once per day

*"Digitalization" represents an initial, loading dose. Maintenance doses are usually only 10–35% of the loading dose, and maintenance doses are typically given orally.

Effects and Mechanism of Action

Mechanical Effects. Digitalis and the other cardiac glycosides increase the mechanical pumping ability of the heart by bringing about an increase in intracellular calcium concentration. Increased intracellular calcium enhances contractility by facilitating the interaction between thick and thin filaments in the myocardial cell.[47] Digitalis probably increases intracellular calcium concentration by several mechanisms that are illustrated in Figure 24–3. Digitalis exerts its primary effect on calcium concentration by inhibiting the sodium-potassium pump on the myocardial cell membrane.[25,26,42] The sodium-potassium pump is an active transport system that normally transports sodium out of the cell and potassium into it. Inhibition of the sodium-potassium pump causes sodium to accumulate within the cell, which then facilitates an increase in intracellular calcium through an effect on the sodium-calcium exchange mechanism (part *1a* of Fig. 24–3).[47] Although the details of this exchange mechanism are complex, increased intracellular sodium basically causes intracellular calcium to increase by directly enhancing calcium entry into the cardiac cell and/or by decreasing calcium extrusion from the cardiac cell.[47] Digitalis may also increase intracellular calcium concentration by increasing calcium entry through membrane calcium channels

FIGURE 24–3. Proposed mechanism of digitalis action on the sarcomere located within the myocardial cell. Digitalis inhibits the Na, K-ATPase (*1*) resulting in increased intracellular sodium (Na). Increased intracellular sodium alters the Na, Ca exchange mechanism (*1a*) so that intracellular Ca also increases. Digitalis may also directly increase intracellular calcium by opening membrane Ca channels (*2*) and by increasing Ca release from the sarcoplasmic reticulum (*3*). The combined effects of these actions causes increased intracellular Ca, which facilitates contractile protein-binding, resulting in increased myocardial contractility. (From Katzung and Parmley,[31] p 179, with permission.)

(Fig. 24–3, part 2) and by increasing calcium release from the sarcoplasmic reticulum (Fig. 24–3, part 3).[31]

Electrophysiologic Effects. In addition to its effects on cardiac contractility, digitalis also improves some electrophysiologic properties of cardiac tissues.[26] Therapeutic levels of digitalis generally stabilize heart rate and slow impulse conduction through the myocardium. In fact, digitalis is used to prevent and treat certain arrhythmias such as atrial tachycardia and atrial fibrillation. Some of these electrical properties are caused by the direct effect of digitalis on the sodium-potassium pump and can be attributed to alterations in sodium, potassium, and calcium fluxes. Digitalis also indirectly affects cardiac electrical function by causing reflex stimulation of the vagus nerve, thus further slowing heart rate and conduction.[26] The electrical properties of digitalis generally complement the mechanical effects of this drug in treating congestive heart failure.

Adverse Side Effects

Digitalis toxicity is a fairly common and potentially fatal side effect. The exact incidence of digitalis toxicity is difficult to determine,[38] but may be as high as 20 to 25 percent in hospitalized patients taking this drug.[26,40] Common signs of toxicity include gastrointestinal distress (nausea, vomiting, diarrhea), and CNS disturbances (drowsiness, fatigue, confusion, visual disturbances). Because digitalis alters the electrophysiologic properties of the heart, abnormalities in cardiac function are also common during digitalis toxicity. Common adverse cardiac effects include arrhythmias such as premature atrial and ventricular contractions, paroxysmal atrial tachycardia, ventricular tachycardia, and high degrees of atrioventricular block. As toxicity increases, severe arrhythmias such as ventricular fibrillation can occur and may result in death.

To prevent digitalis toxicity, drug dosage should be maintained as low as possible. Plasma levels of digitalis should be monitored in suspected cases of toxicity to determine an appropriate decrease in dosage.[4] Health-care personnel should also be encouraged to look for early signs of toxicity so that digitalis can be discontinued before these effects become life-threatening.

DIURETICS

Diuretics increase the excretion of sodium and water. These agents are useful in congestive heart failure primarily because of their ability to decrease vascular fluid volume, thus decreasing the amount of fluid the heart must pump (cardiac preload).[45,56] Diuretics are often used alone in the early stages of heart failure, or later they are combined with digitalis. Diuretic drugs are also used to treat hypertension, and are discussed in more detail in Chapter 21. Diuretics that can be used in the treatment of congestive heart failure and hypertension are listed in Chapter 21, Table 21–3.

Effects and Mechanism of Action

Diuretics all work by inhibiting the reabsorption of sodium from the nephron, which, in turn, decreases the amount of water that is normally reabsorbed with sodium, thus increasing water excretion. Less water in the vascular system decreases cardiac preload, thereby decreasing the workload on the heart. Chapter 21 provides a more detailed discussion on the mechanism of action of diuretic drugs.

Adverse Side Effects

By the very nature of their action, diuretics are often associated with disturbances in fluid and electrolyte balance. Volume depletion, hyponatremia, hypokalemia, and altered pH balance are among the most frequently seen problems.[45,50,56] These electrolyte and pH changes can produce serious consequences by affecting cardiac excitability and precipitating arrhythmias. Patients on diuretics should be monitored closely for symptoms such as fatigue, confusion, and nausea, which may indicate the presence of drug-induced disturbances in fluid/electrolyte balance.

ANGIOTENSIN-CONVERTING ENZYME INHIBITORS

Angiotensin-converting enzyme (ACE) inhibitors have been used successfully to treat hypertension (see Chapter 21) and continue to gain acceptance as beneficial agents in congestive heart failure.[8,34] As discussed previously in this chapter, the renin-angiotensin system is often activated in congestive heart failure. ACE inhibitors interrupt this system and help decrease morbidity and mortality in patients with congestive heart failure by improving the patient's neurohormonal and hemodynamic function.[19,36,43,48,49,52,53] The ACE inhibitors commonly used in congestive heart failure include captopril (Capoten), enalapril (Vasotec), and several similar drugs listed in Table 24–1. In severe congestive heart failure, these drugs are often given in combination with diuretics and digitalis.

Effects and Mechanism of Action

As discussed in Chapter 21, ACE inhibitors suppress the enzyme that converts angiotensin I to angiotensin II in the bloodstream. Angiotensin II is a potent vasoconstrictor. By inhibiting the formation of angiotensin II, ACE inhibitors limit peripheral vasoconstriction. This effect results in a decrease in cardiac workload primarily by decreasing the pressure against which the heart must pump (cardiac afterload).[5,9,22] Decreased cardiac afterload eases the strain on the failing heart, resulting in improved cardiac performance and increased exercise tolerance.[22,46]

By directly inhibiting angiotensin II formation, ACE inhibitors also inhibit aldosterone secretion. Angiotensin II stimulates aldosterone secretion from the adrenal cortex (actually it is probably a by-product of angiotensin II—that is, angiotensin III, which directly stimulates aldosterone secretion). Aldosterone increases renal sodium reabsorption, with a subsequent increase in water reabsorption (i.e., the exact opposite effect produced by a diuretic). Inhibition of aldosterone secretion is beneficial in congestive heart failure in that vascular fluid volume does not increase and overtax the failing heart.[43] Consequently, ACE inhibitors may help decrease cardiac workload in congestive heart failure by both hemodynamic mechanisms (prevention of vasoconstriction by angiotensin II) as well as by fluid/electrolyte mechanisms (inhibition of aldosterone secretion).

Adverse Side Effects

Serious adverse effects with ACE inhibitors are relatively rare. In fact, one of the primary advantages of these drugs over more toxic compounds such as digitalis is the low incidence of serious adverse effects.[1] ACE inhibitors are occasionally associated with bothersome side effects such as skin rashes, gastrointestinal discomfort, dizziness, and a persistent dry cough, but these effects are often transient or can be resolved with an adjustment in dosage.

OTHER DRUGS USED IN CONGESTIVE HEART FAILURE

Because of the problems associated with digitalis and the rather poor prognosis of heart failure even with optimal treatment, there is a continual search for safer and more effective drugs.[15] Some of the other agents found effective in congestive heart failure are briefly discussed here.

Amrinone and Milrinone

These drugs are usually described as positive inotropic agents because they increase myocardial contractility in a relatively selective manner.[16,32] Amrinone and milrinone exert their effects by inhibiting the phosphodiesterase enzyme that breaks down cyclic adenosine monophosphate (cyclic AMP) in cardiac cells. Cyclic AMP is a common second messenger in many cells (see Chapter 4), and drugs that inhibit the phosphodiesterase enzyme allow cyclic AMP concentrations to increase in the cell.[7,14,27] In cardiac cells, cyclic AMP acts on membrane calcium channels to allow more calcium to enter the cell.[12,27] Thus, amrinone and milrinone cause a cyclic AMP–mediated increase in intracellular calcium that subsequently increases the force of contraction within the myocardial cell. These drugs also have some vasodilating properties, and some of their beneficial effects in congestive heart failure may be because of their ability to decrease cardiac preload and afterload.[12,27]

Amrinone and milrinone must be administered parenterally by intravenous infusion; hence they are usually limited to the short-term treatment of patients with severe congestive heart failure. These drugs can, however, be especially helpful in improving cardiac function until a more lasting treatment can be instituted.[2,3]

Dopamine and Dobutamine

Dopamine and dobutamine are sometimes used to stimulate the heart in cases of acute heart failure (see Chapter 20). These drugs have also been used on a limited basis to treat congestive heart failure. Dopamine and dobutamine exert a fairly specific positive inotropic effect, presumably through their ability to stimulate beta-1 receptors on the myocardium.[16] Other beta-1 agonists (epinephrine, prenalterol, etc.) will also increase myocardial contractility, but most of these other beta-1 agonists also increase heart rate or have other side effects that prevent their use in congestive heart failure. Dopamine and dobutamine are usually reserved for patients with advanced cases of congestive heart failure who fail to respond to more conventional drugs (e.g., digitalis and diuretics).

Vasodilators

Drugs that vasodilate peripheral vessels have been used successfully in cases of severe congestive heart failure.[10,45] Such drugs include prazosin, hydralazine, minoxidil, and organic nitrates (e.g., nitroglycerin). Prazosin produces vasodilation by blocking alpha-1 receptors on vascular smooth muscle (see Chapter 20), and hydralazine, minoxidil, and organic nitrates produce vasodilation by a direct effect on the vascular smooth-muscle cells (see Chapters 21 and 22). Although these vasodilators work by different mechanisms, all can decrease cardiac workload by decreasing peripheral vascular resistance. These drugs may be combined with other agents (digoxin, ACE inhibitors) to provide optimal benefits in patients with varying degrees of congestive heart failure.[11,52,57]

SUMMARY OF DRUG THERAPY

Digitalis remains a mainstay in the treatment of congestive heart failure. Digitalis, however, is associated with a number of serious side effects, and there is considerable doubt whether digitalis actually increases the rate of survival of patients with congestive heart failure.[20,21] The use of digitalis in the early stages of failure has been replaced to some extent by drugs that decrease cardiac workload such as the diuretics and ACE inhibitors.[24] Digitalis is often added to these other agents as heart failure becomes more pronounced. Vasodilators (prazosin, hydralazine, organic nitrates) have also been used to decrease the workload on the failing heart, especially in the advanced stages of failure.[28] Regardless of which drugs are used, there is consensus that early intervention in the treatment of congestive heart failure is crucial in providing the best outcome in this disease.[20,51]

SPECIAL CONCERNS IN REHABILITATION PATIENTS

Therapists should be aware of the potential for drugs used to treat congestive heart failure to affect the patient's welfare and response to therapy. Acute congestive heart failure may occur in patients with myocardial disease because of a lack of therapeutic drug effects or because of the toxic effects of some cardiac drugs. Therapists should be alert for signs of acute congestive heart failure such as increased dyspnea, rales, cough, and frothy sputum. Therapists should also be alert for signs of digitalis toxicity such as dizziness, confusion, nausea, and arrhythmias. Early recognition by the therapist may prevent serious or even fatal consequences. Likewise, patients taking diuretics sometimes exhibit excessive fatigue and weakness as early signs of fluid and electrolyte depletion. Therapists may help detect serious metabolic and electrolyte imbalances that result from problems with diuretic drugs. Finally, use of vasodilators often causes hypotension and postural hypotension. Therapists must use caution when patients sit up or stand up suddenly. Also, therapeutic techniques that produce systemic vasodilation (whirlpool, exercise) may produce profound hypotension in patients taking vasodilators, and these modalities should therefore be used cautiously.

CASE STUDY

CONGESTIVE HEART FAILURE

Brief History. D.S. is a 67-year-old woman with a long history of congestive heart failure caused by myocarditis. She has been treated successfully with digitalis glycosides (digoxin, 0.5 mg/day) for several years. Despite some swelling in her ankles and feet and a tendency to become winded, she has maintained a fairly active lifestyle and enjoys gardening and other hobbies. Recently, she developed some weakness and incoordination that primarily affected her right side. Subsequent testing revealed that she had suffered a cerebral vascular accident. She was not admitted to the hospital but remained living at home with her husband. Physical therapy, however, was provided in the home to facilitate optimal recovery from her stroke. The therapist began seeing her three times each week for a program of therapeutic exercise and functional training.

Problem/Influence of Medication. The therapist initially found this patient to be alert, coherent, and eager to begin therapy. Although there was some residual weakness and decreased motor skills, the prognosis for a full recovery appeared good. The therapist was impressed by the patient's enthusiasm and pleasant nature during the first two sessions. By the end of the first week, however, the therapist noted a distinct change in the patient's demeanor. She was confused and quite lethargic. The therapist initially suspected that she might have had another stroke. Physical examination did not reveal any dramatic decrease in strength or coordination, however. Realizing that the patient was still taking digitalis for the treatment of heart failure, the therapist began to suspect the possibility of digitalis toxicity.

Decision/Solution. The therapist immediately notified the physician about the change in the patient's status. The patient was admitted to the hospital, where a blood test confirmed the presence of digitalis toxicity (i.e., blood levels of digitalis were well above the therapeutic range). Apparently, the stroke had sufficiently altered the metabolism and excretion of the digitalis so that the dose that was therapeutic prior to the stroke was now accumulating in the patient's body. The altered pharmacokinetic profile was probably caused in part by the decrease in the patient's mobility and level of activity that occurred after the stroke. The digitalis dosage was reduced, and a diuretic was added to provide management of the congestive heart failure. The patient was soon discharged from the hospital and resumed physical therapy at home. Her rehabilitation progressed without further incident.

SUMMARY

Congestive heart failure is a serious cardiac condition in which the ability of the heart to pump blood becomes progressively worse. Decreased myocardial performance leads to a number of deleterious changes including peripheral edema (i.e., congestion) and increased fatigue during physical activity. Treatment of congestive heart failure consists primarily of drug therapy. Certain drugs such as digitalis and other positive inotropic agents attempt to directly increase cardiac pumping ability. Other drugs such as diuretics, vasodilators, and ACE inhibitors decrease cardiac workload by decreasing vascular fluid volume or dilating peripheral blood vessels. Even with optimal treatment, however, the prognosis for patients with congestive heart failure is often poor. Therapists should be aware of the drugs used to treat this disorder, and that certain side effects may adversely affect rehabilitation or signal a problem with drug treatment.

REFERENCES

1. Alicandri, C, et al: Comparison of captopril and digoxin in mild to moderate heart failure. Postgrad Med 62(suppl 1):170, 1986.
2. Anderson, JL: Hemodynamic and clinical benefits with intravenous milrinone in severe congestive heart failure: Results of a multicenter study in the United States. Am Heart J 121:1956, 1991.
3. Anderson, JL, et al: Efficacy and safety of sustained (48 hour) intravenous infusion of milrinone in patients with severe congestive heart failure: A multicenter study. J Am Coll Cardiol 9:711, 1987.
4. Aronson, JK and Hardman, M: ABC of monitoring drug therapy: Digoxin. Br Med J 305:1149, 1992.
5. Batin, P, et al: Cardiac hemodynamic effects of the non-peptide, angiotensin II–receptor antagonist, DuP-753, in conscious Long Evans and Brattleboro rats. Br J Pharmacol 103:1585, 1991.
6. Braunwald, E: Effects of digitalis on the normal and the failing heart. J Am Coll Cardiol 5:51A, 1985.
7. Brown, L, Nabauer, M, and Erdmann, E: The positive inotropic response to milrinone in isolated human and guinea pig myocardium. Naunyn-Schmied Arch Pharmacol 334:196, 1986.
8. Chobanian, V and Warren, JV (eds): Symposium: Update on the clinical utility of converting enzyme inhibitors in cardiovascular disease. Am J Med 81(suppl 4c):1, 1986.
9. Cleland, JGF, et al: Captopril in heart failure: A double-blind controlled study. Br Heart J 52:530, 1984.
10. Cohn, JN, et al: Effect of vasodilator therapy on mortality in chronic congestive heart failure: Results of a veteran's administration cooperative study. N Engl J Med 314:1547, 1986.
11. Cohn, JN, et al: A comparison of enalapril with hydralazine–isosorbide dinitrate in the treatment of congestive heart failure. N Engl J Med 325:303, 1991.
12. Colucci, WS: Cardiovascular effects of milrinone. Am Heart J 121:1945, 1991.
13. Doherty, JE: Clinical use of digitalis glycosides. An update. Cardiology 72:225, 1985.
14. Endoh, M, et al: Effects of new inotropic agents on cyclic nucleotide metabolism and calcium transients in canine ventricle muscle. Circulation 73:120, 1986.
15. Erhardt, PW: In search of the digitalis replacement. J Med Chem 30:231, 1987.
16. Farah, AE, Alousi, AA, and Schwarz, RP: Positive inotropic agents. Annu Rev Pharmacol Toxicol 24:275, 1984.
17. Ferguson, DW: Sympathetic mechanisms in heart failure: Pathophysiological and pharmacological implications. Circulation 87(suppl 7):68, 1993.
18. Francis, GS and Cohn, JN: The autonomic nervous system in congestive heart failure. Annu Rev Med 37:235, 1986.
19. Francis, GS, Cohn, JN, and Johnson, G: Plasma norepinephrine, plasma renin activity, and congestive heart failure: Relations to survival and effects of therapy in V-HeFT II. Circulation 87(suppl 6):VI-40, 1993.
20. Furberg, CD, Yusuf, S, and Thom, TJ: Potential for altering the natural history of CHF: Need for large clinical trials. Am J Cardiol 55:45A, 1985.
21. Gheorghiade, M and Zarowitz, BJ: Review of randomized trials of digoxin therapy in patients with chronic heart failure. Am J Cardiol 69:G48, 1992.
22. Giles, T: Enalapril in the treatment of congestive heart failure. J Cardiovasc Pharmacol 15(suppl 3):S6, 1990.
23. Goldman, L: Cost-effectiveness perspectives in congestive heart disease. Am Heart J 119:733, 1990.

24. Guyatt, GH: The treatment of heart failure: A methodological review of the literature. Drugs 32:538, 1986.
25. Haustein, K-O: Cardiotoxicity of digitalis. Arch Toxicol 59(suppl 9):197, 1986.
26. Hoffman, BF and Bigger, JT: Digitalis and allied cardiac glycosides. In Gilman, AG, et al (eds): The Pharmacological Basis of Therapeutics, ed 8. Pergamon Press, New York, 1990.
27. Honerjager, P: Pharmacology of bipyridine phosphodiesterase III inhibitors. Am Heart J 121:1939, 1991.
28. Horwitz, LD: Congestive heart failure: An overview of drug therapy. Postgrad Med 76:187, 1984.
29. Jennings, RB, Steenbergen, C, and Hackel, DB: The heart. In Rubin, E and Farber, JL (eds): Pathology, ed 2. JB Lippincott, Philadelphia, 1994.
30. Katz, AM: Heart failure. In Fozzard, HA, et al (eds): The Heart and Cardiovascular System, Scientific Foundations, Vol 1, ed 2. Raven Press, New York, 1991.
31. Katzung, BG and Parmley, WW: Cardiac glycosides and other drugs used in congestive heart failure. In Katzung, BG (ed): Basic and Clinical Pharmacology, ed 5. Appleton & Lange, Norwalk, CT, 1992.
32. Kubo, SH, et al: Acute dose range study of milrinone in congestive heart failure. Am J Cardiol 55:726, 1985.
33. Kulick, DL and Rahimtoola, SH: Current role of digitalis therapy in patients with congestive heart failure. JAMA 265:2995, 1991.
34. Laragh, JH (ed): Symposium: Converting enzyme inhibition for understanding and management of hypertensive disorders and congestive heart failure. Am J Med 77(suppl 2a):1, 1984.
35. Lee, DCS, et al: Heart failure in outpatients: A randomized trial of digoxin versus placebo. N Engl J Med 306:699, 1982.
36. Levine, TB, Olivari, MT, and Cohn, JN: Angiotensin converting enzyme inhibitors in congestive heart failure: Overview of comparison of captopril and enalapril. Am J Med (suppl 4c):36, 1986.
37. Levitt, B and Keefe, DL: Clinical use of digitalis materials. J Clin Pharmacol 25:507, 1985.
38. Mahdyoon, H, et al: The evolving pattern of digitalis intoxication: Observations at a large urban hospital from 1980–1988. Am Heart J 120:1189, 1990.
39. Mancini, DM, et al: Central and peripheral components of cardiac failure. Am J Med 80(suppl 2b): 2, 1986.
40. Mauskopf, JA and Wenger, TL: Cost-effectiveness analysis of the use of digoxin immune Fab(ovine) for treatment of digoxin toxicity. Am J Cardiol 68:1709, 1991.
41. Mulrow, CD, Feussner, JR, and Velez, R: Reevaluation of digitalis efficacy: New light on an old leaf. Ann Intern Med 101:113, 1984.
42. Noble, D: Mechanism of action of therapeutic levels of cardiac glycosides. Cardiovasc Res 14:495, 1980.
43. Pitt, B: Natural history of patients with congestive heart failure: Potential role of converting enzyme inhibitors in improving survival. Am J Med 8(suppl 4c):32, 1986.
44. Pugh, SE, et al: Clinical, haemodynamic, and pharmacological effects of withdrawal and reintroduction of digoxin in patients with heart failure in sinus rhythm after long term treatment. Br Heart J 61:529, 1989.
45. Remme, WJ: Congestive heart failure: Pathophysiology and medical treatment. J Cardiovasc Pharmacol 8(suppl 1):S36, 1986.
46. Riegger, GAJ: The effects of ACE inhibitors on exercise capacity in the treatment of congestive heart failure. J Cardiovasc Pharmacol 15(suppl 2):S41, 1990.
47. Siegl, PKS: Overview of cardiac inotropic mechanisms. J Cardiovasc Pharmacol 8(suppl 9):S1, 1986.
48. SOLVD Investigators: Effect of enalapril on mortality and the development of heart failure in asymptomatic patients with reduced left ventricular ejection fractions. N Engl J Med 327:685, 1992.
49. SOLVD Investigators: Effect of enalapril on survival in patients with reduced left ventricular ejection fractions and congestive heart failure. N Engl J Med 325:293, 1991.
50. Sonnenblick, M, Friedlander, Y, and Rosin, AJ: Diuretic-induced severe hyponatremia: Review and analysis of 129 reported patients. Chest 103:601, 1993.
51. Swan, HJC: Can heart failure be prevented, delayed, or reversed? Am Heart J 120:1540, 1990.
52. Swedberg, K: Reduction in mortality by pharmacological therapy in congestive heart failure. Circulation 87(suppl 4):126, 1993.
53. Sweet, CS, et al: Increased survival in rats with congestive heart failure treated with enalapril. J Cardiovasc Pharm 10:636, 1987.
54. Symposium (various authors): The costs and benefits of congestive heart disease risk factor reduction. Am Heart J 119:711, 1990.
55. Symposium (various authors): Heart failure: Adaptive and maladaptive processes. Circulation 87(suppl 7):1, 1993.
56. Taylor, SH: Diuretics in cardiovascular therapy: Pursuing the past, practicing in the present, preparing for the future. Z Kardiol 74(suppl 2):2, 1985.
57. Tisdale, JE and Gheorghiade, M: Acute hemodynamic effects of digoxin alone or in combination with other vasoactive agents in patients with congestive heart failure. Am J Cardiol 69:34G, 1992.

CHAPTER 25

Treatment of Coagulation Disorders and Hyperlipidemia

Blood coagulation, or *hemostasis*, is necessary to prevent excessive hemorrhage from damaged blood vessels. Under normal conditions, clotting factors in the bloodstream spontaneously interact with damaged vessels to create a blood clot that plugs the leaking vessel. Obviously, inadequate blood clotting is harmful since even minor vessel damage can lead to excessive blood loss. Overactive clotting is also detrimental since it will lead to *thrombogenesis* (i.e., the abnormal formation of blood clots, or thrombi). Thrombus formation may lead directly to vessel occlusion and tissue infarction. Also, a piece of a thrombus may dislodge, creating an embolism that causes infarction elsewhere in the body, for example, in the lungs or brain.

Consequently, normal hemostasis can be regarded as a balance between too much and too little blood coagulation. This balance is often disrupted by a number of factors. Inadequate clotting typically occurs because of insufficient levels of blood clotting factors, as in patients with hemophilia. Excessive clotting often occurs during prolonged bed rest or when blood flow through vessels is partially obstructed, as in coronary atherosclerosis.

Restoration of normal hemostasis is accomplished through pharmacologic methods. Excessive clotting and thrombus formation are rectified by drugs that prevent clot formation (anticoagulants, antithrombotics) or facilitate the removal of previously formed clots (*thrombolytics*). Inadequate clotting is resolved by replacing the missing clotting factors or by drugs that facilitate the synthesis of specific clotting factors.

Hemostasis can also be influenced by *hyperlipidemia*, which is a chronic and excessive increase in plasma lipids. Hyperlipidemia causes cholesterol and other lipids to be progressively deposited onto arterial walls, forming plaquelike lesions indicative of atherosclerosis. These atherosclerotic lesions progressively occlude the arterial lumen, thus leading to thrombosis and infarction. Atherosclerotic heart disease is one of the leading causes of morbidity and mortality in the United States, and pharmacologic methods to lower plasma lipids are often used in conjunction with dietary and lifestyle modifications to help treat hyperlipidemia and prevent atherosclerosis.

Drugs used to normalize blood clotting or reduce hyperlipidemia are among the

348

most common medications used clinically, and rehabilitation specialists will deal with many patients taking these agents. Many patients, in fact, will be treated in therapy for problems relating directly to thrombus formation (e.g., stroke, myocardial infarction, pulmonary embolism). Individuals with inadequate clotting, such as patients with hemophilia, are also seen routinely in rehabilitation because of the intrajoint hemorrhaging and other problems associated with this disease. Consequently, the purpose of this chapter is to acquaint therapists with several common and important groups of drugs used to treat coagulation disorders and hyperlipidemia.

NORMAL MECHANISM OF BLOOD COAGULATION

To understand how various drugs affect hemostasis, a review of the normal way in which blood clots are formed and broken down is necessary. The physiologic mechanisms involved in hemostasis are outlined in Figure 25–1, with clot formation and breakdown illustrated in the upper and lower parts of this figure, respectively.

Clot Formation

Clot formation involves the activation of various clotting factors that are circulating in the bloodstream.[19] These clotting factors are proteolytic enzymes synthesized in the liver that remain in an inactive form until there is some injury to a blood vessel. Blood vessel damage begins a cascade effect whereby the activation of one of the clotting factors leads to the activation of the next factor, and so forth.[19] As shown in Figure 25–1, clot formation occurs through two systems, an intrinsic and an extrinsic system. In the intrinsic system, the direct contact of the first clotting factor (factor XII) with the damaged vessel wall activates the clotting factor and initiates the cascade. In the extrinsic system, some substance, known as *tissue thromboplastin*, is released from the damaged vascular cell. Tissue thromboplastin directly activates clotting factor VII, which then activates subsequent factors in the clotting mechanism. For optimal coagulation to occur in vivo, both the intrinsic and extrinsic systems must be present.

Both the intrinsic and extrinsic systems ultimately lead to the conversion of prothrombin to thrombin. *Thrombin* is an enzyme that quickly converts the inactive fibrinogen molecule to *fibrin*. Individual strands of fibrin bind together to form a mesh-like structure, which ultimately forms the framework for the blood clot. Other cellular components, especially platelets, help reinforce the clot by sticking to the fibrin mesh.

Clot Breakdown

The breakdown of blood clots is illustrated in the lower part of Figure 25–1. *Tissue plasminogen activator* (t-PA) converts plasminogen to plasmin. *Plasmin*, also known as fibrinolysin, is an enzyme that directly breaks down the fibrin mesh, thus destroying the clot.

The balance between clot formation and breakdown is crucial in maintaining normal hemostasis. Obviously, clots should not be broken down as quickly as they are formed because then no coagulation will occur. Likewise, a lack of breakdown would enable clots to proliferate at an excessive rate, leading to thrombus formation.

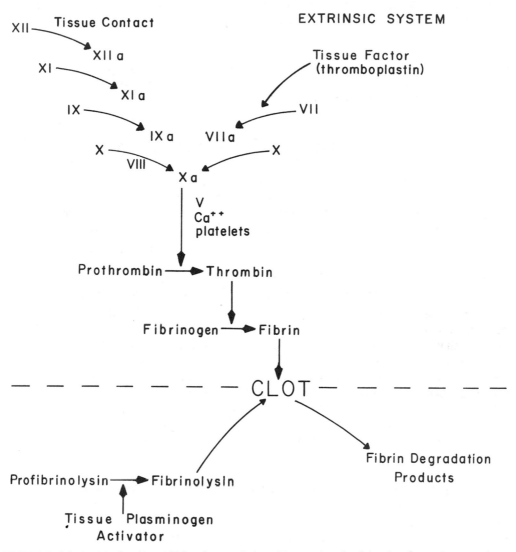

FIGURE 25–1. Mechanism of blood coagulation. Factors involved in clot formation are shown above the dashed line; factors involved in clot breakdown are shown below the dashed line. See text for further discussion.

DRUGS USED TO TREAT OVERACTIVE CLOTTING

Drugs used to treat excessive clot formation can be grouped into three primary categories: anticoagulant, antithrombotic, and thrombolytic agents (Table 25–1). Anti-coagulants exert their effect by controlling the function and synthesis of clotting factors, and these drugs are used primarily to prevent clot formation in the venous system, that is, venous thrombosis. Antithrombotic drugs act primarily by inhibiting platelet function, and these drugs primarily prevent thrombus formation in arteries. Thrombolytic drugs facilitate the destruction of blood clots, and these drugs are used to re-establish blood flow through vessels that have been occluded by thrombi. Specific agents discussed here are listed in Table 25–1.

Anticoagulants

The primary anticoagulants are heparin and a group of orally acting agents including warfarin (Coumadin) and other coumarin derivatives. These drugs are used primarily in the treatment of abnormal clot formation in the venous system. Venous clots typically form in the deep veins of the legs because of the relatively sluggish blood flow through those vessels. Hence, deep vein thrombosis is a primary indication for anticoagulant therapy.[5,28,34] Deep vein thrombosis results in thromboembolism when a piece of the clot breaks off and travels through the circulation to lodge elsewhere in the vascular system. Emboli originating in the venous system typically follow the venous flow back to the right side of the heart, where they are then pumped to the lungs. They finally lodge in the smaller vessels within the lungs, thus creating a pulmonary embolism.[5] Consequently, pulmonary embolism secondary to venous thrombosis is often the pathologic condition that initiates anticoagulant therapy.[31]

Anticoagulant drugs are administered for the acute treatment of venous thrombosis and thromboembolism, or they may be given prophylactically to individuals who are at high risk to develop venous thrombosis. For instance, these drugs are often administered after mechanical heart valve replacement, or following hip surgery and similar situations where patients will be relatively inactive for extended periods of time. Specific anticoagulant drugs are presented here.

HEPARIN

Heparin is usually the primary drug used in the initial treatment of venous thrombosis.[30] The anticoagulant effects of heparin are seen almost instantly after administration. Heparin works by potentiating the activity of a circulating protein

TABLE 25–1 Drugs Used to Treat Overactive Clotting

Drug Category	Primary Effect and Indication
Anticoagulants 　Heparin (Calciparine; Liquaemin) 　Oral anticoagulants 　　Anisindione (Miradon) 　　Dicumarol (generic) 　　Warfarin (Coumadin, Panwarfin)	Inhibit synthesis and function of clotting factors; used primarily to prevent and treat venous thromboembolism
Antithrombotics 　Aspirin 　Dipyridamole (Dipridacot, Persantine) 　Sulfinpyrazone (Anturane)	Inhibit platelet aggregation and platelet-induced clotting; used primarily to prevent arterial thrombus formation
Thrombolytics 　Anistreplase (Eminase) 　Streptokinase (Kabikinase, Streptase) 　Tissue plasminogen activator (t-PA) 　Urokinase (Abbokinase)	Facilitate clot dissolution; used to reopen occluded vessels in arterial and venous thrombosis

known as *antithrombin III.*[9,24] Antithrombin III binds to several of the active clotting factors (including thrombin) and renders the clotting factors inactive. Heparin accelerates the antithrombin III–induced inactivation of these clotting factors, thus reducing the tendency for clotting and thrombogenesis.

Heparin is a large, sugarlike molecule that is poorly absorbed from the gastrointestinal tract. Consequently, heparin must be administered parenterally. Heparin is often given by intravenous infusion or by repeated IV injection through a rubber-capped indwelling needle called a *heparin lock*. Subcutaneous or intrafat injection may also be used, and this route is preferred if heparin must be administered for relatively prolonged periods.[33,35,58] Subcutaneous administration of a specific form of heparin known as *low-molecular-weight heparin* (LMWH) has been advocated recently because this method provides anticoagulant effects similar to traditional (intravenous) administration, but subcutaneous LMWH may be somewhat safer because it causes less bleeding.[22] Subcutaneous administration of LMWH is also easier and more convenient than intravenous administration, which is advantageous for people who are being treated at home or as outpatients.[33]

ORAL ANTICOAGULANTS

Drugs that are structurally and functionally similar to dicumarol constitute a group of orally active anticoagulant agents (see Table 25–1). The primary drug in this group is warfarin. These drugs exert their anticoagulant effects by impairing the hepatic synthesis of several clotting factors.[50,68] The specific mechanism of coumarin drugs is illustrated in Figure 25–2. In the liver, vitamin K acts as a catalyst in the final step of the synthesis of clotting factors II, VII, IX, and X. In the process, vitamin K is oxidized to an altered form known as vitamin K epoxide. For the process to continue,

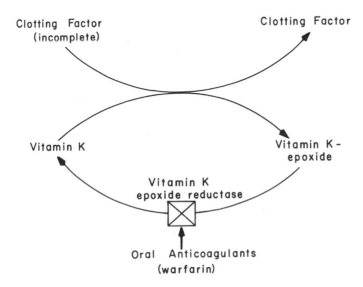

FIGURE 25–2. Role of vitamin K in the synthesis of vitamin K–dependent clotting factors (II, VII, IX, and X). Vitamin K catalyzes the reaction necessary for completion of clotting factor synthesis, but it is oxidized in the process to vitamin K epoxide. Regeneration of vitamin K occurs via vitamin K epoxide reductase. Oral anticoagulants such as warfarin (Coumadin) block the regeneration of the vitamin K, thus halting the further synthesis of the vitamin K–dependent factors.

vitamin K epoxide must be reduced to its original form. As shown in Figure 25–2, coumarin drugs block the conversion of vitamin K epoxide to vitamin K, thus impairing the synthesis of several clotting factors. With time, a decrease in the level of circulating clotting factors results in a decrease in blood coagulation and in thrombogenesis.

Unlike heparin, coumarin drugs can be administered orally. However, because of the nature of their action, there is often a lag time of several days before an anticoagulant effect is appreciated, because several days are required before the decreased production of clotting factors is sufficient to interrupt the clotting cascade. Consequently, anticoagulant therapy often begins with parenteral administration of heparin followed by oral administration of coumarin drugs. Heparin is administered for the first few days to achieve an immediate effect. Coumarin drugs are then initiated, and heparin is discontinued after the coumarin drugs have had time to exert their anticoagulant effect. Oral administration of coumarin drugs may then be continued for several weeks to several months following an incident of thrombosis.[32,64]

Antithrombotic Drugs

Whereas anticoagulants affect the synthesis and function of clotting factors, antithrombotics primarily inhibit the function of platelets.[13,20,51] In the bloodstream, platelets respond to vascular injury by changing their shape and adhering to one another (aggregation) at the site of clot formation. Platelets may sometimes aggregate inappropriately, however, thus forming a thrombus and occluding certain blood vessels. In particular, arterial thrombi are often formed by abnormal platelet aggregation. Hence, the antithrombotic drugs are used primarily to prevent the formation of arterial clots, such as those that cause coronary artery occlusion or cerebral infarction.

ASPIRIN

Aspirin suppresses platelet aggregation by inhibiting the synthesis of prostaglandins and thromboxanes.[20] As discussed in Chapter 15, aspirin exerts virtually all of its effects by inhibiting the cyclooxygenase enzyme that initiates the synthesis of lipidlike hormones known as prostaglandins and thromboxanes. Certain prostaglandins and thromboxanes, especially thromboxane A_2, have a potent ability to induce platelet aggregation. By inhibiting the synthesis of these proaggregation substances, aspirin prevents platelet-induced thrombus formation.

Because of its antithrombotic effects, aspirin has received a great deal of attention regarding its use in preventing myocardial infarction. Long-term aspirin administration following a heart attack may prevent the occurrence of a second infarction in susceptible individuals.[3] Also, very low doses of aspirin (325 mg every other day) have been shown to decrease the incidence of an initial infarction in a population of male physicians with no previous history of myocardial infarction, stroke, or transient ischemic attacks.[67] These rather remarkable findings have prompted a great deal of debate about the chronic use of aspirin and possible side effects such as increased hemorrhage. Indeed, the study that reported a decreased incidence of initial myocardial infarction saw a slight increase in the incidence of stroke because of cerebrovascular hemorrhage.[67] Still, the possibility that aspirin may be successful in preventing coronary thrombosis and myocardial infarction is encouraging.

354 PHARMACOLOGY IN REHABILITATION

Although increasing the risk of hemorrhagic stroke, aspirin may help prevent the type of stroke caused by cerebral ischemia and infarction.[37] The rationale is that aspirin will prevent infarction in cerebral vessels in the same manner that it prevents coronary infarction in heart attacks. The benefits of aspirin in stroke remain somewhat controversial, however. Clearly, the use of aspirin must be limited to only the types of stroke that result from insufficient blood flow, as opposed to hemorrhagic stroke. Even so, the antithrombotic benefits of aspirin in some cerebral vessels must be weighed against possible side effects such as increased bleeding in other vessels. Long-term aspirin therapy is probably beneficial in a certain percentage of stroke patients, but this drug must be used selectively.[37]

Consequently, the role of chronic aspirin administration in helping to prevent myocardial and possibly cerebral infarction remains an area of intense investigation. A great deal of information remains to be determined, however. For instance, the long-term effects of aspirin on other organs such as the liver, kidneys, and gastrointestinal tract must be considered. Likewise, men appear to benefit more than women from aspirin's antithrombotic effects, and the reasons for this gender-related difference need to be determined.[45,66] Hence, continued analysis of this topic promises to be an exciting and productive area of pharmacologic research.

Finally, aspirin has also been used to prevent thromboembolism following surgical procedures such as coronary artery bypass, arterial grafts, endarterectomy, and valve replacement.[10,16,41,47] By preventing platelet-induced thrombogenesis, aspirin helps maintain patency and prevent reocclusion of vessels following these procedures.

OTHER ANTITHROMBOTIC DRUGS

Several other agents have been used to limit platelet aggregation. For the most part, these other drugs have not been proved superior to aspirin. They may, however, be used in patients where aspirin is poorly tolerated or contraindicated. The nonaspirin antiplatelet drugs currently in use are dipyridamole and sulfinpyrazone. Dipyridamole (Dipridacot, Persantine) inhibits platelet aggregation by a mechanism that is poorly understood. This drug may affect platelet function by impairing adenosine metabolism and/or by increasing the concentration of cyclic adenosine monophosphate within the platelet.[20,23] Dipyridamole, which does not appear to be effective when used alone, has traditionally been administered with aspirin or warfarin. Combining dipyridamole with aspirin, however, is not more effective than aspirin used alone, so the use of these two drugs together has essentially been discontinued. Sulfinpyrazone (Anturane) is usually administered to treat gouty arthritis but has also shown some antithrombotic properties because of an ability to decrease platelet function. Sulfinpyrazone decreases platelet aggregation by inhibiting prostaglandin synthesis in a manner similar to aspirin.[13,20] Other antithrombotic platelet inhibitors are currently being investigated and may be available in the future.

Thrombolytic Drugs

Thrombolytics facilitate the breakdown and dissolution of clots that have already formed. These drugs work by converting plasminogen (profibrinolysin) to plasmin (fibrinolysin).[62] As shown in Figure 25–1, plasmin is the active form of an endogenous enzyme that breaks down fibrin clots. Drugs that activate this enzyme by various mechanisms can be used to dissolve clots that have already formed, thus reopening occluded blood vessels.

Thrombolytic drugs have proved extremely valuable in treating acute myocardial infarction.[8,36,39,57,59,61,63,76] When administered within 3 to 6 hours after the onset of symptoms, these drugs can actually re-establish blood flow through occluded coronary vessels, often preventing or reversing myocardial damage, thus decreasing the morbidity and mortality normally associated with a heart attack.[6,27] It was originally believed that thrombolytic drugs had to be administered directly into the coronary arteries to reopen occluded coronary vessels.[2,36] Considerable evidence now indicates that these drugs may produce beneficial effects when injected intravenously into the systemic circulation; that is, the drug can be injected into any accessible vein and eventually reach the coronary clot through the general circulation.[1,11,42,55,57] The intravenous route is a much more practical method of administration because it is easier, faster, and safer than the intracoronary route.

Consequently, thrombolytic drugs offer an attractive method of preventing, or even reversing, myocardial damage during acute myocardial infarction. Not all patients will respond to thrombolytic treatment, and there are some risks involved, including an increased chance of hemorrhage.[1,48] Also, thrombolytic therapy is not curative, but it may buy time for the patient so that a more permanent procedure such as coronary angioplasty or bypass surgery can be performed.[49]

Thrombolytic drugs have also been used for vascular occlusion in other areas of the systemic circulation.[8] Atherosclerotic occlusion in lower-extremity arteries (femoral, popliteal) has been successfully treated by local (intra-arterial) administration of thrombolytic drugs.[46,54,65,69,72] Bypass grafts and shunts that have become occluded because of clot formation may be cleaned out with the use of thrombolytic drugs.[40,53] Systemic administration of these drugs may be used to treat pulmonary embolism, primarily in serious or massive cases.[15,31] Because of the risk of increased intracranial hemorrhage, these drugs are generally *not* used to treat stroke resulting from acute cerebral embolism.[48]

STREPTOKINASE AND UROKINASE

Although they work by somewhat different methods, these agents both bring about the activation of plasmin. Streptokinase indirectly activates plasmin (fibrinolysin) by binding to the precursor molecule plasminogen (profibrinolysin) and facilitating activation by endogenous mechanisms. Urokinase directly converts plasminogen to plasmin by enzymatically cleaving a peptide bond within the plasminogen molecule. Both agents have been used successfully to resolve acute clot formation in the coronary arteries and other peripheral vessels, but, when administered systemically, neither drug seems to have a distinct clinical advantage over the other. Streptokinase tends to be used more frequently, however, because this drug is much cheaper than urokinase.

TISSUE PLASMINOGEN ACTIVATOR

In the endogenous control of hemostasis, plasminogen is activated by an intrinsic substance known as *tissue plasminogen activator* (t-PA) (see Figure 25–1). Intravenous administration of t-PA rapidly and effectively initiates clot breakdown by directly activating plasmin (fibrinolysin). Although extraction of t-PA from human blood is costly and impractical, the commercial synthesis of t-PA has been made possible through the use of recombinant DNA techniques. Consequently, t-PA is now available, along with streptokinase and urokinase, as a thrombolytic agent.

Tissue plasminogen activator has been used successfully to treat acute myocardial infarction and acute pulmonary embolism.[14,21,71,73,74] Preliminary findings suggested that t-PA may also be more effective than streptokinase in reopening coronary arteries in acute myocardial infarction[70] and that t-PA may have a greater ability to dissolve only the harmful clot without impairing normal clot formation elsewhere in the body.[17,18,53,73] More recent studies, however, suggest that the thrombolytic effects of t-PA and streptokinase are basically similar,[27,75] and that t-PA may actually be associated with a slightly higher incidence of hemorrhagic side effects including stroke.[43] Hence, it is not clear at present if t-PA offers any distinct clinical advantages over streptokinase. Tissue plasminogen activator is considerably more expensive than streptokinase, so a clear advantage of t-PA still needs to be established before this drug can be considered superior to the much less expensive form of thrombolysis using streptokinase.[27]

ANISTREPLASE

Anistreplase (Eminase) is a newer thrombolytic that is also known as anisoylated plasminogen-streptokinase activator complex (APSAC). This compound is formed by combining plasminogen with streptokinase and then chemically altering (anisoylating) the catalytic site on this complex so that plasminogen remains inactive until it is administered. When administered systemically, anistreplase binds to fibrin, where it is then chemically activated so that streptokinase can modify plasminogen and initiate clot breakdown. The supposed advantage of using anistreplase is that this compound will be more selective for clots that have already formed with less effect on systemic fibrinolysis. Anistreplase does cause considerable systemic fibrinolysis, however, and the advantages of this compound over streptokinase alone remain to be determined.

Adverse Side Effects of Anticoagulant, Antithrombotic, and Thrombolytic Agents

Predictably, hemorrhage is the primary and most serious problem with drugs used to decrease blood clotting.[5] Increased bleeding is often seen with the anticoagulants (heparin, warfarin) and may be quite severe in some patients. Any unusual bleeding such as blood in the urine or stools, unexplained nosebleeds, or an unusually heavy menstrual flow may indicate a problem. Also, back pain or joint pain may be an indication of abdominal or intrajoint hemorrhage, respectively. To prevent excessive bleeding, laboratory tests that measure hemostasis are used to monitor patients taking anticoagulant drugs. Tests such as partial thromboplastin time and prothrombin time are routinely used to assess the effectiveness of drugs that alter blood coagulation, and adjustments in drug dosage are made based on whether coagulation time falls within an acceptable range.

Other adverse effects occur with specific agents. Heparin is associated with a severe decrease in platelets (thrombocytopenia) in some patients. Heparin may also cause an allergic-like reaction, especially in individuals who are hypersensitive to other substances. Oral anticoagulants (such as warfarin), as well as aspirin, may produce stomach irritation and gastrointestinal distress in some individuals. Streptokinase and anistreplase (but not urokinase or t-PA) are associated with hypersensitivity and a febrile reaction in some individuals.

TREATMENT OF CLOTTING DEFICIENCIES

Hemophilia

Hemophilia is a hereditary disease in which an individual is unable to synthesize adequate amounts of a specific clotting factor. The two most common forms of hemophilia are hemophilia A, which is caused by deficiency of clotting factor VIII, and hemophilia B, which is a deficit in clotting factor IX. In either form of this disease, patients experience a profound inability for hemostasis. Even trivial injuries can produce serious or fatal hemorrhage. Also, patients with hemophilia often develop joint problems because of intra-articular hemorrhage (hemarthrosis).

Treatment of hemophilia consists of replacing the missing clotting factor. Although this seems relatively simple, obtaining sufficient amounts of the missing factor is a very costly procedure. At the present time, the primary source of clotting factors VIII and IX is from human blood extract. Obtaining an adequate supply from this source can cost more than $25,000 per patient per year.

A more serious problem is the potential for clotting factor extract to contain viruses such as hepatitis B or HIV, which causes AIDS. The lack of proper blood screening has resulted in tragic consequences; for example, clotting factors extracted from patients infected with HIV have served as a vehicle for viral transmission to patients with hemophilia. More stringent screening procedures and other techniques such as heat treatment of clotting factor extracts have decreased the risk of AIDS transmission, but patients with hemophilia receiving exogenous factors remain at risk for viral infection. New methods of drug production, such as genetic engineering and recombinant DNA techniques, are currently being used to manufacture specific clotting factors such as factor VIII.[60] It is hoped that these techniques will provide a safer, cheaper source of missing clotting factors for patients with hemophilia.

Deficiencies of Vitamin K–Dependent Clotting Factors

Previously in this chapter, the need for vitamin K in the hepatic synthesis of clotting factors II, VII, IX, and X was noted. As shown in Figure 25–2, vitamin K catalyzes the final steps in the synthesis of these factors. Normally, vitamin K is supplied through the diet or synthesized by intestinal bacteria and subsequently absorbed from the gastrointestinal tract into the body. However, any defect in vitamin K ingestion, synthesis, or absorption may result in vitamin K deficiency. Insufficient vitamin K in the body results in an inadequate hepatic synthesis of the clotting factors listed previously, thus resulting in poor hemostasis and excessive bleeding.

Deficiencies in vitamin K and the related synthesis of the vitamin K–dependent clotting factors are treated by administering exogenous vitamin K. Various commercial forms of this vitamin are available for oral or parenteral (intramuscular or subcutaneous) administration. Specifically, individuals with a poor diet, intestinal disease, or impaired intestinal absorption may require vitamin K to maintain proper hemostasis.

Also, vitamin K is routinely administered to newborn infants to prevent hemorrhage. For the first 5 to 8 days following birth, newborns lack the intestinal bacteria necessary to help synthesize vitamin K. Vitamin K is administered to facilitate clotting factor synthesis until the newborn is able to produce sufficient endogenous vitamin K.

Antifibrinolytics

The excessive bleeding that sometimes occurs following surgery or trauma may be caused by an overactive fibrinolytic system, that is, *hyperfibrinolysis*. Hyperfibrinolysis results in excessive clot destruction and ineffective hemostasis. Likewise, patients with hemophilia who undergo surgery, including dental procedures (tooth extractions, restorations, etc.), will benefit if clot breakdown is inhibited because hemorrhage and the need for additional clotting factors will be reduced. Antifibrinolytic agents such as aminocaproic acid (Amicar) and tranexamic acid (Cyklokapron) are often used in these situations. These drugs appear to inhibit activation of plasminogen (profibrinolysin) to plasmin (fibrinolysin). Plasmin is the enzyme responsible for breaking down fibrin clots (see Fig. 25–1). Antifibrinolytics prevent the activation of this enzyme, thus preserving clot formation.

Aminocaproic acid and tranexamic acid are administered either orally or intravenously for the acute treatment of hyperfibrinolysis or to prevent clot breakdown in patients with hemophilia who are undergoing surgery. Some adverse effects such as nausea, diarrhea, dizziness, and headache may occur when these drugs are administered, but these problems are relatively minor and usually disappear when the drug is discontinued.

AGENTS USED TO TREAT HYPERLIPIDEMIA

Hyperlipidemia, an abnormally high concentration of lipids in the bloodstream, is one of the primary causes of cardiovascular disease in industrialized nations. This condition typically causes deposition of fatty plaquelike lesions on the walls of large and medium-sized arteries (*atherosclerosis*), which can lead to thrombosis and infarction. Hence, elevated plasma lipids are related to some of the events discussed previously in this chapter because atherosclerosis can precipitate increased clotting and thromboembolic disease.

Hyperlipidemia is often caused by poor diet and lifestyle as well as by several genetic conditions that cause disorders in lipid metabolism.[7,44] It is not possible to review here the endogenous control of lipid metabolism or the various pathologic processes involved in hyperlipidemia, and these topics are addressed in other sources.[7,12,44,56] It should be realized, however, that lipids such as cholesterol are transported in the bloodstream as part of a lipid-protein complex known as a *lipoprotein*. Certain lipoproteins are considered beneficial because they may decrease the formation of atherosclerotic plaques by removing cholesterol from the arterial wall. These beneficial complexes are known as high-density lipoproteins (HDL) because of the relatively large amount of protein in the complex. Other lipoproteins are considered harmful because they transport and deposit cholesterol onto the arterial wall. These atherogenic lipoproteins include intermediate-density lipoproteins (IDL), low-density lipoproteins (LDL), and very-low-density lipoproteins (VLDL). Pharmacologic and nonpharmacologic strategies to reduce hyperlipidemia typically focus on reducing these atherogenic lipoproteins and increasing the beneficial HDL.

Drugs that can be used to treat hyperlipidemia are summarized in Table 25–2 and are discussed briefly here. These agents are typically used when plasma lipid levels are not successfully controlled by nonpharmacologic methods such as low-fat diets, weight reduction, regular exercise, and smoking cessation. Likewise, these drugs should be used in conjunction with nonpharmacologic methods, and optimal results are often realized through a combination of drug therapy and various dietary and lifestyle modifications.

HMG-CoA Reductase Inhibitors

This category includes lovastatin (Mevacor), pravastatin (Pravachol), and simvastatin (Zocor). These drugs act by inhibiting an enzyme known as 3-hydroxy-3-methylglutaryl coenzyme A (HMG-CoA) reductase.[25] This enzyme catalyzes one of the early steps of cholesterol synthesis, and drugs that inhibit HMG-CoA reductase decrease cholesterol production, especially in liver cells. Decreased hepatic cholesterol biosynthesis also causes more surface receptors for LDL cholesterol to be synthesized, and this increase in surface receptors triggers an increase in the breakdown of LDL choles-

TABLE 25–2 Drugs Used to Treat Hyperlipidemia

Generic Name	Trade Name(s)	Dosage*	Primary Effect
Cholestyramine	Cholybar, Questran	4 g 1–6 times each day before meals and at bedtime	Decreases plasma LDL-cholesterol levels
Clofibrate	Abitrate, Atromid-S	1.5–2.0 g each day in 2–4 divided doses	Lowers plasma triglycerides by decreasing LDL and IDL levels
Gemfibrozil	Lopid	1.2 g each day in 2 divided doses 30 min before morning and evening meal	Similar to clofibrate
Lovastatin	Mevacor	20–80 mg each day as a single dose or in divided doses with meals	Decreases plasma LDL-cholesterol levels; may also decrease triglycerides and increase HDL somewhat
Niacin	Niacor, Nicobid, others	1–2 g 3 times each day	Lowers plasma triglycerides by decreasing VLDL levels
Pravastatin	Pravachol	10–40 mg once each day at bedtime	Similar to lovastatin
Probucol	Lorelco	500 mg 2 times each day with morning and evening meal	Decreases LDL and HDL cholesterol; may also inhibit deposition of fat into arterial wall
Simvastatin	Zocor	5–40 mg once each day in the evening	Similar to lovastatin

*Doses represent typical adult oral maintenance dose.
HDL = high-density lipoproteins; IDL = intermediate-density lipoproteins; LDL = low-density lipoproteins; VLDL = very-low-density lipoproteins.

terol and a decrease in the synthesis of VLDL, which serves as a precursor for LDL synthesis. Hence, HMG-CoA reductase inhibitors improve plasma lipid profiles by decreasing plasma LDL cholesterol and VLDL concentrations. Moderate decreases in plasma triglycerides and increases in HDL cholesterol levels have also been associated with certain agents such as lovastatin.

Fibric Acids

This category includes clofibrate (Abitrate, Atromid-S) and gemfibrozil (Lopid), and these drugs lower plasma triglyceride levels by increasing the breakdown of triglyceride-rich lipoproteins such as LDL and IDL.[26] The exact mechanism of these drugs is unclear, but they probably work by increasing the activity of the lipoprotein lipase enzyme in peripheral tissues.

Other Lipid-Lowering Agents

Several other agents have beneficial effects on plasma lipid profiles that occur through various cellular mechanisms.[12,44] Cholestyramine (Questran) attaches to bile acids within the gastrointestinal lumen and increases fecal excretion of these acids. This action leads to decreased plasma cholesterol concentrations because cholesterol breakdown is accelerated to replace the bile acids that are lost in the feces. Niacin (nicotinic acid, vitamin B_3, Niacor, Nicolar) decreases LDL synthesis by inhibiting the production of VLDL, which serves as a precursor for LDL. This effect reduces the primary lipoproteins used to transport cholesterol in the bloodstream. Probucol (Lorelco) increases LDL breakdown somewhat, and this drug may also directly inhibit the deposition of cholesterol into arterial walls. This latter effect has received considerable attention recently because this drug may directly reduce atherosclerotic plaque formation in certain individuals.

Adverse Effects of Antihyperlipidemia Agents

Most of the drugs used to treat hyperlipidemia are fairly well tolerated. Some gastrointestinal distress (nausea, diarrhea) is fairly common with most of these drugs, but these problems are usually minor and do not require that drug therapy be discontinued. Other bothersome side effects are related to specific agents. Niacin, for instance, is often associated with cutaneous vasodilation and a sensation of warmth when doses are administered, but these sensations are not usually a problem. Some fairly serious problems including liver dysfunction, gallstones, and pancreatitis can occur with many antihyperlipidemia drugs, but the incidence of these side effects is relatively rare. Other neuromuscular side effects such as myalgia, myositis, and fatigue/weakness have been occasionally noted with the HMG-CoA reductase inhibitors (lovastatin, others) and with the fibric acids (clofibrate, gemfibrozil), and paresthesias may occur with probucol. Cardiovascular problems such as arrhythmias, blood dyscrasias, and angioneurotic syndrome may occur with the fibric acids and probucol.

SPECIAL CONCERNS IN REHABILITATION PATIENTS

Therapists will frequently encounter patients taking drugs to alter hemostasis. Many patients on prolonged bed rest will have a tendency for increased thrombus formation and are particularly susceptible to deep vein thrombosis. These patients will often be given anticoagulant drugs. Heparin followed by warfarin may be administered prophylactically or in response to the symptoms of thrombophlebitis in patients who have undergone hip surgery, heart valve replacement, and so on. Therapists should be aware that the primary problem associated with anticoagulant drugs is an increased tendency for bleeding. Any rehabilitation procedures that deal with open wounds (dressing changes, debridement, etc.) should be carefully administered. Rigorous manual techniques such as deep tissue massage or chest percussion must also be used with caution since these procedures may directly traumatize tissues and induce bleeding in patients taking anticoagulant drugs.

Anticoagulants and antithrombotic drugs (e.g., aspirin) may also be given to rehabilitation patients to prevent the recurrence of myocardial infarction. As discussed previously, aspirin appears to be especially attractive in preventing an initial incident or the recurrence of infarction. Aspirin is relatively free from any serious side effects that may influence the rehabilitation session. Long-term anticoagulant and antithrombotic therapy is also frequently employed in specific cases of cerebrovascular accidents (strokes) that are due to recurrent cerebral embolism and occlusion. Obviously, giving anticoagulant and antithrombotic drugs to patients with a tendency toward the hemorrhagic type of stroke is counterproductive, because these drugs would only exacerbate this condition. However, stroke cases in which hemorrhage has been ruled out may benefit from prolonged anticoagulant or antithrombotic therapy. Again, therapists should be cognizant of the tendency for increased bleeding with these agents. However, the long-term use of these agents, especially aspirin, usually does not create any significant problems in the course of rehabilitation.

Thrombolytic drugs (streptokinase, t-PA, others) usually do not impact directly on physical therapy or occupational therapy. Thrombolytics are typically given in acute situations, immediately following myocardial infarction. Therapists may, however, benefit indirectly from the effects of these drugs because patients may recover faster and more completely from heart attacks. Thrombolytics may also help reopen occluded peripheral vessels, thus improving tissue perfusion and wound healing in rehabilitation patients.

Therapists will often work with individuals having chronic clotting deficiencies, such as patients with hemophilia. Intrajoint hemorrhage (*hemarthrosis*) with subsequent arthropathy is one of the primary problems associated with hemophilia.[4,38] The joints most often affected are the knees, ankles, and elbows.[29] Hemarthrosis is usually treated by replacing the missing clotting factor and by rehabilitating the affected joints. Therapists often employ a judicious program of exercise and cryotherapy to help improve joint function following hemarthrosis.[29,52] Consequently, the therapist often works in conjunction with pharmacologic management to help improve function in hemophiliac-related joint disorders.

Finally, therapists may help encourage patients to comply with pharmacologic and nonpharmacologic methods used to lower plasma lipids. Drugs used to treat hyperlipidemia are typically used in conjunction with diet, exercise, and other lifestyle changes that reduce fat intake and improve plasma lipid profiles. Therapists can help design and implement exercise programs that enable patients to lose weight and increase plasma levels of antiatherogenic components such as HDL, thus maximizing the effects of drug therapy.

CASE STUDY

CLOTTING DISORDERS

Brief History. C.W. is an obese, 47-year-old woman who sustained a compression fracture of the L-1 and L-2 vertebrae during a fall from a second-story window. (There was some suggestion that she may have been pushed during an argument with her husband, but the details remain unclear.) She was admitted to the hospital, where her medical condition was stabilized, and surgical procedures were performed to treat her vertebral fracture. Her injuries ultimately resulted in a partial transection of the spinal cord, with diminished motor and sensory function in both lower extremities. She began an extensive rehabilitation program, including physical therapy and occupational therapy. She was progressing well when she developed shortness of breath and an acute pain in her right thorax. A diagnosis of massive pulmonary embolism was made. Evidently she had developed deep vein thrombosis in both lower extremities, and a large embolism from the venous clots had lodged in her lungs, producing a pulmonary infarction.

Drug Treatment. Because of the extensive nature of the pulmonary infarction, a thrombolytic agent was used to attempt to resolve the clot. An initial dosage of 250,000 units of streptokinase was administered intravenously within 2 hours after the onset of symptoms. Streptokinase was continued via intravenous infusion at a rate of 100,000 units/hr for 24 hours after the initial dose.

To prevent further thromboembolism, streptokinase infusion was followed by heparin. Heparin was administered intravenously, 5000 units every 4 hours. Clotting time was monitored closely by periodic blood tests during the heparin treatment. After 3 days of heparin therapy, C.W. was switched to warfarin. Warfarin was administered orally, and the dosage was adjusted until she was ultimately receiving 5 mg/day. Oral warfarin was continued throughout the remainder of the patient's hospital stay, as well as after discharge.

Impact on Rehabilitation. The drugs used to resolve the thromboembolic episode greatly facilitated the patient's recovery from that incident. The use of a thrombolytic agent (streptokinase) enabled the patient to resume her normal course of rehabilitation within 2 days of the pulmonary embolism. Thus, the use of these drugs directly facilitated physical therapy and occupational therapy by allowing the patient to resume therapy much sooner than if the embolism had been treated more conservatively (i.e., rest and anticoagulants) or more radically (i.e., surgery). Since the patient remained on anticoagulant drugs for an extended period of time, the therapists dealing with the patient routinely looked for signs of excessive bleeding such as skin bruising and hematuria. The patient remained free from any further thromboembolic episodes, however, and was eventually discharged to an extended-care rehabilitation facility to continue her progress.

SUMMARY

Normal hemostasis is a balance between excessive and inadequate blood clotting. Overactive blood clotting is harmful because of the tendency for thrombus formation and occlusion of arteries and veins. Vessels may become directly blocked by the thrombus, or a portion of the thrombus may break off and create an embolism that lodges elsewhere in the vascular system. The tendency for excessive thrombus formation in the venous system is usually treated with anticoagulant drugs such as heparin and warfarin. Prevention of arterial thrombogenesis is often accomplished by platelet inhibitors such as aspirin. Vessels that have suddenly become occluded because of acute thrombus formation may be successfully reopened by thrombolytic drugs (streptokinase, urokinase) that facilitate the dissolution of the harmful clot.

The inadequate blood clotting and excessive bleeding that occur in patients with hemophilia are treated by replacing the missing clotting factor. Other conditions associated with inadequate coagulation may be treated by administering either vitamin K, which helps improve the synthesis of certain clotting factors, or antifibrinolytic agents (aminocaproic acid, tranexamic acid), which inhibit clot breakdown.

Hyperlipidemia can lead to atherosclerosis and subsequent cardiovascular incidents such as thrombosis and infarction. This condition is often treated by a combination of drug therapy and diet/lifestyle modifications. Pharmacologic interventions are typically targeted toward decreasing the synthesis of harmful (atherogenic) plasma components, including certain lipoproteins (IDL, LDL, VLDL) that are associated with atherosclerotic plaque formation.

REFERENCES

1. Acar, J, et al: Thrombolytic treatment in acute myocardial infarction. Semin Thromb Hemost 13:186, 1987.
2. Anderson, JL, et al: A randomized trial of intracoronary streptokinase in the treatment of acute myocardial infarction. N Engl J Med 308:1312, 1983.
3. Antiplatelet Trialists' Collaboration: Secondary prevention of vascular disease by prolonged antiplatelet therapy. Br Med J 296:320, 1988.
4. Aronstram, A, Rainsford, SG, and Painter, MJ: Patterns in bleeding in adolescents with severe hemophilia. Br Med J 17:469, 1979.
5. Baker, WF and Bick, RL: Deep vein thrombosis: Diagnosis and management. Med Clin 78:685, 1994.
6. Bell, WR: Thrombolytic therapy: Agents, indications, and laboratory monitoring. Med Clin 78:745, 1994.
7. Benditt, EP and Schwartz, SM: Blood vessels. In Rubin, E and Farber, JL (eds): Pathology, ed 2. JB Lippincott, Philadelphia, 1994.
8. Benedict, CR, et al: Thrombolytic therapy: A state of the art review. Hosp Pract 27:61, 1992.
9. Bjork, I and Lindahl, U: Mechanism of the anticoagulant action of heparin. Mol Cell Biochem 48:161, 1982.
10. Bollinger, A and Brunner, U: Antiplatelet drugs improve the patency rates after femoro-popliteal endarterectomy. Vasa 14:272, 1985.
11. Bonnier, HJRM, et al: Comparison of intravenous anisoylated plasminogen streptokinase activator complex and intracoronary streptokinase in acute myocardial infarction. Am J Cardiol 62:25, 1988.
12. Brown, MS and Goldstein, JL: Drugs used in the treatment of hyperlipoproteinemias. In Gilman, AG, et al (eds): The Pharmacological Basis of Therapeutics, ed 8. Pergamon Press, New York, 1990.
13. Buckler, P and Douglas, AS: Antithrombotic treatment. Br Med J 287:196, 1983.
14. Califf, RM, Topol, EJ, and George, BS: One-year outcome after therapy with tissue plasminogen activator: Report from the thrombolysis and angioplasty in myocardial infarction trial. Am Heart J 119:777, 1990.
15. Cella, G, Palla, A, and Sasahara, AA: Controversies of different regimens of thrombolytic therapy in acute pulmonary embolism. Semin Thromb Hemost 13:163, 1987.
16. Chesebro, JH, Steele, PM, and Fuster, V: Platelet-inhibitor therapy in cardiovascular disease. Effective defense against thromboembolism. Postgrad Med 78:48, 1985.

17. Collen, D, et al: Analysis of coagulation and fibrinolysis during intravenous infusion of recombinant human tissue-type plasminogen activator in patients with acute myocardial infarction. Circulation 73:511, 1986.
18. Collen, D, Stump, DC, and Gold, HK: Thrombolytic therapy. Annu Rev Med 39:405, 1988.
19. Furie, B and Furie, BC: Molecular and cellular biology of blood coagulation. N Engl J Med 326:800, 1992.
20. Gallus, AS: Aspirin and the other platelet-aggregation inhibiting drugs. Med J Aust 142:41, 1985.
21. Goldhaber, SZ, Markis, JE, and Kessler, GM: Perspectives on treatment of acute pulmonary embolism with tissue plasminogen activator. Semin Thromb Hemost 13:171, 1987.
22. Green, D, Chen, D, and Chmiel, JS: Prevention of thromboembolism in spinal cord injury: Role of low molecular weight heparin. Arch Phys Med Rehabil 75:290, 1994.
23. Gresele, P, et al: Mechanism of the antiplatelet action of dipyridamole in whole blood: Modulation of adenosine concentration and activity. Thromb Haemost 55:12, 1986.
24. Griffith, MJ: Heparin-catalyzed inhibitor/protease reactions: Kinetic evidence for a common mechanism of action of heparin. Proc Natl Acad Sci USA 80:5460, 1983.
25. Grundy, SM: HMG-CoA reductase inhibitors for treatment of hypercholesterolemia. N Engl J Med 319:24, 1988.
26. Grundy, SM and Vega, GL: Fibric acids: Effects on lipids and lipoprotein metabolism. Am J Med 83(suppl 5B):9, 1987.
27. GUSTO Angiographic Investigators: The effects of tissue plasminogen activator, streptokinase, or both on coronary artery patency, ventricular function, and survival after acute myocardial infarction. N Engl J Med 329:1615, 1993.
28. Hattersley, PG, Mitsuoka, JC, and King, JH: Heparin therapy for thromboembolic disorders: A prospective evaluation of 134 cases monitored by active coagulation time. JAMA 250:1413, 1983.
29. Helske, T, et al: Joint involvement in patients with severe haemophilia A in 1957–59 and 1978–79. Br J Haematol 51:643, 1982.
30. Hirsh, J: Drug therapy: Heparin. N Engl J Med 324:1565, 1991.
31. Hirsh, J: Treatment of pulmonary embolism. Annu Rev Med 38:91, 1987.
32. Holmgren, K, et al: One-month versus six-month therapy with oral anticoagulants after symptomatic deep vein thrombosis. Acta Med Scand 218:279, 1985.
33. Hull, RD, Raskob, GE, and Pineo, GF: Subcutaneous low-molecular-weight heparin compared with continuous intravenous heparin in the treatment of proximal-vein thrombosis. N Engl J Med 326:975, 1992.
34. Hull, RD, et al: A comparison of low-molecular-weight heparin with warfarin sodium for prophylaxis against deep-vein thrombosis after hip or knee implantation. N Engl J Med 329:1370, 1993.
35. Kakkar, VV, et al: Antithrombin III and heparin. Lancet I:103, 1980.
36. Kennedy, JW, et al: Western Washington randomized trial of intra-coronary streptokinase in acute myocardial infarction. N Engl J Med 309:1477, 1983.
37. Kistler, JP, Ropper, AH, and Heros, RC: Medical progress: Therapy of ischemic cerebral vascular disease due to atherothrombosis. N Engl J Med 311:27,100, 1984.
38. Koch, B, et al: Hemophiliac knee: Rehabilitation techniques. Arch Phys Med Rehabil 63:379, 1982.
39. Laffel, GL and Braunwald, E: Thrombolytic therapy: A new strategy of the treatment of acute myocardial infarction. N Engl J Med 311:710, 770, 1984.
40. LeBlanc, JG, et al: Treatment of grafts and major vessel thrombosis with low-dose streptokinase in children. Ann Thorac Surg 41:630, 1986.
41. Lorenz, RL, et al: Improved aortocoronary bypass patency by low-dose aspirin (100 mg daily): Effects on platelet aggregation and thromboxane formation. Lancet I:1261, 1984.
42. Losman, JG, et al: Myocardial surgical revascularization after streptokinase treatment for acute myocardial infarction. J Thorac Cardiovasc Surg 89:25, 1985.
43. Maggioni, AP, et al: The risk of stroke in patients with acute myocardial infarction after thrombolytic and antithrombotic treatment. N Engl J Med 327:1, 1992.
44. Malloy, MJ and Kane, JP: Agents used in hyperlipidemia. In Katzung, BG (ed): Basic and Clinical Pharmacology, ed 5. Appleton & Lange, Norwalk, CT, 1992.
45. Manson, JE, et al: A prospective study of aspirin use and primary prevention of cardiovascular disease in women. JAMA 266:521, 1991.
46. McNamara, TO: Role of thrombolysis in peripheral arterial occlusion. Am J Med 83(suppl 2a):6, 1987.
47. Meister, W, et al: Low-dose acetylsalicylic acid (100 mg/day) after aortocoronary bypass surgery: A placebo-controlled trial. Br J Clin Pharmacol 17:703, 1984.
48. O'Connor, CM, et al: Stroke and acute myocardial infarction in the thrombolytic era: Clinical correlates and long-term prognosis. J Am Coll Cardiol 16:533, 1990.
49. O'Neill, W, et al: A prospective randomized trial of intracoronary streptokinase versus coronary angioplasty for acute myocardial infarction. N Engl J Med 314:812, 1986.
50. O'Reilly, RA: Vitamin K and the oral anticoagulant drugs. Annu Rev Med 27:245, 1976.
51. Patrono, C: Drug therapy: Aspirin as an antiplatelet drug. N Engl J Med 330:1287, 1994.
52. Pelletier, JR, Findlay, TW, and Gemma, SA: Isometric exercise for an individual with hemophiliac arthropathy. Phys Ther 67:1359, 1987.
53. Risius, B, et al: Recombinant human tissue-type plasminogen activator for thrombolysis in peripheral arteries and bypass grafts. Radiology 160:183, 1986.

54. Rodriguez, RL, et al: Selective management of arterial occlusion with low-dose streptokinase. Am J Surg 151:343, 1986.
55. Rogers, WJ, et al: Prospective randomized trial of intravenous and intracoronary streptokinase in acute myocardial infarction. Circulation 68:1051, 1983.
56. Ross, R: The pathogenesis of atherosclerosis: An update. N Engl J Med 314:488, 1986.
57. Rovelli, F, et al: Effectiveness of intravenous thrombolytic treatment in acute myocardial infarction. Lancet I:397, 1986.
58. Salzman, EW: Progress in preventing venous thromboembolism. N Engl J Med 309:980, 1983.
59. Schreiber, T: Review of clinical studies of thrombolytic agents in acute myocardial infarction. Am J Med 83(suppl 2a):20, 1987.
60. Schwartz, RS, et al: Human recombinant DNA-derived antihemophiliac factor (factor VIII) in the treatment of hemophilia A. N Engl J Med 323:1800, 1990.
61. Sherry, S: Appraisal of various thrombolytic agents in the treatment of acute myocardial infarction. Am J Med 83(suppl 2a):31, 1987.
62. Sherry, S and Gustafson, E: The current and future use of thrombolytic therapy. Annu Rev Pharmacol Toxicol 25:413, 1985.
63. Sherry, S and Solomon, HA (eds): Symposium: Thrombolytic therapy in cardiovascular diseases. Am J Med 83(suppl 2a):1, 1987.
64. Smith, P, Arnesen, H, and Holme, I: The effect of warfarin on mortality and reinfarction after myocardial infarction. N Engl J Med 323:147, 1990.
65. Sniderman, KW, et al: Low-dose fibrinolytic therapy for recent lower extremity thromboembolism. J Can Assoc Radiol 40:98, 1989.
66. Spranger, M, Aspey, BS, and Harrison, MJG: Sex differences in antithrombotic effect of aspirin. Stroke 20:34, 1989.
67. Steering Committee of the Physicians' Health Study Research Group: Preliminary report: Findings from the aspirin component of the on-going physicians' health study. N Engl J Med 318:262, 1988.
68. Suttie, JW: Warfarin and vitamin K. Clin Cardiol 13(suppl VI):16, 1990.
69. Taylor, LM, et al: Intra-arterial streptokinase infusion for acute popliteal and tibial artery occlusion. Am J Surg 147:583, 1984.
70. TIMI Study Group: The thrombolysis in myocardial infarction (TIMI) trial. N Engl J Med 312:932, 1985.
71. Topol, EJ, Bell, WR, and Weisfeldt, ML: Coronary thrombolysis with recombinant tissue-type plasminogen-activator: A hematological and pharmacological study. Ann Intern Med 103:837, 1985.
72. Verhaeghe, R, Wilms, G, and Vermylen, J: Local low-dose thrombolysis in arterial disease of the limbs. Semin Thromb Hemost 13:206, 1987.
73. Verstraete, M, et al: Randomized trial of intravenous recombinant tissue-type plasminogen activator versus intravenous streptokinase in acute myocardial infarction. Lancet I:842, 1985.
74. Verstraete, M, et al: Double-blind randomized trial of intravenous tissue-type plasminogen activator versus placebo in acute myocardial infarction. Lancet II:965, 1985.
75. White, HD, et al: Effect of intravenous streptokinase as compared with that of tissue plasminogen activator on left ventricular function after first myocardial infarction. N Engl J Med 320:817, 1989.
76. Yusuf, S, et al: Intravenous and intracoronary fibrinolytic therapy in acute myocardial infarction: Overview on results of mortality, reinfarction and side effects from 33 randomized controlled trials. Eur Heart J 6:556, 1985.

SECTION VI

Respiratory and Gastrointestinal Pharmacology

CHAPTER 26

Respiratory Drugs

The respiratory system is responsible for mediating gas exchange between the external environment and the bloodstream. The upper respiratory tract conducts air to the lower respiratory passages and ultimately to the lungs. The upper respiratory tract also humidifies and conditions inspired air, and serves to protect the lungs from harmful substances. In the lungs, gas exchange takes place between the alveoli and the pulmonary circulation.

The drugs discussed in this chapter are directed primarily at maintaining proper airflow through the respiratory passages. Agents that treat specific problems in the lungs themselves are not discussed here, but are covered in other areas of this text. For instance, drugs used to treat infectious diseases of the lower respiratory tract and lungs are presented in Section VIII (Chapters 33 to 35).

The respiratory agents presented here are divided into two primary categories. The first group includes drugs that treat acute and relatively minor problems such as nasal congestion, coughing, and seasonal **allergies**. The second category includes drugs that treat more chronic and serious airway obstructions such as bronchial asthma, chronic bronchitis, and emphysema. Physical therapists and occupational therapists will frequently treat patients with both acute and chronic respiratory conditions. Consequently, the overview of the drugs presented in this chapter should be of interest to rehabilitation specialists.

DRUGS USED TO TREAT RESPIRATORY TRACT IRRITATION AND CONTROL RESPIRATORY SECRETIONS

The drugs presented here are used to treat symptomatic coughing and irritation resulting from problems such as the common cold, seasonal allergies, and upper respiratory tract infections. Many of these drugs are found in over-the-counter preparations. Often, several different agents are combined in the same commercial preparation; for example, a decongestant, an antitussive, and an expectorant may be combined and identified by a specific trade name. Also, agents within a specific category may have some properties that overlap into other drug categories. Certain antihistamines, for instance, may also have antitussive properties.

TABLE 26–1 Common Antitussive Agents

Generic Name	Trade Name(s)*	Method of Action
Benzonatate	Tessalon	Local anesthetic effect on respiratory mucosa
Caramiphen	Tuss-Ornade	Antihistamine
Codeine	Many trade names	Inhibits cough reflex by direct effect on brainstem cough center
Dextromethorphan	Many trade names	Similar to codeine
Diphenhydramine	Benadryl (others)	Antihistamine
Hydrocodone	Hycodan, Hycomine, Triaminic Expectorant DH, many others	Similar to codeine

*Trade names often reflect combination of the antitussive with other agents (i.e., expectorants, decongestants).

Antitussives

Antitussive drugs are used to suppress coughing that is associated with the common cold and other minor throat irritations. When used to treat cold and flu symptoms, these drugs are often combined with aspirin or acetaminophen, as well as with other respiratory tract agents. Antitussives are usually recommended only for short-term use in relieving symptomatic coughing.

Some of the commonly used antitussives are listed in Table 26–1. As shown in the table, codeine and similar opiate derivatives suppress the cough reflex by a central inhibitory effect. Other nonopioid antitussives work by inhibiting the irritant effects of histamine on the respiratory mucosa, or by a local anesthetic action on the respiratory epithelium. The primary adverse effect associated with most antitussives is sedation. Dizziness and gastrointestinal upset may also occur with antitussive use.

Decongestants

Congestion within and mucosal discharge of the upper respiratory tract are familiar symptoms of many conditions. Allergies, the common cold, and various respiratory infections often produce a runny nose and stuffy head sensation. Decongestants used to treat these symptoms are usually alpha-1–adrenergic agonists (see Chapter 20).[40] These agents bind to alpha-1 receptors located on the blood vessels of the nasal mucosa and stimulate vasoconstriction, thus effectively drying up the mucosal vasculature and decreasing local congestion in the nasal passages.

Alpha-1 agonists used as decongestants are listed in Table 26–2. Depending on the preparation, these agents may be taken systemically or applied locally to the nasal mucosa via aerosol sprays. The primary adverse effects associated with decongestants are headache, dizziness, nervousness, nausea, and cardiovascular irregularities (increased blood pressure, palpitations). These adverse effects become more apparent during prolonged or excessive use of these drugs.[40]

TABLE 26–2 Common Nasal Decongestants

Generic Name	Trade Name(s)*	Dosage Forms
Ephedrine	Primatene Tablets	Oral
Epinephrine	Primatene Mist, others	Nasal spray
Naphazoline	Privine	Nasal spray
Oxymetazoline	Afrin, Neo-Synephrine 12 hour	Nasal spray
Phenylephrine	Neo-Synephrine, others	Nasal spray
Phenylpropanolamine	Propagest, Triaminic, others	Oral
Pseudoephedrine	Actifed, Sudafed, many others	Oral
Tetrahydrozoline	Tyzine	Nasal Spray
Xylometazoline	Otrivin	Nasal Spray

*Trade names often reflect combination of the decongestant with other ingredients.

Antihistamines

Antihistamines are used for a number of diverse reasons, ranging from sedation to the treatment of parkinsonism. One of the most common applications of antihistamines, however, is the treatment of the respiratory allergic response to seasonal allergies such as hay fever (hence their inclusion in this chapter).

Histamine is an endogenous chemical that is involved in the normal regulation of certain physiologic functions (gastric secretion, CNS neural modulation), as well as various hypersensitivity (allergic) reactions.[18] Histamine exerts its effects on various cells through two primary receptor subtypes: the H_1 and H_2 receptors.[18,69] H_1 receptors are located on several tissues including vascular, respiratory, and gastrointestinal smooth muscle. H_2 receptors are involved primarily in the regulation of gastric acid secretion. By definition, antihistamines are drugs that specifically block the H_1 subtype of histamine receptors. Drugs that selectively block the H_2 receptor (referred to simply as H_2 antagonists) may help control gastric secretion in conditions such as peptic ulcer; these drugs are discussed in Chapter 27. A third receptor subtype, the H_3 receptor, has also been identified, and this subtype may be involved in the local regulation of histamine release from CNS nerve terminals.[1] The clinical and pharmacologic significance of H_3 receptors remains to be fully determined, however.

Antihistamines used in the symptomatic treatment of hay fever and similar allergies are listed in Table 26–3. By blocking the effects of histamine on the upper respiratory tissues, these drugs help decrease the nasal congestion, mucosal irritation and discharge (rhinitis, sinusitis), and conjunctivitis caused by inhaled allergens.[33,51] Similarly, antihistamines may decrease the coughing and sneezing associated with the common cold. In general, these drugs do not prevent the inflammation-induced bronchospasm associated with asthma (see "Treatment of Bronchial Asthma"). Antihistamines may, however, be used occasionally as an adjunct in patients with asthma to help control rhinitis and sinusitis.

The primary adverse effects associated with antihistamines are sedation, fatigue, dizziness, blurred vision, and incoordination. Gastrointestinal distress (nausea, vomiting) is also quite common. Sedation, which is often the primary side effect that limits the use of certain antihistamines, occurs because these drugs cross the blood-brain barrier. Newer antihistamines such as astemizole (Hismanal), loratadine (Claritin), and terfenadine (Seldane) do not cross the blood-brain barrier, and these drugs provide pe-

TABLE 26–3 Antihistamines

Generic Name	Trade Name(s)	Dosage*	Sedation Potential[†]
Astemizole	Hismanal	10 mg once a day	Low
Azatadine	Optimine	1–2 mg every 8–12 hr	Low
Brompheniramine	Bromphen, Dimetane, others	4 mg every 4–6 hr	Low
Carbinoxamine	Clistin	4–8 mg every 6–8 hr	Low to moderate
Cetirizine	Reactine	5–10 mg once a day	Low
Chlorpheniramine	Chlor-Trimeton, Phenetron, others	4 mg every 4–6 hr	Low
Clemastine	Tavist	1.34 mg twice daily or 2.68 mg 1–3 times daily	Low
Cyproheptadine	Periactin	4 mg every 6–8 hr	Moderate
Dexchlorpheniramine	Polaramine	2 mg every 4–6 hr	Low
Dimenhydrinate	Dramamine, others	50–100 mg every 4 hr	High
Diphenhydramine	Allerdryl, Benadryl, others	25–50 mg every 4–6 hr	High
Diphenylpyraline	Hispril	5 mg every 12 hr	High
Doxylamine	Unisom Nighttime Sleep-Aid	12.5–25 mg every 4–6 hr	High
Hydroxyzine	Atarax, others	25–100 mg 3–4 times a day	Moderate
Loratadine	Claritin	10 mg once a day	Low
Phenindamine	Nolahist	25 mg every 4–6 hr	Low
Pyrilamine	Nisaval	25–50 mg every 8 hr	Moderate
Terfenadine	Seldane	60 mg every 8–12 hr	Low
Tripelennamine	PBZ	25–50 mg every 4–6 hr	Moderate
Triprolidine	Actidil, others	2.5 mg every 6–8 hr	Low

*Normal adult dosage when taken orally for antihistamine effects.
[†]Sedation potential is based on comparison to other antihistamines and may vary considerably from person to person.

riphcral antihistaminergic effects without producing excessive sedation. Several other antihistamines that do not cross the blood-brain barrier are currently under development, and it is hoped that these agents will be available in prescription and over-the-counter preparations in the future.[40]

Mucolytics and Expectorants

Mucolytic drugs attempt to decrease the viscosity of respiratory secretions. **Expectorant** drugs facilitate the production and ejection of mucus. These drugs are used to prevent the accumulation of thick, viscous secretions that can clog respiratory passages and lead to pulmonary problems. Expectorants and mucolytics are used in acute disorders ranging from the common cold to pneumonia, as well as in chronic disorders such as emphysema and chronic bronchitis. These drugs are often used in combination with other agents (e.g., antitussives, decongestants, bronchodilators). Although mucolytics and expectorants are widely used, whether they have specific pharmacologic effects on respiratory secretion remain doubtful. That is, they may not offer any added advantage over inhalation of humidified air or aerosol saline preparations.[66]

The primary mucolytic drug currently in use is acetylcysteine (Mucomyst, Mucosil). This drug is believed to work by splitting the disulfide bonds of respiratory mucoproteins, thus forming a less viscous secretion. Acetylcysteine is usually administered directly to the respiratory mucosa by inhalation or by intratracheal instillation (through a tracheostomy). The primary adverse effects associated with this drug include nausea, vomiting, inflammation of the oral mucosa (stomatitis), and rhinorrhea. Serious adverse effects are relatively rare, however.

Several expectorant agents have been used in the past, but only guaifenesin is currently acknowledged by the FDA to have evidence of therapeutic effects.[39] This drug is administered to increase the production of respiratory secretions, thus encouraging ejection of phlegm and sputum. Exactly how guaifenesin exerts this effect, however, is not fully understood. Guaifenesin, which is usually administered orally in some form of syrup or elixir, is often combined with other agents in over-the-counter preparations, which are known by many different trade names. The primary adverse effect associated with guaifenesin is gastrointestinal upset, which is exacerbated if excessive doses are taken or if this drug is taken on an empty stomach.

DRUGS USED TO MAINTAIN AIRWAY PATENCY IN OBSTRUCTIVE PULMONARY DISEASE

Airway obstruction is a major problem in respiratory disorders such as bronchial asthma, chronic bronchitis, and emphysema. The latter two disorders are usually grouped under the heading of *chronic obstructive pulmonary disease* (COPD).[59,60] Asthma and COPD are characterized by bronchospasm, airway inflammation, and mucous plugging of the airways.[15,36,44,59] One of the primary goals of drug treatment is to prevent or reverse the bronchial constriction and subsequent obstruction of the airways in these disorders by using bronchodilators (beta-adrenergic agonists, xanthine derivatives, anticholinergics) and anti-inflammatory agents (corticosteroids, cromolyn sodium). These agents are discussed in the next section.

Beta-Adrenergic Agonists

RATIONALE FOR USE AND MECHANISM OF ACTION

Respiratory smooth-muscle cells contain the beta-2 subtype of adrenergic receptors.[29,52] (See Chapter 18 for a discussion of adrenergic receptor classifications.) Stimulation of these beta-2 receptors results in relaxation of bronchiole smooth muscle. Hence, drugs that stimulate these beta-2 adrenergic receptors (i.e., beta-adrenergic agonists) produce bronchodilation and can be used to prevent or inhibit airway obstruction during bronchospastic attacks.[7,15,19,33,56]

Beta-adrenergic agonists are believed to induce smooth-muscle relaxation by the mechanism illustrated in Figure 26–1. As shown in the figure, stimulation of the beta-2 receptor increases activity of the adenyl cyclase enzyme. This enzyme increases the production of intracellular cyclic adenosine monophosphate (cAMP). The cAMP acts as an intracellular second messenger, which then increases the activity of other enzymes such as protein kinase. The increased protein kinase activity ultimately inhibits smooth-muscle contraction, probably by adding a phosphate group to specific contractile proteins.

FIGURE 26–1. Mechanism of action of beta agonists on respiratory smooth muscle. Beta agonists facilitate bronchodilation by stimulating adenyl cyclase activity, which in turn increases intracellular cyclic AMP production. Cyclic AMP activates protein kinase, which appears to add an inhibitory phosphate group to contractile proteins, thus causing muscle relaxation and bronchodilation.

SPECIFIC AGENTS AND METHOD OF ADMINISTRATION

Beta-adrenergic agonists that are used to induce bronchodilation are listed in Table 26–4. As shown in Table 26–4, some drugs are nonselective and stimulate alpha and beta receptors fairly equally. Other agonists are more selective and preferentially stimulate the beta-adrenergic receptors. Finally, the beta-2–specific agents are the most selective and tend to bind preferentially to beta-2 receptors. These beta-2–selective agonists offer an advantage when administered systemically because there is less chance of side effects caused by stimulation of other adrenergic receptors located on other tissues (e.g., beta-1 receptors on the myocardium). When administered via inhalation, however, the issue of adrenergic receptor selectivity becomes less important because the drug is applied directly to the respiratory tissues that primarily contain the beta-2 subtype.[52]

Beta-adrenergic drugs can be administered orally, subcutaneously, or by inhalation. Inhalation of these drugs is often the preferred method of administration in treating respiratory disorders. Inhalation allows the drug to be delivered directly to the respiratory tissues, with a minimum of systemic side effects because of absorption into the systemic circulation. The onset of action is also more rapid with inhalation. Oral or subcutaneous administration is usually associated with more side effects. Beta ago-

TABLE 26–4 Beta-Adrenergic Bronchodilators

Drug	Primary Receptor	Route of Administration	Onset of Action (min)	Time to Peak Effect	Duration of Action (hr)
Albuterol	Beta-2	Inhalation	5–15	1–1.5	3–6
		Oral	15–30	2–3	8 or more
Bitolterol	Beta-2	Inhalation	3–4	0.5–1	5–8
Ephedrine	Alpha, beta-1,2	Oral	15–60	—	3–5
		Intramuscular	10–20	—	0.5–1
		Subcutaneous	—	—	0.5–1
Epinephrine	Alpha, beta-1,2	Inhalation	3–5	—	1–3
		Intramuscular	Variable	0.3	<1–4
		Subcutaneous	6–15	—	<1–4
Ethylnorepinephrine	Beta-1,2	Intramuscular	6–12	—	1–2
		Subcutaneous	6–12	—	1–2
Fenoterol	Beta-2	Inhalation	5	0.5–1	2–3
		Oral	30–60	2–3	6–8
Isoetharine	Beta-2	Inhalation	1–6	0.25–1	1–4
Isoproterenol	Beta-1,2	Inhalation	2–5	—	0.5–2
		Intravenous	Immediate	—	<1
		Sublingual	15–30	—	1–2
Metaproterenol	Beta-2	Inhalation (aerosol)	Within 1	1	1–5
		Oral	Within 15–30	Within 1	Up to 4
Pirbuterol	Beta-2	Inhalation	Within 5	0.5–1	5
Procaterol	Beta-2	Inhalation	Within 5	1.5	6–8
Terbutaline	Beta-2	Inhalation	15–30	1–2	3–6
		Oral	Within 60–120	Within 2–3	4–8
		Parenteral	Within 15	Within 0.5–1	1.5–4

nists, however, may reach the more distal branches of the airway to a greater extent when administered orally or subcutaneously rather than by inhalation. This fact makes sense when one considers that the bronchioles are usually constricted during an asthmatic attack, and the drug may simply not reach the distal respiratory passages when administered by inhalation.

When given by inhalation, several beta agonists are available in metered dose inhalers (MDIs). MDIs contain the drug in a small aerosol canister, and a specific amount of the drug is dispensed each time the patient depresses the canister.[26] Although MDIs are convenient because of their small size and portability, there is a certain amount of coördination required on the part of the patient to ensure adequate delivery of the drug. Some patients (e.g., young children) may have trouble timing the inhaled dose with a proper inspiratory effort. In these patients, drug delivery can be facilitated using a spacer or reservoir-like attachment that sequesters the drug between the MDI and the patient's mouth.[26] The patient can first dispense the drug into the reservoir and then take a deep breath, thus improving delivery to the respiratory tissues. The other primary method of inhaling beta agonists is through a *nebulizer*. These devices are not portable and must be used in the home. They are much easier to use, however, and administer the drug over a more prolonged period of time (10 minutes), which allows better delivery to the more distal bronchioles.[4]

ADVERSE SIDE EFFECTS

With prolonged or excessive use, inhaled adrenergic agonists may cause bronchial irritation. Other side effects depend on the relative selectivity and route of administration of specific agents. Adrenergic agonists that also stimulate beta-1 receptors may cause cardiac irregularities if they reach the myocardium through the systemic circulation. Similarly, stimulation of CNS adrenergic receptors may produce symptoms of nervousness, restlessness, and tremor. Severe adverse effects are relatively infrequent, however, when beta-adrenergic agonists are used as directed, especially when they are administered locally via inhalation.

Xanthine Derivatives

RATIONALE FOR USE AND MECHANISM OF ACTION

The xanthine derivatives are a group of chemically similar compounds that exert a variety of pharmacologic effects. Commonly occurring xanthine derivatives include theophylline, caffeine, and theobromine (Fig. 26–2), and these compounds are frequently found in various foods and beverages (tea, coffee, soft drinks). In addition, theophylline and several theophylline derivatives are administered therapeutically to produce bronchodilation in asthma and other forms of reversible airway obstruction (bronchitis, emphysema).[42,43,46,64] Theophylline also increases respiratory muscle strength, accelerates mucociliary transport, decreases pulmonary artery pressure, and limits the release of inflammatory mediators from mast cells.[2,43] These additional effects are also generally helpful in bronchospastic disease. Theophylline and caffeine are also potent CNS stimulants, and some of the more common side effects of these drugs are related to this CNS excitation (see the next "Adverse Side Effects" later in this chapter).

Although the ability of xanthine derivatives to produce bronchodilation has been theophylline

caffeine

FIGURE 26–2. Common xanthine derivatives. Theophylline is often administered therapeutically to produce bronchodilation.

theobromine

recognized for some time, the exact mechanism of action of theophylline and similar agents has been the subject of much debate. Originally these drugs were thought to cause bronchodilation by inhibiting the phosphodiesterase (PDE) enzyme located in bronchial smooth-muscle cells. The PDE breaks down cAMP. Inhibiting this enzyme results in higher intracellular cAMP concentrations. As discussed previously in this section (see "Beta-Adrenergic Agonists"), cAMP is the second messenger that brings about respiratory smooth-muscle relaxation and subsequent bronchodilation. However, more recent evidence indicates that theophylline may act as an adenosine antagonist.[11,57] Adenosine is thought to bind to specific receptors on the smooth-muscle cells and to stimulate contraction. By blocking this effect, theophylline would facilitate smooth-muscle relaxation. Alternatively, theophylline may help produce bronchodilation by other mechanisms such as inhibition of intracellular calcium release or prostaglandin inhibition.[63] In reality, theophylline and similar drugs may induce bronchodilation through a combination of several mechanisms, but the relative importance of each cellular effect remains to be determined.

SPECIFIC AGENTS AND METHOD OF ADMINISTRATION

Xanthine derivatives used in the treatment of bronchospastic disease are listed in Table 26–5. In general, these drugs are administered orally, although certain drugs may be given rectally or by injection if the oral route is not tolerated. When the oral route is used, sustained-release preparations of theophylline are available (see Table 26–5). These preparations enable the patient to take the drug just once or twice each day, thus often improving patient compliance.[13]

ADVERSE SIDE EFFECTS

The most serious limitation in the use of xanthine bronchodilators is the possibility of toxicity.[10,70] Toxicity may appear when plasma levels are between 15 and 20 μg/mL. Because the recommended levels are between 10 and 20 μg/mL, signs of toxicity may occur in some patients even when blood levels are in the therapeutic range. Early signs of toxicity include nausea, confusion, irritability, and restlessness. When blood levels exceed 20 μg/mL, serious toxic effects such as cardiac arrhythmias and seizures may occur. In some patients, the serious toxic effects may be the first indication that there is a problem, because these serious effects are not always preceded by the more innocuous signs of toxicity. Theophylline-induced seizures are a life-threatening phenomenon, with fatalities reported in 50 percent of the patients exhibiting such seizures.[10]

Consequently, during long-term use, care should be taken to avoid a toxic accumulation of theophylline. Patients in whom the metabolism of this drug is altered are especially prone to toxicity. In particular, factors such as liver disease, heart failure, alcohol consumption, cigarette smoking, concomitant use of other drugs (e.g., cimetidine), and patient age (older than 55) have all been identified as possible predisposing factors in theophylline toxicity.[10,32,49] To prevent toxicity, the dosage should be individualized for each patient, and plasma levels should be monitored periodically to ensure that theophylline levels are within the therapeutic range.[24,28,32]

TABLE 26–5 Xanthine Derivative Bronchodilators

Drug	Common Trade Names	Dosage Forms
Aminophylline	Palaron, Phyllocontin	Oral, extended-release oral, rectal, injection
Dyphylline	Dilor, Lufyllin, Neothylline, others	Oral, injection
Oxtriphylline	Choledyl, Novotriphyl	Oral, extended-release oral
Theophylline	Aerolate, Quibron, Theo-Dur, many others	Oral, extended-release oral, injection

Anticholinergic Drugs

RATIONALE FOR USE AND MECHANISM OF ACTION

The lungs receive extensive parasympathetic innervation via the vagus nerve.[5,52] The efferent fibers of the vagus nerve release acetylcholine onto respiratory smooth-muscle cells, which contain muscarinic cholinergic receptors. When stimulated, these receptors mediate bronchoconstriction. Consequently, drugs that block muscarinic cholinergic receptors prevent acetylcholine-induced bronchoconstriction, thus improving airflow in asthma and COPD. Anticholinergics are usually not the first choice as bronchodilators in obstructive pulmonary disease, but these drugs may be useful in certain patients with COPD or in patients who are unable to tolerate other bronchodilator drugs.[15,21,22]

SPECIFIC AGENTS AND ROUTE OF ADMINISTRATION

The anticholinergic bronchodilators include atropine and similar muscarinic receptor blockers. Although atropine is the prototypical muscarinic antagonist, its use in respiratory conditions is somewhat limited because it must be administered through a nebulizer. Atropine is also absorbed easily into the systemic circulation and tends to cause side effects fairly frequently. A newer drug, ipratropium (Atrovent), appears to be more advantageous for several reasons.[20,21] Ipratropium can be administered by an aerosol inhaler, and it is poorly absorbed into the systemic circulation. Thus, inhaled ipratropium is associated with substantially fewer systemic side effects. This drug is often equal to, or slightly more potent than, beta-2 agonists in producing bronchodilation in patients with COPD, but ipratropium is somewhat less effective than other bronchodilators in patients with asthma.[21,33]

ADVERSE SIDE EFFECTS

Systemic side effects associated with atropine include dry mouth, constipation, urinary retention, tachycardia, blurred vision, and confusion. As stated previously, these effects appear to occur much less often with inhaled anticholinergics like ipratropium, which are not absorbed as readily into the systemic circulation.

Corticosteroids

RATIONALE FOR USE AND MECHANISM OF ACTION

Inflammation appears to be a key underlying factor in the exaggerated responsiveness of the respiratory passages in asthma and other obstructive pulmonary disorders.[8,30] Because of their powerful anti-inflammatory effects, corticosteroids are used to control inflammation-mediated bronchospasm and are undoubtedly the most effective agents for controlling asthma.[34,48]

Corticosteroids inhibit the inflammatory response in several different ways.[48,53] These drugs inhibit the production of proinflammatory prostaglandins and leukotrienes. Corticosteroids also reverse increases in vascular permeability and inhibit the migration of neutrophils and monocytes that typically occurs during the inflammatory response. The mechanism of action of corticosteroids and cellular responses mediated by the corticosteroids are discussed in more detail in Chapter 29.

SPECIFIC AGENTS AND ROUTES OF ADMINISTRATION

Corticosteroids used to treat asthma are listed in Table 26–6. During severe, acute episodes of bronchoconstriction (e.g., *status asthmaticus*), corticosteroids are usually administered intravenously. For more prolonged use, corticosteroids are given orally or by inhalation. As with the beta agonists, the inhaled route is preferable because of the decreased chance of systemic side effects.[65] Corticosteroids that are currently available via inhalation include beclomethasone, dexamethasone, flunisolide, and triamcinolone (see Table 26–6). Inhalation of corticosteroids allows the drug to be applied directly to the respiratory mucosa, and any corticosteriod that does happen to be absorbed into the systemic circulation is rapidly metabolized. When these drugs are used appropriately, there are essentially no systemic adverse side effects such as those to be described later.[33,35,55] Patients should rinse their mouth cavities with water after using oral corticosteroid inhalers, however, to prevent local irritation of the oral mucosa.

ADVERSE SIDE EFFECTS

The major limitation of the corticosteroids in any disease is the risk of serious adverse effects. Because of the general catabolic effect of these drugs on supporting tissues, problems with osteoporosis, skin breakdown, and muscle wasting can occur during prolonged systemic use or if excessively high doses (greater than 1000 μg/day) are administered through inhalation.[55] Other adverse effects include cataracts, hyperglycemia, aggravation of diabetes mellitus, and hypertension. Consequently, prolonged systemic administration of these drugs should be avoided, and corticosteroids should be administered by inhalation using the lowest effective dose. Nonetheless, these drugs are extremely effective in treating various types of bronchoconstriction, and they should be used judiciously whenever possible.[33,37]

Cromolyn Sodium

RATIONALE FOR USE AND MECHANISM OF ACTION

Cromolyn sodium is used to prevent bronchospasm in people with asthma. This drug is not a bronchodilator, and it will not reverse bronchoconstriction during an asthmatic attack. Hence, cromolyn must be taken prior to the onset of bronchoconstric-

TABLE 26–6 Corticosteroids Used in Obstructive Pulmonary Disease

Generic Name	Trade Name(s)	Dosage Forms
Beclomethasone	Beclovent, Vanceril	Inhalation
Dexamethasone	Decadron	Inhalation
Flunisolide	AeroBid	Inhalation
Methylprednisolone	Medrol	Intravenous injection
Prednisolone	Hydeltrasol	Intravenous or intramuscular injection
Triamcinolone	Azmacort	Inhalation

tion, and this drug has typically been administered prophylactically to prevent asthma attacks that are initiated by specific, well-defined activities (e.g., exercise, exposure to a friend's pet, etc.).[57] Likewise, the regular use of cromolyn several times each day for several months may decrease airway hyperresponsiveness so that the incidence of asthmatic attacks is decreased.[50]

Cromolyn is believed to prevent bronchoconstriction by inhibiting the release of inflammatory mediators such as histamine and leukotrienes from pulmonary mast cells. The exact way in which cromolyn exerts this effect is unknown, however.[57] Cromolyn is available as a capsule but is administered by inhalation using a special device known as a Spinhaler. This device punctures the cromolyn capsule, thus releasing a powder that is then aerosolized and inhaled directly from the Spinhaler. Cromolyn can also be administered by a power-operated nebulizer or by a nasal spray.

ADVERSE SIDE EFFECTS

Some irritation of the nasal and upper respiratory passages may occur following inhalation, but severe adverse reactions are relatively rare with cromolyn use.

TREATMENT OF BRONCHIAL ASTHMA

Pathophysiology of Bronchial Asthma

Asthma is a disease of the respiratory system characterized by bronchial smooth-muscle spasm, airway inflammation, and mucous plugging of the airways.[36,61] Patients with asthma have an exaggerated bronchoconstrictor response of the airways to various stimuli.[30,59,68] In some patients, the stimuli that trigger an asthmatic attack are well defined (e.g., allergens like dust, pollen, chemicals, or certain drugs). Other factors such as exercise, cold, psychologic stress, and viral infections may trigger an asthmatic attack in some individuals. In other patients, the initiating factor may be unknown.

Although the exact cause of asthma remains to be determined, the basis for the increased airway reactivity in asthma has been elucidated somewhat. Airway inflammation is a critical factor in initiating the exaggerated bronchial reactions associated with this disease.[4,8,41,67] In asthmatic airways, there seems to be a complex interaction between several different cells including macrophages, neutrophils, eosinophils, platelets, and the airway epithelial cells themselves.[6,59] These cells release proinflammatory chemical mediators such as prostaglandins, leukotrienes, bradykinin, histamine, and platelet activating factor.[4,59,67] These chemicals irritate the respiratory epithelium, as well as stimulate contraction of bronchiole smooth muscle. Thus, the localized inflammation appears to sensitize airway structures to asthmatic triggers, and the bronchoconstriction and other features of asthma seem to be related directly to the inflammatory response underlying this disease.

Long-Term Management of Asthma

The primary focus of treating asthma has undergone a definite shift within the past few years. In the past, treatment consisted primarily of bronchodilators such as the beta-adrenergic agonists and the xanthine derivatives, with systemic anti-inflammatory steroids (corticosteroids) being added only in more advanced and severe cases. The use of corticosteroids has increased, however, to where these drugs are now used as first-line agents in many patients, including cases of newly detected, mild asthma.[23,67] The increased use of corticosteroids is partially because certain types of corticosteroids can now be administered by inhalation. As indicated previously, inhaled corticosteroids are not absorbed readily into the systemic circulation, and the risk of serious systemic side effects is therefore substantially reduced. Another reason for the shift toward increased corticosteroid use is the recognition that these drugs directly reduce the inflammation that underlies asthmatic disease, whereas bronchodilators merely treat the secondary manifestations of this disease.[34] Put more simply, corticosteroids directly affect the underlying disease process by decreasing the inflammation that causes airway hyperresponsiveness.

Hence, corticosteroids have assumed a much more prominent role as one of the primary drugs used to prevent asthma attacks. Beta-2 agonists are still used extensively, however, and these drugs remain the primary method of *symptomatically* treating asthma attacks.[33] Many patients routinely inhale beta-2 agonists through MDIs at the onset of a bronchospastic attack, and this technique is a mainstay in managing acute episodes of asthma. Nonetheless, the use of beta-2 agonists has come under scrutiny recently with reports that long-term use of beta-2 agonists may actually *increase* airway hyperresponsiveness, thus leading to increased morbidity and mortality in some patients with asthma.[9,54,62] It is unclear, however, if these patients were experiencing adverse effects from these drugs or if they were merely succumbing to the more advanced stages of asthmatic disease.[62] The current philosophy appears to be that beta-2 agonists should still be used by patients who are experiencing good results with these agents.[45] Use of beta-2 agonists should be reconsidered, however, if asthma is poorly controlled, even when beta-2 agonists are combined with corticosteroids.[45] Likewise, the need for repeated or excessive use of inhaled beta-2 agonists (e.g., more than three or four asthma attacks in a 24-hour period) may indicate a potential problem and the need to alter drug therapy to accommodate a change in the patient's condition.[14]

Consequently, inhaled corticosteroids and beta agonists are currently considered the primary drugs used to manage asthmatic disease in many patients. Once considered the foundation for drug therapy, theophylline has assumed a somewhat secondary role. Systemic theophylline can be added when inhaled beta agonists alone cannot adequately control asthmatic symptoms, but theophylline is often discontinued when symptoms are brought under control by a combination of inhaled corticosteroids and beta agonists.[33] Of course, the specific drug regimen for treating asthma must be determined on a patient-by-patient basis. The optimal combination of corticosteroids, beta agonists, theophylline, and other drugs (i.e., cromolyn and anticholinergics) must be constantly reviewed and adjusted in response to the patient's needs and the clinical course of the asthmatic disease.

Along with drug therapy, several nonpharmacologic interventions should be employed. Efforts should be made to determine the initiating factors of an asthmatic attack, and patients should be taught how to avoid these factors whenever possible. Also, considerable evidence exists that aerobic conditioning may help decrease the incidence of asthmatic attacks and the concomitant need for antiasthmatic drugs in certain patients.[25,64] Of course, exercise itself may be an asthmatic trigger in some individuals.[44] However, certain forms of aerobic exercise such as swimming may be an excellent way to improve the cardiorespiratory status of patients with asthma without causing excessive risk of bronchospastic attacks in these individuals.[16]

TREATMENT OF REVERSIBLE BRONCHOSPASM IN COPD

As indicated previously, bronchospasm is often present in COPD—that is, in chronic bronchitis and emphysema. *Chronic bronchitis* is a clinical diagnosis applied to a long-standing inflammation of the bronchial tree.[59,61,68] *Emphysema* is a pathologic condition marked by destruction of alveolar walls and enlargement of the terminal air spaces.[59,61,68]

Drug therapy for COPD is directed primarily toward maintaining airway patency and preventing airflow restriction.[15] Thus, bronchodilators such as inhaled beta-2 agonists or anticholinergics (ipratropium) are typically the first drugs used, followed by oral theophylline.[15,17,42,43] Corticosteroids have also been used to treat airway inflammation in COPD, but their use in these situations remains controversial. In contrast to their beneficial effects in asthma, corticosteroids have not always produced clear therapeutic benefits in patients with COPD.[67] Hence, these drugs are not typically prescribed on a routine basis but are usually reserved for the more severe cases of COPD-related bronchospasm.[15,47,60]

TREATMENT OF RESPIRATORY PROBLEMS IN CYSTIC FIBROSIS

Cystic fibrosis is one of the most common hereditary diseases in white populations. This autosomal-recessive trait is found in approximately 1 of every 2500 live births.[58] Cystic fibrosis essentially affects all the major exocrine glands, resulting in very thick, viscous secretions. These thickened secretions often form mucous plugs, which obstruct major ducts in various glands and organs.[58,67] For instance, the pancreatic and bile ducts are often obstructed, resulting in problems with nutrient digestion and absorption. Mucous plugging of the bronchioles occurs quite frequently, leading to a number of pulmonary problems such as pneumonia, bronchiectasis, pulmonary fibrosis, and various pulmonary infections (especially *Staphylococcus*). These respiratory problems are usually the primary health threat to individuals with cystic fibrosis.[58,67]

Pharmacologic management of respiratory problems in cystic fibrosis is focused on maintaining airway patency as much as possible. Bronchodilators and mucolytic/expectorant drugs may help limit the formation of mucous plugs. Systemic corticosteroids (e.g., prednisone) may also be beneficial in some patients in limiting airway inflammation and improving pulmonary function.[3] Respiratory infections are treated using appropriate antibiotic agents.[31,67] In addition to drug therapy, daily maintenance of respiratory hygiene (postural drainage, breathing exercises, etc.) is essential in sustaining pulmonary function.[12] Even with optimal medical care, however, the prognosis for this disease remains poor. Individuals with cystic fibrosis often succumb to respiratory-related problems within their second or third decade of life.

Although there is still no cure for cystic fibrosis, several pharmacologic techniques have been developed recently that may help decrease the viscosity of respiratory secretions in patients with this disease. One technique uses aerosol preparations that contain enzymes known as *deoxyribonucleases*. These enzymes can be inhaled to break down the large quantities of DNA that are present in respiratory secretions of patients with cystic fibrosis.[27] Respiratory secretions in these patients often contain large amounts of DNA because the genetic material contained in airway inflammatory cells is deposited into the airway lumen when these cells are destroyed. DNA increases the viscosity and thickness of the respiratory secretions, and preparations that contain deoxyribonuclease can lyse this DNA, thus decreasing the viscosity of these secretions and reducing the chance of atelectasis and infection.

Another new technique consists of inhaling nucleotide compounds such as adenosine triphosphate and uridine triphosphate.[38] These nucleotides stimulate chloride secretion from airway epithelial cells. The increased chloride secretion creates an osmotic force that draws water into the airway, thus hydrating respiratory secretions and decreasing the viscosity of these secretions. These newer procedures that decrease respiratory fluid viscosity are still experimental at the present time, but there is hope that these techniques may someday provide a means to alleviate the primary respiratory complications that often lead to illness and death in patients with cystic fibrosis.

RESPIRATORY DRUGS: SPECIAL CONCERNS IN REHABILITATION PATIENTS

Proper respiratory hygiene is crucial in preventing the serious adverse effects of respiratory infection and obstructive pulmonary disease. The accumulation of bronchial secretions can lead to decreased gas exchange, atelectasis, and additional infection. Rehabilitation specialists often play a critical role in preventing pulmonary mucus accumulation. Therapists can facilitate the pharmacotherapeutic effects of mucolytic and expectorant drugs by performing postural drainage and breathing exercises. Even if patients are not being treated directly with chest physical therapy and respiratory hygiene, rehabilitation specialists should always encourage patients to cough and raise secretions for expectoration. Physical therapists and occupational therapists should also coordinate their treatments with respiratory therapy. Often, mucolytic and expectorant drugs are administered by the respiratory therapist through a nebulizer or positive-pressure ventilator. A program of chest physical therapy may be most effective when administered 30 minutes to 1 hour after these agents are administered (i.e, after these drugs have had some time to exert an effect on respiratory secretions).

Therapists should be aware of which patients are prone to bronchospastic attacks. If patients use some sort of portable aerosol bronchodilator, they should be encouraged to bring their medication to therapy. Rehabilitation procedures that involve exercise may trigger a bronchospastic attack in some individuals, so the medication should be close at hand.

Therapists should also be aware of the potential side effects of bronchodilator drugs. In particular, the cardiac side effects of the beta-adrenergic agonists and xanthine derivatives (theophylline, others) should be considered. Therapists may notice cardiac arrhythmias while monitoring the ECG or taking the patient's pulse, and these cardiac abnormalities may indicate a problem with bronchodilator medications. Other, noncardiac symptoms such as nervousness, confusion, and tremors may also indicate bronchodilator toxicity and should be brought to the physician's attention. Early recognition of toxicity may be lifesaving, especially when xanthine derivatives such as theophylline are used. Finally, patients receiving systemic corticosteroid treatment may be prone to the well-known catabolic effects of these drugs. Therapists should be especially alert for skin breakdown, and care should be taken not to overstress bones and musculotendinous structures that may be weakened by the prolonged use of corticosteroids.

CASE STUDY

RESPIRATORY DRUGS

Brief History. V.C., a 63-year-old man, has a long history of COPD and hypertension. Twelve years ago, he was diagnosed with emphysema. During the past 5 years, his symptoms of shortness of breath, wheezing, and bronchospasm have become progressively worse. He is also a chronic cigarette smoker and has had a cough for many years, which produces large amounts of sputum daily. Although his physician advised him repeatedly to quit smoking, the patient was unable to kick the habit. To control his bronchospasm, the patient self-administers a beta-2 agonist (albuterol) via an MDI. He is also taking a diuretic and beta-1 blocker to control his hypertension. Two days ago, he was admitted to the hospital with weakness and incoordination in his left arm and leg. Subsequent medical tests indicated that he had suffered a cerebral vascular accident. Physical therapy was ordered to begin at the patient's bedside to facilitate optimal recovery from the stroke. The physical therapist began treating the patient with passive and active exercises to encourage motor return. The patient was also being seen by a respiratory therapist. The respiratory therapy treatments included administration of the mucolytic drug acetylcysteine via a nebulizer, three times daily. The patient continued to self-administer the beta-2 agonist at the onset of bronchospasms.

Problem/Influence of Medication. Despite the program of respiratory therapy, bronchial secretions began to accumulate in the patient's airways. The patient had also been instructed in deep-breathing and coughing exercises, and he was told by the respiratory therapist to perform these exercises periodically throughout the day. However, no postural drainage was being performed to encourage ejection of sputum.

Decision/Solution. In addition to the neuromuscular facilitation activities, the physical therapist initiated a program of chest physical therapy including postural drainage and deep-breathing exercises. The physical therapist coordinated these activities with the respiratory therapist so that the patient first received a treatment of the mucolytic agent. Also, the physical therapist had the patient self-administer a dose of the inhaled beta-2 bronchodilator approximately 1 hour prior to the chest therapy session, thus allowing the bronchodilator to produce maximal airway dilation and permit optimal clearance of bronchial secretions.

SUMMARY

The drugs discussed in this chapter are used to control irritation and maintain airflow through the respiratory passages. Drugs such as the antitussives, decongestants, antihistamines, mucolytics, and expectorants are used primarily for the temporary relief of cold, flu, and seasonal allergy symptoms. These agents are frequently found in over-the-counter preparations, and several different agents are often combined together in the same commercial product. Airway obstruction in chronic disorders such as bronchial asthma, chronic bronchitis, and emphysema is treated primarily with bronchodilator agents (beta-adrenergic agonists, xanthine derivatives, anticholinergics) and anti-inflammatory drugs (corticosteroids, cromolyn sodium). Rehabilitation specialists should also be cognizant of which patients suffer from bronchospastic disorders (e.g., asthma) and of what medications are being used to control airway obstruction in each patient. Therapists can also help facilitate the pharmacotherapeutic goals in patients with obstructive pulmonary disease by encouraging proper respiratory hygiene and breathing exercises and by helping improve overall cardiorespiratory endurance whenever possible.

REFERENCES

1. Arrang, J-M, et al: Highly potent and selective ligands for histamine H_3-receptors. Nature 327:117, 1987.
2. Aubier, M: Effects of theophylline on diaphragmatic and other skeletal muscle function. J Allergy Clin Immunol 78(suppl 11):787, 1986.
3. Auerbach, HS, et al: Alternate-day prednisone reduces morbidity and improves pulmonary function in cystic fibrosis. Lancet 2:686, 1985.
4. Barnes, PJ: New concepts in the pathogenesis of bronchial hyperresponsiveness. In Schmitz-Schumann, M, Menz, G, and Page, CP (eds): PAF, Platelets and Asthma. Birkhauser Verlag, Boston, 1987.
5. Bleecker, ER: Cholinergic and neurogenic mechanisms in obstructive airway disease. Am J Med 81(suppl 5a):93, 1986.
6. Bousquet, J, et al: Eosinophilic inflammation in asthma. N Engl J Med 323:1033, 1990.
7. Bukowskyj, M, Nakatsu, K, and Munt, PW: Theophylline reassessed. Ann Intern Med 101:63, 1984.
8. Busse, WW, Calhun, CF, and Segwick, JD: Mechanism of airway inflammation in asthma. Am Rev Resp Dis 147(suppl 6):S20, 1993.
9. Chung, KF: The current debate concerning beta-agonists in asthma: A review. J Royal Soc Med 86:96, 1993.
10. Covelli, HD, Knodel, AR, and Heppner, BT: Predisposing factors to apparent theophylline-induced seizures. Ann Allergy 54:411, 1985.
11. Cushley, MJ, Tattersfield, AE, and Holgate, ST: Adenosine antagonism as an alternative mechanism of action of methylxanthines in asthma. In Morley, J and Rainsford, KD (eds): Pharmacology of Asthma. Birkhauser Verlag, Boston, 1983.
12. DeCesare, JA and Graybill, CA: Physical therapy for the child with respiratory dysfunction. In Irwin, S and Tecklin, JS (eds): Cardiopulmonary Physical Therapy, ed 2. CV Mosby, St Louis, 1990.
13. Dockhorn, RJ, Green, AW, and Green, E: Assessing the efficacy and safety of Q.D. theophylline therapy: A multicenter study. Ann Allergy 55:658, 1985.
14. Executive Committee, American Academy of Allergy and Immunology: Inhaled beta-2 adrenergic agonists in asthma. J Allergy Clin Immunol 91:1234, 1993.
15. Ferguson, GT and Cherniak, RM: Current concepts: Management of COPD. N Engl J Med 328:1017, 1993.
16. Fitch, KD, Morton, AR, and Blanksby, BA: Effect of swimming training on children with asthma. Arch Dis Child 51:190, 1976.
17. Fragoso, CAV and Miller, MA: Review of the clinical efficacy of theophylline in the treatment of chronic obstructive pulmonary disease. Am Rev Resp Dis 147(suppl 6):S40, 1993.
18. Garrison, JC: Histamine, bradykinin, 5-hydroxytryptamine, and their antagonists. In Gilman, AG, et al (eds): The Pharmacological Basis of Therapeutics, ed 8. Pergamon Press, New York, 1990.
19. Grassi, V, et al: Oral beta 2-selective adrenergic bronchodilators. Int J Clin Pharmacol Res 6:93, 1986.
20. Gross, NJ: Ipratropium bromide. N Engl J Med 319:486, 1988.

21. Gross, NJ and Skorodin, MS: Anticholinergic, antimuscarinic bronchodilators. Am Rev Respir Dis 129:856, 1984.
22. Gross, NJ and Skorodin, MS: Role of the parasympathetic system in airway obstruction due to emphysema. N Engl J Med 311:421, 1984.
23. Haahtela, T, et al: Comparison of a beta$_2$-agonist, terbutaline, with an inhaled corticosterioid, budesonide, in newly detected asthma. N Engl J Med 325:388, 1991.
24. Harder, S, Staib, AH, and Stauder, J: Individual theophylline dosage after out-patient determination of theophylline clearance. Prax Klin Pneumol 40:334, 1986.
25. Henriksen, JM and Nielsen, TT: Effect of physical training on exercise-induced bronchoconstriction. Acta Paediatr Scand 72:31, 1983.
26. Hirnle, RW: Agents used to treat bronchial obstruction. In Kuhn, MA (ed): Pharmacotherapeutics: A Nursing Process Approach, ed 3. FA Davis, Philadelphia, 1994.
27. Hubbard, RC, et al: A preliminary study of aerosolized recombinant human deoxyribonuclease I in the treatment of cystic fibrosis. N Engl J Med 326:812, 1992.
28. Hurley, SF, et al: A randomized controlled clinical trial of pharmacokinetic theophylline dosing. Am Rev Respir Dis 134:1219, 1986.
29. Ind, PW and Dollery, CT: Pulmonary adrenoceptors and asthma. In Morley, J and Rainsford, KD (eds): Pharmacology of Asthma. Birkhauser Verlag, Boston, 1983.
30. Ingram, RH: Asthma and airway hyperresponsiveness. Annu Rev Med 42:139, 1991.
31. Jackson, MA, et al: Comparison of piperacillin vs. tricarcillin plus tobramycin in the treatment of acute pulmonary exacerbations of cystic fibrosis. Pediatr Infect Dis 5:440, 1986.
32. Jenne, JW: Effect of disease states on theophylline elimination. J Allergy Clin Immunol 78:727, 1986.
33. Kaliner, M and Lemanske, R: Rhinitis and asthma. JAMA 268:2807, 1992.
34. Kemp, JP: Approaches to asthma management: Realities and recommendations. Arch Intern Med 153:805, 1993.
35. Kerrebijn, KF: Use of topical corticosteroids in the treatment of childhood asthma. Am Rev Resp Dis 141:S77, 1990.
36. Kerrebijn, KF: New developments in the pathophysiology of asthma. In Saxena, PR and Elliott, GR (eds): Pathophysiology and Treatment of Asthma and Arthritis. Birkhauser Verlag, Boston, 1984.
37. Kerstjens, HAM, et al: A comparison of bronchodilator therapy with or without inhaled corticosteroid therapy for obstructive airway disease. N Engl J Med 327:1413, 1992.
38. Knowles, MR, Clarke, LL, and Boucher, RC: Activation of extracellular nucleotides of chloride secretion in the airway epithelia of patients with cystic fibrosis. N Engl J Med 325:533, 1991.
39. Koda-Kimple, MA: Therapeutic and toxic potential of over-the-counter agents. In Katzung, BG (ed): Basic and Clinical Pharmacology, ed 5. Appleton & Lange, Norwalk, CT, 1992.
40. Krause, HF: Antihistamines and decongestants. Otolaryngol Head Neck Surg 107:835, 1992.
41. Lazarus, SC: Role of inflammation and inflammatory mediators in airway disease. Am J Med 81(suppl 5a):2, 1986.
42. Mahler, DA: The role of theophylline in the treatment of dyspnea in COPD. Chest 92(suppl):2S, 1987.
43. McFadden, ER: Introduction: Methylxanthine therapy and reversible airway obstruction. Am J Med (suppl 6a):1, 1985.
44. McFadden, ER and Gilbert, IA: Current concepts: Exercise-induced asthma. N Engl J Med 330:1362, 1994.
45. McFadden, ER and Gilbert, IA: Medical progress: Asthma. N Engl J Med 327:1928, 1992.
46. Milgrom, H and Bender, B: Current issues in the use of theophylline. Am Rev Resp Dis 147(suppl 6):S33, 1993.
47. Mitchell, DM, et al: Effects of prednisolone in chronic airflow limitation. Lancet 2:193, 1984.
48. Morris, HG: Mechanisms of action and therapeutic role of corticosteroids in asthma. J Allergy Clin Immunol 75:1, 1985.
49. Muhlberg, W, et al: Pharmacokinetics and pharmacodynamics of theophylline in geriatric patients with multiple diseases. Klin Wochenschr 65:551, 1987.
50. Murphy, S and Kelly, HW: Cromolyn sodium: A review of mechanisms and clinical use in asthma. Drug Intell Clin Pharm 21:22, 1987.
51. Naclerio, RM: Drug therapy: Allergic rhinitis. N Engl J Med 325:860, 1991.
52. Nadel, JA and Barnes, PJ: Autonomic regulation of the airways. Annu Rev Medicine 35:451, 1984.
53. Nijkamp, FP: The pharmacology of anti-asthmatic drugs. In Saxena, PR and Elliott, GR (eds): Pathophysiology and Treatment of Asthma and Arthritis. Birkhauser Verlag, Boston, 1984.
54. Page, CP: An explanation of the asthma paradox. Am Rev Resp Dis 147(suppl 6):S29, 1994.
55. Pavord, I and Knox, A: Pharmacokinetic optimizaiton of inhaled steroid therapy in asthma. Clin Pharmacokinet 25:126, 1993.
56. Pearlman, DS, et al: A comparison of salmeterol with albuterol in the treatment of mild-to-moderate asthma. N Engl J Med 327:1420, 1992.
57. Rall, TW: Drugs used in the treatment of asthma. In Gilman, AG, et al (eds): The Pharmacological Basis of Therapeutics, ed 8. Pergamon Press, New York, 1990.
58. Rubin, E and Farber, JL: Developmental and genetic diseases. In Rubin, E and Farber, JL (eds): Pathology, ed 2. JB Lippincott, Philadelphia, 1994.

59. Rubin, E and Farber, JL: The respiratory system. In Rubin, E and Farber, JL (eds): Pathology, ed 2. JB Lippincott, Philadelphia, 1994.
60. Skorodin, MS: Pharmacologic management of obstructive lung disease: Current perspectives. Am J Med 81(suppl 5a):8, 1986.
61. Spencer, H: Pathology of the Lung, ed 4. Pergamon Press, New York, 1985.
62. Spitzer, WO, et al: The use of beta-agonists and the risk of death and near death from asthma. N Engl J Med 326:501, 1992.
63. Svedmyr, N: Methylxanthines in asthma. In Morley, J and Rainsford, KD (eds): Pharmacology of Asthma. Birkhauser Verlag, Boston, 1983.
64. Svenonius, E, Kautto, R, and Arborelius, M: Improvement after training of children with exercise induced asthma. Acta Paediatr Scand 72:23, 1983.
65. Taburet, A-M and Schmit, B: Pharmacokinetic optimization of asthma treatment. Clin Pharmacokinet 26:396, 1994.
66. Wardell, SC and Bousard, LB: Mucolytics and expectorants. In Nursing Pharmacology: A Comprehensive Approach to Drug Therapy. Wadsworth Health Sciences, Monterey, CA, 1985.
67. Weinberger, SE: Medical progress: Recent advances in pulmonary medicine. N Engl J Med 328:1389, 1993.
68. West, JB: Pulmonary Pathophysiology: The Essentials, ed 4. Williams & Wilkins, Baltimore, 1992.
69. White, JP, Mills, J, and Eiser, NM: Comparison of the effects of histamine H_1- and H_2-receptor agonists on large and small airways in normal and asthmatic subjects. Br J Dis Chest 81:155, 1987.
70. Woodcock, AA, Johnson, MA, and Geddes, DM: Theophylline prescribing, serum concentrations, and toxicity. Lancet 2:610, 1983.

CHAPTER 27

Gastrointestinal Drugs

This chapter discusses drugs that are used to treat specific problems in the gastrointestinal (GI) system. The GI tract is responsible for the digestion of food and the absorption of nutrients and water. Dietary constituents normally undergo a series of digestive processes as they progress through the GI system. Under normal conditions, the transit time of food and water is adequate to allow the processes of digestion and absorption to take place. Indigestible and nonabsorbable products are eliminated by defecation.

The primary disorders that occur in the GI tract are related to damage from gastric acid secretion and abnormal movement of food through the GI tract. Problems may occur if digestive secretions in the stomach begin to damage the upper GI mucosa and cause a peptic ulcer. Certain drugs attempt to prevent or heal peptic ulcers by controlling gastric acid secretion and protecting the mucosal lining. Problems with gastrointestinal motility may also respond to pharmacologic management. Excessive motility (*diarrhea*) and inadequate bowel evacuation (*constipation*) are treated with various agents that normalize peristalsis and facilitate normal bowel movements. Drugs are also available to treat other problems with digestion and vomiting (*emesis*). The GI system is also susceptible to various infectious and parasitic invasions. The drugs used to treat these disorders are presented in Chapters 33 through 35, which deal with the chemotherapy of infectious diseases.

Rehabilitation specialists will invariably treat patients taking some form of GI agent. These medications are commonly used by the general public as well as by hospitalized individuals and outpatients receiving physical therapy and occupational therapy. Although the direct impact of most GI drugs on physical rehabilitation is relatively small, an understanding of how these drugs are used will help therapists recognize their role in the patient's pharmacotherapeutic regimen.

DRUGS USED TO CONTROL GASTRIC ACIDITY AND SECRETION

The acidic nature of the gastric juices is essential for activating digestive protease activity and controlling intestinal bacteria. The gastric acids, however, can cause severe

389

ulceration and hemorrhage of the stomach lining if excessive amounts of acid are produced or if the normal protection of the stomach mucosa is disturbed.[11,24,36] Consequently, several different types of drugs are available that attempt to control or prevent the detrimental effects of gastric acid. These agents are used to treat *peptic ulcers*, that is, ulcerations of the mucosal lining of the esophagus, stomach, and duodenum.[8] These drugs may also be used to treat the heartburn sensations caused by leakage of gastric acid into the distal esophagus, called *gastroesophageal reflux*.[25] Agents used to control gastric acidity and secretion are presented here.

Antacids

RATIONALE FOR USE AND MECHANISM OF ACTION

Antacids attempt to chemically neutralize stomach acids. These drugs typically contain a base such as carbonate or hydroxide combined with aluminum, magnesium, or calcium.[1] In the stomach, the base combines with excess H^+ to increase intragastric pH. The basic strategy of this chemical neutralization is illustrated in Figure 27–1.

Antacids are frequently used to treat the episodic minor gastric discomfort (indigestion, heartburn) that often accompanies overeating or indulging in certain incompatible foods. One concern regarding antacids is that they may be abused in this respect. The public has come to regard antacids as a panacea for poor eating habits. Antacids are also used in more serious and chronic conditions of peptic ulcer and gastroesophageal reflux.[3,24] In treating ulcers, these agents may not only help relieve gastric pain, but they may actually facilitate ulcer healing as well.[3] Fairly large doses of antacids must be taken fairly frequently, however, to achieve this healing effect. Consequently, more convenient drugs such as the H_2 blockers are often the initial agents used in treating ulcers. Antacids remain a suitable alternative, however, if other drugs are ineffective or poorly tolerated.[3]

Basic Strategy:

antacid + hydrochloric acid ---> salt + water

Examples:

aluminum hydroxide
$$Al(OH)_3 + 3\ HCl\ ---> \quad AlCl_3 + 3\ H_2O$$

magnesium hydroxide
$$Mg(OH)_2 + 2\ HCl\ ---> \quad MgCl_2 + 2\ H_2O$$

calcium carbonate
$$CaCO_3 + 2\ HCl\ \quad ---> \quad CaCl_2 + H_2O + CO_2$$

sodium bicarbonate
$$NaHCO_3 + HCl\ \quad ---> \quad NaCl + H_2O + CO_2$$

FIGURE 27–1. Neutralization of hydrochloric acid (HCl) by the primary forms of antacids. In each reaction, the antacid combines with HCl to form a salt and water. Carbon dioxide (CO_2) is also produced by calcium carbonate and sodium bicarbonate antacids.

SPECIFIC AGENTS

Antacids are identified by many trade names and frequently appear in over-the-counter products. There is such a plethora of antacids on the market that even a partial listing of commercial preparations is difficult. The primary antacids are classified as aluminum-containing, magnesium-containing, calcium carbonate–containing, sodium bicarbonate–containing, or virtually any combination of these classifications. These drugs are typically taken orally, either as tablets or as a liquid oral suspension.

ADVERSE SIDE EFFECTS

Constipation is the most common side effect associated with the aluminum-containing antacids, whereas diarrhea often occurs with magnesium-containing preparations. A common problem with all antacids is the acid-rebound phenomenon.[18] Antacids increase the pH of the gastric fluids, which serves as the normal stimulus for increased acid secretion. This situation does not present a problem while the antacid is in the stomach, because most of the excess acid will be neutralized. Gastric secretion may remain elevated, however, even after the antacid effects diminish and stomach pH returns to normal levels. The unopposed rebound of acid secretion may then cause increased gastric distress.

H_2 Receptor Blockers

RATIONALE FOR USE AND MECHANISM OF ACTION

The regulation of gastric acid secretion involves the complex interaction of many endogenous chemicals including histamine.[13,39] Histamine stimulates specific receptors on stomach parietal cells to increase gastric acid secretion. These histamine receptors are classified as H_2 receptors, to differentiate them from the H_1 receptors located on vascular, respiratory, and gastrointestinal smooth muscle.[13] Drugs have been developed that selectively bind to H_2 receptors without activating the receptor. These H_2 antagonists or blockers prevent the histamine-activated release of gastric acid under basal conditions and during stimulation by food and other factors.[13,36]

H_2 blockers are currently used for both acute and long-term management of peptic ulcer.[23,33,34] These drugs appear to be especially effective in patients who have excessive acid secretion (as opposed to patients with a problem in the gastric mucosal barrier under normal or low gastric secretion).[19]

SPECIFIC AGENTS

The primary H_2 blockers used to control gastric secretions are listed in Table 27–1. Cimetidine was the first H_2 blocker to be widely used as an antiulcer agent. Newer drugs such as famotidine, nizatidine, and ranitidine appear to be at least as effective as cimetidine, but they are more potent and may be better tolerated than cimetidine in some patients.[15,20,26] Likewise, some of the newer agents, famotidine and nizatidine in particular, appear to have a lower potential for interacting with other drugs, hence their preferential use in patients taking several different types of medications.[10]

TABLE 27-1 H$_2$ Receptor Blockers

Generic Name	Trade Name	Adult Oral Dosage
Cimetidine	Tagamet	300 mg 4 times each day
Famotidine	Pepcid	40 mg once daily at bedtime
Nizatidine	Axid	300 mg once daily at bedtime
Ranitidine	Zantac	100-150 mg twice daily

ADVERSE SIDE EFFECTS

These drugs are generally well tolerated in most patients, and serious adverse effects are rare. Problems that may occur include headache and dizziness. Mild, transient GI problems (nausea, diarrhea, constipation) may also occur with the H$_2$ blockers, and arthralgia and myalgia have been reported with cimetidine use.

Other Agents Used to Control and Treat Gastric Ulcers

Several other agents besides the antacids and H$_2$ blockers have proved successful in preventing or treating problems associated with gastric acidity and mucosal breakdown. Some of the more frequently used agents are discussed here.

Anticholinergics. The role of muscarinic cholinergic antagonists in treating peptic ulcers was discussed in Chapter 19. Cholinergic stimulation of the gut via vagal efferent fibers produces a general increase in GI motility and secretion. Drugs that block the effects of acetylcholine on stomach parietal cells will decrease the release of gastric acid. Atropine and similar anticholinergics are used occasionally as adjuncts to antacids or H$_2$ blockers to help control gastric acid secretion. Widespread use of these drugs is limited, however, because most cholinergic muscarinic inhibitors cause many side effects such as dry mouth, constipation, urinary retention, and confusion.[36] One notable exception is the antimuscarinic drug pirenzepine (Gastrozepin). Pirenzepine, which is fairly selective for muscarinic receptors located on the stomach mucosa, effectively decreases gastric secretion at a dose that does not cause excessive side effects.[14,36] Hence, this drug may be a viable alternative to the other agents currently available to treat excessive gastric secretions.

Metoclopramide (Clopra, Maxolon, Reglan). This drug is officially classified as a dopamine receptor antagonist but also appears to enhance the peripheral effects of acetylcholine. Primarily because of this latter effect, metoclopramide stimulates motility in the upper GI tract, which may be useful in moving the stomach contents toward the small intestine, thus preventing mucosal irritation caused by acidic gastric juices. This drug is used primarily in treating gastric ulcers (as opposed to duodenal ulcers) and may also help prevent gastroesophageal reflux. The primary side effects associated with metoclopramide are related to its antagonistic effects on CNS dopamine receptors. Restlessness, drowsiness, and fatigue are fairly common. Some extrapyramidal symptoms (i.e., parkinsonism-like tremor and rigidity) may also occur because of the central antidopamine effects.

Omeprazole (Prilosec, Losec). This drug inhibits the H$^+$, K$^+$- ATPase enzyme that is ultimately responsible for secreting acid from gastric parietal cells into the lumen of the stomach.[30] This enzyme is also known as the "proton pump"; hence this drug is often referred to as a proton pump inhibitor. Omeprazole is extremely effective at inhibiting the proton pump, and therapeutic doses can virtually eliminate gastric acid secretion.[1] Omeprazole is used to treat gastric and duodenal ulcers as well as gastroesophageal reflux. This drug is fairly well tolerated, although bacterial colonization can occur in the stomach if gastric acid secretion is completely inhibited for prolonged periods. Hence, doses may need to be adjusted to prevent excessive secretion, while still allowing a small amount of acid secretion for digestive and antibacterial purposes.

Prostaglandins. There is little doubt that certain prostaglandins such as PGE_2 and PGI_2 inhibit gastric secretion and help protect the stomach mucosa by stimulating gastric mucus secretion.[4,16,28,32] The problem has been determining exactly how the prostaglandins are involved, and whether exogenous prostaglandin analogs can be used to help treat peptic ulcer. Two prostaglandin analogs, enprostil and misoprostol, have been studied as possible treatments for peptic ulcer.[2,17,31,38] The general consensus from clinical trials has been that these drugs are successful in treating ulcers, but they do not seem to offer any advantages over the more traditional antiulcer drugs such as cimetidine.[31,40] Also, prostaglandin analogs may only be effective at doses that also cause other GI effects such as diarrhea.[31,40]

Consequently, prostaglandin analogs have not gained overwhelming acceptance as antiulcer drugs. Currently, only misoprostol (Cytotec) is available for clinical use, and this drug is typically reserved for the treatment of gastric damage caused by aspirin and similar nonsteroidal anti-inflammatory drugs (NSAIDs).[9,37] The use of misoprostol to reduce or prevent NSAID-induced gastropathy is discussed in more detail in Chapter 15.

Sucralfate (Carafate, Sulcrate). Sucralfate is a disaccharide that exerts a cytoprotective effect on the stomach mucosa.[12,29] Although the exact mechanism is unclear, sucralfate may form a protective gel within the stomach that adheres to ulcers and shields them from the stomach contents. The protective barrier formed by the drug prevents further erosion and permits healing of duodenal and gastric ulcers. Sucralfate is fairly well tolerated, although constipation may occur in some patients.

ANTIDIARRHEAL AGENTS

Normal propulsion of food through the GI tract is crucial for proper absorption of nutrients and water. If transit time is too fast, diarrhea occurs, resulting in poor food absorption and dehydration. Diarrhea is often a temporary symptom of many relatively minor GI disorders. Diarrhea may also occur with more serious conditions such as **dysentery,** ulcerative colitis, and cholera. If diarrhea is sustained for even a few days, the resulting dehydration can be a serious problem, especially in infants or debilitated patients. Consequently, efforts should be made to control diarrhea as soon as possible. Antidiarrheal agents are listed in Table 27–2, and their pharmacology is discussed in the following sections.

Opioid Derivatives

RATIONALE FOR USE AND MECHANISM OF ACTION

The constipating effects of morphine and certain other opioid derivatives have been recognized for some time. These drugs produce a general decrease in GI motility and prevent excessive propulsion. The exact manner in which opioids slow intestinal

TABLE 27–2 Antidiarrheal Agents

Generic Name	Trade Names	Dosage
Adsorbents		
Kaolin	Kaopectate, Kao-tin,	60–120 mL regular-strength suspension after each
Pectin	Kapectolin*	loose bowel movement
Bismuth salicylate	Pepto-Bismol	525 mg every half hour to 1 hour or 1050 mg every hour if needed
Opioid derivatives		
Diphenoxylate	Diphenatol, Lomotil, others†	2.5–5 mg 3 or 4 times daily
Loperamide	Imodium	4 mg initially, 2 mg after each unformed stool
Opium tincture	—	0.3–1.0 mL 1–4 times daily
Paregoric	—	5–10 mL 1–4 times daily

*Commercial products typically contain both kaolin and pectin.
†Commercial products often combine diphenoxylate (an opioid) with atropine (an anticholinergic).

peristalsis is not known. Opioid derivatives are believed to exert a local effect on the GI tract, probably at the level of intrinsic neural control within the gut wall.[5] Some of the antidiarrheal effects, however, may be caused by a central inhibitory effect on the brain as well.[6,21]

SPECIFIC AGENTS

Opioid derivatives used to treat diarrhea are listed in Table 27–2. Opium tincture (laudanum) and camphorated opium tincture (paregoric) are naturally occurring opiates that are very potent inhibitors of peristalsis. These natural agents are still available for treating diarrhea, but they have essentially been replaced by newer opioids such as diphenoxylate and loperamide. These newer opioids are somewhat less potent but may produce fewer side effects.

ADVERSE SIDE EFFECTS

The primary side effects with these drugs are nausea, abdominal discomfort, constipation, and other GI disturbances. Drowsiness, fatigue, and dizziness have also been reported. Although addiction is a potential problem when opioids are administered, the risk of tolerance and physical dependence is fairly small when these drugs are used in recommended dosages for the short-term treatment of diarrhea.

Adsorbents

RATIONALE FOR TREATMENT AND MECHANISM OF ACTION

Adsorbents are administered to take up and hold harmful substances such as bacteria and toxins in the intestinal lumen. Theoretically, these adsorbents sequester the harmful products causing the diarrhea. These products are used frequently in minor diarrhea, although there is some doubt as to whether they really help decrease stool production and water loss.

SPECIFIC AGENTS

Adsorbents used to treat diarrhea are listed in Table 27–2. These agents frequently appear as the active ingredients in over-the-counter products and may be combined with each other or with other drugs such as antacids.

ADVERSE SIDE EFFECTS

Adsorbents are essentially free from side effects, although constipation may occur following prolonged or excessive use.

Bismuth Salicylate

RATIONALE FOR TREATMENT AND MECHANISM OF ACTION

Bismuth salicylate has a number of properties that contribute to its antidiarrheal effects. This drug may stimulate water and electrolyte absorption from the lower GI tract, thus decreasing fecal fluid loss. In addition, the bismuth component of this compound may have antibacterial effects, and the salicylate component may inhibit the production of prostaglandins that irritate the intestinal lining. The combination of these properties makes this drug fairly effective in treating mild-to-moderate diarrhea.[7] Bismuth salicylate also decreases gastric acid secretion and exerts antacid effects, hence its use in stomach upset and minor gastric irritation.

SPECIFIC AGENTS

Bismuth salicylate is the active ingredient in Pepto-Bismol, a fairly inexpensive and readily available over-the-counter commercial product.

ADVERSE SIDE EFFECTS

This drug is relatively free from serious side effects. Problems with salicylate intoxication may occur during overdose or in people who are sensitive to aspirin and other salicylates.

LAXATIVES AND CATHARTICS

Rationale for Use

Laxatives are used to promote evacuation of the bowel and defecation. **Cathartics**, or purgatives, are also used to promote lower GI evacuation, but in a somewhat more rapid fashion than with typical laxatives. For this discussion, the term "laxative" will be used to include both the relatively slow-acting and fast-acting agents.

Laxatives are typically used whenever normal bowel movements have been impaired but no obstruction exists in the GI system. For instance, laxatives may benefit patients on prolonged bed rest, patients with infrequent or painful bowel movements, individuals with spinal cord injuries, or patients who should avoid straining during defecation (e.g., postpartum patients and those recovering from surgical procedures).

Laxatives are also indicated for bowel evacuation prior to surgical or diagnostic procedures.

The problem with laxatives is that they are frequently abused. The long-term, chronic use of laxatives is usually unnecessary and often unhealthy. These agents are often self-administered by individuals who are obsessed with maintaining daily bowel movements. Such individuals may have the misconception that daily bowel evacuation is needed to maintain normal GI function. Also, laxatives are often relied upon instead of other factors that promote normal bowel evacuation such as a high-fiber diet, adequate hydration, and physical activity. Consequently, laxatives serve an important but finite role in GI function, and their role in helping maintain routine daily evacuation should be de-emphasized.

Specific Agents and Mechanism of Action

There are many different types of laxatives available that are usually classified by their apparent mode of action.[35] Often, two different laxatives, either from the same class or from two different classes, will be combined in the same commercial preparation. Some of the more common laxatives are listed in Table 27–3 according to their apparent mechanisms of action. The major laxative classes and the rationale for their use are also outlined in the next few sections.

Bulk-Forming Laxatives. These agents absorb water and swell within the lower GI tract. The increased size of the water-laden laxative stretches the bowel, thus stimulating peristalsis. Bulk laxatives commonly contain natural and semisynthetic dietary fiber such as bran, psyllium, and methylcellulose.

Stimulant Laxatives. The precise mechanism of stimulant laxatives is not known. They may activate peristalsis by a direct irritant effect on the intestinal mucosa, or by stimulating the nerve plexus within the gut wall. Some evidence suggests that they

TABLE 27–3 Laxatives*

Bulk-forming	
Methylcellulose	Citrucel, Cologel
Psyllium	Fiberall, Metamucil
Stimulants	
Bisacodyl	Dulcolax
Castor oil	Purge
Phenolphthalein	Correctol, Ex-Lax, Feen-A-Mint
Hyperosmotic	
Glycerin	Sani-Supp
Lactulose	Chronulac
Magnesium hydroxide	Phillips' Milk of Magnesia
Magnesium sulfate	Epsom salts
Sodium phosphate	Fleet Enema
Lubricants and stool softeners	
Docusate	Colace, Disonate
Mineral oil	Agoral, Nujol

*Some of the more common agents are listed as examples in each laxative category. Common trade names are listed in the right-hand column. Many other preparations are available that combine two or more laxatives in the same commercial product.

may work by increasing fluid accumulation within the small intestine. Common stimulant laxatives are castor oil, bisacodyl, and phenolphthalein.

Hyperosmotic Laxatives. Administration of osmotically active substances produces a gradient that draws water into the bowel and small intestine. This gradient increases stool fluid content and stimulates peristalsis. A variety of hyperosmotic substances, including magnesium salts, sodium salts, potassium salts, lactulose, and glycerin, can be used to achieve this effect.

Lubricants and Stool Softeners. Agents like mineral oil and docusate facilitate entry of water into the fecal mass, thus softening the stool and permitting easier defecation. These agents may also exert a laxative effect because of the increased pressure in the bowel secondary to the increased stool size.

Adverse Effects

Disturbances in the GI system, such as nausea and cramps, may occur with laxative use. With prolonged use, serious lower GI irritation, including spastic colitis, may occur. Fluid and electrolyte abnormalities are also a potential problem. Excessive loss of water and the concomitant loss of electrolytes may transpire, resulting in dehydration and possible acid-base imbalances. These fluid and electrolyte abnormalities are especially significant in older or debilitated patients. Finally, chronic administration may result in a laxative dependence, where bowel evacuation has become so subservient to laxative use that the normal mechanisms governing evacuation and defecation are impaired.

MISCELLANEOUS GASTROINTESTINAL DRUGS

Several other types of drugs are administered for specific purposes in controlling GI function. These other drugs are introduced here only to alert the reader to their existence. For a more detailed description of the use of any of these agents, one of the drug indices such as the *Physician's Desk Reference* (*PDR*) should be consulted.

Digestants

These agents are administered to help aid in the digestion of food. The primary digestant preparations contain pancreatic enzymes or bile salts. Pancreatic enzymes such as amylase, trypsin, and lipase are responsible for digestion of carbohydrates, proteins, and lipids, respectively. These enzymes are normally synthesized in the pancreas and secreted into the duodenum via the pancreatic duct. Bile salts are synthesized in the liver, stored in the gallbladder, and released into the duodenum via the common bile duct. Bile salts serve to emulsify lipids in the intestinal tract and are important in lipid digestion and absorption.

Digestant preparations are used to replace digestive constituents in the stomach and upper small intestine whenever the endogenous production of these constituents is impaired. In particular, digestants are often administered to individuals with cystic fibrosis.[7] As discussed in Chapter 26, cystic fibrosis is a hereditary disease that affects all the major exocrine glands, resulting in thick, viscous secretions.[27] These thickened secretions may form mucous plugs that obstruct certain ducts such as the pancreatic and bile ducts. This condition leads to a chronic deficiency of pancreatic enzymes and bile salts, and, as a result, patients cannot digest and absorb nutrients from the GI tract. Preparations containing these digestants may be administered orally to replace these missing compounds, thus improving digestion and nutrient absorption.

Emetics

Emetics are used to induce vomiting and are frequently administered to help empty the stomach of poisons or ingested toxins. The two primary emetics are apomorphine and ipecac. Both agents seem to work by stimulating the medullary emetic center, and ipecac also exerts a direct emetic effect on the stomach.

Antiemetics

Antiemetics are used to decrease the nausea and vomiting that are associated with motion sickness and recovery from surgery, or in response to other medical treatments, such as cancer chemotherapy and radiation treatments. Antiemetic agents include antihistamines (dimenhydrinate, meclizine, others), phenothiazines (prochlorperazine, thiethylperazine), anticholinergics (scopolamine), and several other drugs that act at various sites in the CNS to suppress nausea and vomiting. Other antiemetic drugs such as antacids and adsorbents act locally to soothe the gastric mucosa and decrease the irritation that may cause vomiting.

Cholelitholytic Agents

Certain types of gallstones can be dissolved by drugs like chenodiol. This drug decreases the cholesterol content of bile and may help dissolve the types of gallstones that are supersaturated with cholesterol, but chenodiol does not appear effective in the treatment of calcified gallstones.

SPECIAL CONCERNS IN REHABILITATION PATIENTS

Drugs affecting the GI system are important in rehabilitation patients by virtue of their frequent use. About 60 to 100 percent of critically ill patients will suffer some degree of stress-related damage to the stomach mucosa.[22] This stress ulceration syndrome appears to be especially prevalent in patients with burns, multiple trauma, renal failure, and CNS trauma. Drugs such as the H_2 receptor blockers (cimetidine, ranitidine, others) are often helpful in controlling gastric acid secretions, thus preventing damage to the mucosal lining in these patients. Patients seen in rehabilitation are often relatively inactive and suffer from many adverse effects of prolonged bed rest, including constipation. Constipation and fecal impaction may also be a recurrent and serious problem in patients with spinal cord injuries. Laxatives are used routinely in these patients to facilitate adequate bowel evacuation. Patients receiving cancer chemotherapy often have problems with nausea and vomiting, and antiemetic drugs may be helpful in these individuals. Various other GI disorders including diarrhea and chronic indigestion occur frequently in many rehabilitation patients and are often treated effectively with the appropriate agents.

Despite their frequent use, most GI drugs do not produce any significant side effects that will impair rehabilitation procedures. Some dizziness and fatigue may occur with agents such as the opiates used to treat diarrhea or the antiulcer H_2 blockers, but this is fairly mild. Other problems with GI drugs are generally related to transient GI disturbances. In general, GI drugs are well tolerated and fairly safe in most patients. In effect, these drugs indirectly facilitate physical rehabilitation by resolving annoying and uncomfortable GI symptoms, thus allowing the patient to participate more readily in the rehabilitation program.

CASE STUDY

GASTROINTESTINAL DRUGS

Brief History. M.B. is a 48-year-old insurance sales representative with a long history of back pain. He has had recurrent episodes of sciatica because of a herniated disk at the L5-S1 interspace. Currently, he is being seen as an outpatient in a private physical therapy practice. Despite several treatments, his back pain did not improve. In fact, his pain was recently exacerbated when he was straining to pass a stool during a period of constipation. Evidently, this occurrence had been repeated often, and the patient's back problems had been increased by bowel-related problems causing straining during defecation.

Decision/Solution. The physical therapist consulted with the patient's physician and recommended that a brief trial with a bulk-forming laxative might be helpful during the acute episode of back pain in this patient. The therapist also explained to the patient that straining during defecation exacerbated his back problems. To prevent the recurrence of this problem, the patient was encouraged to ingest a high-fiber diet and adequate amounts of water to prevent constipation. M.B. was also informed that the short-term use of a laxative might be necessary to avoid constipation and straining. The therapist warned the patient, however, about the laxative dependence that can occur during chronic laxative use.

SUMMARY

A variety of pharmacologic agents are used to maintain proper function in the GI system. Drugs such as antacids and H_2 receptor antagonists help control gastric acid secretion and protect the stomach mucosa. These agents are widely used to prevent and treat peptic ulcer. Specific drugs are used to control GI motility. Drugs that inhibit excessive peristalsis (i.e., diarrhea) include the opiate derivatives, adsorbents, and bismuth salicylate. Decreased motility (constipation) is usually treated with various laxatives. Other GI agents attempt to treat specific problems such as poor digestion, emesis, or gallstones. GI drugs are used frequently in rehabilitation patients and, it is hoped, will produce beneficial effects that will allow the patient to participate more actively in the rehabilitation program.

REFERENCES

1. Altman, DF: Drugs used in gastrointestinal diseases. In Katzung, BG (ed): Basic and Clinical Pharmacology, ed 5. Appleton & Lange, Norwalk, CT, 1992.
2. Bader, JP (ed): Symposium: Advances in prostaglandins and gastroenterology: Focus on misoprostol. Am J Med 83(suppl 1a):1, 1987.
3. Becker, U, et al: Antacid treatment of duodenal ulcer. Acta Med Scand 221:95, 1987.
4. Befrits, R and Johansson, C: Oral PGE_2 inhibits gastric secretion in man. Prostaglandins 29:143, 1985.
5. Bianchi, G, et al: Morphine tissue levels and reduction of gastrointestinal transit in rats: Correlation supports primary action site in gut. Gastroenterology 85:852, 1983.
6. Borody, TJ and Quigley, EMM: Effects of morphine and atropine on motility and transit in the human ileum. Gastroenterology 89:522, 1985.
7. Brunton, LL: Agents affecting gastrointestinal water flux and motility, digestants, and bile acids. In Gilman, AG, et al (eds): The Pharmacological Basis of Therapeutics, ed 8. Pergamon Press, New York, 1990.
8. Burt, MJ: The management of peptic ulceration. NZ Med J 106:107, 1993.
9. Day, RO, et al: Non-steroidal anti-inflammatory induced upper gastrointestinal haemorrhage and bleeding. Med J Aust 157:810, 1992.
10. Feldman, M and Burton, ME: Drug therapy: Histamine$_2$-receptor antagonists: Standard therapy for acid-peptic diseases. N Engl J Med 323:1672, 1990.
11. Fromm, D: Mechanisms involved in gastric mucosal resistance to injury. Annu Rev Med 38:119, 1987.
12. Garnett, WR: Sucralfate: Alternative therapy for peptic-ulcer disease. Clin Pharm 1:307, 1982.
13. Garrison, JC: Histamine, bradykinin, 5-hydroxytryptamine, and their antagonists. In Gilman, AG, et al (eds): The Pharmacological Basis of Therapeutics, ed 8. Pergamon Press, New York, 1990.
14. Giorgi-Conciato, M, et al: Efficacy and safety of pirenzipine in peptic ulcer and nonulcerous gastroduodenal disease: A multicenter controlled clinical trial. Scand J Gastroenterol 17(suppl 81):1, 1982.
15. Gough, KR, et al: Ranitidine and cimetidine in prevention of duodenal ulcer relapse: A double-blind, randomized, multicenter, comparative trial. Lancet 2:659, 1984.
16. Hawkey, CJ and Rampton, DS: Prostaglandins and the gastrointestinal mucosa: Are they important in its function, disease, or treatment? Gastroenterology 89:1162, 1985.
17. Herting, RL and Nissen, CH: Overview of misoprostol clinical experience. Dig Dis Sci 31(suppl):47S, 1986.
18. Holtermuller, KH and Dehdaschti, M: Antacids and hormones. Scand J Gastroenterol 17(suppl 75):24, 1982.
19. Lewis, JH: Treatment of gastric ulcer: What is old and what is new. Arch Intern Med 143:264, 1983.
20. Liedberg, G, et al: Ulcer healing and relapse prevention by ranitidine in peptic ulcer disease. Scand J Gastroenterol 20:941, 1985.
21. Manara, L and Bianchetti, A: The central and peripheral influences of opioids on gastrointestinal propulsion. Annu Rev Pharmacol Toxicol 25:249, 1985.
22. Peura, DA and Freston, JW: Introduction: Evolving perspectives on parenteral H$_2$-receptor antagonist therapy. Am J Med 83(suppl 6a):1, 1987.
23. Piper, DW: Drugs for the prevention of peptic ulcer recurrence. Drugs 26:439, 1983.
24. Richardson, CT: Pathogenetic factors in peptic ulcer disease. Am J Med 79(suppl 2c):1, 1985.
25. Richter, JE and Castell, DO: Gastroesophageal reflux: Pathogenesis, diagnosis, and therapy. Ann Intern Med 97:93, 1982.
26. Rohner, H-G and Gugler, R: Treatment of active duodenal ulcers with famotidine: A double-blind comparison with ranitidine. Am J Med 81(suppl 4b):13, 1986.
27. Rubin, E and Farber, JL: Developmental and genetic diseases. In Rubin, E and Farber, JL (eds): Pathology, ed 2. JB Lippincott, Philadelphia, 1994.
28. Russel, RI: Protective effects of the prostaglandins on the gastric mucosa. Am J Med 81(suppl 2a):2, 1986.
29. Sabesin, SM and Lam, SK (eds): Symposium: International sucralfate research conference. Am J Med 83(suppl 3b):1, 1987.
30. Sachs, G, et al: Gastric H^+, K^+−ATPase as a therapeutic target. Annu Rev Pharmacol Toxicol 28:269, 1988.
31. Shield, MJ: Interim results of a multicenter international comparison of misoprostol and cimetidine in the treatment of out-patients with benign gastric ulcers. Dig Dis Sci 30(suppl):178S, 1985.
32. Sontag, SJ: Prostaglandins in peptic ulcer disease: An overview of current status and future directions. Drugs 32:445, 1986.
33. Strom, M, et al: Results of short- and long-term cimetidine treatment in patients with juxtapyloric ulcers, with special reference to gastric acid and pepsin secretion. Scand J Gastroenterol 21:521, 1986.

34. Strum, WB: Prevention of duodenal ulcer recurrence. Ann Intern Med 105:757, 1986.
35. Tedesco, FJ: Laxative use in constipation. Am J Gastroenterol 80:303, 1985.
36. Voirin, J: Drug therapy for peptic ulcer disease. Am Fam Physician 30:154, 1984.
37. Walt, RP: Drug therapy: Misoprostol for the treatment of peptic ulcer and anti-inflammatory-drug induced gastroduodenal ulceration. N Engl J Med 327:1575, 1992.
38. Waterbury, LD, Mahoney, JM, and Peak, TM: Stimulatory effect of enprostil, an anti-ulcer prostaglandin, on gastric mucus secretion. Am J Med 81(suppl 2a):30, 1986.
39. Whitehead, WE and Schuster, MM: Gastrointestinal Disorders: Behavioral and Physiological Basis for Treatment. Academic Press, New York, 1985.
40. Winters, L: Comparison of enprostil and cimetidine in active duodenal ulcer disease: Summary of pooled European studies. Am J Med 81(suppl 2a):69, 1986.

Endocrine Pharmacology

CHAPTER 28

Introduction to Endocrine Pharmacology

The endocrine system helps maintain internal homeostasis through the use of endogenous chemicals known as hormones. A *hormone* is typically regarded as a chemical messenger that is released into the bloodstream to exert an effect on target cells located some distance from the site of hormonal release.[2] Various endocrine glands manufacture and release specific hormones that help regulate such physiologic processes as reproduction, growth and development, energy metabolism, fluid and electrolyte balance, and the response to stress and injury.[18,39]

The use of drugs to help regulate and control endocrine function is an important area of pharmacology. In one sense, hormones can be considered drugs that are manufactured by the patient's body. This situation presents an obvious opportunity to use exogenous chemicals to either mimic or attenuate the effects of specific hormones during endocrine dysfunction.

Drugs can be used as replacement therapy during hormonal deficiency, for example, insulin administration in diabetes mellitus. Likewise, exogenous hormone analogs can be administered to accentuate the effects of their endogenous counterparts, such as using corticosteroids to help treat inflammation. Conversely, drugs can be administered to treat endocrine hyperactivity; for example, the use of antithyroid drugs in treating hyperthyroidism. Finally, drugs can be used to regulate normal endocrine function to achieve a desired effect, as is seen through inhibition of ovulation by oral contraceptives.

The purpose of this chapter is to review the basic aspects of endocrine function, including the primary hormones and their effects. The factors regulating hormonal release and cellular mechanisms of hormone action are also briefly discussed. Finally, the basic ways in which drugs can be used to alter endocrine function are presented. This overview is intended to provide rehabilitation specialists with a general review of endocrine and hormone activity, with subsequent chapters dealing with specific endocrine drugs and the problems they are used to treat.

405

PRIMARY ENDOCRINE GLANDS AND THEIR HORMONES

The primary endocrine glands and the hormones they produce are briefly discussed here. These glands and the physiologic effects of their hormones are also summarized in Tables 28–1 and 28–2. For the purpose of this chapter, only the primary endocrine glands and their respective hormones are discussed. Substances such as prostaglandins and kinins, which are produced locally by a variety of different cells, are not discussed here, but are referred to elsewhere in this text (e.g., see Chapter 15). Also, chemicals such as norepinephrine, which serve a dual purpose as hormones and neurotransmitters, are discussed in this chapter only with regard to their endocrine function.

Hypothalamus and Pituitary Gland

The pituitary gland is a small, pea-shaped structure located within the sella turcica at the base of the brain. The pituitary lies inferior to the hypothalamus and is attached to the hypothalamus by a thin stalk of tissue known as the *infundibulum*. The structural and functional relationships between the hypothalamus and pituitary gland are briefly discussed further on in this section. A more detailed presentation of the anatomic and physiologic function of the hypothalamus and pituitary gland can be found in several sources listed at the end of this chapter.[12,18,19,31]

The pituitary can be subdivided into an anterior, an intermediate, and a posterior

TABLE 28–1 Hypothalamic and Pituitary Hormones

Hypothalamic Hormones and Releasing Factors	Effect
Growth hormone–releasing hormone (GHRH)	↑ GH release
Growth hormone–inhibitory hormone (GHIH)	↓ GH release
Gonadotropin-releasing hormone (GnRH)	↑ LH and FSH release
Thyrotropin-releasing hormone (TRH)	↑ TSH release
Corticotropin-releasing hormone (CRH)	↑ ACTH release
Prolactin-inhibitory factor (PIF)	↓ Pr release

Pituitary Hormones	*Principal Effects*
Anterior lobe	
Growth hormone (GH)	↑ tissue growth and development
Luteinizing hormone (LH)	Female: ↑ ovulation; ↑ estrogen and progesterone synthesis from corpus luteum Male: ↑ spermatogenesis
Follicle-stimulating hormone (FSH)	Female: ↑ follicular development and estrogen synthesis Male: Enhance spermatogenesis
Thyroid-stimulating hormone (TSH)	↑ synthesis of thyroid hormones (T_3, T_4)
Adrenocorticotropic hormone (ACTH)	↑ adrenal steroid synthesis (e.g., cortisol)
Prolactin (Pr)	Initiates lactation
Posterior lobe	
Antidiuretic hormone (ADH)	↑ renal reabsorption of water
Oxytocin	↑ uterine contraction; ↑ milk ejection during lactation

TABLE 28-2 Other Primary Endocrine Glands

Gland	Hormone(s)	Principal Effects
Thyroid	Thyroxine (T_4) Triiodothyronine (T_3)	Increase cellular metabolism; facilitate normal growth and development
Parathyroids	Parathormone (PTH)	Increase blood calcium
Pancreas	Glucagon	Increase blood glucose
	Insulin	Decrease blood glucose; increase carbohydrate, protein, and fat storage
Adrenal cortex	Glucocorticoids	Regulate glucose metabolism; enhance response to stress
	Mineralocorticoids	Regulate fluid and electrolyte levels
Adrenal medulla	Epinephrine Norepinephrine	Vascular and metabolic effects that facilitate increased physical activity
Testes	Testosterone	Spermatogenesis; male sexual characteristics
Ovaries	Estrogens Progesterone	Female reproductive cycle and sexual characteristics

lobe. These subdivisions and their respective hormones are listed in Table 28-1 and are briefly discussed here.

Anterior Lobe. The anterior pituitary, or adenohypophysis, secretes six important peptide hormones. Hormones released from the anterior pituitary are growth hormone (GH), luteinizing hormone (LH), follicle-stimulating hormone (FSH), thyroid-stimulating hormone (TSH), adrenocorticotropic hormone (ACTH), and prolactin (Pr). The physiologic effects of these hormones are listed in Table 28-1.

Hormonal release from the anterior pituitary is controlled by specific hormones or releasing factors from the hypothalamus.[38] Basically, a releasing factor is sent from the hypothalamus to the anterior pituitary via local vascular structures known as the hypothalamic-hypophysial portal vessels. For example, to increase the secretion of growth hormone, the hypothalamus first secretes growth hormone–releasing hormone (GHRH) into the portal vessels. The GHRH travels the short distance to the anterior pituitary via the hypothalamic-hypophysial portal system. Upon arriving at the pituitary, the GHRH causes the anterior pituitary to release growth hormone into the systemic circulation, where it can then travel to various target tissues in the periphery. Other hypothalamic-releasing factors that have been identified are listed in Table 28-1. Specific releasing factors are still being investigated, and the identification of additional releasing factors (including factors that inhibit anterior pituitary hormone release) will undoubtedly be forthcoming.

Intermediate Lobe. In mammals, there is a small intermediate lobe of the pituitary that may secrete melanocyte-stimulating hormone (MSH). Although it can influence skin pigmentation in lower vertebrates, MSH is not produced in meaningful amounts in humans, and human skin does not have receptors that mediate MSH responses similar to those seen in other animals.[19] Hence, MSH does not have any apparent physiologic or pharmacologic significance in humans.

Posterior Lobe. The posterior pituitary, or neurohypophysis, secretes two hormones: antidiuretic hormone (ADH) and oxytocin. ADH exerts its effect primarily on the kidney, where it increases the reabsorption of water from the distal renal tubules. Oxytocin, which is important in parturition, stimulates the uterus to contract. It also promotes lactation by stimulating the ejection of milk from the mammary glands.

The hypothalamic control of the posterior pituitary is quite different than in the anterior and intermediate lobes. Specific neurons have their cell bodies in certain hypothalamic nuclei. Cell bodies in the paraventricular nuclei manufacture oxytocin, whereas the supraoptic nuclei contain cell bodies that synthesize ADH. The axons from these cells extend downward through the infundibulum to terminate in the posterior pituitary. The hormones synthesized in the hypothalamic cell bodies are transported down the axon to be stored in neurosecretory granules in their respective nerve terminals located in the posterior pituitary. When an appropriate stimulus is present, these neurons fire an action potential, which causes the hormones to be released from their pituitary nerve terminals. The hormones are ultimately picked up by the systemic circulation and transported to their target tissues.

Thyroid Gland

The thyroid gland is located in the anterior neck region approximately at the level of the fifth cervical to first thoracic vertebrae. This gland consists of bilateral lobes that lie on either side of the trachea and are connected by a thin piece of the gland known as the isthmus. The thyroid synthesizes and secretes two hormones: thyroxine (T_4) and triiodothyronine (T_3). The synthesis of these hormones is controlled by the hypothalamic-pituitary system via thyroid-releasing hormone from the hypothalamus, which causes thyroid-stimulating hormone release from the anterior pituitary. Thyroid-stimulating hormone increases T_3 and T_4 synthesis and release from the thyroid gland.

The primary effect of the thyroid hormones is to increase cellular metabolism in most body tissues.[12,21] These hormones stimulate virtually all aspects of cellular function, including protein, fat, and carbohydrate metabolism. By exerting a stimulatory effect on the cellular level, the thyroid hormones play a crucial role in helping maintain and regulate body heat (*thermogenesis*) in the whole organism. T_3 and T_4 also play an important role in growth and development, especially in the growth and maturation of normal bone. Finally, thyroid hormones play a permissive role in allowing other hormones such as steroids to exert their effects. Physiology and pharmacology of the thyroid hormones are further discussed in Chapter 31.

Parathyroid Gland

The parathyroid glands are small, egg-shaped structures embedded in the posterior surface of the thyroid gland. There are usually four parathyroid glands, with two glands located on each half of the thyroid gland. The parathyroids synthesize and release parathyroid hormone (PTH). PTH is essential in maintaining normal calcium homeostasis in the body, and the primary effect of PTH is to increase the concentration of calcium in the bloodstream.[1,12] PTH increases circulating calcium levels primarily by mobilizing calcium from storage sites in bone.

The primary factor regulating PTH release is the level of calcium in the bloodstream.[29] Parathyroid gland cells appear to act as calcium sensors that monitor circulating calcium levels. As circulating calcium levels fall below a certain level, PTH secretion is increased. Conversely, elevated plasma calcium titers inhibit PTH secretion. The pituitary gland may also influence PTH secretion to some extent, but the presence of a specific hormone that stimulates parathyroid function in humans remains to be determined.[22]

Pancreas

The pancreas is located behind the stomach in the lower left area of the abdomen. This gland is unique in that it serves both endocrine and exocrine functions.[9,12] The exocrine aspect of this gland involves digestive enzymes that are excreted into the duodenum. As an endocrine gland, the pancreas primarily secretes two peptide hormones: insulin and glucagon. These hormones are synthesized and secreted by cells located in specialized clusters known as the *islets of Langerhans*. In the islets of Langerhans, glucagon and insulin are synthesized by A (alpha) and B (beta) cells, respectively.

Pancreatic hormones are involved in the regulation of blood glucose, and the glucose concentration in the blood serves as the primary stimulus for the release of these hormones. As blood glucose levels fall—for example, following a fast—glucagon is released from pancreatic alpha cells. Glucagon mobilizes the release of glucose from storage sites in the liver, thus bringing blood glucose levels back to normal. An increase in blood glucose after eating a meal stimulates insulin release from the beta cells. Insulin facilitates the storage of glucose in liver and muscle, thus removing glucose from the bloodstream and returning blood glucose back to normal levels. Insulin also exerts a number of other effects on protein and lipid metabolism. The effects of insulin and the pharmacologic replacement of insulin in diabetes mellitus are discussed in more detail in Chapter 32.

Adrenal Gland

The adrenal glands are located at the superior poles of each kidney. Each adrenal gland is composed of an outer cortex and an inner medulla. The hormones associated with the adrenal cortex and adrenal medulla are described in the following sections.

Hormones of the Adrenal Cortex. The adrenal cortex synthesizes and secretes two primary groups of steroidal hormones: the **glucocorticoids** and the **mineralocorticoids**.[28] Small amounts of sex steroids (estrogens, androgens, progesterone) are also produced, but these amounts are essentially insignificant during normal adrenal function.

Glucocorticoids such as cortisol have a number of physiologic effects.[13] Glucocorticoids are involved in the regulation of glucose metabolism and are important in enhancing the body's ability to handle stress. Glucocorticoids also have significant anti-inflammatory and immunosuppressive properties and are often used therapeutically to control inflammation or suppress the immune response in various clinical situations. Glucocorticoid synthesis is controlled by the hypothalamic-pituitary system. Corticotropin-releasing hormone (CRH) from the hypothalamus stimulates ACTH release from the anterior pituitary, which in turn stimulates the synthesis of glucocorticoids.

Mineralocorticoids are involved in controlling electrolyte and fluid levels.[30] The primary mineralocorticoid produced by the adrenal cortex is *aldosterone*. Aldosterone increases the reabsorption of sodium from the renal tubules. By increasing sodium reabsorption, aldosterone facilitates the reabsorption of water. Aldosterone also inhibits the renal reabsorption of potassium, thus increasing potassium excretion. Mineralocorticoid release is regulated by fluid and electrolyte levels in the body and by other hormones such as the renin-angiotensin system.

The pharmacologic aspects of the glucocorticoids and mineralocorticoids are discussed in more detail in Chapter 29.

Hormones of the Adrenal Medulla. The adrenal medulla synthesizes and secretes epinephrine and norepinephrine.[20] These hormones have a number of physiologic effects, which are discussed in Chapters 18 and 20. Small amounts of epinephrine and norepinephrine are released under resting, basal conditions. The primary significance of these hormones, however, seems to be in helping prepare the body for sudden physical activity. The classic function of the adrenal medulla is illustrated by the fight-or-flight reaction, where a stressful challenge is presented to the individual and is interpreted as requiring either defense or a need to flee from the challenge.

The release of epinephrine and norepinephrine from the adrenal medulla is controlled by the sympathetic division of the autonomic nervous system. As discussed in Chapter 18, sympathetic cholinergic preganglionic neurons directly innervate this gland. An increase in sympathetic activity causes increased firing in these neurons, which in turn stimulates the release of epinephrine and norepinephrine from the adrenal medulla.

Gonads

The reproductive organs are the primary source of steroid hormones, which influence various aspects of sexual and reproduction function. In men, the testes produce *testosterone* and similar **androgens** that are responsible for spermatogenesis and the secondary sexual characteristics of adult males.[7,34] In women, sexual maturation and reproductive function are governed by the production of **estrogens** and **progestins** from the ovaries.[14,25] The release of male and female sex steroids is controlled by hormones from the hypothalamus and anterior pituitary.[6,7,32] The control of male and female hormone activity and the pharmacologic implications of these hormones are discussed in Chapter 30.

ENDOCRINE PHYSIOLOGY AND PHARMACOLOGY

Hormone Chemistry

Hormones can be divided into several primary categories according to their basic chemical structure. *Steroid hormones* share a common chemical framework that is derived from lipids such as cholesterol.[24] Examples of steroids include the sex hormones (androgens, estrogens, progesterone), the glucocorticoids, and the mineralocorticoids. *Peptide hormones* consist of amino acids linked together in a specific sequence. These peptide chains can range in length anywhere from 3 amino acids to 180 amino acids. Primary examples of peptide hormones are the hypothalamic releasing factors and the pituitary hormones. Finally, several hormones are modified from a single amino acid. For instance, the thyroid hormones (T_3 and T_4) are manufactured from the amino acid tyrosine. Also, hormones from the adrenal medulla (epinephrine, norepinephrine) are synthesized from either phenylalanine or tyrosine.

The basic chemical structure of various hormones is significant in determining how the hormone will exert its effects on target tissues (see "Hormone Effects on the

Target Cell"). Also, different hormones that are fairly similar in structure can often have similar physiologic and pharmacologic effects. This is especially true for the steroids, in which one category of steroidal agents may have some of the properties of a different category.[24] For instance, the endogenous glucocorticoids—for example, cortisol—also exert some mineralocorticoid effects, presumably because of their similar chemical structure. These overlapping effects and their consequences are discussed in more detail in Chapters 29 through 32, which deal with specific endocrine systems.

Synthesis and Release of Hormones

Hormones are typically synthesized within the cells of their respective endocrine glands. Most hormones are synthesized and packaged in storage granules within the gland. When the gland is stimulated, the storage granule fuses with the cell membrane and the hormone is released by exocytosis. Notable exceptions to this are the thyroid and steroid hormones, which are not stored to any great extent, but are synthesized on demand when an appropriate stimulus is present.[21]

Hormone synthesis and release can be initiated by both extrinsic and intrinsic factors.[2] Extrinsic factors include various environmental stimuli such as pain, temperature, light, smell, and so on. Intrinsic stimuli include various humoral and neural factors. For instance, release of a hormone can be initiated by other hormones. These occurrences are particularly true of the anterior pituitary hormones, which are controlled by releasing hormones from the hypothalamus. Hormonal release can be influenced by neural input; a primary example is the sympathetic neural control of epinephrine and norepinephrine release from the adrenal medulla. Other intrinsic factors that affect hormone release are the levels of ions and metabolites within the body. For instance, parathyroid hormone release is directly governed by the calcium concentration in the bloodstream, and the release of glucagon from pancreatic alpha cells is dependent on blood glucose levels.

Feedback Control Mechanisms in Endocrine Function

As mentioned previously, the endocrine system is concerned with maintaining homeostasis within the body. When a disturbance in physiologic function occurs, hormones are released to rectify the disturbance. As function returns to normal, hormone release is attenuated and homeostasis is resumed. For example, an increase in the blood glucose level initiates the release of insulin from pancreatic beta cells. Insulin increases the incorporation into and storage of glucose in liver, skeletal muscle, and other tissues. Blood glucose levels then return to normal, and insulin release is terminated.

Hormonal release is also frequently regulated by some form of negative feedback system.[8,12] In these feedback systems, increased release of a specific hormone ultimately serves to inhibit its own release, thus preventing the amount of the released hormone from becoming excessively large. An example of a negative feedback system involving the hypothalamic-pituitary axis is illustrated in Figure 28–1. The endocrine hormone ultimately inhibits its own release by inhibiting the secretion of specific hypothalamic releasing factors and pituitary hormones. Numerous examples of such negative feedback loops are present in various endocrine pathways.

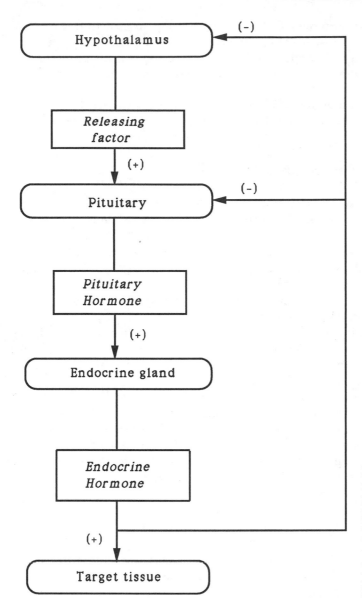

FIGURE 28–1. Negative feedback control in the hypothalamic–pituitary–endocrine pathways. Excitatory and inhibitory effects are indicated by (+) and (−), respectively. Negative feedback loops occur owing to inhibition of the endocrine hormone on the pituitary and hypothalamus.

There are also a few examples of positive feedback mechanisms in the endocrine system. In a positive feedback loop, rising concentrations of one hormone cause an increase in other hormones, which, in turn, facilitates increased production of the first hormone. The primary example of this type of feedback occurs in the female reproductive system, where low levels of estrogen production increase the release of pituitary hormones (LH, FSH).[14,17] Increased LH and FSH then facilitate further estrogen production, which further increases pituitary hormone secretion and so on (see Chapter 30). Positive feedback mechanisms are relatively rare, however, compared with negative feedback controls in the endocrine system.

The presence of feedback systems in endocrine function is important from a pharmacologic perspective. Drugs can be administered that act through the intrinsic feedback loops to control endogenous hormone production. A primary example is the use of oral contraceptives, where exogenous estrogen and progesterone are administered in controlled amounts to inhibit ovulation (see Chapter 30). Therapeutic administration of hormonal agents may create problems, however, due to these negative feedback effects. For instance, glucocorticoid administration may act as negative feedback to suppress the normal endogenous production of adrenal steroids.[33] If the body is unable to produce its own supply of adrenal steroids, abrupt withdrawal of the exogenous compounds can result in severe or even fatal consequences. Adrenocortical suppression is discussed in more detail in Chapter 29.

Hormone Transport

Hormones are usually carried from their site of origin to the target cell via the systemic circulation.[2] During transport in the bloodstream, certain hormones such as steroids are bound to specific plasma proteins. These protein carriers appear to help prolong the half-life of the hormone and prevent premature degradation. Other protein carriers may be important in the local effects of hormone function. For instance, the testes produce androgen-binding protein, which helps transport and concentrate testosterone within the seminiferous tubules of the testes (see Chapter 30).

Hormone Effects on the Target Cell

Most hormones affect their target cell by interacting with a specific receptor. Hormone receptors are usually located at one of the three locations shown in Figure 28–2. These primary locations are on the surface membrane of the cell, within the cytosol of the cell, or within the cell's nucleus.[10] Receptors at each location tend to be specific for different types of hormones and also tend to affect cell function in a specific manner. Each type of receptor is briefly discussed here.

Surface Membrane Receptors. These receptors are located on the outer surface of the plasma membrane (see Fig. 28–2.)[16] Surface receptors tend to recognize the peptide hormones and some amino acid derivatives (e.g., pituitary hormones, catecholamines). Surface receptors are typically linked to specific intracellular enzymes. When stimulated by a peptidelike hormone, the receptor initiates some change in the enzymatic machinery located within the cell. This event usually results in a change in the production of some intracellular chemical second messenger such as cyclic adenosine monophosphate (cAMP).[12]

An example of a hormone that exerts its effects through a surface receptor–second messenger system is ACTH.[36] ACTH is a polypeptide that binds to a surface receptor on adrenal cortex cells. The surface receptor then stimulates the adenylate cyclase enzyme to increase production of cAMP. The cAMP acts as a second messenger (the hormone was the first messenger), which then increases the activity of other enzymes within the cell to synthesize adrenal steroids such as cortisol. For a more detailed description of surface receptor–second messenger systems, see Chapter 4.

Cytosolic Hormone Receptors. The steroid hormones typically bind to protein receptors, which are located directly within the cytosol (see Fig. 28–2.)[5,23] Of course, this means that the hormone must first enter the cell, which is easily accomplished by

FIGURE 28–2. Primary cellular locations of hormone receptors. Peptide hormones tend to bind to surface membrane receptors (site I); steroid hormones bind to cytosolic receptors (site II); and thyroid hormones bind to receptors in the cell nucleus (site III).

the steroid hormones because they are highly lipid soluble. After entering the cell, the hormone initiates a series of events that are depicted in Figure 28–3. Basically, the hormone and receptor form a large activated steroid–receptor complex.[26,35] This complex then travels to the cell's nucleus, where it binds to specific genes located within the DNA sequence.[3,4,11] This process initiates gene expression and transcription of messenger RNA units, which go back to the cytosol and are translated into specific proteins by the endoplasmic reticulum.[4] These newly manufactured proteins are usually enzymes or structural proteins that change cell function in a specific manner. For instance, **anabolic steroids** increase muscle size by facilitating the production of more contractile proteins. Thus, steroids tend to exert their effects on target cells by directly affecting the cell's nucleus and subsequently altering the production of certain cellular proteins.

Nuclear Hormone Receptors. Receptors located directly on the chromatin within the cell nucleus are specific for the thyroid hormones (see Fig. 28–2.)[15,27] Thyroid hormones (T_3 and T_4) that reach these nuclear receptors invoke a series of changes similar to those caused by the steroid–cytosolic receptor complex; that is, the nucleus begins to transcribe messenger RNA, which ultimately is translated into specific proteins. In the case of the thyroid hormones, these new proteins usually alter the cell's metabolism. The thyroid hormones are discussed in more detail in Chapter 31.

Hormone receptors have some obvious and important pharmacologic distinction. Drugs that can bind to and activate specific hormonal receptors (agonists) will mimic the effects of the endogenous compounds. Drugs that block the receptors (antagonists) will attenuate any unwanted hormonal effects. In fact, drugs may be produced that are

Steroid-responsive Cell

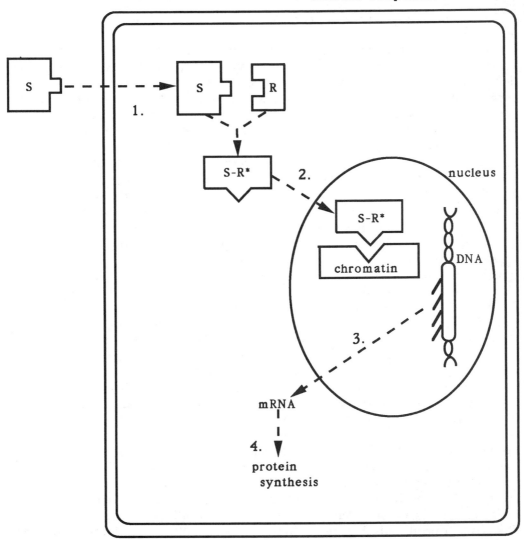

FIGURE 28–3. Sequence of events of steroid hormone action. (1) Steroid hormone enters the cell, binds to a cytosolic receptor, and creates an activated steroid-receptor complex (S-R). (2) S-R complex travels to the cell's nucleus, where it binds to specific gene segments on nuclear chromatin. (3) DNA undergoes transcription into messenger RNA (mRNA) units. (4) mRNA undergoes translation in the cytosol into specific proteins that alter cell function.

even more specific for hormonal receptors that their endogenous counterparts. For instance, synthetic glucocorticoids, such as dexamethasone, exert anti-inflammatory effects in a manner similar to that of endogenous glucocorticoids, but with diminished mineralocorticoid-like side effects such as water and sodium retention. This increased specificity is presumably brought about by a more precise action of the synthetic compound on the glucocorticoid rather than the mineralocorticoid receptors.

CLINICAL USE OF ENDOCRINE DRUGS

The general ways in which pharmacologic agents can be used to alter endocrine activity are as follows.

Replacement Therapy. If the endogenous production of a hormone is deficient or absent, therapeutic administration of the hormone can be used to restore normal endocrine function.[37] The exogenous hormone can be obtained from natural sources, such as extracts from animal tissues, or from chemical synthesis. In addition, new recombinant DNA techniques are being used to produce hormones from cell cultures, and these techniques have shown great promise in being able to generate hormones like human insulin.

Hormone substitution is sometimes referred to as simple replacement therapy. The use of exogenous hormones to replace normal endocrine function is sometimes a complicated task, however. Problems such as regulation of optimal dosage, interaction of the exogenous drug with other endogenous hormone systems, and drug-induced side effects are frequently encountered.

Diagnosis of Endocrine Disorders. Hormones or their antagonists can be administered to determine the presence of excess endocrine function or endocrine hypofunction. For example, hormones or their synthetic analogs can be administered that either increase or decrease pituitary secretion to determine if pituitary function is normal. Likewise, antagonists to specific hormones can be administered to see if symptoms are caused by excessive production of these hormones. Specific examples of how hormones are used to diagnose endocrine abnormalities are presented in subsequent chapters.

Treatment of Excessive Endocrine Function. Hyperactive or inappropriate endocrine function is often treated pharmacologically. Inhibition of hormone function can occur at several levels. For instance, drugs may be administered that directly inhibit the synthesis of the hormone or inhibit its release through various negative feedback mechanisms (see "Feedback Control Mechanisms in Endocrine Function"). Also, hormone antagonists, drugs that block hormone receptors, may be used for prolonged periods to attenuate the effects of excessive hormone production.

Exploitation of Beneficial Hormone Effects. Hormones and their synthetic analogs are often administered to exaggerate the beneficial effects of their endogenous counterparts. The classic example is the use of glucocorticoids to treat inflammation. Doses of glucocorticoids that are much higher than the physiologic levels produced by the body can be very effective in decreasing inflammation in a variety of clinical conditions (e.g., rheumatoid arthritis, allergic reactions). Of course, the use of high doses of hormones to accentuate beneficial effects may also cause some adverse side effects and impair various aspects of endocrine function. The short-term use of hormones in this capacity is often a useful therapeutic intervention, however.

Use of Hormones to Alter Normal Endocrine Function. Because of the intrinsic control mechanisms in the endocrine system, administration of exogenous hormones can often affect the normal release of hormones. This fact can be exploited in certain situations to cause a desired change in normal endocrine function. For instance, oral contraceptives containing estrogen and progesterone inhibit ovulation by inhibiting the release of LH and FSH from the anterior pituitary.

Use of Hormones in Nonendocrine Disease. There are many examples of how various hormones and hormone-related drugs can be used to treat conditions that are not directly related to the endocrine system. For instance, certain forms of cancer respond to treatment with sex steroids (see Chapter 36). Drugs that block the cardiac beta-1 receptors may help control angina and hypertension by preventing excessive stimulation from adrenal medulla hormones (epinephrine, norepinephrine) (see Chapters 21 and 22).

SUMMARY

The endocrine glands regulate a variety of physiologic processes through the release of specific hormones. Hormones are the equivalent of endogenously produced drugs that usually travel through the bloodstream to exert an effect on specific target tissues. Hormones typically alter cell function by binding to receptors located at specific sites on or within the target cell. Pharmacologic agents can be administered to mimic or exaggerate hormonal effects, inhibit excessive hormonal activity, and produce other desirable changes in endocrine activity. The use of hormones and hormone-related substances in the pharmacologic management of specific disorders is discussed in Chapters 29 through 32.

REFERENCES

1. Aurbach, GD, Marx, SJ, and Spiegel, AM: Parathyroid hormone, calcitonin, and the calciferols. In Wilson, JD and Foster, DW (eds): Textbook of Endocrinology, ed 8. WB Saunders, Philadelphia, 1992.
2. Baulieu, EE: Hormones, a complex communications network. In Baulieu, EE and Kelly, PA (eds): Hormones: From Molecule to Disease. Chapman & Hall, New York, 1990.
3. Becker, PB, et al: In vivo protein-DNA interactions in a glucocorticoid response element require the presence of the hormone. Nature 324:686, 1986.
4. Burnstein, KL and Cidlowski, JA: Regulation of gene expression by glucocorticoids. Annu Rev Physiol 51:683, 1989.
5. Clark, JH, Schrader, WT, and O'Malley, BW: Mechanisms of action of steroid hormones. In Wilson, JD and Foster, DW (eds): Textbook of Endocrinology, ed 8. WB Saunders, Philadelphia, 1992.
6. Conn, PM, et al: Mechanism of action of gonadotropin releasing hormone. Annu Rev Physiol 48:495, 1986.
7. Dufau, ML: Endocrine regulation and communicating functions of the Leydig cell. Annu Rev Physiol 50:483, 1988.
8. Genuth, SM: General principles of endocrine physiology. In Berne, RM and Levy, MN (eds): Physiology, ed 3. Mosby Year Book, St Louis, 1993.
9. Genuth, SM: Hormones of the pancreatic islets. In Berne, RM and Levy, MN (eds): Physiology, ed 3. Mosby Year Book, St Louis, 1993.
10. Goth, A: Medical Pharmacology: Principles and Concepts, ed 11. CV Mosby, St Louis, 1984.
11. Groner, B, et al: DNA sequences involved in the regulation of gene expression by glucocorticoid hormones. Biochem Biophys Acta 781:1, 1984.
12. Guyton, AC: Textbook of Medical Physiology, ed 8. WB Saunders, Philadelphia, 1991.
13. Haynes, RC: Adrenocorticotropic hormone; adrenocortical steroids and their synthetic analogs; inhibitors of the synthesis and actions of adrenocortical hormones. In Gilman, AG, et al (eds): The Pharmacological Basis of Therapeutics, ed 8. Pergamon Press, New York, 1990.
14. Hotchkiss, J and Knobil, E: The menstrual cycle and its neuroendocrine control. In Knobil, E and Neill, JD (eds): The Physiology of Reproduction, Vol 2, ed 2. Raven Press, New York, 1994.
15. Jaffe, RD: Thyroid hormone receptors. In Conn, PM (ed): The Receptors, Vol 1. Academic Press, New York, 1984.
16. Kahn, CR, Smith, RJ, and Chin, WW: Mechanism of action of hormones that act at the cell surface. In Wilson, JD and Foster, DW (eds): Textbook of Endocrinology, ed 8. WB Saunders, Philadelphia, 1992.
17. Karsch, FJ: Central actions of ovarian steroids in the feedback regulation of pulsatile secretion of luteinizing hormone. Annu Rev Physiol 49:365, 1990.
18. Klonoff, DC and Karam, JH: Hypothalamic and pituitary hormones. In Katzung, BG (ed): Basic and Clinical Pharmacology, ed 5. Appleton & Lange, Norwalk, CT, 1992.
19. Kuret, JA and Murad, F: Adenohypophyseal hormones and related substances. In Gilman, AG, et al (eds): The Pharmacological Basis of Therapeutics, ed 8. Pergamon Press, New York, 1990.

20. Landsberg, L and Young, JB: Catecholamines and the adrenal medulla. In Wilson, JD and Foster, DW (eds): Textbook of Endocrinology, ed 8. WB Saunders, Philadelphia, 1992.
21. Larsen, PR and Ingbar, SH: The thyroid gland. In Gilman, AG, et al (eds): The Pharmacological Basis of Therapeutics, ed 8. Pergamon Press, New York, 1990.
22. Latman, NS: Pituitary stimulation of parathyroid hormone secretion: Evidence in cattle for a parathyroid stimulating hormone. J Exp Zool 212:313, 1980.
23. Litwack, G, et al: Steroid receptor activation: The glucocorticoid receptor as a model system. In Chrousos, GP, Loriaux, DL, and Lipsett, MB (eds): Steroid Hormone Resistance: Mechanisms and Clinical Aspects. Plenum Press, New York, 1986.
24. Milgrom, E: Steroid hormones. In Baulieu, EE and Kelly, PA (eds): Hormones: From Molecule to Disease. Chapman & Hall, New York, 1990.
25. Murad, F and Kuret, JA: Estrogens and progestins. In Gilman, AG, et al (eds): The Pharmacological Basis of Therapeutics, ed 8. Pergamon Press, New York, 1990.
26. O'Malley, BW, Schrader, WT, and Tsai, M-J: Molecular actions of steroid hormones. In Chrousos, GP, Loriaux, DL, and Lipsett, MB (eds): Steroid Hormone Resistance: Mechanisms and Clinical Aspects. Plenum Press, New York, 1986.
27. Oppenheimer, JH: Thyroid hormone action at the nuclear level. Ann Intern Med 102:374, 1985.
28. Orth, DN, Kovacs, WJ, and DeBold, CR: The adrenal cortex. In Wilson, JD and Foster, DW (eds): Textbook of Endocrinology, ed 8. WB Saunders, Philadelphia, 1992.
29. Papapoulos, SE, et al: Effects of decreasing serum calcium on circulating parathyroid hormone and vitamin D metabolites in normocalcaemic and hypercalcaemic patients treated with APD. Bone Miner 1:69, 1986.
30. Quinn, SJ and Williams, GH: Regulation of aldosterone secretion. Annu Rev Physiol 50:409, 1988.
31. Racadot, J: The hypothalamus-pituitary system: An overview. In Baulieu, EE and Kelly, PA (eds): Hormones: From Molecule to Disease. Chapman & Hall, New York, 1990.
32. Richards, JS and Hedin, L: Molecular aspects of hormone action in ovarian follicular development, ovulation, and luteinization. Annu Rev Physiol 50:441, 1988.
33. Schlaghecke, R, et al: The effect of long-term glucocorticoid therapy on pituitary-adrenal responses to exogenous corticotropin-releasing hormone. N Engl J Med 326:226, 1992.
34. Sharpe, RM: Regulation of spermatogenesis. In Knobil, E and Neill, JD (eds): The Physiology of Reproduction, Vol 2, ed 2. Raven Press, New York, 1994.
35. Sherman, MR: Structure of mammalian steroid receptors: Evolving concepts and methodological developments. Annu Rev Physiol 46:83, 1984.
36. Simpson, ER and Waterman, MR: Regulation of the synthesis of steroidogenic enzymes in adrenal cortical cells by ACTH. Annu Rev Physiol 50:427, 1988.
37. Symposium (various authors): Hormone replacement therapy. Br Med Bull 48:249, 1992.
38. Thorner, MO, et al: The anterior pituitary. In Wilson, JD and Foster, DW (eds): Textbook of Endocrinology, ed 8. WB Saunders, Philadelphia, 1992.
39. Wilson, JD and Foster, DW: Introduction. In Wilson, JD and Foster, DW (eds): Textbook of Endocrinology, ed 8. WB Saunders, Philadelphia, 1992.

CHAPTER 29

Adrenocorticosteroids

This chapter discusses the pharmacology of the steroid hormones produced by the adrenal cortex. The two primary types of adrenal steroids are the glucocorticoids and mineralocorticoids. Small amounts of other steroids such as the sex hormones (androgens, estrogens, and progestins) are also produced by the adrenal cortex. These steroids are discussed in Chapter 30.

The **adrenocorticosteroids** have several important physiologic and pharmacologic functions. The **glucocorticoids** (cortisol, corticosterone) are primarily involved in the control of glucose metabolism and the body's ability to deal with stress. Glucocorticoids have other attributes such as their ability to decrease inflammation and suppress the immune system. **Mineralocorticoids** such as aldosterone are involved in maintaining fluid and electrolyte balance in the body.

Adrenal steroids and their synthetic analogs can be administered pharmacologically to mimic the effects of their endogenous counterparts. This approach is frequently undertaken as replacement therapy in various hormonal deficiencies. The quantity administered during hormonal replacement is roughly equivalent to the normal endogenous production and is often referred to as a **physiologic dose.** In higher doses, adrenal steroids can be used to capitalize on a particular beneficial effect, such as using glucocorticoids as anti-inflammatory agents. The larger quantity used to obtain a particular effect is typically referred to as a **pharmacologic dose** to differentiate it from the amount used to maintain normal endocrine function.

Physical therapists and occupational therapists will encounter many patients who are receiving adrenal steroids for replacement of missing hormones or for various other therapeutic reasons. This chapter first discusses the biosynthesis of the adrenal steroids in an effort to show some of the structural and functional similarities between various steroid groups. The basic physiologic and pharmacologic properties of the glucocorticoids are then addressed, followed by a description of mineralocorticoid function. This discussion should provide therapists with a better understanding of the pharmacotherapeutic as well as toxic characteristics of these compounds.

STEROID SYNTHESIS

The primary pathways involved in steroid biosynthesis are shown in Figure 29–1. These hormones are manufactured by enzymes located in the cytosol of adrenocortical cells. As shown in Figure 29–1, there are three primary pathways, each leading to one of the major types of steroid hormone.[36] The mineralocorticoid pathway synthesizes

FIGURE 29–1. Pathways of adrenal steroid biosynthesis. Cholesterol is the precursor for the three steroid hormone pathways. Note the similarity between the structures of the primary mineralocorticoid (aldosterone), the primary glucocorticoid (cortisol), and the sex hormones (testosterone, estradiol). See text for further discussion.

aldosterone, the glucocorticoid pathway synthesizes cortisol, and the androgen/estrogen pathway leads to synthesis of the sex hormones. Although all three pathways are present in the adrenal cortex, the mineralocorticoid and glucocorticoid pathways predominate. The appropriate enzymes for sex hormone biosynthesis are also present in the gonads, and the primary site for synthesis of these hormones is in the testes (men) or ovaries (women).

The steroid hormones bear a remarkable structural similarity to one another (see Fig. 29–1). The precursor for steroid biosynthesis is cholesterol. Consequently, all of the steroid hormones share the same basic chemical configuration as their parent compound. This fact has several important physiologic and pharmacologic implications. First, only relatively minor changes in the side chains of the parent compound create steroids with dramatically different physiologic effects. For instance, the addition of only one hydrogen atom in the sex steroid pathway changes testosterone (the primary male hormone) to estradiol (one of the primary female hormones). Second, the structural similarity between different types of steroids helps explain why there is often some crossover in the physiologic effects of each major category. One can readily understand how aldosterone has some glucocorticoid-like activity and cortisol has some mineralocorticoid-like effects when one considers the similarity in their organic configuration. Corticosterone (a glucocorticoid) is even the precursor to aldosterone (a mineralocorticoid).

Steroid structure and biosynthesis has been used from a pharmacologic standpoint. Pharmacologists have tried to develop more effective and less toxic synthetic steroids by manipulating the chemical side groups of these compounds. An example is the synthetic glucocorticoid prednisolone, which is four times more potent in reducing inflammation than cortisol but has less of a tendency to cause sodium retention than the naturally occurring glucocorticoid.[21] Also, excessive steroid synthesis can be rectified in certain situations by using drugs that inhibit specific enzymes shown in the biosynthetic pathways.

GLUCOCORTICOIDS

Role of Glucocorticoids in Normal Function

The primary glucocorticoid released in humans is *cortisol* (also known as hydrocortisone). Cortisol synthesis and secretion are under the control of specific hypothalamic and pituitary hormones.[29,44,48,51] Corticotropin-releasing hormone (CRH) from the hypothalamus stimulates the release of adrenocorticotropic hormone (ACTH) from the anterior pituitary. ACTH travels in the systemic circulation to reach the adrenal cortex, where it stimulates cortisol synthesis. Cortisol then travels in the bloodstream to various target tissues to exert a number of physiologic effects (see "Physiologic Effects of Glucocorticoids").

Cortisol also plays a role in controlling the release of CRH and ACTH from the hypothalamus and pituitary, respectively. As illustrated in Figure 29–2, the relationship between plasma cortisol and CRH/ACTH release is a classic example of a negative feedback control system. Increased plasma cortisol levels serve to inhibit subsequent release of CRH and ACTH, thus helping to maintain homeostasis by moderating glucocorticoid activity.

Under normal conditions, cortisol release occurs on a cyclic basis, as shown in Figure 29–3. In an unstressed human, plasma cortisol levels rise slowly throughout the early morning hours and peak at approximately 8 AM. This type of physiologic event is often referred to as a *circadian rhythm*, indicating that the cycle is repeated over a 24-hour period. The fact that plasma cortisol levels progressively increase as the individual is preparing to arise suggests that cortisol helps prepare the organism for increased activity. Indeed, this belief is supported by the observation that in the rat, plasma glucocorticoid levels peak at around midnight, which corresponds to the time when nocturnal animals are becoming active.

In addition to their normal circadian release, glucocorticoids are also released in response to virtually any stressful stimulus. For instance, trauma, infection, hemorrhage, temperature extremes, food and water deprivation, and any perceived psycho-

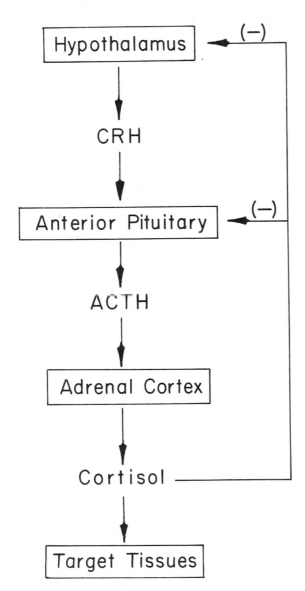

FIGURE 29–2. Negative feedback control of glucocorticoid synthesis. Cortisol limits its own synthesis by inhibiting the release of corticotropin-releasing hormone (CRH) from the hypothalamus and adrenocorticotropic hormone (ACTH) from the anterior pituitary.

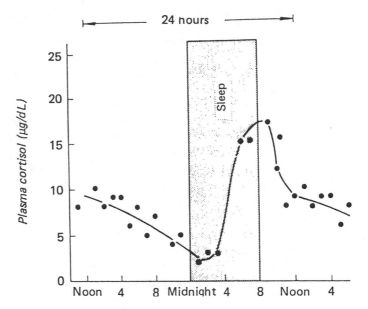

FIGURE 29-3. Circadian rhythm of cortisol production in humans. Peak plasma cortisol levels normally occur at approximately the time an individual awakens (6 to 8 AM). (Reproduced, with permission, from Katzung, BG: Basic and Clinical Pharmacology, copyright Lange Medical Publications, 1982; after Liddle, 1966.)

logic stress can serve to increase cortisol release.[38] Various stressful events generate afferent input to the hypothalamus, thus evoking CRH and ACTH release from the hypothalamus and anterior pituitary, respectively.

Mechanism of Action of Glucocorticoids

Glucocorticoids affect various cells in a manner characteristic of steroid hormones (see Chapter 28, Fig. 28–3). In general, steroids alter protein synthesis in responsive cells through a direct effect on the cell's nucleus. These hormones alter the transcription of specific DNA genes, which results in subsequent changes in RNA synthesis and the translation of RNA into cellular proteins.[9,40]

Specifically, glucocorticoids exert their cellular effects by first entering the target cell and binding to a receptor located in the cytosol.[33,40,49] Binding the glucocorticoid to the receptor creates an activated hormone-receptor complex. This activated complex then travels to the nucleus of the cell, where it binds directly to specific DNA gene segments.[2,20] Binding of the hormone-receptor complex modulates the transcription of DNA into messenger RNA units.[7] These messenger RNA units ultimately lead to increased protein synthesis in the cell. Newly formed proteins can alter cell function by acting as enzymes, membrane carriers, structural proteins, and so on. Consequently, glucocorticoids induce changes in protein synthesis on the cellular level that ultimately lead to the physiologic effects of these hormones.

Physiologic Effects of Glucocorticoids

Glucocorticoids exert a number of diverse physiologic effects, which are briefly discussed here.

EFFECTS ON GLUCOSE, PROTEIN, AND LIPID METABOLISM

Cortisol and other glucocorticoids increase blood glucose and liver glycogen.[21,38] This fact is somewhat of a metabolic paradox because circulating levels of glucose are increased at the same time that glucose storage is enhanced. This situation is analogous to being able to draw money out of a savings account while at the same time increasing the amount of money in the savings account. The withdrawn money is available to be spent (i.e., the increased blood glucose is readily available as an energy source), while the savings account accrues additional funds (i.e., liver glycogen is increased).

Glucocorticoids accomplish this paradox by affecting the metabolism of glucose, fat, and protein, as shown in Figure 29–4. Cortisol facilitates the breakdown of muscle into amino acids and lipids into free fatty acids, which can be transported to the liver for gluconeogenesis. Glucose that is synthesized in the liver can either be stored as glycogen or released back into the bloodstream to increase blood glucose levels. Cortisol also inhibits the uptake of glucose into muscle and fat cells, thus allowing more glucose to remain available in the bloodstream.

Consequently, one of the primary effects of glucocorticoids is to maintain blood

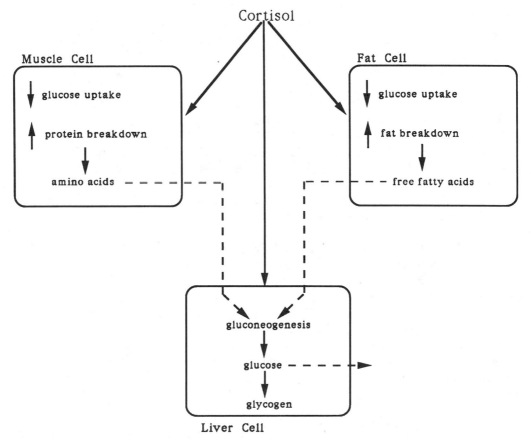

FIGURE 29–4. Effects of cortisol on muscle, fat, and liver cells. Cortisol causes breakdown of muscle and fat into amino acids and free fatty acids, which can be used by the liver to produce glucose.

glucose and liver glycogen levels to enable a supply of this energy substrate to be readily available for increased activity. This effect occurs during the daily basal release of cortisol and to even a greater extent when high levels of cortisol are released in response to stress. The beneficial effects on glucose titers occur largely at the expense of muscle breakdown, however. This muscle catabolism is one of the primary problems that occurs when glucocorticoids are administered for long periods as a therapeutic agent (see "Adverse Effects of Glucocorticoids").

ANTI-INFLAMMATORY EFFECTS

Glucocorticoids are effective and potent anti-inflammatory agents. Regardless of the cause of the inflammation, glucocorticoids attenuate the heat, erythema, swelling, and tenderness of the affected area. The exact way that these agents intervene in the inflammatory process is complex and not completely understood. Some of the primary anti-inflammatory mechanisms are addressed here.

Inhibition of Eicosanoid Biosynthesis

Glucocorticoids inhibit the production of proinflammatory substances such as prostaglandins and leukotrienes.[32,45] The role of these substances in mediating the inflammatory response was discussed in Chapter 15. Glucocorticoids promote the synthesis of a protein or family of proteins known as *lipocortins*.[4,12,24,25] Lipocortins inhibit the phospholipase A_2 enzyme, which is the enzyme responsible for liberating phospholipids from cell membranes so that they can be transformed into prostaglandins and leukotrienes (see Chapter 15, Fig. 15–1). By inhibiting this enzyme, glucocorticoids eliminate the precursor for prostaglandin and leukotriene biosynthesis, thus preventing the production of these proinflammatory substances.

Inhibition of Cellular Components of the Inflammatory Reaction

Glucocorticoids impair the function of a number of cells involved in the inflammatory response. These agents inhibit the release of chemicals (chemotactic factors) that attract leukocytes and macrophages to the site of inflammation,[11] and glucocorticoids limit the ability of macrophages to phagocytize and destroy invading microorganisms in inflamed tissues.[19,41] Glucocorticoids also inhibit the ability of various inflammatory cells to synthesize and release inflammatory mediators such as platelet activating factor, tissue necrosis factor, interleukin-1, and other chemicals produced locally by leukocytes and macrophages.[21] These inflammatory mediators are normally responsible for initiating local biochemical changes that cause the typical symptoms of the inflammatory response (i.e., swelling, tenderness, etc.).[15] By inhibiting the release of these mediators from leukocytes and macrophages, glucocorticoids blunt the local tissue damage and vascular changes that are characteristic of an inflammatory response.

Other Anti-Inflammatory Mechanisms

At higher doses, glucocorticoids appear to stabilize lysosomal membranes, thereby making them less fragile and susceptible to rupture.[19] Lysosomes are subcellular organelles that contain a variety of degradative enzymes. When lysosomes are ruptured, these enzymes begin to digest cellular components, thus contributing to the local damage present at a site of inflammation. Glucocorticoids may help prevent lysosomal rupture and the subsequent damage that contributes to the inflammatory response. Glucocorticoids also decrease vascular permeability by either directly causing vasoconstriction or by suppressing the local release of vasoactive substances such as histamine, kinins, and other chemicals that cause increased capillary permeability.[19] This reduction in vascular permeability helps control swelling and erythema at the site of inflammation.

IMMUNOSUPPRESSION

Glucocorticoids have long been recognized for their ability to inhibit hypersensitivity reactions, especially the delayed or cell-mediated allergic reactions. The exact way in which this immunosuppression occurs is unclear, but many of the immunosuppressive effects are mediated by the same actions that explain the anti-inflammatory effects of these drugs. As indicated previously, glucocorticoids inhibit the migration of leukocytes and macrophages to the location of a foreign tissue or antigen.[21] These drugs also suppress the ability of these cells to synthesize or respond to certain chemical mediators such as interleukins and interferons.[3,28,30,31] Chemicals such as interleukin-1, gamma interferon, and related substances normally mediate the communication between immune system cells such as T cells, B cells, and other lymphocytes.[13] By suppressing the synthesis and effects of these mediators, glucocorticoids interrupt cellular interaction and inhibit activation of key cellular components that cause the immune response. The effects of glucocorticoids on the immune response and the clinical applications of glucocorticoid-induced immunosuppression are discussed further in Chapter 37.

OTHER EFFECTS OF GLUCOCORTICOIDS

Cortisol and similar glucocorticoids affect a variety of other tissues.[21] These hormones affect renal function by enhancing sodium and water reabsorption and by impairing the ability of the kidneys to excrete a water load. They alter CNS function, with abnormal glucocorticoid levels (either too high or too low) producing changes in behavior and mood. Glucocorticoids alter the formed elements in the blood by facilitating an increase in erythrocytes, neutrophils, and platelets while decreasing the number of lymphocytes, eosinophils, monocytes, and basophils. Adequate amounts of glucocorticoids are needed for normal cardiac and skeletal muscle function. Vascular reactivity diminishes and capillary permeability increases if glucocorticoids are not present. Clearly, these hormones are involved in regulating a number of diverse and important physiologic functions.

THERAPEUTIC GLUCOCORTICOID AGENTS

The primary glucocorticoids used pharmacologically are listed in Table 29–1. These drugs are either chemically identical to the naturally occurring hormones, or they are synthetic analogs of cortisol. The clinical choice of a particular agent depends on the problem being treated and the desired effect in each patient.

As indicated in Table 29–1, glucocorticoids are available in various preparations that correspond to specific routes of administration. For instance, systemic preparations can be administered either orally or parenterally to treat systemic disorders (such as collagen diseases and adrenocortical insufficiency). In more localized problems,

TABLE 29–1 Therapeutic Glucocorticoids

Generic Name	Common Trade Name(s)	Type of Preparation Available					
		Systemic	Topical	Inhalation	Ophthalmic	Otic	Nasal
Alclometasone	Aclovate		X				
Amcinonide	Cyclocort		X				
Beclomethasone	Beclovent, Vanceril			X			X
Betamethasone	Celestone, Uticort	X	X		X	X	
Clobetasol	Dermovate, Temovate		X				
Clocortolone	Cloderm		X				
Cortisone	Cortone	X					
Desonide	DesOwen, Tridesilon		X				
Desoximetasone	Topicort		X				
Dexamethasone	Decadron, Dexasone	X	X	X	X	X	X
Diflorasone	Florone, Maxiflor		X				
Flumethasone	Locacorten		X				
Flunisolide	AeroBid, Nasalide			X			X
Fluocinolone	Fluonid, Flurosyn		X				
Fluocinonide	Lidex		X				
Fluorometholone	FML S.O.P., Fluor-Op				X		
Flurandrenolide	Cordran		X				
Fluticasone	Cultivate		X				
Halcinonide	Halog		X				
Halobetasol	Ultravate		X				
Hydrocortisone	Cortaid, Hydrocortone	X	X		X	X	
Medrysone	HMS Liquifilm				X		
Methylprednisolone	Medrol	X					
Mometasone	Elocon		X				
Paramethasone	Haldrone	X					
Prednisolone	Hydeltrasol, Prelone	X					
Prednisone	Deltasone, Meticorten	X				X	
Triamcinolone	Azmacort, Aristocort	X	X	X			

these agents may be applied directly to a specific area using other preparations (e.g., topical, ophthalmic). Glucocorticoids are sometimes injected into a specific tissue or anatomic space to treat a localized problem. For instance, certain types of back and neck pain may be treated by injection into the epidural space,[6,50] and local glucocorticoid injections have been used to treat problems such as carpal tunnel syndrome.[18] Likewise, glucocorticoids may be injected directly into a joint to treat severe acute inflammation that is isolated to that joint. The repeated intra-articular administration of glucocorticoids is not advisable, however, because of the catabolic effect of these hormones on supporting tissues (see "Adverse Effects of Glucocorticoids"). Also, the repeated injection of glucocorticoids in and around tendons is not recommended since glucocorticoids can cause breakdown and rupture of these structures.[10,34] Hence, a general rule of thumb is to limit the number of glucocorticoid injections into a specific joint to four or fewer per year.[42]

CLINICAL USES OF GLUCOCORTICOIDS

Glucocorticoids are used in two primary situations: to evaluate and treat endocrine disorders and to help resolve the symptoms of a variety of nonendocrine problems. These two major applications are discussed here.

Glucocorticoid Use in Endocrine Conditions

REPLACEMENT THERAPY

Glucocorticoids are administered to help restore normal function in conditions of adrenal cortical hypofunction. Glucocorticoid replacement is instituted in both primary and secondary adrenal insufficiency. In primary insufficiency (Addison's disease), glucocorticoid production is deficient because of destruction of the adrenal cortex. In secondary insufficiency, adrenal cortex function is diminished because of other factors such as a lack of adequate ACTH release from the anterior pituitary. Replacement therapy can also be initiated after the removal of the adrenals or pituitary gland because of disease and tumors. For instance, adrenalectomy or destruction of the pituitary to resolve adrenal cortical hypersecretion (Cushing's syndrome) is typically followed by long-term glucocorticoid administration. Replacement therapy is needed to maintain optimum health whenever normal physiologic function of the adrenal cortex is disrupted.

EVALUATION OF ENDOCRINE DYSFUNCTION

Glucocorticoids may be given for diagnostic purposes when trying to evaluate hormonal disorders. Exogenous glucocorticoids (especially the synthetic hormones such as dexamethasone) are potent inhibitors of ACTH secretion from the anterior pituitary. By suppressing the secretion of ACTH, glucocorticoids can help determine whether an endocrine imbalance is influenced by ACTH secretion. Favorable changes in the endocrine profile during ACTH suppression indicate that ACTH and ACTH-related hormones have a role in mediating the abnormality.

Use in Nonendocrine Conditions

Glucocorticoids are used primarily for their anti-inflammatory and immunosuppressive effects to treat a long and diverse list of nonendocrine conditions. Some of the approved indications for glucocorticoid administration are listed in Table 29–2. Of particular interest to rehabilitation specialists is the use of these agents in treating collagen diseases and rheumatic disorders, including rheumatoid arthritis.

As indicated in Table 29–2, these drugs are generally used to control inflammation or suppress the immune system for relatively short periods of time, regardless of the underlying pathology. The very fact that these drugs are successful in such a wide range of disorders illustrates that glucocorticoids do not cure the underlying problem. In a sense they treat only a symptom of the original disease—that is, inflammation. This fact is important because the patient may appear to be improving, having de-

TABLE 29–2 Nonendocrine Disorders Treated with Glucocorticoids

General Indication	Principal Desired Effect of Glucocorticoids	Examples of Specific Disorders
Allergic disorders	Decreased inflammation	Anaphylactic reactions, drug-induced allergic reactions, severe hay fever, serum sickness
Collagen disorders	Immunosuppression	Acute rheumatic carditis, dermatomyositis, systemic lupus erythematosus
Dermatologic disorders	Decreased inflammation	Alopecia areata, dermatitis (various forms), keloids, lichens, mycosis fungoides, pemphigus, psoriasis
Gastrointestinal disorders	Decreased inflammation	Inflammatory bowel disease, Crohn's disease, ulcerative proctosigmoiditis
Hematologic disorders	Immunosuppression	Autoimmune hemolytic anemia, congenital hypoplastic anemia, erythroblastopenia, thrombocytopenia
Nonrheumatic inflammation	Decreased inflammation	Bursitis, tenosynovitis
Neoplastic disease	Immunosuppression	Leukemias, lymphomas, nasal polyps, cystic tumors
Neurologic disease	Decreased inflammation and immunosuppression	Tuberculous meningitis, multiple sclerosis, myasthenia gravis
Neurotrauma	Decreased edema*	Brain surgery, closed head injury, certain brain tumors
Ophthalmic disorders	Decreased inflammation	Chorioretinitis, conjunctivitis, herpes zoster, iridocyclitis, keratitis, optic neuritis
Respiratory disorders	Decreased inflammation	Bronchial asthma, berylliosis, aspiration pneumonitis, symptomatic sarcoidosis, pulmonary tuberculosis
Rheumatic disorders	Decreased inflammation and immunosuppression	Ankylosing spondylitis, psoriatic arthritis, rheumatoid arthritis, gouty arthritis, osteoarthritis

*Efficacy of glucocorticoid use in decreasing cerebral edema has not been conclusively proved.

creased symptoms of inflammation, while the disease continues to worsen. Also, glucocorticoids are often administered in fairly high dosages to capitalize on their anti-inflammatory and immunosuppressive effects. These high dosages may create serious adverse effects when given for prolonged periods (see the next section, "Adverse Effects of Glucocorticoids"). Despite these limitations, glucocorticoids can be extremely helpful and even lifesaving in the short-term control of severe inflammation and various allergic responses.

ADVERSE EFFECTS OF GLUCOCORTICOIDS

The effectiveness and extensive clinical use of natural and synthetic glucocorticoids must be tempered by the serious side effects produced by these agents. Some of the more common problems associated with glucocorticoid use are described here.

Adrenocortical Suppression

Adrenocortical suppression occurs because of the negative feedback effect of the administered glucocorticoids on the hypothalamic/anterior pituitary system and the adrenal glands.[46] Basically, the patient's normal production of glucocorticoids is shut down by the exogenous hormones. The magnitude and duration of this suppression are related to the dosage and duration of glucocorticoid therapy. Some degree of adrenocortical suppression can even occur after a single large systemic dose.[52] This suppression will become more pronounced as systemic administration is continued for longer periods. Also, topical glucocorticoid administration over an extensive area of the body (especially in infants) may provide enough systemic absorption to suppress adrenocortical function.[17,47] Adrenocortical suppression can be a serious problem when glucocorticoid therapy is terminated. Patients who have experienced complete suppression will not be able to immediately resume production of glucocorticoids. Because abrupt withdrawal can be life-threatening in these patients, glucocorticoids must be withdrawn slowly by tapering the dose.

Drug-Induced Cushing's Syndrome

In drug-induced Cushing's syndrome, patients begin to exhibit many of the symptoms associated with the adrenocortical hypersecretion that occurs during naturally occurring Cushing's syndrome. These patients commonly exhibit symptoms of roundness and puffiness in the face, fat deposition and obesity in the trunk region, muscle wasting in the extremities, hypertension, osteoporosis, increased body hair (*hirsutism*), and glucose intolerance. These changes are all caused by the metabolic effects of the glucocorticoids. These adverse effects can be alleviated somewhat by reducing the glucocorticoid dosage. Some of the Cushing's syndrome effects must often be tolerated, however, to allow the glucocorticoids to maintain a therapeutic effect (decreased inflammation or immunosuppression).

Breakdown of Supporting Tissues

Glucocorticoids exert a general catabolic effect not only on muscle (as described previously), but also on other tissues. Bone, ligaments, tendons, and skin are also subject to a wasting effect from prolonged glucocorticoid use. Glucocorticoids weaken these supporting tissues by inhibiting collagen formation. Glucocorticoids appear to bind directly to the genes that are responsible for collagen production and to prevent transcription of these genes.[39] The molecular basis for the effects of glucocorticoids on skeletal muscle is complex and somewhat unclear, but glucocorticoids probably interfere with muscle protein synthesis by altering the muscle's ability to retain and use amino acids.[1,5] Thus, these drugs cause atrophy of skeletal muscle by increasing the rate of protein breakdown and decreasing the rate of protein synthesis.[23]

The magnitude of the wasting effect caused by systemic glucocorticoids is dependent on many factors including the patient's overall health and the duration and dosage of drug therapy. Although some evidence exists that low doses of these drugs can be given for prolonged periods without excessive bone loss,[37] other sources believe that significant bone and muscle loss can occur in some women even when these drugs are given in low doses.[8,24] Likewise, moderate-to-high doses will almost certainly cause some degree of muscle and bone loss in a variety of patients when glucocorticoids are administered continuously for more than a few weeks. Hence, the potential for tissue breakdown must always be considered during rehabilitation of patients taking these drugs, and therapists must be especially careful to avoid overstressing tissues that are weakened by the prolonged use of systemic glucocorticoids.

Other Adverse Effects

Several other problems can occur during prolonged glucocorticoid use. Peptic ulcer may occur because of either the breakdown of supporting proteins in the stomach wall or direct mucosal irritation by the drugs. An increased susceptibility to infection often occurs because of the immunosuppressive effect of glucocorticoids. These drugs may retard growth in children because of an inhibition of growth hormone. Glucocorticoids may cause glaucoma by impairing the normal drainage of aqueous fluid from the eye, and cataract formation is also associated with prolonged use. Mood changes and even psychoses have been reported, but the reasons for these occurrences are not clear. Glucocorticoids with some mineralocorticoid-like activity may cause hypertension because of sodium and water retention. Some of the newer synthetic drugs have fewer mineralocorticoid effects, however, and hypertension occurs less frequently with these.

DRUGS THAT INHIBIT ADRENOCORTICAL HORMONE BIOSYNTHESIS

Occasionally the production of adrenal steroids should be inhibited. Two agents are available that block specific enzymes in the glucocorticoid biosynthetic pathway. Aminoglutethimide (Cytadren) inhibits the first step in adrenal corticoid synthesis by blocking the conversion of cholesterol to subsequent hormone precursors (see Fig. 29–1). Metyrapone (Metopirone) inhibits the hydroxylation reaction of several intermediate compounds in the adrenal corticoid pathway. Both drugs essentially eliminate the endogenous production of glucocorticoids and mineralocorticoids.

Aminoglutethimide and metyrapone are sometimes used to decrease adrenal corticoid hypersecretion in conditions such as adrenal tumors. Adrenal hypersecretion caused by increased pituitary ACTH release (Cushing's syndrome of pituitary origin) may also be resolved temporarily by these drugs. However, a longer-term solution to pituitary ACTH hypersecretion, such as pituitary irradiation, is usually desirable.[21] Metyrapone is also used to test hypothalamic–anterior pituitary function. Specifically, this drug is used to evaluate the ability of the anterior pituitary to release ACTH. When the production of adrenal glucocorticoids is attenuated by this drug, the anterior pituitary should respond by secreting ACTH into the bloodstream. If the ACTH response is too low, pituitary hypofunction is indicated. Pituitary hyperfunction, Cushing's syndrome of pituitary origin, is indicated if the ACTH response is exaggerated.

MINERALOCORTICOIDS

Mineralocorticoids are also steroid hormones that are produced by the adrenal cortex. The principal mineralocorticoid in humans is *aldosterone*. Aldosterone is primarily involved in maintaining fluid and electrolyte balance in the body. This hormone works on the kidneys to increase sodium and water reabsorption and potassium excretion.

Regulation of Mineralocorticoid Secretion

Aldosterone release is regulated by several factors that are related to the fluid and electrolyte status in the body.[43] A primary stimulus for aldosterone release is increased levels of *angiotensin II*. Angiotensin II is part of the renin-angiotensin system, which is concerned with maintaining blood pressure (see Chapter 21). Basically, a sudden fall in blood pressure initiates a chain of events that generates increased circulating levels of angiotensin II. Angiotensin II helps maintain blood pressure by vasoconstricting peripheral vessels. Angiotensin II (and probably also its metabolic by-product angiotensin III) also helps exert a more prolonged antihypotensive effect by stimulating aldosterone secretion from the adrenal cortex. Aldosterone can then facilitate sodium and water retention, thus maintaining adequate plasma volume.

In addition to the angiotensin II effects, aldosterone secretion is regulated by increased plasma potassium levels.[43] Presumably, elevated plasma potassium serves as a stimulus to increase aldosterone release, thus causing increased potassium excretion and a return to normal plasma levels. Finally, there is evidence that ACTH may also play a role in aldosterone release. Although ACTH is primarily involved in controlling glucocorticoid secretion, this hormone may also stimulate mineralocorticoid release to some extent.[43]

Mechanism of Action and Physiologic Effects of Mineralocorticoids

Aldosterone exerts its effects on the kidneys by binding to specific receptors in epithelial cells that line the distal tubule of the nephron.[16] These receptors have a high affinity for mineralocorticoid hormones. They also have a moderate affinity for many of the natural glucocorticoid hormones (e.g., cortisol) and a low affinity for the newer synthetic glucocorticoids, like dexamethasone. This accounts for the finding that certain glucocorticoids exert some mineralocorticoid-like effects, while others have relatively minor effects on electrolyte and fluid balance.[16]

Mineralocorticoids are believed to increase sodium reabsorption by the mechanism illustrated in Figure 29–5. These hormones first bind to receptors in the tubule cell and create an activated hormone-receptor complex. This complex then travels to the nucleus to initiate transcription of messenger RNA units, which are translated into specific membrane-related proteins. These proteins in some way either create or help open sodium pores on the cell membrane, thus allowing sodium to leave the tubule and enter the epithelial cell by passive diffusion.[35] Sodium is then actively transported out of the cell and reabsorbed into the bloodstream. Water reabsorption is increased as water follows the sodium movement back into the bloodstream. As sodium is reab-

FIGURE 29–5. Effect of aldosterone on renal tubule cells. (1) Aldosterone (A) enters the cell and binds to a cytosolic receptor (R), creating an activated hormone–receptor complex (A–R). (2) A–R complex travels to the cell's nucleus, where it induces mRNA synthesis. (3) mRNA units undergo translation in the cytosol. (4) Specific proteins are synthesized that increase membrane permeability to sodium (Na^+). (5) Na^+ leaves the nephron lumen and enters the cell down an electrochemical gradient. (6) Na^+ is actively reabsorbed into the body, and potassium (K^+) is actively secreted from the bloodstream by the cellular Na^+–K^+ pump.

sorbed, potassium is secreted by a sodium-potassium exchange, thus increasing potassium excretion (see Fig. 29–5).

Therapeutic Use of Mineralocorticoid Drugs

Drugs with mineralocorticoid-like activity (aldosterone agonists) are frequently administered as replacement therapy whenever the natural production of mineralocorticoids is impaired. Mineralocorticoid replacement is usually required in patients with chronic adrenocortical insufficiency (Addison's disease), following adrenalectomy, or in other forms of adrenal cortex hypofunction. These conditions usually require both mineralocorticoid and glucocorticoid replacement.

Fludrocortisone (Florinef) is the primary aldosterone-like agent that is used in replacement therapy. This compound is chemically classified as a glucocorticoid, but it has high levels of mineralocorticoid activity and is used exclusively as a mineralocorticoid. Fludrocortisone is administered orally.

The primary problem associated with mineralocorticoid agonists is hypertension. Because these drugs increase sodium and water retention, blood pressure may increase if the dosage is too high. Other adverse effects may include peripheral edema, weight gain, and hypokalemia. These problems are also caused by the effects of these drugs on electrolyte and fluid balance, and they are usually resolved by adjusting the dosage.

Mineralocorticoid Antagonists

Spironolactone (Aldactone) is a competitive antagonist of the aldosterone receptor. This drug binds to the receptor but does not activate it. When bound to the receptor, spironolactone blocks the effects of endogenous mineralocorticoids by preventing them from binding. Consequently, spironolactone antagonizes the normal physiologic effects of aldosterone, resulting in increased sodium and water excretion and decreased potassium excretion.

Spironolactone is used primarily as a diuretic in treating hypertension. This drug is classified as a potassium-sparing diuretic because it helps increase sodium and water excretion without increasing the excretion of potassium (see Chapter 21). Spironolactone is also used to help diagnose hyperaldosteronism. The drug is given for several days to antagonize the effects of excessive aldosterone production. When the drug is discontinued, serum potassium levels will decrease sharply if hyperaldosteronism is present; that is, plasma potassium levels will fall when aldosterone is again permitted to increase potassium excretion.

SPECIAL CONCERNS OF ADRENAL STEROID USE IN REHABILITATION PATIENTS

Adrenal steroids play an important role in the pharmacologic management of many patients seen in rehabilitation. As indicated in Table 29–2, systemic conditions such as rheumatoid arthritis, ankylosing spondylitis, and lupus erythematosus are often treated with glucocorticoid drugs. More localized musculoskeletal conditions, such as acute bursitis and tenosynovitis, may also be treated for short periods with glucocorticoids. Because these problems are often being treated simultaneously in a rehabilitation setting, therapists must be especially cognizant of the effects and implications of glucocorticoids.

The primary aspect of glucocorticoid administration that should concern therapists is the catabolic effect of these hormones on supporting tissues. As discussed previously, glucocorticoids cause a general breakdown in muscle, bone, skin, and other collagenous structures. The glucocorticoid-induced catabolism of these tissues can be even greater than expected in the presence of other contributing factors such as inactivity, poor nutrition, and the effects of aging. For instance, a certain amount of osteoporosis would be expected in an elderly, sedentary woman with rheumatoid arthritis. The use of glucocorticoids, however, may greatly accelerate the bone dissolution in such a patient, even when these drugs are used for relatively limited periods.[37]

Therapists can help attenuate some of the catabolic effects of these drugs. Strengthening activities help maintain muscle mass and prevent severe wasting of the musculotendinous unit.[22,23,26,27] Various strengthening and weight-bearing activities may also reduce bone loss to some extent. In general, any activities that promote mobility and ambulation will be beneficial during and after glucocorticoid therapy. Therapists must use caution, however, to avoid injuring structures that are weakened by glucocorticoid use. The load placed on the musculoskeletal system must be sufficient to evoke a therapeutic response, but not excessive so that musculoskeletal structures are damaged. The difference between a therapeutic stress and a harmful stress may be rather small in some patients taking glucocorticoids. Therapists must use sound clinical judgment when developing and implementing exercise routines in these patients. Because glucocorticoids also cause thinning and wasting of skin, therapists should also ensure that extra efforts are made to prevent skin breakdown in patients on prolonged glucocorticoid therapy.

Other aspects of prolonged adrenocorticoid administration also concern physical therapists and occupational therapists. Therapists should be aware of the sodium- and water-retaining properties of both glucocorticoids and mineralocorticoids. When used in acute situations or in long-term replacement therapy, both groups of adrenal steroids may cause hypertension. Therapists should routinely monitor blood pressure in patients taking either type of agent. Because of their immunosuppressive effects, glucocorticoids increase patients' susceptibility to infection. Therapists must be especially cautious about exposing these patients to any possible sources of infection. Finally, therapists should be alert for any other signs of toxicity to adrenal steroids, such as mood changes or psychoses. Therapists may recognize the early stages of such toxic reactions and prevent serious consequences by alerting the medical staff.

CASE STUDY

ADRENOCORTICOSTEROIDS

Brief History. E.M. is a 58-year-old woman with a history of rheumatoid arthritis. She has involvement of many joints in her body, but her knees are especially affected by this disease. Her symptoms of pain, swelling, and inflammation are controlled fairly well by nonsteroidal anti-inflammatory drugs. She does experience periods of exacerbation and remission, however. During periods of exacerbation, she receives physical therapy as an outpatient at a physical therapy private practice. Physical therapy typically consists of heat, ultrasound, range of motion, and strengthening activities to both knees. During a recent exacerbation, her symptoms were more severe than usual, and the patient began to develop flexion contractures in both knees. The therapist suggested that she consult her physician. Upon noting the severe inflammation, the physician elected to inject both knees with a glucocorticoid agent. Prednisolone (Hydeltra TBA Suspension) was injected into the knee joints. The patient was advised to continue physical therapy on a daily basis.

Problem/Influence of Medication. Glucocorticoid administration produced a dramatic decrease in the swelling and inflammation in both knees. The therapist was tempted to begin aggressive stretching activities to resolve the knee flexion contractures and restore normal range of motion. The therapist was aware, however, that glucocorticoids may weaken ligaments, tendons, and other supporting structures because of an inhibitory effect on collagen formation. The therapist also realized that this effect may be present for some time after glucocorticoid administration. Even though only a single intra-articular injection was used, the drug may be retained locally within fat and other tissues because of the high degree of lipid solubility of steroid agents. Consequently, the injected glucocorticoid may continue to exert a catabolic effect on knee joint structures for some time.

Decision/Solution. The therapist was especially careful to use low-intensity, prolonged-duration stretching forces when trying to resolve the knee flexion contractures. Gentle stretching, massage, and other manual techniques were continued until full active and passive knee extension was achieved.

SUMMARY

The two principal groups of adrenal steroids are the glucocorticoids and mineralocorticoids. These hormones are synthesized from cholesterol within cells of the adrenal cortex. The primary glucocorticoid produced in humans is cortisol (hydrocortisone), and the primary mineralocorticoid is aldosterone. Glucocorticoids exert a number of effects such as regulation of glucose metabolism, attenuation of the inflammatory response, and suppression of the immune system. Mineralocorticoids are involved primarily in the control of fluid and electrolyte balance.

Pharmacologically, natural and synthetic adrenal steroids are often used as replacement therapy to resolve a deficiency in adrenal cortex function. The glucocorticoids are also administered primarily for their anti-inflammatory and immunosuppressive effects in a diverse group of clinical problems. These agents can be extremely beneficial in controlling the symptoms of various rheumatic and allergic disorders. Prolonged glucocorticoid use, however, is limited by a number of serious adverse effects such as adrenocortical suppression and breakdown of muscle, bone, and other tissues. Physical therapists and occupational therapists should be especially aware of the potential side effects of glucocorticoids, since these hormonal drugs are used in many disorders that are seen in a rehabilitation setting.

REFERENCES

1. Almon, RR and Dubois, DC: Fiber-type discrimination in disease and glucocorticoid-induced atrophy. Med Sci Sports Exerc 22:304, 1990.
2. Becker, PB, et al: In vivo protein-DNA interactions in a glucocorticoid response element require the presence of the hormone. Nature 324:686, 1986.
3. Besedovsky, H, et al: Immunoregulatory feedback between interleukin-1 and glucocorticoid hormones. Science 233:652, 1986.
4. Blackwell, GJ, et al: Macrocortin: A polypeptide causing the anti-phospholipase effect of glucocorticoids. Nature 287:147, 1980.
5. Block, KP and Buse, MG: Glucocorticoid regulation of muscle branched-chain amino acid metabolism. Med Sci Sports Exerc 22:316, 1990.
6. Bowman, SJ, et al: Outcome assessment after epidural corticosteroid injection for low back pain and sciatica. Spine 18:1345, 1993.
7. Burnstein, KL and Cidlowski, JA: Regulation of gene expression by glucocorticoids. Annu Rev Physiol 51:683, 1989.
8. Caldwell, JR and Furst, DE: The efficacy and safety of low-dose corticosteroids for rheumatoid arthritis. Semin Arthritis Rheum 21:1, 1991.
9. Clark, JH, Schrader, WT, and O'Malley, BW: Mechanisms of action of steroid hormones. In Wilson, JD and Foster, DW (eds): Textbook of Endocrinology, ed 8. WB Saunders, Philadelphia, 1992.
10. Cox, JS: Current concepts in the role of steroids in the treatment of sprains and strains. Med Sci Sports Exerc 16:216, 1984.
11. Cunha, FQ and Ferreira, SH: The release of a neutrophil chemotactic factor from peritoneal macrophages by endotoxin: Inhibition by glucocorticoids. Eur J Pharmacol 129:65, 1986.
12. Davidson, FF and Dennis, EA: Biological relevance of lipocortins and related proteins as inhibitors of phospholipase A_2. Biochem Pharmacol 38:3645, 1989.
13. Dinarello, CA and Mier, JW: Lymphokines. N Engl J Med 317:940, 1987.
14. Durant, S: In vivo effects of catecholamines and glucocorticoids on mouse thymic cAMP content and thymolysis. Cell Immunol 102:136, 1986.
15. Fantone, JC and Ward, PA: Inflammation. In Rubin, E and Farber, JL (eds): Pathology, ed 2. JB Lippincott, Philadelphia, 1994.
16. Funder, JW: Aldosterone receptors. In Chrousos, GP, Loriaux, DL, and Lipsett, MD (eds): Steroid Hormone Resistance: Mechanism and Clinical Aspects. Plenum Press, New York, 1986.
17. Garden, JM and Freinkel, RK: Systemic absorption of topical steroids: Metabolic effects as an index of mild hypercortisolism. Arch Dermatol 122:1007, 1986.
18. Giannini, F, et al: Electrophysiologic evaluation of local steroid injection in carpal tunnel syndrome. Arch Phys Med Rehabil 72:738, 1991.
19. Goldfien, A: Adrenocorticosteroids and adrenocortical antagonists. In Katzung, BG (ed): Basic and Clinical Pharmacology, ed 5. Appleton & Lange, Norwalk, CT, 1992.
20. Groner, B, et al: DNA sequences involved in the regulation of gene expression by glucocorticoid hormones. Biochem Biophys Acta 781:1, 1984.
21. Haynes, RC: Adrenocorticotropic hormone; adrenocortical steroids and their synthetic analogs; inhibitors of the synthesis and actions of adrenocortical hormones. In Gilman, AG, et al (eds): The Pharmacological Basis of Therapeutics, ed 8. Pergamon Press, New York, 1990.
22. Hickson, RC, et al: Glucocorticoid antagonism by exercise and androgenic-anabolic steroids. Med Sci Sports Exerc 22:331, 1990.
23. Hickson, RC and Marone, JR: Exercise and inhibition of glucocorticoid-induced muscle atrophy. Exerc Sport Sci Rev 21:135, 1993.
24. Hirata, F: Glucocorticoids and head injury: A possible participation of lipocortin (lipomodulin) in actions of steroid hormones. Neurochem Pathol 7:33, 1987.
25. Hirata, F, et al: A phospholipase A_2 inhibitory protein in rabbit neutrophils induced by glucocorticoids. Proc Natl Acad Sci 77:2533, 1980.
26. Horber, FF, et al: Impact of physical training on the ultrastructure of midthigh muscle in normal subjects and in patients treated with glucocorticoids. J Clin Invest 79:1181, 1987.
27. Horber, FF, et al: Evidence that prednisone-induced myopathy is reversed by physical training. J Clin Endocrinol Metab 61:83, 1985.
28. Horst, H-J and Flad, HD: Corticosteroid-interleukin 2 interactions: Inhibition of binding of interleukin 2 to interleukin 2 receptors. Clin Exp Immunol 68:156, 1987.
29. Klonoff, DC and Karam, JH: Hypothalamic and pituitary hormones. In Katzung, BG (ed): Basic and Clinical Pharmacology, ed 5. Appleton & Lange, Norwalk, CT, 1992.
30. Lee, SW, et al: Glucocorticoids selectively inhibit the transcription of the interleukin 1-beta gene and decrease stability of interleukin 1-beta messenger RNA. Proc Natl Acad Sci 85:1204, 1988.
31. Lew, W, Oppenheim, JJ, and Matsushima, K: Analysis of the suppression of IL-1 alpha and IL-1 beta

products in human peripheral blood mononuclear adherent cells by a glucocorticoid hormone. J Immunol 140:1895, 1988.

32. Lewis, GD, Campbell, WB, and Johnson, AR: Inhibition of prostaglandin synthesis of glucocorticoids in human endothelial cells. Endocrinology 119:62, 1986.

33. Litwack, G, et al: Steroid receptor activation: The glucocorticoid receptor as a model system. In Chrousos, GP, Loriaux, DL, and Lipsett, MD (eds): Steroid Hormone Resistance: Mechanism and Clinical Aspects. Plenum Press, New York, 1986.

34. Mahler, F and Fritschy, D: Partial and complete ruptures of the Achilles tendon and local corticosteroid injections. Br J Sports Med 26:7, 1992.

35. Marver, D: Models of aldosterone action on sodium transport: Emerging concepts. In Chrousos, GP, Loriaux, DL, and Lipsett, MD (eds): Steroid Hormone Resistance: Mechanism and Clinical Aspects. Plenum Press, New York, 1986.

36. Milgrom, E: Steroid hormones. In Baulieu, EE and Kelly, PA (eds): Hormones: From Molecules to Disease. Chapman & Hall, New York, 1990.

37. Mitchell, DR and Lyles, KW: Minireview: Glucocorticoid-induced osteoporosis: Mechanisms for bone loss; evaluation of strategies for prevention. J Gerontol 45:M153, 1990.

38. Munck, A and Guyre, PM: Glucocorticoid physiology, pharmacology, and stress. In Chrousos, GP, Loriaux, DL, and Lipsett, MD (eds): Steroid Hormone Resistance: Mechanism and Clinical Aspects. Plenum Press, New York, 1986.

39. Oikarinen, AI, et al: Modulation of collagen metabolism by glucocorticoids: Receptor-mediated effects of dexamethasone on collagen biosynthesis in chick embryo fibroblasts and chondrocytes. Biochem Pharmacol 37:1451, 1988.

40. O'Malley, BW, Schrader, WT, and Tsai, M-J: Molecular actions of steroid hormones. In Chrousos, GP, Loriaux, DL, and Lipsett, MD (eds): Steroid Hormone Resistance: Mechanism and Clinical Aspects. Plenum Press, New York, 1986.

41. Parillo, JE and Fauci, AS: Mechanisms of glucocorticoid action on immune processes. Annu Rev Pharmacol Toxicol 19:179, 1979.

42. Porter, DR and Sturrock, RD: Fortnightly review: Medical management of rheumatoid arthritis. Br Med J 307:425, 1993.

43. Quinn, SJ and Williams, GH: Regulation of aldosterone secretion. Annu Rev Physiol 50:409, 1988.

44. Rivier, CL and Plotsky, PM: Mediation by corticotropin releasing factor (CRF) of adenohypophyseal hormone secretion. Annu Rev Physiol 48:475, 1986.

45. Robinson, DR: Prostaglandins and the mechanism of action of anti-inflammatory drugs. Am J Med 75(suppl 4b):26, 1983.

46. Schlaghecke, R, et al: The effect of long-term glucocorticoid therapy on pituitary-adrenal responses to exogenous corticotropin-releasing hormone. N Engl J Med 326:226, 1992.

47. Shohat, M, et al: Adrenocortical suppression by topical application of glucocorticoids in infants with seborrheic dermatitis. Clin Pediatr 25:209, 1986.

48. Simpson, ER and Waterman, MR: Regulation of the synthesis of steroidogenic enzymes in adrenal cortical cells by ACTH. Annu Rev Physiol 50:427, 1988.

49. Slater, EP, et al: Mechanisms of glucocorticoid hormone action. In Chrousos, GP, Loriaux, DL, and Lipsett, MD (eds): Steroid Hormone Resistance: Mechanism and Clinical Aspects. Plenum Press, New York, 1986.

50. Stav, A, et al: Cervical epidural steroid injection for cervicobrachialgia. Acta Anaesth Scand 37:562, 1993.

51. Thorner, MO, et al: The anterior pituitary. In Wilson, JD and Foster, DW (eds): Textbook of Endocrinology, ed 8. WB Saunders, Philadelphia, 1992.

52. Zora, JA, et al: Hypothalamic-pituitary axis suppression after short-term, high-dose glucocorticoid therapy in children with asthma. J Allergy Clin Immunol 77:9, 1986.

CHAPTER 30

Male and Female Hormones

In this chapter the pharmacology of the male and female hormones is discussed. The male hormones such as testosterone are usually referred to collectively as **androgens**. The female hormones consist of two principal groups: the **estrogens**, such as estradiol, and the **progestins**, such as progesterone. Androgens, estrogens, and progestins are classified as **steroid** hormones, and their chemical structure is similar to those of the other primary steroid groups, the glucocorticoids and mineralocorticoids (see Chapter 29). The principal functions, however, of the male and female hormones are control of reproductive function and secondary sexual characteristics in their respective gender groups.

Male and female hormones are produced primarily in the gonads. Androgens are synthesized in the testes in the male. In the female, the ovaries are the principal site of estrogen and progestin production. As discussed in Chapter 29, small amounts of the sex-related hormones are also produced in the adrenal cortex in both sexes, accounting for the fact that small amounts of the opposite sex hormones are seen in females and males; that is, low testosterone levels are seen in females, and males produce small quantities of estrogen. However, under normal conditions, the amounts of sex-related hormones produced by the adrenal cortex are usually too small to produce significant physiologic effects.

This chapter first discusses the physiologic role of the male hormones and the pharmacologic use of natural and synthetic androgens. The physiologic and pharmacologic characteristics of the female hormones are then addressed. As these discussions indicate, there are several aspects of the male and female hormones that should concern physical therapists and occupational therapists. These agents may be used by rehabilitation patients for approved purposes, for example, female hormones as oral contraceptives. These agents may also be used for illicit reasons, such as the use of male hormones to enhance athletic performance. Hence, rehabilitation specialists should be aware of the therapeutic and potential toxic effects of these drugs.

ANDROGENS

Source and Regulation of Androgen Synthesis

In adult males, *testosterone* is the principal androgen produced by the testes.[19,53] Testosterone is synthesized by Leydig's cells located in the interstitial space between the seminiferous tubules (Fig. 30–1). The *seminiferous tubules* are convoluted ducts within the testes in which sperm production (*spermatogenesis*) takes place. Testosterone produced by the Leydig's cells exerts a direct effect on the seminiferous tubules as well as systemic effects on other physiologic systems (see "Physiologic Effects of Androgens").

Production of testosterone by the Leydig's cells is regulated by the pituitary **gonadotropins** *luteinizing hormone* (LH) and *follicle-stimulating hormone* (FSH). LH and FSH appear to control spermatogenesis, as shown in Figure 30–1. LH is the primary hormone that stimulates testosterone production. LH released from the anterior pituitary binds to receptors on the surface of Leydig's cells and directly stimulates testosterone synthesis. The exact role of FSH is less clear. Although it does not directly increase steroidogenesis, FSH may augment the effects of LH by increasing Leydig's cell differentiation and function.[19] For instance, FSH appears to increase the number of LH binding sites on Leydig's cells.[53] However, FSH is believed to exert its primary effects on the Sertoli's cells, which line the seminiferous tubules (see Fig. 30–1). FSH stimulates the Sertoli's cells to produce a polypeptide known as androgen-binding protein (ABP). ABP may concentrate testosterone within the seminiferous tubules and help transport testosterone to the epididymis.[49,53]

Consequently, both pituitary gonadotropins are required for optimal androgen function. LH acts on the Leydig's cells to stimulate testosterone synthesis, whereas FSH acts on the Sertoli's cells to stimulate production of ABP, which enables testosterone to reach target tissues within the seminiferous tissues. Other hormones may also play a synergistic role in steroidogenesis in the male; for instance, growth hormone and prolactin may also increase the effects of LH on testosterone synthesis.[19]

Release of the pituitary gonadotropins (LH, FSH) is regulated by gonadotropin-releasing hormone (GnRH) from the hypothalamus.[17] A classic negative feedback system exists between the GnRH/pituitary gonadotropins and testosterone synthesis. Increased plasma levels of testosterone inhibit the release of GnRH, LH, and FSH, thus maintaining testosterone levels within a relatively finite range. Also, testosterone production is fairly tonic in normal men. Although wide fluctuations may occur in the amount of testosterone produced over a given period of time, androgen production does not correspond to a regular cycle. Testosterone is produced more or less constantly, whereas the female hormones usually are produced according to the stages of the menstrual cycle (see "Estrogen and Progesterone").

Physiologic Effects of Androgens

Testosterone and other androgens are involved in the development of the sexual characteristics in males and in the stimulation of spermatogenesis. These two primary effects are described here.

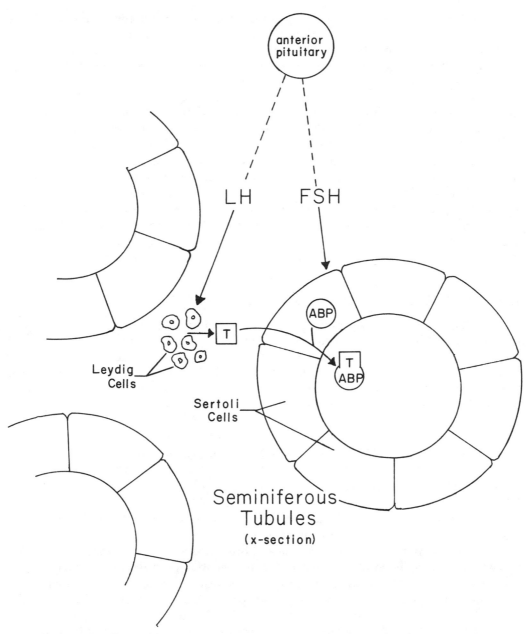

FIGURE 30–1. Effects of pituitary gonadotropins on spermatogenesis. Luteinizing hormone (LH) stimulates testosterone (T) production from Leydig's cells. Follicle-stimulating hormone (FSH) acts primarily on Sertoli's cells to increase synthesis of androgen-binding protein (ABP). ABP appears to bind with T and facilitate transport into the seminiferous tubule, where spermatogenesis takes place.

DEVELOPMENT OF MALE CHARACTERISTICS

The influence of testosterone on sexual differentiation begins in utero. In the fetus, the testes produce small amounts of testosterone that affect the development of the male reproductive organs. Androgen production then remains relatively unimportant until puberty. At the onset of puberty, a complex series of hormonal events stimulates the testes to begin to synthesize significant amounts of testosterone. The production of testosterone brings about the development of most of the physical characteristics associated with men. Most notable are the increased body hair, increased skeletal muscle mass, voice change, and maturation of the external genitalia.

These changes are all caused by the effect of androgenic steroids on their respective target tissues. Like other steroids, the androgens enter the target cell and bind to a cytoplasmic receptor.[29,54] The activated steroid-receptor complex then travels to the cell's nucleus, where it binds to specific chromatin units. Binding of the activated complex to DNA gene segments increases protein synthesis through the transcription/translation of RNA. The proteins produced then cause a change in cellular function, which is reflected as one of the maturational effects of the androgens. For instance, testosterone increases protein synthesis in skeletal muscle, thus increasing muscle mass in certain situations, such as at the onset of puberty. This particular androgenic effect (increased muscle mass) as it relates to androgen abuse in athletes is discussed in more detail under "Androgen Abuse" later in this chapter.

ROLE IN SPERMATOGENESIS

As discussed previously, androgens are essential for the production and development of normal sperm.[49,53] Testosterone is produced by the Leydig's cells located in the interstitial space between the seminiferous tubules. LH serves as the primary stimulus to increase androgen production from Leydig's cells. Testosterone then enters the tubules to directly stimulate the production of sperm through an effect on protein synthesis within the tubule cells.

PHARMACOLOGIC USE OF ANDROGENS

Clinical Use of Androgens

Androgens and their synthetic derivatives are approved for administration in several clinical situations,[55] which are given here.

Replacement Therapy. Testosterone and other androgens are administered as replacement therapy in conditions where the endogenous production of testosterone is impaired. Such conditions include removal of the testes (orchiectomy), various intrinsic forms of testicular failure (cryptorchidism, orchitis), and problems in the endocrine regulation of testosterone production such as lack of LH production.

Catabolic States. Androgens can be administered for their anabolic properties in conditions in which there is substantial muscle catabolism and protein loss. Such conditions include chronic infections, severe trauma, and recovery from extensive surgery. However, the use of androgens in these situations is somewhat controversial. These agents are not typically used as the primary treatment, but they are used as adjuncts to more conventional treatments such as dietary supplementation and exercise.

Delayed Puberty. In males, androgens may be administered on a limited basis to accelerate the normal onset of puberty. These drugs are typically used when puberty is anticipated to occur spontaneously but at a relatively late date—that is, when puberty is not delayed because of some pathologic condition.

Breast Cancer. Androgens are used to treat a limited number of hormone-sensitive tumors such as certain cases of breast cancer in women. These agents are typically combined with other antineoplastic treatments, and their role in the treatment of cancer is discussed in more detail in Chapter 36.

Anemia. Testosterone and similar compounds are potent stimulators of erythropoietin synthesis from the kidneys and other tissues. Erythropoietin, in turn, stimulates production of red blood cell synthesis in bone marrow. Hence, androgens can be used in certain types of anemia caused by renal failure or in congenital conditions such as aplastic anemia, hypoplastic anemia, and myelofibrotic anemias. Androgens may also be helpful in certain anemias caused by other medications such as cancer chemotherapy drugs.

Hereditary Angioedema. This hereditary disorder is characterized by a defect in the control of clotting factors that ultimately leads to increased vascular permeability. Loss of vascular fluid from specific capillary beds causes localized edema in various tissues such as the skin, upper respiratory tract, and gastrointestinal tract. Certain androgens act on the liver to restore production of several clotting factors and to increase production of a glycoprotein that inhibits the initial stages of the clotting sequence that leads to increased vascular permeability. Hence, androgens are typically given prophylactically to decrease the frequency and severity of angioedema attacks.

Specific Agents

Androgens that are used clinically are listed in Table 30–1. As indicated, specific agents are usually administered orally or intramuscularly to replace endogenous androgen production or to treat various medical problems. Androgens can also be classified according to their relative androgenic and anabolic properties. That is, certain androgens are given primarily to mimic the male sexual characteristics (androgenic effects), whereas other androgens are given primarily to enhance tissue metabolism (anabolic effects) (see Table 30–1). This distinction is not absolute, however, because

TABLE 30–1 Clinical Use of Androgens

Generic Name	Trade Name(s)	Primary Indication(s)	Routes of Administration
Fluoxymesterone	Halotestin	Androgen replacement, breast cancer, delayed puberty in males, anemia	Oral
Methyltestosterone	Android, Oreton, Testred, Virilon	Androgen replacement, breast cancer, delayed puberty in males	Oral
Nandrolone	Androlone, Durabolin	Anemia, breast cancer	Intramuscular
Oxandrolone	Anavar	Catabolic states	Oral
Oxymetholone	Anadrol	Anemia, angioedema	Oral
Stanozolol	Winstrol	Angioedema	Oral
Testosterone*	Histerone, Testaqua, Andro-Cyp, De-potest, Testex, others	Anemia, androgen replacement, delayed puberty in males, breast cancer	Intramuscular

*Testosterone is available as testosterone sterile suspension, testosterone cypionate, testosterone enanthate, and testosterone propionate; specific trade names and indications depend on the specific form of testosterone administered.

all compounds given to produce anabolism will also produce some androgenic effects. Many other androgenic/anabolic steroids exist and can be acquired relatively easily on a black market by individuals engaging in androgen abuse (see "Androgen Abuse"). Nonetheless, the agents listed in Table 30–1 are the principal androgens approved for clinical use, and these drugs are used to treat catabolic states, anemias, and similar conditions.

Adverse Effects of Clinical Androgen Use

The primary problems associated with androgens are related to the masculinizing effects of these drugs. In women, androgen administration can produce hirsutism, hoarseness or deepening of the voice, and changes in the external genitalia (enlarged clitoris). Irregular menstrual periods and acne may also occur in women undergoing androgen therapy. In men, these drugs may produce bladder irritation, breast swelling and soreness, and frequent or prolonged erections. When used in children, androgens may cause accelerated sexual maturation and impairment of normal bone development because of premature closure of epiphyseal plates. Consequently, these drugs are used very cautiously in children.

The adverse effects just described are related to the dose and duration of androgen use, with problems seen more frequently during prolonged androgen administration at relatively high doses. In adults, most of these adverse effects are reversible, and symptoms will diminish with discontinued use. A few effects, however, such as vocal changes in females, may persist even after the drugs are withdrawn. Skeletal changes are irreversible, and permanent growth impairment may occur if these drugs are used in children.

Other serious side effects of long-term, high-dose androgen use include liver damage and hepatic carcinoma. Hypertension may occur because of the salt-retaining and water-retaining effects of these drugs. Although these hepatic and cardiovascular problems may occur during therapeutic androgen use, their incidence is even more prevalent when extremely large doses of androgens are used to enhance athletic performance. The use and abuse of androgens in athletes is discussed in "Androgen Abuse."

Antiandrogens

Antiandrogens are drugs that inhibit the synthesis or effects of endogenous androgen production.[26] These agents can be helpful in conditions such as prostate cancer and other conditions aggravated by excessive androgen production. Specific antiandrogens affect endogenous male hormones in several different ways. Finasteride (Proscar) inhibits the conversion of testosterone to dihydrotestosterone. Dihydrotestosterone accelerates the growth and development of the prostate gland, and finasteride may be helpful in attenuating this effect in conditions such as benign prostate hypertrophy. Flutamide (Eulexin) and cyproterone (Berlex) act as antagonists (blockers) of the cellular androgen receptor, and these drugs are used to decrease hirsutism in women or to help treat prostate cancer.

Advanced prostate cancer is also treated with a number of drugs that mimic the effects of GnRH. These GnRH analogs include buserelin (Suprefact), goserelin (Zoladex), leuprolide (Lupron), and nafarelin (Synarel). When first administered, these agents cause an increase in pituitary LH release, which, in turn, stimulates testicular androgen production. However, continued administration of GnRH analogs desensitizes pituitary GnRH receptors, thus decreasing LH and testosterone production from the pituitary and testes, respectively.[33]

ANDROGEN ABUSE

Nature of Androgen Abuse

The use of androgens or **anabolic steroids** to increase athletic performance is an issue of controversy and concern. The fact that certain athletes self-administer large doses of androgens in an effort to increase muscle size and strength has been known for some time. Typically, androgen use has been associated with athletes involved in strength and power activities such as weight lifting, bodybuilding, shot put, and the like. Androgen abuse, however, has infiltrated many aspects of athletic competition at both the amateur and professional levels.

Individuals who admit to using anabolic steroids or who test positive for androgen abuse represent some of the top performers in their respective sports.[9] Also, the use of anabolic steroids among the general athletic population may be reaching alarming proportions. A comprehensive survey of male high school seniors indicated that almost 7 percent of the athletes were using or had previously used anabolic steroids.[11] Clearly, androgen abuse is one of the major problems affecting the health and welfare of athletes of various ages and athletic pursuits.

Athletes engaging in androgen abuse usually obtain these drugs from various illicit but readily available sources.[4] Some examples of anabolic steroids that are used by athletes are listed in Table 30–2. Several different androgens are often taken simultaneously for a combined dose that is 10 to 40 times greater than the therapeutic dose.[34,41,42] This "stacking" of different anabolic steroids often consists of combining oral and injectable forms of these drugs (see Table 30–2). Athletes often self-administer these drugs in cycles that last between 7 and 14 weeks, and the dosage of each drug is progressively increased during the cycle. An example of a dosing cycle using stacked anabolic steroids is shown in Table 30–3.

TABLE 30–2 Examples of Anabolic Androgens That Are Abused by Athletes

Generic Name	Trade Name
Orally active androgens	
Ethylestrenol	Maxibolin
Fluoxymesterone	Android-F, Halotestin
Methandrostenolone	Dianabol
Oxandrolone	Anavar
Oxymetholone	Anadrol-50
Stanozolol	Winstrol
Androgens administered by intramuscular injection	
Nandrolone phenpropionate	Durabolin
Nandrolone decanoate	Deca-Durabolin
Testosterone cypionate	Depo-Testosterone
Testosterone enanthate	Delatestryl

TABLE 30-3 Example of a Steroid Dosing Cycle Used
During Androgen Abuse*

Drug Name	Dosage (mg)							
	Week							
	1	2	3	4	5	6	7	8
Testosterone cypionate	200	400	600	1200	2400	4200	4200	4200
Nandrolone (Deca-Durabolin)	100	100	100	200	400	600	600	600
Oxymetholone (Anadrol)	100	150	200	250	300	500	750	1000
Methandrostenolone (Dianabol)	25	30	35	50	60	75	100	125
Methandrostenolone (Dianabol injectable)	25	25	50	50	100	100	100	100
Oxandrolone (Anavar)	25	30	35	50	50	50	50	50

*This regimen was used by a bodybuilder who went through three of these cycles each year for 8 years.
The subject also reported taking 600 mg of testosterone per week between cycles. This subject ultimately developed avascular necrosis in both femoral heads.
From Pettine,[43] p 96, with permission.

To help control anabolic steroid abuse, drug testing at the time of a specific competition has been instituted in many sports. To prevent detection, the athlete will also employ a complex pattern of high-dosage androgen administration followed by washout periods. Washouts are scheduled a sufficient period of time prior to the competition, thus allowing the drug to be eliminated from the body prior to testing. The practice of planned schedules can be negated to some extent, however, through randomized drug testing that subjects the athlete to testing at any point in the training period as well as at the time of the competition.

Two primary questions usually arise concerning anabolic steroids: Do these agents really enhance athletic performance, and what are the adverse effects of androgen abuse? Definitive answers to these questions are difficult because of the illicit nature of androgen abuse and because of the ethical and legal problems of administering large doses of androgens to healthy athletes as part of controlled research studies. The effects of androgens on athletic performance and the potential adverse effects of these drugs are discussed briefly here.

Effects of Androgens on Athletic Performance

There is little doubt that androgens can promote skeletal muscle growth and increase strength in people who do not synthesize meaningful amounts of endogenous androgens (women, prepubescent males). The question has often been whether large amounts of exogenous androgens can increase muscle size, strength, and athletic performance in healthy men. For example, certain athletic men taking androgens during strength training may experience greater increments in lean body mass and muscle strength than athletes training without androgens.[2-5,10,27] Increased muscle strength with steroid use has not been consistently reported in all research studies, however. In one review, approximately half of the investigations observed a significant effect of steroid administration on muscle strength, whereas the other half of the studies were inconclusive.[34] Some of this discrepancy was undoubtedly caused by differences in dosage and types of androgens used.

The magnitude of any strength gains that can be directly attributed to anabolic steroids also remains unclear. For instance, the anabolic effects of the steroids cannot be easily isolated from the other factors that produce increments in strength and muscle size (e.g., weight training). In particular, androgens appear to increase aggressiveness, and individuals taking these drugs may train longer and more intensely than athletes who are not taking anabolic steroids.[3] Consequently, strength increments in the athlete taking androgens may be brought about by the enhanced quality and quantity of training rather than as a direct effect of anabolic steroids on muscle protein synthesis.

Thus, the effects of androgens on athletic performance in men remain unclear. These drugs may produce some increments in muscle strength and size in some athletes, but whether these increments can be directly attributed to a physiologic effect of the androgens is uncertain. We may never know the exact ergogenic effects of these drugs in men because of the illicit nature of androgen abuse and the ethical problems involved in performing clinical studies of these drugs in humans.

Adverse Effects of Androgen Abuse

Virtually any drugs that are taken at extremely high dosages can be expected to produce some serious side effects. Exactly how harmful androgen abuse is in an athletic population remains somewhat uncertain, however. The illicit nature of androgen abuse and the various dosage regimens have made it difficult to determine the precise incidence and type of adverse effects. Also, the long-term effects of androgen abuse may not be known for some time; that is, pathologies may not be fully realized until several years after discontinuing the drugs. Nonetheless, there is considerable evidence, often in the form of individual reports and case studies, that androgen abuse can have severe and possibly fatal consequences. Some of the more common adverse effects associated with androgen administration are presented here. Further discussion of the potential adverse effects in athletes can be found in several reviews listed at the end of this chapter.[3,4,9,32,34]

High doses of androgens can produce liver damage, including the formation of hepatic tumors and peliosis hepatis (blood-filled cysts within the liver).[4,18] In some individuals, these liver abnormalities have proved fatal. Androgens also produce unfavorable changes in blood lipid profiles such as decreased high-density lipoprotein cholesterol levels.[61] These effects on plasma lipids can predispose the athlete to atherosclerotic lesions and subsequent vessel occlusion, and specific cases of stroke and myocardial infarction in athletes using androgens have been attributed to the atherogenic effects of these drugs.[23,36] Androgens also cause hypertension because of the salt-retaining and water-retaining properties of these drugs. Problems with glucose metabolism brought about by insulin resistance have also been reported.[15]

Androgens can affect bone metabolism, and avascular necrosis of the femoral heads has been documented in a weight lifter using these drugs.[43] Androgens also accelerate closure of epiphyseal plates and can lead to impaired skeletal growth in young children. This effect on skeletal development is important because athletes may begin to self-administer anabolic steroids at a relatively young age (i.e., prior to age 16).[11] As previously mentioned, androgens may produce behavioral changes including increased aggression, leading to radical mood swings and violent episodes in some individuals.[3,44,45]

Androgens can produce changes in reproductive function and secondary sexual characteristics. In males, high levels of androgens act as negative feedback and lead to testicular atrophy and impaired sperm production. This occurrence can produce infertility in males because of an inability to form sperm (*azoospermia*).[30] In females, androgens produce certain masculinizing effects such as increased body hair, deepening of the voice, and changes in the external genitalia. Androgens may also impair the normal female reproductive (menstrual) cycle. Some changes in male and female sexual/reproductive function appear to be reversible, but changes such as male infertility/azoospermia may take 4 months or longer to return to normal levels.[30] Other effects such as vocal changes in females may be permanent.

In summary, anabolic steroids may produce some ergogenic benefits in a limited subset of athletes, but rather serious consequences may occur. Nonetheless, athletes may be so driven to succeed that the adverse effects are disregarded. Also, athletes may suspect that their competitors are using steroids and feel that they must also take these drugs to remain competitive. Clearly, there is a need for governing agencies to try to eliminate the illicit use of these substances from athletic competition. Health-care professionals can also discourage androgen abuse by informing athletes that the risks of androgen abuse exceed any potential benefits.

ESTROGEN AND PROGESTERONE

In women, the ovaries produce two major categories of steroid hormones: estrogens and progestins. The primary estrogen produced in humans is *estradiol* and the primary progestin is *progesterone*. For simplicity, the terms "estrogen" and "progesterone" will be used to indicate these two primary forms of female hormones. Small amounts of male hormones (androgens) are also produced by the ovaries, and these androgens may play a role in the development of some secondary sexual characteristics in the female during puberty, for example, increased body hair and growth spurts. Nonetheless, the hormones that exert the major influence on sexual development and reproduction in the female are estrogen and progesterone. The physiologic effects of these hormones are presented here.

Effects of Estrogen and Progesterone on Sexual Maturation

Estrogen and progesterone play a primary role in promoting sexual differentiation in the developing female fetus. These hormones also become important in completing female sexual maturation during puberty. At the onset of puberty, a complex series of hormonal events stimulate the ovaries to begin producing estrogen and progesterone. Ovarian production of these hormones initiates the maturation of reproductive function and development of secondary sexual characteristics in the female.

Estrogen is the primary hormone that initiates the growth and development of the female reproductive system during puberty. Changes in the external genitalia and maturation of the internal reproductive organs (e.g., uterus, oviducts, vagina) are primarily brought about by the influence of estrogen. Estrogen also produces several other characteristic changes of female sexual maturation such as breast development, deposition of subcutaneous fat stores, and changes in the skeletal system (for example, closure of epiphyseal plates, widening of the pelvic girdle). Progesterone is less important in sexual maturation but is involved to a greater extent in facilitating and maintaining pregnancy.

Regulation and Effects of Hormonal Synthesis During the Menstrual Cycle

In the nonpregnant, postpubescent female, production of estrogen and progesterone is not tonic in nature but follows a pattern or cycle of events commonly referred to as the *menstrual cycle*. The menstrual cycle involves a sequence of events usually occurring over a 28-day period. The primary function of this cycle is to stimulate the ovaries to produce an ovum that is available for fertilization, while simultaneously preparing the endometrium of the uterus for implantation of the ovum should fertilization occur. The primary events of the menstrual cycle are illustrated in Figure 30–2. This cycle is characterized by several specific phases and events that are briefly outlined here. A more detailed description of the regulation of female reproduction can be found in several sources listed at the end of this chapter.[25,31,39,48]

Follicular Phase. The first half of the menstrual cycle is influenced by hormonal release from a developing ovarian follicle, hence the term *follicular phase*. In the follicular phase, FSH is released by the anterior pituitary. As its name implies, FSH stimulates the maturation of several follicles within the ovary. Usually, one such follicle undergoes full maturation and ultimately yields an ovum. Because of the effect of FSH, the developing follicle also begins to secrete increasing amounts of estrogen. Estrogen produced by the ovarian follicle causes a proliferation and thickening of the endometrial lining of the uterus. The follicular phase is also referred to as the *proliferative phase*. Endometrial vascularization is also increased, and glandular structures begin to develop in the uterine wall. The uterine glands, however, do not begin to function (secrete mucus) to any great extent during the follicular phase.

Ovulation. Just prior to the midpoint of the cycle, the anterior pituitary secretes a sudden, large burst of LH. A smaller burst of FSH secretion also occurs around the midpoint of the cycle, as seen in Figure 30–2. The LH surge is the primary impetus for ovulation. During ovulation, the mature follicle ruptures, releasing the ovum from the ovary. At this point, the ovum should begin to travel toward the uterus via the fallopian tubes. The ruptured follicle remains in the ovary and continues to play a vital role in the reproductive cycle. After releasing the ovum, the follicle becomes infiltrated with lipids and is referred to as the *corpus luteum* (yellow body). The role of the corpus luteum is described here.

Luteal Phase. The *luteal phase* refers to the fact that the corpus luteum governs the events in the second half of the menstrual cycle. In response to the residual effects of the LH/FSH surge, the corpus luteum continues to grow and develop for approximately 1 week after ovulation. During this time, the corpus luteum secretes both estrogen and progesterone. The combined effects of estrogen and progesterone cause a further thickening in the uterine lining, as well as an increase in the vascularization and glandular secretion of the endometrium. During the luteal phase, progesterone is the primary stimulus that causes the uterine glands to fully develop and secrete a mucous substance that provides a favorable environment for implantation of the fertilized egg. Hence, the luteal phase is also referred to as the *secretory phase* because of the enhanced function of the uterine glands.

Corpus Luteum Regression and Termination of the Cycle. If the egg is not fertil-

FIGURE 30–2. The menstrual cycle, showing changes in follicular development, uterine endometrium, pituitary gonadotropins (LH, FSH), and ovarian hormones. (Reproduced, with permission, from Katzung, BG: Basic and Clinical Pharmacology, ed 5, copyright Appleton & Lange, 1992.)

ized or implantation does not occur, the corpus luteum begins to regress, primarily because of a lack of continued support for the corpus luteum from the pituitary gonadotropins (LH, FSH). Because the corpus luteum regresses, it can no longer produce adequate amounts of estrogen and progesterone to maintain the endometrium of the uterus. Consequently, the endometrium begins to slough off, creating the menstrual bleeding that typifies the female reproductive cycle. The onset of menstrual bleeding marks the end of one reproductive cycle and the beginning of the next.

In summary, the menstrual cycle is primarily regulated by the interaction between pituitary and ovarian hormones. Also, releasing hormones from the hypothalamus play a role in controlling female reproduction through their effects on LH and FSH release from the anterior pituitary.[17] A complex series of positive and negative feedback mechanisms exist that control the cyclic release of various female hormones.[25,48] For instance, increased estrogen secretion in the follicular phase stimulates the LH surge that evokes ovulation. This event is considered an example of positive feedback because low estrogen levels increase LH release, which further increases estrogen secretion, thus further increasing LH release, and so on. Conversely, secretion of the pituitary gonadotropins (LH, FSH) is inhibited toward the latter part of the luteal phase, presumably because of the negative feedback influence of high levels of estrogen and progesterone.

Pharmacologic intervention can take advantage of these complex feedback systems in certain situations. Most notable is the use of estrogen and progesterone as oral contraceptives. By altering the normal control between pituitary/ovarian hormones and uterine function, preparations containing these two steroids are an effective means of birth control. This particular pharmacologic use of female hormones is discussed in more detail in "Pharmacologic Use of Estrogen and Progesterone."

Female Hormones in Pregnancy and Parturition

Estrogen and progesterone also play a significant role in pregnancy and childbirth. For successful implantation and gestation of the fertilized egg, synthesis of these two steroids must be maintained to prevent the onset of menstruation. As just mentioned, menstruation begins when the corpus luteum is no longer able to produce sufficient estrogen and progesterone to sustain the endometrium. When fertilization does occur, however, some hormonal response must transpire to maintain steroid production from the corpus luteum and ensure that the endometrium remains ready for implantation. This response is caused by the release of human chorionic gonadotropin (HCG) from the fertilized ovum. HCG takes over the role of LH and rescues the corpus luteum from destruction.[33] The corpus luteum then continues to produce steroids (especially progesterone), which maintain the uterine lining in a suitable state for implantation and gestation of the fertilized egg.

Eventually the corpus luteum does begin to degenerate between the 9th and 14th week of gestation. By that point, estrogen and progesterone production has been assumed by the placenta. Generally speaking, maternal progesterone helps to maintain the uterus and placenta throughout the rest of the pregnancy. Progesterone also increases the growth and development of the maternal mammary glands in preparation for lactation. Although the role of estrogen is less clear, increased estrogen production may play a pivotal part in setting the stage for parturition. Clearly, both steroids are needed for normal birth and delivery.

PHARMACOLOGIC USE OF ESTROGEN AND PROGESTERONE

The most frequent and prevalent use of the female hormones is in oral contraceptive preparations (see "Oral Contraceptives"). The other primary indications for estrogen and progesterone are the replacement of endogenous hormone production and subsequent resolution of symptoms related to hormonal deficiencies. This replacement can be especially important following menopause, that is, when the female reproductive cycle ceases and the associated cyclic production of the ovarian hormones ends.

Specific clinical conditions that may be resolved by estrogen and progesterone are listed here.

Conditions Treated with Estrogen and Progesterone

Replacement Therapy. Estrogen and progesterone are often used to replace the endogenous production of these hormones following menopause or in women who have had an ovariectomy. In particular, estrogens are often very effective in reducing some of the severe symptoms associated with menopause.[8,24,38,52] These include symptoms such as atrophic vaginitis, atrophic dystrophy of the vulva, and vasomotor effects such as hot flashes. Estrogens may also help prevent the osteoporosis associated with loss of estrogens following menopause.[14,16,22,28] Bone mineral loss may be decreased by estrogen administration, especially when combined with calcium supplements and physical activity.[1,21]

Estrogen replacement also appears to decrease the risk of coronary heart disease in postmenopausal women.[37,47,56,57] Low doses of estrogen cause favorable changes in plasma lipid profiles, including decreased levels of low-density lipoproteins and increased levels of high-density lipoproteins.[40,60] These effects on plasma lipoproteins decrease the risk of atherosclerotic lesions, thus reducing the incidence of coronary heart disease.

Hypogonadism. Estrogens or a combination of estrogen and progesterone may be used to treat abnormally low ovarian function. Appropriate use of these hormones induces the uterine changes and cyclic bleeding associated with the normal female reproductive cycle.

Failure of Ovarian Development. Occasionally, the ovaries fail to undergo normal development because of hypopituitarism or other disorders. Estrogens may be given at the time of puberty to encourage development of the secondary sexual characteristics (e.g., breast development).

Menstrual Irregularities. Various problems with normal menstruation are treated by estrogen and progesterone. These hormones are used either separately or in combination to resolve amenorrhea, dysmenorrhea, and other types of functional uterine bleeding that are caused by a hormonal imbalance.

Endometriosis. Endometriosis is a condition characterized by growths of uterine-like tissue that occur at various locations within the pelvic cavity. Progesterone and estrogen-progesterone combinations help suppress bleeding from these tissues and may help regress the size of these growths.

Carcinoma. Estrogen has been used to treat metastatic breast cancer in men and postmenopausal women. Advanced prostate cancer in men may also respond to estrogen treatment. Progesterone is helpful in treating uterine cancer and several other types of metastases such as breast, renal, and endometrial carcinoma.

Specific Agents

Types of estrogens and progestins that are used therapeutically are listed in Tables 30–4 and 30–5. Both types of hormones can be administered in their natural form (estradiol and progesterone), and several synthetic derivatives of each type are also available. Most of the drugs listed in Tables 30–4 and 30–5 are available as oral prepa-

TABLE 30–4 Clinical Use of Estrogens

Generic Name	Trade Name(s)	Primary Indication(s)
Chlorotrianisene	TACE	Estrogen replacement, antineoplastic
Dienestrol	Ortho Dienestrol	Estrogen replacement (vaginal)
Diethylstilbestrol	Honvol, Stilphostrol	Antineoplastic
Estradiol	Depo-Estradiol, Estrace, Estradiol L.A., Estraderm, many others	Estrogen replacement, antineoplastic, prevention of osteoporosis
Conjugated estrogens	Premarin	Estrogen replacement, antineoplastic, prevention of osteoporosis, prevention of abnormal uterine bleeding
Esterified estrogens	Estratab, Menest	Estrogen replacement, antineoplastic, prevention of osteoporosis
Estrone	Estronol, Gynogen, Unigen, many others	Estrogen replacement, antineoplastic, prevention of abnormal uterine bleeding
Estropipate	Ogen	Estrogen replacement
Ethinyl estradiol	Estinyl	Estrogen replacement, antineoplastic
Quinestrol	Estrovis	Estrogen replacement

rations, and many conditions can be conveniently treated by oral administration. Estrogens may also be administered transdermally in certain conditions, such as replacement therapy, and the transdermal route may offer certain advantages, such as decreased liver problems.[13,20] Finally, several preparations are also available for injection, and parenteral routes may be used in some situations, such as severe uterine bleeding.

Adverse Effects of Estrogen and Progesterone

Therapeutic use of estrogen may cause nausea, which is usually transient. Swelling of the feet and ankles may also occur because of sodium and water retention. Higher doses of estrogen have been associated with serious cardiovascular problems including myocardial infarction and thromboembolism. These problems are significant when relatively large doses are administered to men for the treatment of breast and prostate cancer. Estrogen replacement in postmenopausal women may increase the risk of endometrial and breast cancer, especially if estrogen is given for prolonged periods without concomitant progesterone therapy.[7] The primary problems associated

TABLE 30–5 Clinical Use of Progestins

Generic Name	Trade Name(s)	Primary Indication(s)
Hydroxyprogesterone	Duralutin, Hyprogest, others	Amenorrhea, functional uterine bleeding, adenocarcinoma of uterine corpus
Medroxyprogesterone	Cycrin, Provera, others	Amenorrhea, functional uterine bleeding, endometrial or renal carcinoma
Megestrol	Megace	Breast or endometrial carcinoma
Norethindrone	Aygestin, Micronor, Norlutin, others	Amenorrhea, functional uterine bleeding, endometriosis
Progesterone	Gesterol, Progestaject, others	Amenorrhea, functional uterine bleeding

with progesterone also involve abnormal blood clotting, which may lead to thrombophlebitis, pulmonary embolism, and cerebral infarction. Progesterone may alter the normal menstrual cycle, leading to unpredictable changes in the bleeding pattern.

Antiestrogens

Many hormones including androgens and progesterone tend to diminish the effects of estrogens. In addition, a limited number of drugs directly antagonize the effects of estrogen and are considered to be true antiestrogens. These antiestrogens appear to bind to estrogen receptors in the cytosol but do not cause any subsequent changes in cellular function. Hence, these drugs block the effects of estrogen by occupying the estrogen receptor and preventing estrogen from exerting a response. The principal antiestrogens used clinically are tamoxifen (Nolvadex) and clomiphene (Clomid, Serophene). Tamoxifen is used primarily in treating certain forms of estrogen-sensitive tumors (see Chapter 36). Clomiphene is administered to women to treat infertility. The mechanism of clomiphene as a fertility drug is somewhat complex. Relatively high levels of estrogen normally produce an inhibitory or negative feedback effect on the release of pituitary gonadotropins (LH and FSH). As an antiestrogen, clomiphene blocks this inhibitory effect, thus facilitating gonadotropin release.[39] Increased gonadotropins (especially LH) promote ovulation, thus improving the chance of fertilization. The primary adverse effects associated with clomiphene are vascular hot flashes. Enlarged ovaries may also occur because of the stimulatory effect of increased gonadotropin release.

ORAL CONTRACEPTIVES

During the 1960s, oral contraceptives containing estrogens and progestins were approved for use in preventing pregnancy. The introduction of these birth control pills provided a relatively easy and effective method of contraception. Today approximately 10 million women in the United States and 60 million women worldwide take some type of oral contraceptive,[39] making oral contraceptives one of the most frequently prescribed pharmacologic agents.

Types of Contraceptive Preparations

The most common form of oral contraceptive contains a fixed amount of estrogen and progesterone in the same pill. Examples of some common estrogen/progestin contraceptives are listed in Table 30–6. When taken appropriately, these preparations appear to be 99 to 100 percent effective in preventing pregnancy.[39] Typically, the contraceptive pill is taken each day for 3 weeks, beginning at the onset of menstruation. This intake is followed by 1 week in which either no pill is taken or a "blank" pill that lacks the hormones is taken. For convenience and improved compliance, these preparations are usually packaged in some form of dispenser that encourages the user to remember to take one pill each day.

Other versions of oral contraceptives are available that contain only a progestin (norethindrone, norgestrel) (see Table 30–6). These "minipills" were developed to

TABLE 30–6 Oral Contraceptives

Estrogen Component	Progestin Component	Common Trade Name(s)
Estrogen and progestin combinations		
Ethinyl estradiol	Ethynodiol diacetate	Demulen
Ethinyl estradiol	Levonorgestrel	Levlen, Nordette, Triphasil
Ethinyl estradiol	Norethindrone acetate	Loestrin, Norlestrin
Ethinyl estradiol	Norethindrone	Brevicon, Genora 1/35, Ortho-Novum 10-11, others
Mestranol	Norethindrone	Genora 1/50, Norinyl 1+50, Ortho-Novum 1/50, others
Ethinyl estradiol	Norgestrel	Lo/Ovral, Ovral
Preparations containing only progestins		
NA*	Norethindrone	Micronor, Norlutin, Nor-Q.D.
NA	Norgestrel	Ovrette

*NA = not applicable.

avoid the adverse effects normally attributed to estrogen. Progestin-only minipills are somewhat less attractive as an oral contraceptive because these preparations are only about 97 to 98 percent effective and because they tend to cause irregular and unpredictable menstrual cycles. An implantable form of a progestin-only preparation (Norplant) has also been developed, whereby small, semipermeable tubes containing levonorgestrel are inserted subcutaneously in the arm. The progestin is delivered in a slow, continuous fashion, allowing effective contraception for up to 5 years. These implants appear to have contraceptive efficacy that is better than progestin-only pills and only slightly less effective than combined estrogen-progestin oral contraceptives. Progestin-only implants can be replaced at the end of 5 years to continue this method of contraception, or they can be removed at any time because of side effects or other reasons. These implants are still relatively new, and it will be interesting to see how this form of contraception is received by the general public.

Oral contraceptives that contain only estrogen are sometimes used to prevent conception following sexual intercourse, especially in specific situations such as rape. These "morning-after pills" are not meant to be an alternative to traditional birth control methods, however. Also, the use of estrogen-only preparations as morning-after pills has generally been replaced by estrogen-progestin combinations that are somewhat safer (e.g., ethinyl estradiol combined with norgestrel).

Mechanism of Contraceptive Action

Oral contraceptives exert their effects primarily by inhibiting ovulation and by impairing the normal development of the uterine endometrium. As discussed previously, the normal menstrual cycle is governed by the complex interaction between endogenous ovarian hormones and the pituitary gonadotropins. High levels of estrogen and progesterone in the bloodstream act as negative feedback and inhibit the release of LH and FSH from the anterior pituitary. Oral contraceptives maintain fairly high plasma levels of estrogen and progestin, thus limiting the release of LH and FSH through this negative feedback system. Since ovulation is normally caused by the midcycle LH surge (see Fig. 30–2), inhibition of LH release prevents ovulation. This event prevents an ovum from being made available for fertilization.

The estrogen and progestin supplied by the contraceptive also affect the development of the uterine lining. Oral contraceptives promote a certain amount of growth and proliferation of the uterine endometrium. The endometrium, however, does not develop to quite the same extent or in quite the same manner as it would if controlled by normal endogenous hormonal release. Consequently, the endometrial environment is less than optimal for implantation even if ovulation and fertilization should take place. Also, there is an increase in the thickness and viscosity of the mucous secretions in the uterine cervix, thus impeding the passage of sperm through the cervical region, which adds to the contraceptive efficacy of these preparations.

Through the effects on the endometrium, oral contraceptive administration can be used to mimic a normal menstrual flow. When the contraceptive hormones are withdrawn at the end of the third week, the endometrium undergoes a sloughing similar to that in the normal cycle. Of course, the endometrium is being regulated by the exogenous hormones rather than the estrogen and progesterone normally produced by the ovaries. Still, this method of administration and withdrawal can produce a more or less normal pattern of uterine activity, with the exception that chances of conception are dramatically reduced.

Adverse Effects of Oral Contraceptives

Although oral contraceptives provide an easy and effective means of birth control, their use has been limited somewhat by potentially serious side effects. In particular, the pill has been associated with cardiovascular problems such as thrombophlebitis, stroke, and myocardial infarction. However, the incidence of these side effects may be diminished with the newer forms of oral contraceptives, which contain relatively less estrogen than their predecessors.

Over the years, the amount of estrogen contained in the combined estrogen/progesterone preparations has been reduced without sacrificing the contraceptive efficacy of these drugs.[6,58] Evidently, the lower estrogen content reduces the risk of cardiovascular problems. This does not mean that oral contraceptives are devoid of cardiovascular side effects. The pill may impair normal hemostasis and lead to thromboembolism and stroke.[46,59] This risk is relatively modest, however, with the current low-estrogen preparations. Still, oral contraceptives should not be used by women with any preexisting cardiovascular problems (hypertension, recurrent thrombosis) or any conditions or situations that may lead to cardiovascular disease (e.g., diabetes mellitus and cigarette smoking).[46]

There has been some indication that oral contraceptives may lead to certain forms of cancer. Some early versions of the pill were believed to cause tumors of the endometrium of the uterus. This effect may have been caused by early forms that were sequential in nature; that is, they provided only estrogen for the first half of the menstrual cycle and estrogen combined with progesterone for the second half. The newer, combined forms that supply both hormones throughout the cycle do not appear to increase the risk of uterine cancer, however. In fact, it appears that the form of oral contraceptive commonly used may actually *decrease* the risk of endometrial cancer, as well as prevent other forms of cancer including ovarian cancer.[6,12,35,51] The carcinogenic properties of oral contraceptives have not been totally ruled out, however. The effects on breast cancer remain controversial, and the possibility exists that certain subgroups of women may have an increased risk of breast cancer, depending on factors such as how long they used the pill prior to their first full-term pregnancy.[50] There is also considerable evidence that prolonged use of oral contraceptives (more than 8 years) may increase the risk of liver cancer.[6]

There are a number of other less serious but bothersome side effects associated with oral contraceptives. Problems such as nausea, loss of appetite, abdominal cramping, headache, dizziness, weight gain, and fatigue are fairly common. These symptoms are often transient and may diminish following continued use.

Consequently, the serious risks associated with oral contraceptives have diminished somewhat since their initial appearance on the market. These drugs are not without some hazards, however. In general, it is a good policy to reserve this form of birth control for relatively young, healthy women who do not smoke. Avoiding continuous, prolonged administration to diminish the risk of liver cancer may also be prudent. Finally, any increase in the other side effects associated with oral contraceptives, such as headache and abdominal discomfort, should be carefully evaluated to rule out a more serious underlying problem.

SPECIAL CONCERNS OF SEX HORMONE PHARMACOLOGY IN REHABILITATION PATIENTS

Therapists should be cognizant of the adverse effects related to the estrogens/progesterones and androgens so that they may help recognize problems related to these compounds. For instance, therapists should routinely monitor blood pressure during therapeutic administration of the sex hormones. These compounds tend to promote salt and water retention (mineralocorticoid-like properties), which may promote hypertension. Therapists may also play an important role in educating patients about the dangers of androgen abuse. When dealing with an athletic population, physical therapists may serve as a source of information about anabolic steroids. Therapists should advise athletes about the potential side effects such as liver, cardiovascular, and reproductive abnormalities. Therapists can also monitor blood pressure in athletes who appear to be using androgenic steroids. This interaction may help prevent a hypertensive crisis as well as illustrate to the athlete the harmful effects of these drugs.

CASE STUDY

MALE AND FEMALE HORMONES

Brief History. B.P. is a 72-year-old woman who sustained a compression fracture of the L-1 vertebral body. Evidently, the fracture occurred as she twisted sideways and leaned forward to get out of her daughter's car. X-ray films revealed generalized bone demineralization, and the compression fracture was apparently caused by osteoporosis. The patient was admitted to the hospital and confined to bed rest. Physical therapy was ordered, and heat and gentle massage were initiated at the bedside to decrease pain. To help attenuate bone demineralization, the patient was started on oral conjugated estrogen tablets (Premarin), at a dosage of 0.625 mg/day. A calcium supplement of 1500 mg/day was also added to the pharmacotherapeutic regimen.

Problem/Influence of Medication. The therapist realized that a program of exercise and general conditioning would augment the effects of the estrogen and calcium supplements. The combined effects of physical activity with pharmacologic management would offer the best chance at preventing further bone demineralization and osteoporosis.

Decision/Solution. Upon consultation with the referring physician, the physical therapist began a gradual strengthening and conditioning program. After the acute pain subsided, sitting and progressive ambulation activities were instituted at the bedside. Vertebral extension and abdominal strengthening exercises were also initiated as tolerated by the patient. This exercise and conditioning program was continued after the patient was discharged from the hospital, and a home program was supervised by periodic home visits from a physical therapist. Ambulation and exercise activities were gradually increased over the course of the next few weeks. The fracture had fully healed approximately 3 months following the initial incident. By that time, a formal exercise program had been established, consisting of daily ambulation and active range-of-motion activities. The therapist encouraged the patient to continue the exercise program indefinitely to help maintain bone mineral content and prevent subsequent fractures.

SUMMARY

The male hormones are the androgens, and the female hormones are the estrogens and progestins. These steroid hormones are primarily involved in the control of reproduction and sexual maturation. Male and female hormones also serve several important pharmacologic functions. These agents are often used as replacement therapy to resolve deficiencies in endogenous endocrine function. Androgens and estrogens/progestins are administered for a variety of other therapeutic reasons including the control of some neoplastic diseases. Estrogens and progestins can also be administered to women as an effective means of birth control, and these hormones are used extensively as oral contraceptive agents. Finally, androgens are sometimes used in high doses by athletes in an attempt to increase muscle strength and performance. Although these drugs may produce increments in muscle strength in some individuals, the dangers of using high doses of anabolic steroids outweigh any potential ergogenic benefits.

REFERENCES

1. Aisenbrey, JA: Exercise in the prevention and management of osteoporosis. Phys Ther 67:1100, 1987.
2. Alen, M and Hakkinen, K: Androgenic steroid effects on serum hormones and on maximal force development in strength athletes. J Sports Med Phys Fitness 27:38, 1987.
3. American College of Sports Medicine: Position stand on the use of anabolic-androgenic steroids in sports. Med Sci Sports Exerc 19:534, 1987.
4. American Medical Association Council on Scientific Affairs: Medical and nonmedical uses of anabolic-androgenic steroids. JAMA 264:2923, 1990.
5. American Medical Association Council on Scientific Affairs: Drug abuse in athletes: Anabolic steroids and human growth hormone. JAMA 259:1703, 1988.
6. Baird, DT and Glasier, AF: Hormonal contraception. N Engl J Med 328:1543, 1993.
7. Barrett-Connor, E: Hormone replacement and cancer. Br Med Bull 48:345, 1992.

8. Belchetz, PE: Drug therapy: Hormonal treatment of post-menopausal women. N Engl J Med 330:1062, 1994.

9. Bergman, R and Leach, RE: The use and abuse of anabolic steroids in Olympic-caliber athletes. Clin Orthop 198:169, 1985.

10. Bierly, JR: Use of anabolic steroids by athletes: Do the risks outweigh the benefits? Postgrad Med 82:67, 1987.

11. Buckley, WE, et al: Estimated prevalence of anabolic steroid use among male high school seniors. JAMA 260:3441, 1988.

12. Cancer and Steroid Hormone Study of the Center for Disease Control and the National Institute of Child Health and Human Development: Combination oral contraceptive use and the risk of endometrial cancer. JAMA 257:796, 1987.

13. Chetkowski, RJ, et al: Biologic effects of transdermal estradiol. N Engl J Med 314:1615, 1986.

14. Christiansen, C, et al: Uncoupling of bone formation and resorption by combined oestrogen and progestagin therapy in postmenopausal osteoporosis. Lancet 2:800, 1985.

15. Cohen, JC and Hickman, R: Insulin resistance and diminished glucose tolerance in powerlifters ingesting anabolic steroids. J Clin Endocrinol Metab 64:960, 1987.

16. Compston, JE: Hormone replacement therapy and osteoporosis. Br Med Bull 48:309, 1992.

17. Conn, PM, et al: Mechanism of action of gonadotropin releasing hormone. Annu Rev Physiol 48:495, 1986. .

18. Creagh, TM, Rubin, A, and Evans, DJ: Hepatic tumors induced by anabolic steroids in an athlete. J Clin Pathol 41:441, 1988.

19. Dufau, ML: Endocrine regulation and communicating functions of the Leydig cell. Annu Rev Physiol 50:483, 1988.

20. Ellerington, MC, Whitcroft, SIJ, and Whitehead, MI: Hormone replacement therapy: Developments in therapy. Br Med Bull 48:401, 1992.

21. Ettinger, B, Genant, HK, and Cann, CE: Postmenopausal bone loss is prevented by treatment with low-dosage estrogen with calcium. Ann Intern Med 106:40, 1987.

22. Felson, DT, et al: The effect of postmenopausal estrogen therapy on bone density in elderly women. N Engl J Med 329:1141, 1993.

23. Frankle, MA, Eichberg, R, and Zachariah, SB: Anabolic androgenic steroids and a stroke in an athlete: Case report. Arch Phys Med Rehabil 69:632, 1988.

24. Gambrell, RD: The role of progestogens in the treatment of the postmenopausal patient. Female Patient 10:59, 1985.

25. Gibori, G and Miller, J: The ovary: Follicle development, ovulation, and luteal function. In Zaneveld, LJD and Chatterton, RT (eds): Biochemistry of Mammalian Reproduction. John Wiley & Sons, New York, 1982.

26. Goldfien, A: The gonadal hormones and inhibitors. In Katzung, BG: Basic and Clinical Pharmacology, ed 5. Appleton & Lange, Norwalk, CT, 1992.

27. Haupt, HA: Anabolic steroids and growth hormone. Am J Sports Med 21:468, 1993.

28. Horsman, A, et al: The effect of estrogen doses on postmenopausal bone loss. N Engl J Med 309:1405, 1983.

29. Janne, OA and Bardin, CW: Androgen and antiandrogen receptor binding. Annu Rev Physiol 46:107, 1984.

30. Jarow, JP and Lipshultz, LI: Anabolic steroid-induced hypogonadotropic hypogonadism. Am J Sports Med 18:429, 1990.

31. Keyes, PL and Wiltbank, MC: Endocrine regulation of the corpus luteum. Annu Rev Physiol 50:465, 1988.

32. Kibble, MW and Ross, MB: Adverse effects of anabolic steroids in athletes. Clin Pharm 6:686, 1987.

33. Kuret, JA and Murad, F: Adenohypophyseal hormones and related substances. In Gilman, AG, et al (eds): The Pharmacological Basis of Therapeutics, ed 8. Pergamon Press, New York, 1990.

34. Lamb, DR: Anabolic steroids in athletes: How well do they work and how dangerous are they? Am J Sports Med 12:31, 1984.

35. Lee, NC, et al: The reduction in risk of ovarian cancer associated with oral contraceptive use. N Engl J Med 316:650, 1987.

36. McNutt, RA, et al: Acute myocardial infarction in a 22-year-old world class weight lifter. Am J Cardiol 62:164, 1988.

37. Meade, TW and Berra, A: Hormone replacement therapy and cardiovascular disease. Br Med Bull 48:276, 1992.

38. Montgomery, JC, et al: Effect of oestrogen and testosterone implants on psychological disorders in the climacteric. Lancet 1:297, 1987.

39. Murad, F and Kuret, JA: Estrogens and progestins. In Gilman, AG, et al (eds): The Pharmacological Basis of Therapeutics, ed 8. Pergamon Press, New York, 1990.

40. Nabulsi, AA, et al: Association of hormone replacement therapy with various cardiovascular risk factors in postmenopausal women. N Engl J Med 328:1069, 1993.

41. Perlumutter, G and Lowenthal, DT: Use of anabolic steroids by athletes. Am Fam Physician 32:208, 1985.

42. Perry, PJ, Andersen, KH, and Yates, WR: Illicit anabolic steroid use in athletes: A series of case analyses. Am J Sports Med 18:422, 1990.

43. Pettine, KA: Association of anabolic steroids and avascular necrosis of femoral heads. Am J Sports Med 19:96, 1991.

44. Pope, HG and Katz, DL: Affective and psychotic symptoms associated with anabolic steroid abuse. Am J Psychiatry 145:487, 1988.

45. Pope, HG and Katz, DL: Homocide and near-homocide by anabolic steroid users. J Clin Psychiatry 51:28, 1990.

46. Porter, JB, et al: Oral contraceptives and non-fatal vascular disease. Obstet Gynecol 66:1, 1985.

47. Psaty, BM, et al: A review of the association of estrogens and progestins with cardiovascular disease in postmenopausal women. Arch Intern Med 153:1421, 1993.

48. Richards, JS and Hedin, L: Molecular aspects of hormone action in ovarian follicular development, ovulation, and luteinization. Annu Rev Physiol 50:441, 1988.

49. Rodriguez-Rigau, LJ and Steinberger, E: The testis and spermatogenesis. In Zaneveld, LJD and Chatterton, RT (eds): Biochemistry of Mammalian Reproduction. John Wiley & Sons, New York, 1982.

50. Romieu, I, Berlin, JA, and Colditz, G: Oral contraceptives and breast cancer. Review and meta-analysis. Cancer 66:2253, 1990.

51. Rosner, D and Lane, WW: Oral contraceptive use has no adverse effect on the prognosis of breast cancer. Cancer 57:591, 1986.

52. Schwartz, M, Anwah, I, and Levy, RN: Variations in the treatment of postmenopausal osteoporosis. Clin Orthop 192:180, 1985.

53. Sharpe, RM: Regulation of spermatogenesis. In Knobil, E and Neill, JD (eds): The Physiology of Reproduction, Vol 1, ed 2. Raven Press, New York, 1994.

54. Sherman, MR and Stevens, J: Structure of mammalian steroid receptors. Annu Rev Physiol 46:83, 1984.

55. Snyder, PJ: Clinical use of androgens. Annu Rev Med 35:207, 1984.

56. Stampfer, MJ, et al: Postmenopausal estrogen therapy and cardiovascular disease: Ten-year follow-up from the Nurse's Health Study. N Engl J Med 325:756, 1991.

57. Stampfer, MJ, et al: A prospective study of postmenopausal estrogen therapy and coronary heart disease. N Engl J Med 313:1044, 1985.

58. Szarewski, A and Guillebaud, J: Regular review: Contraception. Br Med J 302:1224, 1991.

59. Vessey, MP, Lawless, M, and Yeates, D: Oral contraceptives and stroke: Findings in a large prospective study. Br Med J 289:530, 1984.

60. Walsh, BW, et al: Effects of postmenopausal estrogen replacement on the concentrations and metabolism of plasma lipoproteins. N Engl J Med 325:1196, 1991.

61. Webb, OL, Laskarzewski, PM, and Clueck, CJ: Severe depression of high density lipoprotein cholesterol levels in weight-lifters and bodybuilders by self-administered exogenous testosterone and anabolic-androgenic steroids. Metabolism 33:971, 1984.

CHAPTER 31

Thyroid and Parathyroid Drugs: Agents Affecting Bone Mineralization

---

This chapter discusses the function and pharmacologic aspects of two important endocrine structures: the thyroid and parathyroid glands. Hormones secreted from the thyroid gland are involved in controlling metabolism and also work synergistically with other hormones to promote normal growth and development. The parathyroid glands are essential in regulating calcium homeostasis and are important in maintaining proper bone mineralization.

Problems in the function of the thyroid or parathyroid glands are often treated by pharmacologic methods. Pharmacologic management of thyroid and parathyroid function should be of interest to rehabilitation specialists because physical therapists and occupational therapists often treat patients with disorders in bone healing and other endocrine problems related to these glands. This chapter first discusses normal physiologic function of the thyroid gland, followed by the types of drugs used to treat hyperthyroidism and hypothyroidism. Then the function of the parathyroid glands is covered, discussing the role of the parathyroid glands and other hormones in maintaining bone mineral homeostasis. Finally, drugs used to regulate bone calcification are presented.

FUNCTION OF THE THYROID GLAND

The thyroid gland lies on either side of the trachea in the anterior neck region and consists of bilateral lobes that are connected by a central isthmus. The entire gland weighs approximately 15 to 20 g and receives a rich vascular supply as well as extensive innervation from the sympathetic nervous system.

The thyroid gland synthesizes two primary hormones: thyroxine and triiodothyronine. Discussion of the synthesis and function of these hormones follows.

Synthesis of Thyroid Hormones

The chemical structures of thyroxine and triiodothyronine are shown in Figure 31–1. As shown in this figure, thyroid hormones are synthesized by first adding iodine to residues of the amino acid *tyrosine*. Addition of one iodine creates monoiodotyrosine, and the addition of a second iodine creates diiodotyrosine. Two of these iodinated tyrosines are then combined to complete the thyroid hormone. The combination of a monoiodotyrosine and a diiodotyrosine yields triiodothyronine, and the combination of two diiodotyrosines yields thyroxine.

Because thyroxine contains four iodine residues, this compound is also referred to by the abbreviation T_4. Triiodothyronine contains three iodine residues, hence the abbreviation T_3. There has been considerable discussion about which hormone exerts the primary physiologic effects. Plasma levels of T_4 are much greater than T_3, but T_3 may exert most of the physiologic effects on various tissues, suggesting that T_4 is primarily a precursor to T_3 and that conversion of T_4 to T_3 occurs in peripheral tissues.[19,36] Regardless of which hormone ultimately affects cellular metabolism, both T_4 and T_3 are needed for normal thyroid function.

The primary steps in thyroid hormone biosynthesis are shown schematically in Figure 31–2. Thyroid follicle cells take up and concentrate iodide from the bloodstream, which is significant because there must be a sufficient amount of iodine in the diet to provide the iodide needed for thyroid hormone production. The thyroid cells also manufacture a protein known as thyroglobulin (TGB), which contains tyrosine residues. The TGB molecule is manufactured within the follicle cell and stored in the central lumen of the thyroid follicle (see Fig. 31–2). During hormone synthesis, iodide is oxidized and covalently bonded to the tyrosine residues of the TGB molecule. Two iodinated tyrosine residues combine within the TGB molecule to form T_4 (primarily),

FIGURE 31–1. Structure of the thyroid hormones triiodothyronine (T_3) and thyroxine (T_4). Addition of one iodine (I) to tyrosine produces monoiodotyrosine; addition of a second iodine produces diiodotyrosine. A monoiodotyrosine and diiodotyrosine combine to form triiodothyronine (T_3). Coupling of two diiodotyrosines forms thyroxine (T_4).

Blood Stream

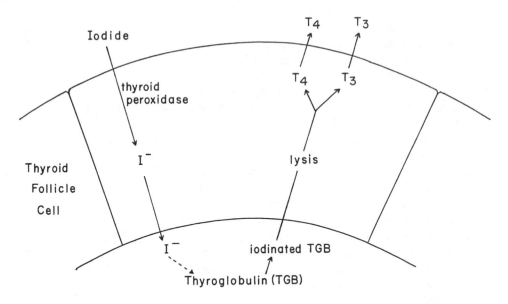

Follicle Lumen

FIGURE 31–2. Thyroid hormone biosynthesis. Iodide is taken into the follicle cell where it is converted by thyroid peroxidase to an oxidized form of iodine (I^-). I^- is transported to the follicle lumen, where it is bonded to tyrosine residues of the thyroglobulin (TGB) molecule. Iodinated TGB is incorporated back into the cell, where it undergoes lysis to yield the thyroid hormones T_3 and T_4. See text for further discussion.

with smaller amounts of T_3 also being produced. At this point, the hormones are still incorporated within the large TGB molecule. Hence, the iodinated TGB molecule (TGB containing the iodinated tyrosines) is absorbed back into the follicle cell, where the large molecule is lysed to yield the thyroid hormones. The hormones are then secreted into the systemic circulation, where they can reach various target tissues.

Regulation of Thyroid Hormone Release

Production of the thyroid hormones is controlled by the hypothalamic-pituitary system (see Chapter 28). Thyrotropin-releasing hormone (TRH) from the hypothalamus stimulates the release of thyroid-stimulating hormone (TSH) from the anterior pituitary. TSH then travels via the systemic circulation to the thyroid gland to stimulate the production of thyroxine and triiodothyronine.

Thryoid hormone release is subject to the negative feedback strategy that is typical of endocrine systems controlled by the hypothalamic-pituitary axis. Increased circulating levels of the thyroid hormones (T_4, T_3) serve to limit their own production by inhibiting TSH release from the anterior pituitary.[21,25] The thyroid hormones do not directly inhibit TRH release from the hypothalamus, but rather the primary negative feedback control is at the level of the pituitary gland.[25] This negative feedback control prevents peripheral levels of thyroid hormones from becoming excessively high.

Physiologic Effects of Thyroid Hormones

Thryoid hormones affect a wide variety of peripheral tissues throughout the entire life of the individual. In some situations, these hormones exert a direct effect on cellular function (e.g., T_4 and T_3 appear to increase cellular metabolism by directly increasing oxidative enzyme activity). In other instances, thyroid hormones appear to play a permissive role in facilitating the function of other hormones. For instance, thyroid hormones must be present for growth hormone to function properly. The principal effects of the thyroid hormones are listed here.

Thermogenesis. T_4 and T_3 increase the basal metabolic rate and subsequent heat production from the body, which are important in maintaining adequate body temperature during exposure to cold environments. Increased thermogenesis is achieved by thyroid hormone stimulation of cellular metabolism in various tissues such as skeletal muscle, cardiac muscle, and liver and kidney cells.

Growth and Development. Thyroid hormones facilitate normal growth and development by stimulating the release of growth hormone and by enhancing the effects of growth hormone on peripheral tissues. Thyroid hormones also directly enhance the development of many physiologic systems, especially the skeletal system and CNS. If thyroid hormones are not present, severe growth restriction and mental retardation (**cretinism**) ensue.

Cardiovascular Effects. Thyroid hormones appear to increase heart rate and myocardial contractility, thus leading to an increase in cardiac output. It is unclear, however, if this occurrence is a direct effect of these hormones or if the thyroid hormones increase myocardial sensitivity to other hormones (norepinephrine and epinephrine).

Metabolic Effects. Thyroid hormones affect energy substrate utilization in a number of ways. For instance, these hormones increase intestinal glucose absorption and increase the activity of several enzymes involved in carbohydrate metabolism. Thyroid hormones enhance lipolysis by increasing the response of fat cells to other lipolytic hormones. In general, these and other metabolic effects help increase the availability of glucose and lipids for increased cellular activity.

Mechanism of Action of Thyroid Hormones

The preponderance of evidence indicates that the thyroid hormones enter the cell and bind to specific receptors located within the cell's nucleus.[19,23,27] Binding of the thyroid hormone then induces transcription of specific DNA gene segments, which ultimately results in altered protein synthesis within the cell. Most, if not all, of the physiologic effects of the thyroid hormones are related to this alteration in cellular protein production. For instance, thyroid hormones may act through nuclear DNA transcription to stimulate the synthesis of a particular enzymatic protein. Such a protein may increase the transport of specific substances (e.g., amino acids, glucose, sodium) across the cell membrane, or the newly synthesized protein may be directly involved in a metabolic pathway (e.g., glycolysis or lipid oxidation).

TREATMENT OF THYROID DISORDERS

Thyroid disorders can basically be divided into two primary categories: conditions that increase thyroid function (hyperthyroidism) and conditions that decrease thyroid function (hypothyroidism). There are several different types of hyperthyroidism and hypothyroidism, depending on the apparent etiology, symptoms, and age of onset of each type. Types of hyperthyroidism and hypothyroidism are listed in Table 31–1. Although we cannot review the causes and effects of all the various forms of thyroid dysfunction at this time, this topic is dealt with extensively elsewhere.[4,5,11,21,25,43]

The clinical manifestations of hyperthyroidism and hypothyroidism are listed in Table 31–2. From a pharmacotherapeutic standpoint, hyperthyroidism is treated with drugs that attenuate the synthesis and effects of the thyroid hormones. Hypothyroidism is usually treated by thyroid hormone administration (replacement therapy). The general aspects and more common forms of hyperthyroidism and hypothyroidism are discussed here, along with the drugs used to resolve these primary forms of thyroid dysfunction.

Hyperthyroidism

Hyperthyrodism (**thyrotoxicosis)** results in the increased secretion of thyroid hormones. This condition may occur secondarily to a number of reasons including thyroid tumors and problems in the endocrine regulation of thyroid secretion—for example, excess TSH secretion (see Table 31–1). Hyperthyroidism is usually associated with enlargement of the thyroid gland, or goiter. One of the more common causes of hyperthyroidism is diffuse toxic goiter (Graves' disease). Graves' disease is believed to be caused by a problem in the immune system. Because of a genetic defect, antibodies are synthesized that directly stimulate the thyroid gland, resulting in exaggerated thyroid hormone production.[25,43,44] There are several other types of hyperthyroidism based on different causes and clinical features (see Table 31–1).[11,21]

The principal manifestations of hyperthyroidism are listed in Table 31–2. The treatment of this condition often consists of ablation of the thyroid gland, accomplished by direct surgical removal of the thyroid or by administering radioactive iodine. Several pharmacologic agents may also be used in the management of hyperthyroidism in various situations.[17] These drugs and their clinical applications are discussed in the following sections.

TABLE 31–1 Primary Types of Hyperthyroidism and Hypothyroidism

Hyperthyroidism (Thyrotoxicosis)	Hypothyroidism (Hypothyroxinemia)

Primary hyperthyroidism
  Graves' disease
  Thyroid adenoma/carcinoma
Secondary hyperthyroidism
  Hyperthyroidism induced by excessive
    hypothalamic or pituitary stimulation
	Primary hypothyroidism
	  Genetic deficiency of enzymes that synthesize
	    thyroid hormones
	Secondary hypothyroidism
	  Hypothyroidism induced by hypothalamic or
	    pituitary deficiencies
	Cretinism (childhood hypothyroidism)
	Myxedema (adult hypothyroidism)
	Other forms of hypothyroidism
	  Hypothyroidism induced by peripheral insensitivity
	    to thyroid hormones, inadequate hormone
	    transport, other causes

TABLE 31–2 Primary Symptoms of
Hyperthyroidism and Hypothyroidism

Hyperthyroidism	Hypothyroidism
Nervousness	Lethargy/slow cerebration
Weight loss	Weight gain (in adult hypothyroidism)
Diarrhea	Constipation
Tachycardia	Bradycardia
Insomnia	Sleepiness
Increased appetite	Anorexia
Heat intolerance	Cold intolerance
Oligomenorrhea	Menorrhagia
Muscle wasting	Weakness
Goiter	Dry, coarse skin
Exophthalmos	Facial edema

Adapted from Kuhn, MA: Thyroid and Parathyroid Glands. In Kuhn, MA (ed): Pharmacotherapeutics: A Nursing Process Approach, ed 3. FA Davis, Philadelphia, 1994, p 981.

Antithyroid Agents. Antithyroid drugs directly inhibit thyroid hormone synthesis. The antithyroid agents currently in use are propylthiouracil (Propyl-Thyracil) and methimazole (Tapazole).[8,17] These drugs inhibit the thyroid peroxidase enzyme necessary for preparing iodide for addition to tyrosine residues (see Fig. 31–2).[15,39] These agents also prevent coupling of tyrosine residues within the thyroglobulin molecule.[9,17] Propylthiouracil also inhibits the effects of the thyroid hormones by blocking the conversion of T_4 to T_3 in peripheral tissues.[9,17] The most common adverse effect of antithyroid drugs is skin rash and itching, although this effect is usually mild and transient. More serious problems involving formed blood elements (agranulocytosis and aplastic anemia) may occur, but the incidence of such problems is relatively small. Finally, excessive inhibition of thyroid hormone synthesis brought about by drug overdosage may cause symptoms resembling hypothyroidism such as coldness and lethargy.

Iodide. Relatively large doses of iodide (exceeding 6 mg/day) cause a rapid and dramatic decrease in thyroid function. In sufficient amounts, iodide inhibits virtually all the steps involved in thyroid hormone biosynthesis. For instance, high iodide levels limit the uptake of iodide into thyroid follicle cells, inhibit the formation of T_4 and T_3, and decrease the secretion of the completed hormones from the thyroid cell.

Although iodide is effective in treating hyperthyroidism for short periods, the effects of this drug begin to diminish after about 2 weeks of administration.[17] Consequently, iodide is used in limited situations, such as in the temporary control of hyperthyroidism prior to thyroidectomy. Also, iodide may cause a severe hypersensitive reaction in susceptible individuals. Therefore, the use of iodide has been replaced somewhat by other agents such as the antithyroid drugs and beta blockers.

Radioactive Iodine. A radioactive isotope of iodine (^{131}I) is often used to selectively destroy thyroid tissues in certain forms of hyperthyroidism, like Graves' disease.[17,20] A specific dose of radioactive iodine is administered orally and is rapidly sequestered within the thyroid gland. The isotope then begins to emit beta radiation, which selectively destroys the thyroid follicle cells. Essentially no damage occurs to surrounding tissues because the radioactivity is contained within the thyroid gland. Thus, administration of radioactive iodine is a simple, relatively safe method of permanently ablating the thyroid gland and reducing excess thyroid hormone function.[20]

Of course, patients who undergo radioactive destruction of the thyroid gland (or surgical thyroidectomy) must often be given thyroid hormones as replacement therapy.[17]

Beta-Adrenergic Blockers. Beta-adrenergic blockers are usually associated with the treatment of cardiovascular problems such as hypertension and angina pectoris. Beta blockers may also be helpful as an adjunct in thyrotoxicosis.[17] Although these drugs do not directly lower plasma levels of thyroid hormones, they may help suppress symptoms such as tachycardia, palpitations, fever, and restlessness. Consequently, beta blockers are usually not the only drugs used in the long-term control of hyperthyroidism but serve as adjuncts to other medications such as the antithyroid drugs. Beta blockers may be especially helpful in severe, acute exacerbations of thyrotoxicosis (thyroid storm). These drugs are also administered preoperatively to control symptoms until a more permanent means of treating thyrotoxicosis (thyroidectomy) can be implemented.[1,26] Some beta blockers that have been used effectively in thyrotoxicosis are acebutolol, atenolol, metoprolol, nadolol, oxprenolol, propranolol, and timolol. The pharmacology and adverse effects of these compounds are described in Chapter 20.

Hypothyroidism

There are many forms of hypothyroidism, differing in their cause and age of onset (see Table 31–1). Severe adult hypothyroidism (**myxedema**) may occur idiopathically or may be caused by specific factors such as autoimmune lymphocytic destruction (Hashimoto's disease). In the child, thyroid function may be congenitally impaired, and cretinism will result if this condition is untreated. Hypothyroidism may result at any age if the dietary intake of iodine is extremely low. Several other forms of hypothyroidism that have a genetic or familial basis also exist.[4,11,21,25]

The primary physiologic effects of decreased thyroid function are listed in Table 31–2. Although enlargement of the thyroid gland (*goiter*) is usually associated with hyperthyroidism, goiter may also be present in some forms of hypothyroidism, although for different reasons. For instance, thyroid enlargement occurs during hypothyroidism when there is a lack of dietary iodine (endemic goiter). Under the influence of TSH, the thyroid manufactures large quantities of thyroglobulin. Thyroid hormone synthesis is incomplete, however, because no iodine is available to add to the tyrosine residues. If no thyroid hormones are produced, there is no negative feedback to limit the secretion of TSH. Consequently, the thyroid gland increases in size because of the unabated production of thyroglobulin.

The primary method of treating hypothyroidism is to administer thyroid hormones as replacement therapy. Long-term administration of thyroid hormones is usually a safe, effective means of maintaining optimal patient health in hypothyroidism. Replacement therapy using thyroid hormone preparations is described here.

Thyroid Hormones. Replacement of deficient thyroid hormones with natural and synthetic analogs is necessary in most forms of hypothyroidism.[42] Preparations containing T_3, T_4, or both hormones are administered to mimic normal thyroid function whenever the endogenous production of these hormones is impaired. Thyroid hormone replacement is often necessary following thyroidectomy or pharmacologic ablation of the thyroid gland using radioactive iodine. Thyroid hormones may also be used to prevent and treat cancer of the thyroid gland and to prevent enlargement of the thyroid gland (goiter) caused by other drugs such as lithium. Thyroid hormone mainte-

TABLE 31–3 Thyroid Hormones Used to Treat Hypothyroidism

Generic Name	Trade Name(s)	Thyroid Hormone Content	Source
Levothyroxine	Levothroid, Synthroid	T_4	Synthetic
Liothyronine	Cytomel	T_3	Synthetic
Liotrix	Euthroid, Thyrolar	T_3 and T_4	Synthetic
Thyroglobulin	Proloid	T_3 and T_4	Natural
Thyroid	—	T_3 and T_4	Natural

T_3 = triiodothyronine; T_4 = thyroxine.

nance may be beneficial in patients who are in the preliminary or subclinical phase of hypothyroidism. Administering these hormones in the early stages may prevent the disease from developing to its full extent.[10,40]

Thyroid hormone preparations used clinically are listed in Table 31–3. The primary problems associated with these agents occur during overdosage. Symptoms of excess drug levels are similar to the symptoms of hyperthyroidism (see Table 31–2). Presence of these symptoms is resolved by decreasing the dosage or changing the medication.

FUNCTION OF THE PARATHYROID GLANDS

In humans, there are usually four parathyroid glands, which are embedded on the posterior surface of the thyroid gland. Each parathyroid gland is a small, pea-sized structure weighing about 50 mg. Despite their diminutive size, the parathyroids serve a vital role in controlling calcium homeostasis.[2,21] Because calcium is crucial in such physiologic processes as synaptic transmission, muscle contraction, and bone mineralization, the importance of parathyroid function is obvious. In fact, removal of the parathyroid glands soon results in convulsions and death because of inadequate plasma calcium levels. The parathyroids control calcium homeostasis through the synthesis and secretion of *parathyroid hormone* (PTH), and the regulation and function of PTH is discussed here.

Parathyroid Hormone

PTH is a polypeptide hormone that is synthesized within the cells of the parathyroid glands. The primary factor controlling the release of PTH is the amount of calcium in the bloodstream.[28] Evidently, parathyroid cells are able to monitor plasma calcium titers. A decrease in plasma calcium stimulates the release of PTH. As blood calcium levels increase, PTH release is reduced.

The primary effect of PTH is to increase blood calcium levels by altering calcium metabolism in three primary tissues: bone, kidneys, and the gastrointestinal tract. PTH directly affects skeletal tissues by increasing bone resorption, thus liberating calcium from skeletal stores.[2,31] High levels of PTH appear to enhance the development and action of cells (osteoclasts) that break down skeletal tissues.[2,7,18] Increased osteoclast activity degrades the collagen matrix within the bone, thus releasing calcium into the bloodstream. PTH also increases plasma calcium levels by increasing renal reabsorption of calcium. As renal calcium reabsorption is increased, PTH produces a simultaneous increase in phosphate excretion. Thus, PTH produces a rise in plasma calcium that is accompanied by a decrease in plasma phosphate levels.

Finally, PTH helps increase the absorption of calcium from the gastrointestinal tract. This effect appears to be caused by the interaction between PTH and vitamin D metabolism. PTH increases the conversion of vitamin D to 1,25-dihydroxycholecalciferol (calcitriol). Calcitriol directly stimulates calcium absorption from the intestine.

Consequently, PTH is crucial to maintaining adequate levels of calcium in the body. In addition, PTH works with two other primary hormones—calcitonin and vitamin D—in regulating calcium homeostasis. These three hormones, as well as several other endocrine factors, are involved in controlling calcium levels for various physiologic needs. Of particular interest to rehabilitation professionals is how these hormones interact in controlling normal bone formation and resorption. Regulation of bone mineral homeostasis and the principal hormones involved in this process are presented in the following section.

REGULATION OF BONE MINERAL HOMEOSTASIS

Bone serves two primary functions: to provide a rigid framework for the body and to provide a readily available and easily interchangeable calcium pool. To serve both functions simultaneously, an appropriate balance must exist between bone formation and bone resorption. As already discussed, bone resorption (breakdown) can supply calcium for various physiologic processes. Mineral resorption, however, occurs at the expense of bone formation. The primary minerals that enable bone to maintain its rigidity are calcium and phosphate. Excessive resorption of these minerals will result in bone demineralization, and the skeletal system will undergo failure (fracture). Also, bone is continually undergoing specific changes in its internal architecture. This process of remodeling allows bone to adapt to changing stresses and optimally resist applied loads.

Consequently, bone is a rather dynamic tissue that is constantly undergoing changes in mineral content and internal structure. The balance between bone resorption and formation is controlled by the complex interaction of local and systemic factors. In particular, there are several hormones that regulate bone formation and help maintain adequate plasma calcium levels. The primary hormones involved in regulating bone mineral homeostasis are described here.

Parathyroid Hormone. The role of the parathyroid gland and PTH in controlling calcium metabolism was discussed previously. Increased secretion of PTH increases blood calcium levels by several methods, including increased resorption of calcium from bone. High levels of PTH accelerate bone breakdown to mobilize calcium for other physiologic needs. Low or normal PTH levels may actually enhance bone formation, however.[2] Thus, PTH plays an integral role in bone metabolism. Increased PTH secretion favors bone breakdown, whereas decreased or normal PTH release encourages bone synthesis and remodeling.

Vitamin D. Vitamin D is a steroidlike hormone that can be either obtained from dietary sources or synthesized in the skin from cholesterol derivatives in the presence of ultraviolet light. Vitamin D produces several metabolites that are important in bone mineral homeostasis.[14,18] In general, vitamin D derivatives increase serum calcium and phosphate levels by increasing intestinal calcium and phosphate absorption and by decreasing renal calcium and phosphate excretion.[13] The effects of vitamin D metabolites on bone itself are somewhat unclear. Some metabolites seem to promote bone resorption, while others favor bone formation.[2] The overall influence of vitamin D, however, is to enhance bone formation by increasing the supply of the two primary minerals needed for bone formation (calcium and phosphate).

Calcitonin. Calcitonin is a hormone secreted by cells located in the thyroid gland. These calcitonin-secreting cells (also known as *parafollicular* or *"C" cells*) are interspersed between the follicles that produce the thyroid hormones. Basically, calcitonin can be considered to be the physiologic antagonist of PTH.[3] Calcitonin lowers blood calcium by stimulating bone formation and increasing the incorporation of calcium into skeletal storage. Incorporation of phosphate into bone is also enhanced by the action of calcitonin. Renal excretion of calcium and phosphate is increased by a direct effect of calcitonin on the kidneys, thus further reducing the levels of these minerals in the bloodstream. The effects of calcitonin on bone mineral metabolism, however, are relatively minor compared to PTH, and calcitonin is not essential for normal bone mineral homeostasis.[3] In contrast, PTH is a much more dominant hormone, and the absence of PTH produces acute disturbances in calcium metabolism resulting in death. Calcitonin does have an important therapeutic function, and pharmacologic doses of calcitonin may be helpful in preventing bone loss in certain conditions (see "Pharmacologic Control of Bone Mineral Homeostasis").

Other Hormones. A number of other hormones influence bone mineral content.[31] Glucocorticoids produce a general catabolic effect on bone and other supporting tissues (see Chapter 29). Certain prostaglandins are also potent stimulators of bone resorption. Bone formation is generally enhanced by a number of hormones such as estrogens, androgens, growth hormone, insulin, and the thyroid hormones. In general, the effects of these other hormones are secondary to the more direct effects of PTH, vitamin D, and calcitonin. Nonetheless, all the hormones that influence bone metabolism interact with one another to some extent in the regulation of bone formation and breakdown. Also, disturbances in any of these secondary endocrine systems may produce problems that are manifested in abnormal bone formation, including excess glucocorticoid activity and growth hormone deficiency.

PHARMACOLOGIC CONTROL OF BONE MINERAL HOMEOSTASIS

Satisfactory control of the primary bone minerals is important in both acute and long-term situations. Blood calcium levels must be maintained within a fairly limited range to ensure an adequate supply of free calcium for various physiologic purposes. The normal concentration of calcium in the blood is 9.4 mg/100 mL.[21] If plasma calcium levels fall to below 6 mg/100 mL, tetanic muscle convulsions quickly ensue. Excess plasma calcium (blood levels greater than 12 mg/100 mL) depresses nervous function, leading to sluggishness, lethargy, and possibly coma.

Chronic disturbances in calcium homeostasis can also produce problems in bone calcification. Likewise, various metabolic bone diseases can alter blood calcium levels, leading to hypocalcemia or **hypercalcemia**. Some of the more common metabolic diseases affecting bone mineralization are listed in Table 31–4. Various problems in bone metabolism may produce abnormal plasma calcium levels, thus leading to the aforementioned problems.

TABLE 31–4 Examples of Metabolic Bone Disease

Disease	Pathophysiology	Drug Treatment
Hypoparathyroidism	Decreased parathyroid hormone secretion; leads to impaired bone resorption and hypocalcemia	Calcium supplements, vitamin D
Hyperparathyroidism	Increased parathyroid hormone secretion; leads to excessive bone resorption and hypercalcemia	Usually treated surgically
Osteoporosis	Generalized bone demineralization; often associated with effects of aging and hormonal changes in postmenopausal women	Calcium supplements, vitamin D, calcitonin, estrogen (see Chapter 30)
Rickets	Impaired bone mineralization in children caused by a deficiency of vitamin D	Calcium supplements, vitamin D
Osteomalacia	Adult form of rickets	Calcium supplements, vitamin D
Paget's disease	Excessive bone formation and resorption (turnover) leads to ineffective remodeling and structural abnormalities within the bone	Calcitonin, etidronate
Renal osteodystrophy	Chronic renal failure induces complex metabolic changes resulting in excessive bone resorption	Vitamin D, calcium supplements
Gaucher's disease	Excessive lipid storage in bone leads to impaired remodeling and excessive bone loss	No drugs are effective
Hypercalcemia of malignancy	Many forms of cancer accelerate bone resorption, leading to hypercalcemia	Calcitonin, etidronate

Consequently, pharmacologic methods to help control bone mineral levels in the bloodstream and maintain adequate bone mineralization must often be used. Specific drugs used to control bone mineralization and the clinical conditions in which they are used are discussed subsequently.

Calcium Supplements

Calcium preparations are often administered to ensure that adequate calcium levels are available in the body for various physiologic needs including bone formation. Specifically, calcium supplements can be used to help prevent bone loss in conditions such as osteoporosis, osteomalacia, rickets, and hypoparathyroidism. For instance, calcium supplements alone cannot prevent osteoporosis in postmenopausal women,[6] but these supplements are certainly helpful when combined with other treatments such as estrogen replacement.[32] The use of oral calcium supplements appears to be especially important in individuals who do not receive sufficient amounts of calcium in their diet.

Types of calcium supplements used clinically are listed in Table 31–5. Typical dosages range between 1000 and 1500 mg of calcium per day. Excessive doses may produce symptoms of hypercalcemia, including constipation, drowsiness, fatigue, and headache. As hypercalcemia becomes more pronounced, confusion, irritability, cardiac arrhythmias, hypertension, nausea and vomiting, skin rashes, and pain in bones and muscle may occur. Hypercalcemia is a cause for concern since severe cardiac irregularities may prove fatal.

Vitamin D

Vitamin D is a precursor for a number of compounds that increase intestinal absorption and decrease renal excretion of calcium and phosphate. Metabolites of vitamin D and their pharmacologic analogs are typically used to increase blood calcium

TABLE 31–5 Drugs Used to Control Bone Mineral Homeostasis

General Category	Examples*	Treatment Rationale and Principal Indications
Calcium supplements	Calcium carbonate (Biocal, Os-Cal 500, Tums) Calcium citrate (Citracal) Calcium glubionate (Neo-Calglucon) Calcium gluconate Calcium lactate Dibasic calcium phosphate Tribasic calcium phosphate (Posture)	Provide an additional source of calcium to prevent calcium depletion and encourage bone formation in conditions such as osteoporosis, osteomalacia, rickets, and hypoparathyroidism
Vitamin D analogs	Calcifediol (Calderol) Calcitriol (Rocaltrol) Dihydrotachysterol (DHT, Hytakerol) Ergocalciferol (Calciferol, Drisdol)	Generally enhance bone formation by increasing the absorption and retention of calcium and phosphate in the body; useful in treating disorders caused by vitamin D deficiency, including hypocalcemia, hypophosphatemia, rickets, and osteomalacia
Diphosphonates	Etidronate (Didronel) Pamidronate (Aredia)	Appears to block excessive bone resorption and formation; is used to normalize bone turnover in conditions such as Paget's disease and to prevent hypercalcemia resulting from excessive bone resorption in certain forms of cancer
Calcitonin	Human calcitonin (Cibacalcin) Salmon calcitonin (Calcimar, Miacalcin)	Mimic the effects of endogenous calcitonin and increase bone formation in conditions such as Paget's disease and osteoporosis; also are used to lower plasma calcium levels in hypercalcemic emergencies

*Common trade names are shown in parentheses.

and phosphate levels and to enhance bone mineralization in conditions such as osteodystrophy and rickets. Certain vitamin D analogs such as calcitriol have also been used experimentally to help treat postmenopausal osteoporosis.[41] Specific vitamin D–related compounds and their clinical applications are listed in Table 31–5.

Vitamin D is a fat-soluble vitamin, and excessive doses can accumulate in the body, leading to toxicity. Some early signs of vitamin D toxicity include headache, increased thirst, decreased appetite, metallic taste, fatigue, and gastrointestinal disturbances (nausea, vomiting, constipation, or diarrhea). Increased vitamin D toxicity is associated with hypercalcemia, high blood pressure, cardiac arrhythmias, renal failure, mood changes, and seizures. Vitamin D toxicity is a serious problem, since death may occur because of cardiac and renal failure.

Diphosphonates

The diphosphonates (also called *bisphosphonates*) are a group of inorganic compounds that include etidronate (Didronel), pamidronate (Aredia), and several similar agents. Although their exact mechanism is unclear, these compounds appear to adsorb directly to calcium crystals in the bone and to reduce bone resorption by inhibiting osteoclast activity.[29] Thus, diphosphonates are often used in Paget's disease to help prevent exaggerated bone turnover and promote adequate mineralization.[16,24] These agents can also be used to inhibit abnormal bone formation in conditions such as heterotopic ossification and to prevent hypercalcemia resulting from increased bone resorption in neoplastic disease.[22,38] Diphosphonates have been used experimentally to reduce bone loss in osteoporosis, and preliminary studies suggest that these agents may be helpful in osteoporotic disease.[29] Additional research, however, is needed to confirm that these agents are a safe, effective treatment for osteoporosis.

The primary adverse effect associated with etidronate is tenderness and pain occurring over the sites of bony lesions in Paget's disease,[24] leading to fractures if excessive doses are taken for prolonged periods. Pamidronate may cause fever and localized pain and redness at the injection site, but these effects usually last for only a day or two. Diphosphonates may produce other relatively minor side effects including gastrointestinal disturbances such as nausea and diarrhea.

Calcitonin

Calcitonin derived from synthetic sources can be administered to mimic the effects of the endogenous hormone. As described previously, endogenous calcitonin decreases blood calcium levels and promotes bone mineralization. Consequently, synthetically derived calcitonin is used to treat hypercalcemia and to decrease bone resorption in Paget's disease.[12] Calcitonin has also been used to help prevent bone loss in a variety of other conditions including rheumatoid arthritis,[37] postmenopausal osteoporosis,[30] and glucocorticoid-induced osteoporosis.[35] In the past, calcitonin was administered by injection (intramuscular or subcutaneous), but aerosolized versions of calcitonin are now available that allow delivery in the form of nasal sprays.[37] Hence, calcitonin has emerged as an effective and easy way to treat a variety of conditions that are characterized by increased bone resorption.[33]

Calcitonin preparations used clinically are either identical to the human form of this hormone (Cibacalcin) or chemically identical to salmon calcitonin (Calcimar, Miacalcin). Redness and swelling may occur locally when these agents are administered by injection. Other side effects include gastrointestinal disturbances (stomach pain, nausea, vomiting, and diarrhea), loss of appetite, and flushing/redness in the head, hands, and feet.

Estrogen

Estrogen replacement is the primary method used to prevent and treat bone loss in women who lack endogenous estrogen production, that is, following menopause or ovariectomy.[6,32,34] Estrogen is critical in maintaining adequate bone mineralization in women, and low doses of estrogen alone or estrogen combined with a progestin are often administered whenever endogenous estrogen production is lost. Replacement of estrogen following menopause has been shown to be especially effective, and this treatment can return the rate of bone formation and bone resorption to premenopausal levels.[6] Hence, estrogen replacement combined with other adjunct treatments (calcium supplements, calcitonin, calcitriol) provides some excellent pharmacologic strategies for preventing the rather devastating effects of osteoporosis in postmenopausal women. The pharmacology and adverse effects of estrogen are discussed in more detail in Chapter 30.

SPECIAL CONCERNS IN REHABILITATION PATIENTS

Physical therapists and occupational therapists should generally be concerned about potential side effects of the drugs discussed in this chapter. With regard to the treatment of thyroid disorders, excessive doses of drugs used to treat either hyperthyroidism or hypothyroidism tend to produce symptoms of the opposite disorder; that is, overdose of antithyroid drugs can produce signs of hypothyroidism, and vice versa. Therapists should be aware of the signs of thyroid dysfunction (see Table 31–2) and should be able to help detect signs of inappropriate drug dosage. Therapists should also avoid using rehabilitation techniques that may exacerbate any symptoms of thyroid dysfunction. For instance, care should be taken not to overstress the cardiovascular system in a patient with decreased cardiac output and hypotension caused by hypothyroidism (see Table 31–2).

Likewise, physical therapists and occupational therapists should be aware of the potential adverse effects of the drugs that regulate calcium homeostasis. For instance, excessive doses of calcium supplements may alter cardiovascular function, resulting in cardiac arrhythmias. Therapists may help detect these arrhythmias while monitoring pulses or ECG recordings. Finally, therapists may enhance the effects of bone-mineralizing drugs by employing exercise and weight-bearing activities to stimulate bone formation. Also, certain modalities may enhance the effects of bone mineralizing agents. In particular, ultraviolet light increases endogenous vitamin D biosynthesis, thus facilitating calcium absorption and bone formation (see the Case Study in this chapter).

CASE STUDY

AGENTS AFFECTING BONE MINERAL METABOLISM

Brief History. R.D. is a 74-year-old woman with a history of generalized bone demineralization caused by osteomalacia brought on primarily by poor diet; that is, total caloric intake and dietary levels of calcium and vitamin D have been very low. The patient is also rather reclusive, spending most of her time indoors. Consequently, she virtually lacks any exposure to natural sunlight. To treat her osteomalacia, she was placed on a regimen of oral calcium supplements and vitamin D. However, she has been reluctant to take these supplements because when she did, she occasionally experienced problems with diarrhea. Recently, she sustained a fracture of the femoral neck during a fall. She was admitted to the hospital, and the fracture was stabilized by open reduction and internal fixation. The patient was referred to physical therapy for strengthening and pre–weight-bearing activities.

Problem/Influence of Medication. During the postoperative period, calcium and vitamin D supplements were reinstituted to facilitate bone formation. The patient, however, soon began to experience bouts of diarrhea, apparently as a side effect of the vitamin D supplements. Consequently, the vitamin D supplements were withdrawn, and only the calcium supplement was continued. Because metabolic by-products of vitamin D accelerate the absorption of calcium from the gastrointestinal tract, both agents should be administered together. This patient, however, was apparently unable to tolerate vitamin D (or its analogs), possibly because of hypersensitivity to these compounds.

Decision/Solution. The physical therapist working with this patient realized that ultraviolet radiation stimulates the production of endogenous vitamin D. Ultraviolet light catalyzes the conversion of a cholesterol-like precursor (7-dehydrocholesterol) to vitamin D_3 within the skin. Vitamin D_3 then undergoes conversions in the liver and kidneys to form specific vitamin D metabolites (i.e., 1,25-dihydroxyvitamin D), which enhance intestinal calcium absorption. After conferring with the physician, the therapist incorporated a program of therapeutic ultraviolet radiation into the treatment regimen. The appropriate dose of ultraviolet exposure was first determined, followed by daily application of whole-body irradiation. Ultraviolet therapy was continued throughout the remainder of the patient's hospitalization, and callus formation at the fracture site was progressing well at the time of discharge.

SUMMARY

The thyroid and parathyroid glands serve a number of vital endocrine functions. The thyroid gland synthesizes and secretes the thyroid hormones T_4 and T_3. These hormones are important regulators of cellular metabolism and metabolic rate. Thyroid hormones also interact with other hormones to facilitate normal growth and development. The parathyroid glands control calcium homeostasis through the release of PTH. This hormone is crucial in maintaining normal blood calcium levels and in regulating bone formation and resorption. PTH also interacts with other hormones such as vitamin D and calcitonin in the control of bone mineral metabolism. Acute and chronic problems in thyroid and parathyroid function are often treated quite successfully with various pharmacologic agents. Rehabilitation specialists should be aware of the general strategies for treating thyroid and parathyroid disorders and of the basic pharmacotherapeutic approach to these problems.

REFERENCES

1. Adlerberth, A, Stenstrom, G, and Hasselgren, P-O: The selective beta-1 blocking agent metoprolol compared with antithyroid drug and thyroxine as preoperative treatment of patients with hyperthyroidism: Results of a prospective, randomized study. Ann Surg 205:182, 1987.
2. Aurbach, GD, Marx, SJ, and Spiegel, AM: Parathyroid hormone, calcitonin, and the calciferols. In Wilson, JD and Foster, DW (eds): Textbook of Endocrinology, ed 8. WB Saunders, Philadelphia, 1992.
3. Austin, LA and Heath, H: Calcitonin. N Engl J Med 304:269, 1981.
4. Bottazzo, GF and Doniach, D: Autoimmune thyroid disease. Annu Rev Med 37:353, 1986.
5. Boyages, SC: Iodine deficiency disorders. J Clin Endocrinol Metab 77:587, 1993.
6. Christiansen, C: Prevention and treatment of osteoporosis: A review of current modalities. Bone 13:S35, 1992.
7. Coccia, PF: Cells that resorb bone. N Engl J Med 310:456, 1983.
8. Cooper, DS: Which anti-thyroid drug? Am J Med 80:1165, 1986.
9. Cooper, DS: Antithyroid drugs. N Engl J Med 311:1353, 1984.
10. Cooper, DS, et al: L-thyroxine therapy in subclinical hypothyroidism: A double-blind, placebo-controlled study. Ann Intern Med 101:18, 1984.
11. Cotran, RS, Kumar, V, and Robbins, SL (eds): Pathologic Basic of Disease, ed 4. WB Saunders, Philadelphia, 1994.
12. Deftos, LJ and First, BP: Calcitonin as a drug. Ann Intern Med 95:192, 1981.
13. DeLuca, HF: The metabolism and functions of vitamin D. In Chrousos, GP, Loriaux, DL, and Lipsett, MB (eds): Steroid Hormone Resistance: Mechanism and Clinical Aspects. Plenum Press, New York, 1986.
14. DeLuca, HF and Schnoes, HK: Vitamin D: Recent advances. Annu Rev Biochem 52:411, 1983.
15. Engler, H, Taurog, A, and Nakashima, T: Mechanism of inactivation of thyroid peroxidase by thioureylene drugs. Biochem Pharmacol 31:3801, 1982.
16. Fleisch, H: Bisphosphonates: Pharmacology. Semin Arthritis Rheum 23:261, 1994.
17. Franklyn, JA: Drug therapy: The management of hyperthyroidism. N Engl J Med 330:1731, 1994.
18. Genuth, SM: Endocrine regulation of calcium and phosphate metabolism. In Berne, RM and Levy, MN (eds): Physiology, ed 3. Mosby Year Book, St Louis, 1993.
19. Genuth, SM. The thyroid gland. In Berne, RM and Levy, MN (eds): Physiology, ed 3. Mosby Year Book, St Louis, 1993.
20. Graham, GD and Burman, KD: Radioactive treatment of Graves' disease: An assessment of its potential risks. Ann Intern Med 105:900, 1986.
21. Guyton, AC: Textbook of Medical Physiology, ed 8. WB Saunders, Philadelphia, 1991.
22. Hasling, C, Charles, P, and Mosekilde, L: Etidronate disodium in the management of malignancy-related hypercalcemia. Am J Med 82(suppl 2A):51, 1987.
23. Jaffe, RC: Thyroid hormone receptors. In Conn, PM (ed): The Receptors, Vol 1. Academic Press, New York, 1984.
24. Krane, SM: Etidronate in the treatment of Paget's disease of bone. Ann Intern Med 96:619, 1982.
25. Larsen, SM and Ingbar, SH: The thyroid gland. In Wilson, JD and Foster, DW (eds): Textbook of Endocrinology, ed 8. WB Saunders, Philadelphia, 1992.
26. Lennquist, S, et al: Beta blockers compared with antithyroid drugs as preoperative treatment in hyperthyroidism: Drug tolerance, complications, and postoperative thyroid function. Surgery 98:1141, 1985.
27. Oppenheimer, JH: Thyroid hormone action at the nuclear level. Ann Intern Med 102:374, 1985.
28. Papapoulos, SE, et al: Effects of decreasing serum calcium on circulating parathyroid hormone and vitamin D metabolites in normocalcaemic and hypercalcaemic patients treated with APD. Bone Mineral 1:69, 1986.
29. Papapoulos, SE, et al: The use of bisphonates in the treatment of osteoporosis. Bone 13:S41, 1992.
30. Prelevic, GM and Adashi, EY: Postmenopausal osteoporosis: Prevention and treatment with calcitonin. Gynecol Endocrinol 6:141, 1992.
31. Raisz, LG and Kream, BE: Regulation of bone formation. N Engl J Med 309:29, 1983.
32. Recker, RR: Current therapy for osteoporosis. J Clin Endocrinol Metab 76:14, 1993.
33. Reginster, J-Y: Management of high-turnover osteoporosis with calcitonin. Bone 13:S37, 1992.

34. Riggs, BL and Melton, LJ: Drug therapy: The prevention and treatment of osteoporosis. N Engl J Med 327:620, 1992.
35. Sambrook, P, et al: Prevention of corticosteroid osteoporosis: A comparison of calcium, calcitriol, and calcitonin. N Engl J Med 328:1747, 1993.
36. Schimmel, M and Utiger RD: Thyroidal and peripheral production of thyroid hormones. Ann Intern Med 87:760, 1977.
37. Sileghem, A, Geusens, P, and Dequeker, J: Intranasal calcitonin for the prevention of bone erosion and bone loss in rheumatoid arthritis. Ann Rheum Dis 51:761, 1992.
38. Singer, FR and Fernandez, M: Therapy of hypercalcemia of malignancy. Am J Med 82(suppl 2A):34, 1987.
39. Taurog, A: The mechanism of action of thioureylene antithyroid drugs. Endocrinology 98:1031, 1976.
40. Tibaldi, J and Barzel, US: Thyroxine supplementations: Method for the prevention of clinical hypothyroidism. Am J Med 79:241, 1985.
41. Tilyard, MW, et al: Treatment of postmenopausal osteoporosis with calcitriol or calcium. N Engl J Med 326:357, 1992.
42. Toft, AD: Drug therapy: Thyroxine therapy. N Engl J Med 331:174, 1994.
43. Walfish, PG, Wall, JR, and Volpe, R (eds): Autoimmunity and the Thyroid. Academic Press, New York, 1985.
44. Wilkin, TJ: Mechanisms of disease: Receptor autoimmunity in endocrine disorders. N Engl J Med 323:1318, 1990.

CHAPTER **32**

Pancreatic Hormones and the Treatment of Diabetes Mellitus

The pancreas functions rather uniquely as both an endocrine and an exocrine gland. The exocrine role of this gland consists of excretion of digestive enzymes into the duodenum via the pancreatic duct. Pancreatic endocrine function consists of the secretion of two principal hormones—insulin and glucagon—into the bloodstream. Insulin and glucagon are involved primarily with the regulation of blood glucose. Insulin also plays a role in protein and lipid metabolism and is important in several aspects of growth and development. Problems with the production and function of insulin cause a fairly common and clinically significant disease known as **diabetes mellitus**.

The purpose of this chapter is to review the normal physiologic roles of the pancreatic hormones and to describe the pathogenesis and treatment of diabetes mellitus. As will be indicated, diabetes mellitus has many sequelae that influence patients' neuromuscular and cardiovascular function. Patients with diabetes mellitus will often undergo physical rehabilitation for problems related to their condition. Consequently, the nature of diabetes mellitus and the pharmacotherapeutic treatment of this disease are important to physical therapists and occupational therapists.

STRUCTURE AND FUNCTION OF THE ENDOCRINE PANCREAS

The cellular composition of the pancreas has been described in great detail.[13,14,23,82] The bulk of the gland consists of acinar cells that synthesize and release the pancreatic digestive enzymes (thereby providing the exocrine function). Interspersed within the acinar tissues are smaller clumps of tissue known as the *islets of Langerhans*. These islets contain cells that synthesize and secrete the pancreatic hormones, thus constituting the endocrine portion of the gland.

478

The pancreatic islets consist of three primary cell types: A (alpha) cells, which produce glucagon; B (beta) cells, which produce insulin; and D (delta) cells, which produce somatostatin. As previously mentioned, this chapter focuses on the functions of insulin and glucagon. *Somatostatin* is a polypeptide hormone that appears to affect several physiologic systems, including regulation of gastrointestinal absorption. Although the exact role of pancreatic somatostatin is still somewhat unclear, this hormone may help coordinate the function and effects of glucagon and insulin.[23,81]

INSULIN

Insulin is a large polypeptide consisting of 51 amino acids arranged in a specific sequence and configuration. The primary effect of insulin is to lower blood glucose levels by facilitating the entry of glucose into peripheral tissues. The effects of insulin on energy metabolism and specific aspects of insulin release and mechanism of action are discussed here.

Effects of Insulin on Carbohydrate Metabolism. Following a meal, blood glucose increases sharply. Insulin is responsible for facilitating the movement of glucose out of the bloodstream and into the liver and other tissues, where it can be stored for future needs. Most tissues in the body (including skeletal muscle cells) are relatively impermeable to glucose and require the presence of some sort of transport system or carrier to help convey the glucose molecule across the cell membrane.[27,82] The carrier-mediated transport of glucose into muscle cells is believed to be a form of facilitated diffusion (see Chapter 2). Insulin appears to directly stimulate this facilitated diffusion, resulting in a 15- to 20-fold increase in the rate of glucose influx.[27] Possible ways in which insulin affects glucose transport on the cellular level are discussed later in "Cellular Mechanisms of Insulin Action."

Insulin affects uptake and use of glucose in the liver somewhat differently than in skeletal muscle and other tissues. Hepatic cells are relatively permeable to glucose, and glucose enters these cells quite easily, even when insulin is not present. Glucose, however, is also free to leave liver cells just as easily, unless it is trapped in the cells in some manner. Insulin stimulates the activity of the glucokinase enzyme, which phosphorylates glucose and subsequently traps the glucose molecule in the hepatic cell. Insulin also increases the activity of enzymes that promote glycogen synthesis and inhibits enzymes that promote glycogen breakdown. Thus, the primary effect of insulin on the liver is to promote sequestration of the glucose molecule and to increase storage of glucose in the form of hepatic glycogen.

Effects of Insulin on Protein and Lipid Metabolism. Although insulin is normally associated with regulating blood glucose, this hormone also exerts significant effects on proteins and lipids. In general, insulin promotes storage of protein and lipid in muscle and adipose tissue, respectively.[23,27,82] Insulin encourages protein synthesis in muscle cells by stimulating amino acid uptake, increasing DNA/RNA activity related to protein synthesis, and inhibiting protein breakdown. In fat cells, insulin stimulates the synthesis of triglycerides (the primary form of lipid storage in the body), as well as inhibiting the enzyme that breaks down stored lipids (hormone-sensitive lipase). Consequently, insulin is involved in carbohydrate, protein, and lipid metabolism, and disturbances in insulin function (diabetes mellitus) will affect storage and use of all the primary energy substrates.

Cellular Mechanism of Insulin Action

Insulin exerts its effects by first binding to a receptor located on the surface membrane of target cells.[34,82] This receptor is a glycoprotein that is highly specific for insulin. The complete insulin receptor consists of two matching or paired units, with each unit consisting of an alpha and a beta subunit (Fig. 32–1). The alpha subunit is the binding site for insulin. The beta subunit appears to be an enzyme that functions as a tyrosine kinase, which means that the beta subunit catalyzes the addition of phosphate groups to tyrosine residues within the beta subunit.[15,38] Thus, binding insulin to the alpha subunit causes the beta subunit to undergo *autophosphorylation*; that is, the receptor adds phosphate groups to itself. This autophosphorylation of the insulin receptor then initiates a series of biochemical changes within the cell.

The exact way that the insulin-receptor interaction triggers subsequent changes in cellular activity remains speculative. A possible sequence of postreceptor events is illustrated in Figure 32–1. Insulin binding and receptor autophosphorylation initiate the production of intracellular chemicals known as *insulin mediators*.[9,20,35,44,69] These insulin mediators act as second messengers that cause changes in cell function such as increased glucose uptake, increased protein synthesis, and so on. In particular, these mediators somehow stimulate movement (*translocation*) of glucose carriers from intracellular storage sites to the cell membrane of skeletal muscle cells and other peripheral tissues (see Fig. 32–1).[42] These glucose carriers are probably proteins that are synthesized and stored within the Golgi system of the cell. Insulin causes these carriers to travel to the cell membrane, where they can then promote the facilitated diffusion of glucose into the cell.

The postreceptor events depicted in Figure 32–1 are still largely theoretical, and the exact chemical nature of the insulin mediators is still unknown. Some possible mediators include small peptides, peptidelike molecules, and phospholipids.[9,20,44] Appropriate levels of intracellular calcium may also be important in mediating the cellular effects of insulin.[18] In reality, insulin may exert its effects by stimulating the production of a number of different chemical mediators that exert different effects in different target tissues (i.e., muscle, liver, or fat). Also, binding insulin to the surface receptor has been reported to cause internalization or movement of the entire insulin-receptor complex to within the cell.[3] The significance of this internalization process, however, is unknown.

Consequently, the manner in which insulin binds to a specific receptor and exerts its effects on target cells has become somewhat clearer, but a great deal of information remains to be determined. Knowledge of exactly how insulin interacts with target tissues is important because defects in receptor binding and problems in the subsequent postreceptor events may be responsible for some of the changes seen in certain forms of diabetes mellitus. The possible role of these receptor-mediated problems in diabetes is discussed in "Type II Diabetes."

GLUCAGON

Glucagon is considered to be the hormonal antagonist of insulin.[27, 83] The primary effect of glucagon is to increase blood glucose to maintain normal blood glucose levels and prevent hypoglycemia.[23,27,85] Glucagon produces a rapid increase in glycogen breakdown (*glycogenolysis*) in the liver, thus liberating glucose into the bloodstream

FIGURE 32–1. Possible mechanism of insulin action on cellular glucose metabolism. An insulin receptor located on the cell's surface consists of 2 alpha (α) and 2 beta (β) subunits. Binding of insulin to the α subunits causes addition of phosphate groups (PO_4) to the β subunits. This receptor autophosphorylation initiates synthesis of 1 or more intracellular chemical mediators that promote translocation of glucose carriers to the cell membrane, where they increase facilitated diffusion of glucose (Glu) into the cell. Mediators also increase the activity of enzymes that promote glucose storage.

from hepatic glycogen stores. Glucagon then stimulates a more prolonged increase in hepatic glucose production (*gluconeogenesis*). This gluconeogenesis sustains blood glucose levels even after hepatic glycogen has been depleted.[27]

Glucagon appears to exert its effects on liver cells by a classic adenyl cyclase–cyclic adenosine monophosphate (cAMP) second-messenger system (see Chapter 4). Glucagon binds to a specific receptor located on the hepatic cell membrane. This stimulates the activity of the adenyl cyclase enzyme that transforms adenosine triphosphate (ATP) into cAMP. Then, cAMP acts as an intracellular second messenger that activates specific enzymes to increase glycogen breakdown and stimulate gluconeogenesis.

CONTROL OF INSULIN AND GLUCAGON RELEASE

An adequate level of glucose in the bloodstream is necessary to provide a steady supply of energy for certain tissues, especially the brain. Normally, blood glucose is maintained between 80 and 90 mg of glucose per 100 mL of blood.[27] A severe drop in blood glucose (*hypoglycemia*) is a potentially serious problem that can result in coma and death. Chronic elevations in blood glucose (**hyperglycemia**) have been implicated in producing pathologic changes in neural and vascular structures. Consequently, insulin and glucagon play vital roles in controlling glucose levels, and release of these hormones must be closely regulated.

The level of glucose in the bloodstream is the primary factor affecting release of the pancreatic hormones. As blood glucose rises (following a meal), insulin secretion from pancreatic B cells is increased. Insulin then promotes movement of glucose out of the bloodstream and into various tissues, thus reducing plasma glucose back to normal levels. As blood glucose levels fall (during a sustained fast), glucagon is released from the A cells in the pancreas. Glucagon resolves this hypoglycemia by stimulating the synthesis and release of glucose from the liver.

Release of insulin and glucagon may also be governed to some extent by other energy substrates (lipids and amino acids), other hormones (thyroxine, cortisol), and autonomic neural control.[23,83] Nonetheless, the major factor influencing pancreatic hormone release is blood glucose. Cells located in the pancreatic islets are bathed directly by the blood supply reaching the pancreas. These cells act as glucose sensors, which directly monitor plasma glucose levels. In particular, the B or insulin-secreting cells act as the primary glucose sensors, and adequate control of insulin release seems to be a somewhat higher priority than control of glucagon function.[72]

An important interaction between insulin and glucagon may also take place directly within the pancreas, and insulin appears to be the dominant hormone controlling this interaction.[72] When the B cells sense an increase in blood glucose, they release insulin, which in turn inhibits glucagon release from the A cells. When insulin release diminishes, the inhibition of glucagon production is removed, and glucagon secretion is free to increase. This intraislet regulation between insulin and glucagon is important during normal physiologic function as well as in pathologic conditions, like diabetes mellitus.[72] A deficiency of insulin production permits an increase in glucagon release, and the effects of increased glucagon may contribute to some of the metabolic changes in diabetes mellitus (although the exact role of increased glucagon in diabetes remains controversial).[83,85]

Consequently, insulin and glucagon serve to maintain blood glucose within a fairly finite range. If the endocrine portion of the pancreas is functioning normally, blood glucose levels remain remarkably constant even in situations such as exercise and prolonged fasting. However, any abnormalities in pancreatic endocrine function can alter the regulation of blood glucose. In particular, problems associated with the production and effects of insulin can produce serious disturbances in glucose metabolism as well as a number of other metabolic problems. Such problems in insulin production and function are characteristic of a disease known as diabetes mellitus. The pathogenesis and treatment of this disease is presented in the following section.

DIABETES MELLITUS

Diabetes mellitus is a disease caused by insufficient insulin secretion or a decrease in the peripheral effects of insulin. This disease is characterized by a primary defect in the metabolism of carbohydrates and other energy substrates. These metabolic defects can lead to serious acute and chronic pathologic changes. The term "diabetes mellitus" differentiates this disease from an unrelated disorder known as diabetes insipidus. **Diabetes insipidus** is caused by a lack of antidiuretic hormone (ADH) production or insensitivity to ADH. Consequently, the full terminology of "diabetes mellitus" should be used when referring to the insulin-related disease. In the vernacular of the layperson, however, diabetes mellitus is often referred to as simply "diabetes."

Diabetes mellitus is a fairly common disease affecting approximately 10 million people in the United States. This disease is a serious problem in terms of the increased morbidity and mortality associated with it.[76] It is estimated that diabetes mellitus is directly responsible for 61,000 deaths each year and is a contributing factor in an additional 140,000 deaths annually. Diabetes mellitus is the leading cause of new cases of blindness in adults and is the primary factor responsible for 30 percent of the cases of end-stage renal failure. Consequently, this disease is a serious problem affecting the lives of many individuals.

Diabetes mellitus is apparently not a single, homogeneous disease but rather a disease existing in at least two primary forms.[13,14,58,82] Patients with diabetes mellitus are usually classified as having either type I or type II diabetes, depending on the pathogenesis of their disease. The primary characteristics of type I and type II diabetes mellitus are summarized in Table 32–1. Specific aspects of these two primary forms of diabetes mellitus are discussed in more detail here.

TABLE 32–1 Comparison of Type I and Type II Diabetes Mellitus

Characteristic	Type I	Type II
Age at onset	Usually before 20	Usually after 30
Type of onset	Abrupt; often severe	Gradual; usually subtle
Usual body weight	Normal	Overweight
Blood insulin	Markedly reduced	Normal or increased
Peripheral response to insulin	Normal	Decreased
Clinical management	Insulin and diet	Diet; insulin or oral hypoglycemics if diet control alone is ineffective

Adapted from Craighead,[13] p 1150, 1994.

Type I Diabetes

Type I diabetes accounts for approximately 10 percent of the individuals with diabetes mellitus. Patients with type I diabetes are unable to synthesize any appreciable amounts of insulin. There appears to be an almost total destruction of pancreatic B cells in these individuals. Because these patients are unable to produce insulin, type I diabetes is also referred to as *insulin-dependent diabetes mellitus* (IDDM); that is, administration of exogenous insulin is necessary for survival. The onset of type I diabetes is usually during childhood, so this form of diabetes is sometimes referred to as "juvenile diabetes." The term "juvenile diabetes," however, has largely been replaced by the other terms mentioned (i.e., type I or IDDM). Patients with type I diabetes are typically close to normal body weight or slightly underweight.

The exact cause of type I diabetes remains unknown. There is considerable evidence, however, that the B-cell destruction characteristic of this disease may be caused by an autoimmune reaction.[13,21,52,55] Specifically, a virus or some other antigen may trigger an autoimmune reaction that selectively destroys the insulin-secreting B cells in susceptible individuals.[65] The susceptibility of certain patients to such viral-initiated immunodestruction may be because of genetic predisposition, environmental factors, or other factors that remain to be determined.[13,40,65,68,82] The idea that type I diabetes may have an autoimmune basis has led to the use of immunosuppressant agents in the early stages of this disease (see "Cyclosporine").

Type II Diabetes

Type II or *non−insulin-dependent diabetes mellitus* (NIDDM) accounts for the other 90 percent of people with diabetes mellitus. This form of diabetes usually occurs in adults, especially in older individuals.[13,14,48] Although the specific factors responsible for this disease are not known, a genetic predisposition combined with poor diet, obesity, and lack of exercise all seem to contribute to the onset of type II diabetes.[13,33] Increased body weight is fairly common in people with type II diabetes.

Whereas type I diabetics simply do not produce any insulin, the problem in type II diabetes is somewhat more complex.[61] In most patients with type II diabetes, pancreatic B cells remain intact and are capable of producing insulin. In fact, insulin levels in the bloodstream of type II patients may be normal or even slightly elevated compared to those of nondiabetic patients. The primary problem in type II diabetes, however, is a decreased sensitivity of peripheral tissues to circulating insulin; this is referred to as *insulin resistance*.[50,63,66] For instance, tissues such as the liver and skeletal muscle fail to respond adequately to insulin in the bloodstream.[17,54] Thus, peripheral uptake and use of glucose is blunted even when insulin is present.

The exact cellular mechanisms responsible for insulin resistance are unknown. This resistance may be caused by a primary (intrinsic) defect at the target cell that results in decreased function of the insulin receptor. For example, insulin resistance could be caused by a decreased binding of insulin to the receptor or by a decrease in the total number of functioning insulin receptors on the cell's surface.[54,62,64] Likewise, insulin resistance could occur because of changes in the way the cell responds after insulin binds to the surface receptor. Problems such as decreased protein phosphorylation, impaired production of chemical mediators, and a lack of glucose transporters have all been suggested as intracellular events that could help explain insulin resistance.[17,54,62,64] Therefore, even when insulin does bind to the receptor, the cellular response is inadequate. Thus, insulin resistance appears to be a complex phenomenon that may involve a number of changes at the cellular level. The exact changes in receptor or postreceptor function that cause this problem remain to be determined.

Consequently, because of insulin resistance in peripheral tissues, greater than normal amounts of insulin are needed to evoke an adequate response in type II diabetes. A defect in pancreatic B-cell function may also contribute to the manifestations of this disease.[39] B cells in type II diabetics often produce large amounts of insulin, and their blood insulin levels may even appear normal compared to nondiabetics. The type II patient, however, needs *greater* than normal amounts of circulating insulin to evoke a normal response. Consequently, B cells fail to increase insulin release in proportion to the increased needs of the type II diabetic patient.[17,39] Hence, the combination of peripheral tissue resistance and inadequate B-cell response creates a *relative* lack of insulin in type II diabetes.

Finally, insulin resistance is present in several disease states other than type II diabetes mellitus. Patients with conditions such as hypertension, obesity, and certain hyperlipidemias are also found to have decreased tissue sensitivity to circulating insulin.[7,54,77] Although the causes of insulin resistance in nondiabetic conditions are not completely understood, they probably involve a complex series of changes at the systemic, cellular, and subcellular levels.[54] There is consensus, however, that therapeutic strategies for resolving insulin resistance should be considered as an important part of the management of various conditions that exhibit this phenomenon.[7,77]

Effects and Complications of Diabetes Mellitus

The most common symptom associated with diabetes mellitus is a chronic elevation of blood glucose (hyperglycemia). Hyperglycemia results from a relative lack of insulin-mediated glucose uptake and use by peripheral tissues. Hyperglycemia then initiates a number of complex and potentially serious acute metabolic changes. For example, hyperglycemia is usually accompanied by increased glucose excretion by the kidneys (**glycosuria**). Glycosuria is caused by an inability of the kidneys to adequately reabsorb the excess amount of glucose reaching the nephron. Increased glucose excretion causes an osmotic force that promotes fluid and electrolyte excretion, thus leading to dehydration and electrolyte imbalance.[74] Also, the loss of glucose in the urine causes a metabolic shift toward the mobilization of fat and protein as an energy source. Increased use of fats and protein leads to the formation of acidic ketone bodies in the bloodstream. Excessive accumulation of ketones lowers plasma pH, producing acidosis (*ketoacidosis*), which can lead to coma and death.[74]

Diabetes mellitus is associated with several other long-term complications involving vascular and neural structures. Perhaps the most devastating complications associated with this disease result from the development of small-blood-vessel abnormalities (*microangiopathy*). Small vessels may undergo a thickening of the basement membrane, which can progress to the point of vessel occlusion.[13,75] The progressive ischemia caused by small-vessel disease is particularly damaging to certain structures such as the retina (leading to blindness) and the kidneys (leading to nephropathy and renal failure).[11,28,56,71,80] Problems with large blood vessels (*macroangiopathy*) occur in diabetic patients as a result of atherosclerotic lesions.[12,13] Macroangiopathy is a principal contributing factor in hypertension, myocardial infarction, and cerebral vascular accident in diabetic patients. Finally, peripheral neuropathies are quite common among patients with long-standing diabetes mellitus.[11]

The neurovascular complications described previously are directly related to the severity and duration of hyperglycemia in diabetic patients.[8,87] Although the details are somewhat unclear, prolonged elevations in blood glucose may promote structural and functional changes in vascular endothelial cells and peripheral neurons. These cellular changes are ultimately responsible for the gross pathologic abnormalities characteristic of poorly controlled diabetes mellitus.

Consequently, the primary goal in the treatment of both type I and type II diabetes mellitus is to control blood glucose levels. Maintenance of blood glucose at or close to normal levels will prevent acute metabolic derangements and greatly reduce the risk of chronic neurovascular complications associated with this disease[8,57,87] The pharmacologic agents used to treat diabetes mellitus are described in the next sections.

USE OF INSULIN IN DIABETES MELLITUS

Therapeutic Effects and Rationale for Use

Exogenous insulin is administered to replace normal pancreatic hormone production in type I diabetes (insulin-dependent diabetes mellitus). Since B-cell function is essentially absent in type I patients, exogenous insulin is crucial in maintaining normal glucose levels and proper metabolic function. Without exogenous insulin, the general health of type I patients is severely compromised, and these patients often succumb to the metabolic and neurovascular derangements associated with this disease.

Insulin may also be administered in some cases of type II diabetes to complement other drugs (oral hypoglycemics) and to supplement endogenous insulin release.[86] In type II diabetes (non–insulin-dependent diabetes mellitus), exogenous insulin basically makes up the difference between the patients' endogenous hormone production and their specific insulin requirement. Type II patients, however, may not require any exogenous insulin if their condition is adequately controlled by dietary management and other drugs such as oral hypoglycemics.

Insulin Preparations

There are many different forms of insulin, depending on the source of the hormones and the length of pharmacologic effects. Insulin used in the treatment of diabetes mellitus is derived from three sources: beef insulin, pork insulin, and human insulin. Beef and pork insulin are obtained by extracting the hormone from the pancreas of the respective host animal. These animal forms of insulin are effective in controlling glucose metabolism in humans even though they have some chemical differences from their human counterpart; that is, the amino acid sequence of beef insulin has three amino acids that differ from human insulin, and pork insulin has one amino acid that is different from the human insulin sequence.[29] More recently, insulin that is identical to human insulin has been produced through the use of cell cultures and recombinant DNA techniques.[31]

Insulin produced by biosynthetic techniques appears to have some advantages over the animal forms, including more rapid absorption after subcutaneous injection.[26,29] Human insulin is also associated with a lower risk of immunologic reactions than insulin derived from animals.[22] Apparently, beef and pork insulin are sufficiently dissimilar from the human form to evoke antibody production, which can lead to allergic reactions in some individuals. Because insulin obtained from recombinant DNA biosynthesis is identical to the endogenous human hormone, the risk of antibody production is minimal.

Insulin preparations used in the treatment of diabetes mellitus are listed in Table 32–2, which shows preparations classified according to their length of action. In general, rapid-acting preparations must be administered frequently and are used when control of diabetes is difficult and must be managed closely. Intermediate-acting and long-acting preparations offer the advantage of requiring less frequent administration (only once each day). These preparations are usually reserved for individuals who require less stringent control of blood glucose levels, for example, those who are helping to manage their condition through dietary and weight control. Also, combinations of different preparations may be used to manage diabetes in specific situations. For instance, a long-acting preparation may be supplemented by occasional administration of a rapid-acting agent to provide optimal glycemic control.

Administration of Insulin

Insulin, a large polypeptide, is not suitable for oral administration. Even if the insulin molecule survived digestion by proteases in the stomach and small intestine, this

TABLE 32–2 Insulin Preparations

Type of Insulin	Effects (hr)			Examples*	
	Onset	Peak	Duration	Animal	Human
Rapid-acting					
Regular insulin	0.5–1	2–4	5–7	Regular Iletin I Regular Iletin II Velosulin	Humulin R Novolin R Velosulin Human
Prompt insulin zinc	1–3	2–8	12–16	Semilente Insulin Semilente Iletin I	—
Intermediate-acting					
Isophane insulin	3–4	6–12	18–28	Insulatard NPH NPH Insulin NPH Iletin I NPH Iletin II	Humulin N Insulatard NPH Human Novolin N
Insulin zinc	1–3	8–12	18–28	Lente Insulin Lente Iletin I Lente Iletin II	Humulin L Novolin L
Long-Acting					
Extended insulin zinc	4–6	18–24	36	Ultralente Insulin Ultralente Iletin I	—
Protamine zinc insulin	4–6	14–24	36	Protamine Zinc and Iletin I Protamine Zinc and Iletin II	—

*Examples are trade names of preparations derived from animal sources (beef, pork, or mixed beef and pork) and synthetic human insulin derived from recombinant DNA techniques.

compound is much too large to be absorbed through the gastrointestinal wall. Consequently, insulin is usually administered through subcutaneous injection. In emergency situations (e.g., diabetic coma), insulin may be administered by the intravenous route.

Patients on long-term insulin therapy are usually trained to administer their own medication. Important factors in safe insulin use include adequate (refrigerated) storage of the preparation, maintenance of sterile syringes, accurate dose measurement and filling of the syringe, and proper injection technique. Patients should rotate the sites of administration (abdomen, upper thighs, upper arms, back, and buttocks) to avoid local damage caused by repeated injection.

The optimal dosage of insulin varies greatly from patient to patient, as well as within each patient. Factors such as exercise and dietary modification can change the insulin requirements for each individual. Consequently, the dose of insulin is often adjusted periodically by monitoring the patient's blood glucose level. Adjustment of insulin dosage in poorly controlled diabetes mellitus is usually done under the close supervision of a physician. Advancements in glucose monitoring devices that can be used in the home, however, now permit patients to routinely check their own blood glucose levels. Many patients can make their own insulin adjustments based on periodic blood glucose measurement. This process of glucose self-monitoring and insulin dose adjustment permits optimal management of blood glucose levels on a day-to-day basis.

To avoid some of the problems of repeated subcutaneous injection, implantable insulin delivery systems or pumps have been employed in some diabetic patients. These pumps are usually implanted subcutaneously and provide a slow, steady supply of insulin for prolonged periods of time. The response to the use of insulin pumps has been mixed. Although improved glycemic control has been reported in some diabetic patients, other investigations did not notice a distinct advantage of insulin pumps over subcutaneous injection.[5,16,47] At present, implantable insulin delivery systems will probably not replace more traditional methods of insulin administration.

Intensive Insulin Therapy

As indicated previously, the ultimate goal in the treatment of diabetes mellitus is to maintain blood glucose in the normal physiologic range as much as possible. To achieve this goal, an administration strategy known as intensive insulin therapy has been developed for people who require exogenous insulin.[60] The idea of intensive insulin therapy is that the patient frequently monitors his or her blood glucose level and self-administers several (three or more) doses of insulin per day, with each dose adjusted carefully to meet the patient's needs throughout the day.[79] Basically, several relatively small doses of insulin are able to maintain blood glucose in the appropriate range much better than one or two relatively large doses.

Of course, intensive insulin therapy requires more motivation and compliance on the part of the patient. There is considerable evidence, however, that this strategy reduces the long-term complications associated with diabetes, including a lower incidence of neuropathies, renal disease, and other complications related to microangiopathy.[67,79] Hence, intensive insulin therapy may be worth the extra effort because this strategy can help prevent the devastating complications that are typically associated with poorly controlled diabetes mellitus.

Adverse Effects of Insulin Therapy

The primary problem associated with insulin administration is *hypoglycemia*.[78] Since insulin lowers blood glucose, exogenous insulin may produce a dramatic fall in blood glucose levels. Hypoglycemia may occur during insulin therapy if the dose of insulin is too high for the patient's particular needs. Missing a meal or receiving a delayed meal may also precipitate hypoglycemia. During insulin treatment, insulin is not released exclusively after a meal as it would be during normal function. Insulin administered from an exogenous source may be present in the bloodstream even if the patient fails to provide glucose by eating. Hence, insulin may reduce blood glucose to below normal levels because of the lack of a periodic replenishment of blood glucose from dietary sources.

Strenuous physical activity may promote hypoglycemia during insulin therapy. Exercise generally produces an insulin-like effect, meaning that exercise accelerates the movement of glucose out of the bloodstream and into peripheral tissues (skeletal muscle) where it is needed. The combined effects of exercise and insulin may produce an exaggerated decrease in blood glucose, thus leading to hypoglycemia. To avoid exercise-induced hypoglycemia, the insulin dose should be decreased by 30 to 35 percent.[4] Careful measurement of blood glucose before and after exercise can help predict how much the insulin dose should be adjusted in each patient.

Initial symptoms of hypoglycemia include headache, fatigue, hunger, tachycardia, sweating, anxiety, and confusion. Symptoms progressively worsen as blood glucose continues to decrease, and severe hypoglycemia may lead to loss of consciousness, convulsions, and death. Consequently, early detection and resolution of hypoglycemia are imperative. In the early stages, hypoglycemia can usually be reversed if the patient ingests foods containing glucose (soft drinks, fruit juice, glucose tablets, etc.). Typically, administration of the equivalent of 20 g of D-glucose is recommended to restore blood glucose in the early stages of hypoglycemia.[6]

Other problems that may be encountered are related to the immunologic effects of insulin use. Certain forms of insulin may evoke an immune reaction and stimulate antibody production. These anti-insulin antibodies may cause an allergic reaction in some individuals as well as resistance to the exogenous insulin molecule. As discussed previously, the incidence of these immunologic reactions seems to be greater when animal (beef and pork) forms of insulin are used. Consequently, these problems are often resolved by switching the patient to another type of preparation, preferably biosynthetic human insulin.

ORAL HYPOGLYCEMIC DRUGS

Mechanism of Action and Rationale for Use

The term "oral hypoglycemic" refers to a group of chemically related compounds that can be administered by mouth and help promote a decrease in blood glucose. Hence, these drugs are named for their effect rather than for the condition they are used to treat (they are used to lower blood glucose, not to treat low blood sugar). Oral hypoglycemics are used to help control blood glucose levels in type II (NIDDM) diabetes mellitus. These agents are not effective in the treatment of type I diabetes.

The efficacy of oral hypoglycemics in type II (but not type I) diabetes is brought about by the apparent mechanism of action of these drugs. Although the exact details are unclear, oral hypoglycemics appear to increase both the release of insulin from B cells in the pancreas and the sensitivity of peripheral tissues to insulin.[41,46,53,73] These drugs are therefore most effective if some endogenous insulin production is present but insulin secretion is relatively inadequate and the peripheral tissues are resistant to the effects of the endogenous insulin. Because type I diabetics do not produce any insulin, oral hypoglycemics will not benefit these patients.

Oral hypoglycemics are effective in the long-term control of glucose metabolism in only about half the type II patients in whom they are used.[24,45] These drugs, however, can reduce or in some cases replace the requirement for exogenous insulin in these patients.[19,70] Oral hypoglycemics seem to be especially useful when combined with a controlled diet and proper caloric intake.[49] Consequently, oral hypoglycemic drugs offer an additional pharmacologic approach to the management of a significant portion of the patients with type II diabetes mellitus.

Specific Agents

Oral hypoglycemics that are in widespread clinical use are members of a group of chemical agents known as *sulfonylureas*. Specific oral hypoglycemics used clinically are listed in Table 32–3. These agents are all fairly similar in their pharmacologic efficacy and are distinguished from one another primarily by individual potencies and pharmacokinetic properties (rate of absorption, duration of action, etc.).

Adverse Effects

Since the principal effect of these drugs is to lower blood glucose, hypoglycemia is a potential problem. As with insulin therapy, hypoglycemia may be precipitated by oral hypoglycemics if the dose is excessive, if a meal is skipped, or if the patient increases his or her level of activity. Consequently, patients should be observed for any indications of low blood glucose, such as anxiety, confusion, headache, and sweating.

Other side effects that may occur during oral hypoglycemic therapy include heartburn, gastrointestinal distress (nausea, vomiting, stomach pain, and diarrhea),

TABLE 32–3 Oral Hypoglycemic Agents

Generic Name	Trade Name	Time to Peak Plasma Concentration (hr)	Duration of Effect (hr)
Acetohexamide	Dymelor	1–3	12–24
Chlorpropamide	Diabinese, Glucamide	2–4	24–48
Glipizide	Glucotrol	1–3	12–24
Glyburide	DiaBeta, Micronase	4	24
Tolazamide	Tolamide, Tolinase	3–4	10
Tolbutamide	Oramide, Orinase	3–4	6–12

headache, dizziness, skin rashes, and hematologic abnormalities (e.g., leukopenia, agranulocytosis). These side effects are usually fairly mild and transient but may require attention if they are severe or prolonged.

OTHER DRUGS USED IN THE MANAGEMENT OF DIABETES MELLITUS

Glucagon

Glucagon is sometimes used to treat acute hypoglycemia induced by insulin or oral hypoglycemic agents. As discussed previously, the initial effect of glucagon is to mobilize the release of glucose from hepatic glycogen stores. Consequently, the patient must have sufficient liver glycogen present in order for glucagon to be effective.

When used to treat hypoglycemia, glucagon is administered by injection (intravenous, intramuscular, or subcutaneous). Glucagon should reverse symptoms of hypoglycemia (including coma) within 5 to 20 minutes after administration. The primary adverse effects associated with glucagon are nausea and vomiting (although these effects may result directly from hypoglycemia). Glucagon may also cause an allergic reaction (skin rash, difficulty breathing) in some individuals.

Cyclosporine

Cyclosporine (Sandimmune) is a powerful immunosuppressant drug that is often used to prevent tissue rejection following organ transplants (see Chapter 37). There is also some indication that this drug may help attenuate the autoimmune reaction that appears to be responsible for B-cell destruction in type I diabetes mellitus.[2,21,36] If administered soon after the onset of symptoms, cyclosporine may promote remission and decrease the subsequent need for exogenous insulin in type I diabetic patients. The use of cyclosporine in the early treatment of type I diabetes is relatively new, and future clinical trials will be needed to determine the long-term benefits (or adverse effects) of this drug.

Aldose Reductase Inhibitors

Drugs that selectively inhibit the aldose reductase enzyme represent a relatively new approach to the treatment of diabetes mellitus.[10] This enzyme, which is located in neurons and vascular endothelial cells, is responsible for converting glucose to another sugar known as sorbitol. The excessive accumulation of sorbitol within the cell may lead to structural and functional changes that are ultimately responsible for the complications associated with diabetes mellitus (neuropathy and angiopathy).[25,37] Consequently, aldose reductase inhibitors may be useful in preventing these complications by inhibiting the formation and accumulation of sorbitol within vascular endothelial cells and peripheral neurons. The clinical use of these drugs is still fairly experimental, however, and their full potential in preventing diabetic complications remains to be determined.

NONPHARMACOLOGIC INTERVENTION IN DIABETES MELLITUS

Dietary Management and Weight Reduction

Despite advancements in the pharmacologic treatment of diabetes mellitus, the most important and effective factor in controlling this disease is still proper nutrition.[1,84] In both type I and type II diabetes, total caloric intake as well as the percentage of calories from specific sources (carbohydrates, fats, or proteins) is important in controlling blood glucose. Also, weight loss is a significant factor in decreasing the patient's need for drugs such as insulin and the oral hypoglycemic agents. By losing weight, the patient may reduce the amount of tissue that requires insulin, thereby reducing the need for exogenous drugs. Because obesity is quite prevalent in type II diabetics, weight loss seems to be especially effective in reducing drug requirements in these individuals.[51]

Exercise

Exercise appears to be beneficial in diabetes mellitus for several reasons. Physical training may help facilitate weight loss, thus helping to decrease body mass and drug requirements. Regular exercise also appears to increase the sensitivity of peripheral tissues to insulin; that is, training helps overcome insulin resistance.[30,32] The exact reason for this training effect is not clear. Finally, a program of physical training will improve the general health and well-being in diabetic patients, making them less susceptible to various problems such as cardiovascular disease.[4] Of course, patients beginning a program of regular exercise should first undergo a complete physical examination, and the frequency and intensity of the exercise should be closely monitored.

Islet Cell Transplants and Gene Therapy

A relatively new approach in treating diabetes mellitus is the transplantation of islet cells into patients with this disease.[43] Islet tissues containing functioning B cells can be harvested from adult, neonatal, or fetal pancreatic tissues and surgically transplanted into the pancreas of patients who lack adequate insulin production (type I diabetics). Likewise, new molecular strategies are being investigated that could re-establish insulin production by transplanting insulin-related genes into the cells of patients with diabetes mellitus.[59] Although techniques such as islet transplants and gene therapy are still relatively experimental, these techniques may eventually be developed to provide a more permanent means of treating diabetes mellitus.

SIGNIFICANCE OF DIABETES MELLITUS IN REHABILITATION

Patients often undergo rehabilitation for complications arising from diabetes mellitus. For instance, peripheral neuropathies may produce functional deficits that require physical therapy and occupational therapy. Small-vessel angiopathy may cause decreased peripheral blood flow, resulting in tissue ischemia and ulceration. This ischemia can lead to tissue necrosis and subsequent amputation, especially in the lower extremities. In advanced stages of diabetes, general debilitation combined with specific conditions (e.g., end-stage renal failure) creates multiple problems that challenge the health of the individual. Consequently, rehabilitation specialists will be involved in the treatment of various sequelae of diabetes mellitus throughout the course of this disease.

Physical therapists and occupational therapists must be aware of the possibility that acute metabolic derangements exist in their patients who have diabetes mellitus. Therapists should realize that patients on insulin and oral hypoglycemic medications may experience episodes of hypoglycemia because of an exaggerated lowering of blood glucose by these drugs. Hypoglycemia may be precipitated if the patient has not eaten or is engaging in relatively strenuous physical activity. Therapists must ensure that patients are maintaining a regular dietary schedule and have not skipped a meal prior to the therapy session. Likewise, therapists should be especially alert for any signs of hypoglycemia during and after exercise in diabetic patients.

Therapists should note any changes (confusion, fatigue, sweating, nausea) in the patient that may signal the onset of hypoglycemia. If these symptoms are observed, administration of a high-glucose snack is typically recommended. Therapists working with diabetic patients should have sources of glucose on hand to reverse these hypoglycemic symptoms. Some sources of glucose include soft drinks, fruit juices, and tablets containing D-glucose.[6]

Finally, physical therapists and occupational therapists may help reinforce the importance of patient compliance during pharmacologic management of diabetes mellitus. Therapists can question whether patients have been taking their medications on a routine basis. Regular administration of insulin is essential in preventing a metabolic shift toward ketone body production and subsequent ketoacidosis, especially in the type I patient. Also, therapists can help explain that adequate control of blood glucose not only prevents acute metabolic problems but also seems to decrease the incidence of the neurovascular complications associated with this disease. Likewise, rehabilitation specialists can encourage patient compliance in the nonpharmacologic management of their disease. Therapists can emphasize the importance of an appropriate diet and adequate physical activity in both type I and type II diabetes. Therapists may also play an important role in preventing the onset of diabetic foot ulcers and infection by educating the patient in proper skin care and footwear.

CASE STUDY

DIABETES MELLITUS

Brief History. W.S. is an 18-year-old woman who began experiencing problems with glucose metabolism following a viral infection when she was 12. She was subsequently diagnosed as having type I diabetes mellitus. Since that time, her condition has been successfully managed by insulin administration combined with dietary control. Once-daily administration of intermediate-acting insulin usually provides optimal therapeutic effects. She is also very active athletically and was a member of her high school soccer team. Currently, she is entering her first year of college and is beginning preseason practice with the college's soccer team. The physical therapist who serves as the team's athletic trainer was apprised of her condition.

Problem/Influence of Medication. Exercise produces an insulin-like effect; that is, it lowers blood glucose by facilitating the movement of glucose out of the bloodstream and into peripheral tissues. Because insulin also lowers blood glucose, the additive effects of insulin and exercise may produce profound hypoglycemia. As a result, a lower dose of insulin is usually required on days that involve strenuous activity. The physical therapist was aware of this and other potential problems in the diabetic athlete.

Decision/Solution. The therapist reminded the athlete to monitor her blood glucose levels before and after each practice session and to adjust her insulin dosage accordingly. During some of the initial practice sessions, blood glucose was also monitored during practice to ensure that insulin doses were adequate. On practice days, insulin was injected into abdominal sites rather than around exercising muscles (thighs), in order to prevent the insulin from being absorbed too rapidly from the injection site. The therapist also reminded the athlete to eat a light meal before each practice and to be sure to eat again afterward. The therapist maintained a supply of glucose tablets and fruit juice on the practice field. The athlete was questioned periodically to look for early signs of hypoglycemia (confusion, nausea, etc.), and ingestion of carbohydrates was encouraged whenever appropriate. Finally, the therapist assigned a teammate to check on the athlete within an hour after practice ended to ensure that no delayed effects of hypoglycemia were apparent. With these precautions, the athlete successfully completed preseason training as well as the entire soccer season without any serious incident.

SUMMARY

The islet cells of the pancreas synthesize and secrete insulin and glucagon. These hormones are important in regulating glucose uptake and use, as well as other aspects of energy metabolism. Problems in the production and effects of insulin are typical of a disease known as diabetes mellitus. Diabetes mellitus can be categorized into two primary forms: type I diabetes, which is caused by an absolute deficiency of insulin; and type II diabetes, which is caused by decreased peripheral insulin effects combined with a relative deficiency of insulin release. Administration of exogenous insulin is required in the treatment of type I diabetes mellitus. Patients with type II diabetes may be treated with insulin or with oral hypoglycemic drugs, depending on the severity of their disease. In both forms of diabetes mellitus, dietary control and adequate physical activity may help reduce the need for drug treatment as well as improve the general health and well-being of the patient. Physical therapists and occupational therapists play an important role in helping treat the complications of diabetes mellitus and in promoting good patient compliance in the management of this disease. Therapists must be cognizant of the potential problems that may occur when working with diabetic patients (hypoglycemia) and should be able to recognize and deal with these problems before a medical emergency arises.

REFERENCES

1. Anderson, JW and Geil, PB: New perspectives in nutrition management of diabetes mellitus. Am J Med 85(suppl 5A):159, 1988.
2. Assan, R, et al: Metabolic and immunologic effects of cyclosporine in recently diagnosed type I diabetes mellitus. Lancet 1:67, 1985.
3. Bergeron, JJM, et al: Uptake of insulin and other ligands into receptor-rich endocytic components of target cells: The endosomal apparatus. Annu Rev Physiol 47:383, 1985.
4. Brannon, FJ, Geyer, MJ, and Foley, MW: Cardiac Rehabilitation: Basic Theory and Application. FA Davis, Philadelphia, 1988.
5. Brink, SJ and Stewart, C: Insulin pump treatment in insulin-dependent diabetes mellitus: Children, adolescents, and young adults. JAMA 255:617, 1986.
6. Brodows, RG, Williams, C, and Amatruda, JM: Treatment of insulin reactions in diabetics. JAMA 252:3378, 1984.
7. Buhler, FR, Julius, S, and Reaven, GM: A new dimension in hypertension: Role of insulin resistance. J Cardiovasc Pharmacol 15(suppl 5):S1, 1990.
8. Camerini-Davalos, RA, et al: Drug-induced reversal of early diabetic microangiopathy. N Engl J Med 309:1551, 1983.
9. Cheng, K and Larner, J: Intracellular mediators of insulin action. Annu Rev Physiol 47:405, 1985.
10. Clements, RS (ed): Symposium: Diabetic complications and the role of aldose reductase inhibition. Am J Med 79(suppl 5A):1, 1985.
11. Clements, RS and Bell, DSH: Complications of diabetes: Prevalence, detection, current treatment, and prognosis. Am J Med 79(suppl 5A):2, 1985.
12. Colwell, JA and Lopes-Virella, MF: A review of the development of large-vessel disease in diabetes mellitus. Am J Med 85(suppl 5A):113, 1988.
13. Craighead, JE: Diabetes. In Rubin, E and Farber, JL (eds): Pathology, ed 2. JB Lippincott, Philadelphia, 1994.
14. Crawford, JM and Cotran, RS: The pancreas. In Cotran, RS, Kumar, V, and Robbins, SL (eds): The Pathologic Basis of Disease, ed 5. WB Saunders, Philadelphia, 1994.
15. Czech, MP: The nature and regulation of the insulin receptor: Structure and function. Annu Rev Physiol 47:357, 1985.
16. Davies, AG, et al: Continuous subcutaneous insulin infusion in diabetes mellitus: A year's prospective trial. Arch Dis Child 59:1027, 1984.
17. DeFronzo, R, Ferrannini, A, and Koivisto, V: New concepts in the pathogenesis and treatment of non-insulin-dependent diabetes mellitus. Am J Med 74(suppl 1A):52, 1983.
18. Draznin, B: Intracellular calcium, insulin secretion, and action. Am J Med 85(suppl 5A):44, 1988.
19. Falko, JM and Osei, K: Combination insulin/glyburide therapy in type II diabetes mellitus. Am J Med 79(suppl 3B):92, 1985.
20. Farese, RV: Phospholipid signaling systems in insulin action. Am J Med 85(suppl 5A):36, 1988.
21. Feutren, G, et al: Cyclosporin increases the rate of remissions in insulin-dependent diabetes of recent onset: Results of a multicentre double-blind trial. Lancet 2:119, 1986.
22. Fineberg, SE, et al: Immunologic improvement resulting from the transfer of animal insulin treated diabetic subjects to human insulin (recombinant-DNA). Diabetes Care 5(suppl 2):107, 1982.
23. Genuth, SM: Hormones of the pancreatic islets. In Berne, RM and Levy, MN (eds): Physiology, ed 3. Mosby Year Book, St. Louis, 1993.
24. Gerich, JE: Sulfonylureas in the treatment of diabetes mellitus—1985. Mayo Clin Proc 60:439, 1985.
25. Greene, DA and Lattimer, SA: Recent advances in the therapy of diabetic peripheral neuropathy by means of an aldose reductase inhibitor. Am J Med 79(suppl 5A):13, 1985.
26. Gulan, M, Gottesman, IS, and Zinman, B: Biosynthetic human insulin improves postprandial glucose excursions in type I diabetes. Ann Intern Med 107:506, 1987.
27. Guyton, AC: Textbook of Medical Physiology, ed 8. WB Saunders, Philadelphia, 1991.
28. Harati, Y: Diabetic peripheral neuropathies. Ann Intern Med 107:546, 1987.
29. Heinemann, L and Richter, B: Clinical pharmacology of human insulin. Diabetes Care 16:90, 1993.
30. Helmrich, SP, et al: Physical activity and reduced occurrence of non-insulin dependent diabetes mellitus. N Engl J Med 325:147, 1991.
31. Home, PH and Alberti, KGMM: The new insulins: Their characteristics and clinical implications. Drugs 24:401, 1982.
32. Horton, ES: Metabolic aspects of exercise and weight reduction. Med Sci Sports Exerc 18:10, 1986.
33. Horton, ES: Role of environmental factors in the development of noninsulin-dependent diabetes mellitus. Am J Med 75(suppl 5B):32, 1983.
34. Jacobs, S and Cuatrecasas, P: Insulin receptors. Annu Rev Pharmacol Toxicol 23:461, 1983.
35. Jarett, L, et al: The chemical mediators of insulin action: Possible targets for postreceptor defects. Am J Med 74(suppl 1A):31, 1983.
36. Jaworski, MA, et al: Immunosuppression in autoimmune disease: The double-edged sword. Clin Invest Med 10(suppl):488, 1987.

37. Kador, PF and Kinoshita, JH: Role of aldose reductase in the development of diabetes-associated complications. Am J Med 79(suppl 5A):8, 1985.
38. Kahn, CR: The molecular mechanism of insulin action. Annu Rev Med 36:429, 1985.
39. Kahn, SE and Porte, D: Islet dysfunction in non–insulin-dependent diabetes mellitus. Am J Med 85(suppl 5A):4, 1988.
40. Karjalainen, J, et al: A bovine albumin peptide as a possible trigger of insulin-dependent diabetes mellitus. N Engl J Med 327:302, 1992.
41. Kolterman, OG, et al: The acute and chronic effects of sulfonylurea therapy to type II diabetic subjects. Diabetes 33:346, 1984.
42. Kono, T, et al: Evidence that translocation of the glucose transport activity is the major mechanism of insulin action on glucose transport in fat cells. J Biol Chem 257:10942, 1982.
43. Lacy, PE and Scharp, DW: Islet transplantation in treating diabetes. Annu Rev Med 37:33, 1986.
44. Larner, J: Mediators of postreceptor action of insulin. Am J Med 74(suppl 1A):38, 1983.
45. Lebovitz, HE: Clinical utility of oral hypoglycemic agents in the management of patients with noninsulin-dependent diabetes mellitus. Am J Med 75(suppl 5B):94, 1983.
46. Lebovitz, HE and Feinglos, MN: Mechanism of action of the second-generation sulfonylurea glypizide. Am J Med 75(suppl 5B):46, 1983.
47. Leichter, SB, et al: Long-term follow-up of diabetic patients using insulin infusion pumps: Considerations for future clinical application. Arch Intern Med 145:1409, 1985.
48. Lipson, LG: Diabetes in the elderly: Diagnosis, pathogenesis, and therapy. Am J Med 80(suppl 5A):10, 1986.
49. Liu, GC, et al: Moderate weight loss and sulfonylurea treatment of non–insulin-dependent diabetes mellitus: Combined effects. Arch Intern Med 145:665, 1985.
50. Lockwood, DH and Amatruda, JM: Cellular alterations responsible for insulin resistance in obesity and type II diabetes mellitus. Am J Med 74(suppl 5B):23, 1983.
51. Lucas, CP, et al: Achieving therapeutic goals in insulin-using diabetic patients with non–insulin-dependent diabetes mellitus. Am J Med 83(suppl 3A):3, 1987.
52. Maclaren, NK: Viral and immunological bases of beta cell failure in insulin-dependent diabetes. Am J Dis Child 131:1149, 1977.
53. Marchetti, P and Navalesi, R: Pharmacokinetic-pharmacodynamic relationships of oral hypoglycaemic agents: An update. Clin Pharmacokinet 16:100, 1989.
54. Moller, DE and Flier, JS: Mechanisms of disease: Insulin resistance—mechanisms, syndromes, and implications. N Engl J Med 325:938, 1991.
55. Muir, A, Schartz, DA, and Maclaren, NK: The pathogenesis, prediction, and prevention of insulin-dependent diabetes mellitus. Endocrinol Metal Clin 21:199, 1992.
56. Nathan, DM: Medical progress: Long-term complications of diabetes mellitus. N Engl J Med 328:1676, 1993.
57. Nathan, DM: The rationale for glucose control in diabetes mellitus. Endocrinol Metab Clin 21:221, 1992.
58. National Diabetes Data Group: Classification and diagnosis of diabetes mellitus and other categories of glucose intolerance. Diabetes 28:1039, 1979.
59. Newgard, CB: Cellular engineering and gene therapy strategies for insulin replacement in diabetes. Diabetes 43:341, 1994.
60. Nolte, MS: Insulin therapy in insulin-dependent (type I) diabetes mellitus. Endocrinol Metab Clin 21:281, 1992.
61. Olefsky, JM: Pathogenesis of insulin resistance and hyperglycemia in non–insulin-dependent diabetes mellitus. Am J Med 79(suppl 3B):1, 1985.
62. Olefsky, JM, Ciaraldi, TP, and Kolterman, OG: Mechanisms of insulin resistance in non–insulin-dependent (type II) diabetes. Am J Med 79(suppl 3B):12, 1985.
63. Olefsky, JM, et al: Cellular mechanisms of insulin resistance in non–insulin-dependent (type II) diabetes. Am J Med 85(suppl 5A):86, 1988.
64. Pollet, RJ: Insulin receptors and action in clinical disorders of carbohydrate tolerance. Am J Med 75(suppl 5B):15, 1983.
65. Powers, AC and Eisenbarth, GS: Autoimmunity to islet cells in diabetes mellitus. Annu Rev Med 36:533, 1985.
66. Reaven, GM (ed): Symposium: The role of insulin resistance in the pathogenesis and treatment of noninsulin-dependent diabetes mellitus. Am J Med 74(suppl 1A):1, 1983.
67. Reichard, P, Nilsson, B-Y, and Rosenquist, U: The effect of long-term intensified insulin treatment on the development of microvascular complications of diabetes mellitus. N Engl J Med 329:304, 1993.
68. Riley, WJ, et al: A prospective study of the development of diabetes in relatives of patients with insulin dependent diabetes mellitus. N Engl J Med 323:1167, 1990.
69. Romero, G and Larner, J: Insulin mediators and the mechanism of insulin action. Adv Pharmacol 24:21, 1993.
70. Rosenstock, J, Meisel, A, and Raskin, P: Conversion from low-dose insulin therapy to glipizide in patients with non–insulin-dependent diabetes mellitus. Am J Med 83(suppl 3A):10, 1987.
71. Rosenstock, J and Raskin, P: Early diabetic neuropathy: Assessment and potential therapeutic interventions. Diabetes Care 9:529, 1986.

72. Samols, E and Stagner, JI: Intra-islet regulation. Am J Med 85(suppl 5A):31, 1988.
73. Shuman, CR: Glipizide: An overview. Am J Med 75(suppl 5B):55, 1983.
74. Siperstein, MD: Diabetic ketoacidosis and hyperosmolar coma. Endocrinol Metab Clin 21:415, 1992.
75. Siperstein, MD: Diabetic microangiopathy, genetics, environment, and treatment. Am J Med 85(suppl 5A):119, 1988.
76. Sussman, KE: Introduction: New horizons in diabetes: A Veteran's Administration Medical Research Service symposium. Am J Med 85(suppl 5A):1, 1988.
77. Symposium (various authors): Insulin sensitivity: Cardioprotection versus metabolic disorders. J Cardiovasc Pharmacol 20(suppl 11):S1, 1992.
78. Tamborlane, WV, and Amiel, SA: Hypoglycemia in the treated diabetic patient: A risk of intensive insulin therapy. Endocrinol Metab Clin 21:313, 1992.
79. The Diabetes Control and Complications Trial Research Group: The effect of intensive treatment of diabetes on the development and progression of long-term complications in insulin-dependent diabetes mellitus. N Engl J Med 329:977, 1993.
80. Tung, P and Levin, SR: Nephropathy in non–insulin-dependent diabetes mellitus. Am J Med 85(suppl 5A):131, 1988.
81. Unger, RH, Dobbs, RE, and Orci, L: Insulin, glucagon, and somatostatin secretion in the regulation of metabolism. Annu Rev Physiol 40:307, 1978.
82. Unger, RH and Foster, DW: Diabetes mellitus. In Wilson, JD and Foster, DW (eds): Textbook of Endocrinology, ed 8. WB Saunders, Philadelphia, 1992.
83. Unger, RH and Orci, L: Glucagon and the A cell. N Engl J Med 304:1518, 1575, 1981.
84. Vinik, AI and Wing, RR: The good, the bad, and the ugly in diabetic diets. Endocrinol Metab Clin 21:237, 1992.
85. Von Schenck, H: Glucagon: Biochemistry, physiology, and pathophysiology. Acta Med Scand 209:145, 1981.
86. Yki-Jarvinen, H, et al: Comparison of insulin regimens in patients with non–insulin-dependent diabetes mellitus. N Engl J Med 327:1426, 1992.
87. Young, CW: Rationale for glycemic control. Am J Med 79(suppl 3B):8, 1985.

Chemotherapy of Infectious and Neoplastic Diseases

CHAPTER 33

Treatment of Infections I: Antibacterial Drugs

This chapter and the next two chapters in this text address drugs used to treat infections caused by pathogenic microorganisms and parasites. Microorganisms such as bacteria, viruses, and protozoa as well as other, larger multicellular parasites frequently invade human tissues and are responsible for various afflictions ranging from mild, annoying symptoms to life-threatening disease. Often, the body's natural defense mechanisms are unable to deal with these pathogenic invaders, and pharmacologic treatment is essential in resolving infections and promoting recovery. Drugs used to treat infection represent one of the most significant advances in medical history, and these agents are among the most important and widely used pharmacologic agents throughout the world.

Drugs used to treat infectious diseases share a common goal of **selective toxicity**, meaning they must selectively kill or attenuate the growth of the pathogenic organism without causing excessive damage to the host (human) cells. In some cases, the pathogenic organism may have some distinctive structural or biochemical feature that allows the drug to selectively attack the invading cell. For instance, drugs that capitalize on certain differences in membrane structure, protein synthesis, or other unique aspects of cellular metabolism in the pathogenic organism will be effective and safe anti-infectious agents. Of course, selective toxicity is a relative term, since all of the drugs discussed in the following chapters will exert some adverse effects on human tissues. However, drugs used to treat various infections generally impair function in the pathogenic organism to a much greater extent than in human tissues.

Several other general terms are also used to describe the drugs used to treat infectious disease. Agents used specifically against small, unicellular organisms (e.g., bacteria, viruses) are often referred to as *antimicrobial drugs*. Antimicrobial agents are also commonly referred to as *antibiotics*, indicating that these substances are used to kill other living organisms (i.e., anti-"bios," or life). To avoid confusion, various drugs in this text are classified and identified according to the primary type of infectious organism they are used to treat—that is, whether they are antibacterial, antiviral, antifungal, and so on.

501

This chapter discusses the drugs used to treat bacterial infections. Drugs used to treat and prevent viral infections are presented in Chapter 34, followed by the pharmacologic management of other parasitic infections (antifungal, antiprotozoal, and anthelmintic drugs) in Chapter 35. Because infectious disease represents one of the most common forms of illness, many patients undergoing physical rehabilitation will be taking one or more of these drugs. Physical therapists and occupational therapists will undoubtedly deal with patients undergoing chemotherapy for infectious disease on a routine basis. The pharmacotherapeutic management of infectious disease presented in Chapters 33 through 35 should be of interest to all rehabilitation specialists.

BACTERIA: BASIC CONCEPTS

Bacterial Structure and Function

Bacteria are unicellular microorganisms, ranging in size from 0.2 to 10.0 μm in diameter.[13] Bacteria are distinguished from other microorganisms by several features, including a rigid cell wall that surrounds the bacterial cell and the lack of a true nuclear membrane (i.e., the genetic material within the bacterial cell is not confined by a distinct membrane). Bacteria usually contain the basic subcellular organelles needed to synthesize proteins and maintain cellular metabolism, including ribosomes, enzymes, and cytoplasmic storage granules. Bacteria, however, must depend on some kind of nourishing medium to provide metabolic substrates to maintain function. Hence, these microorganisms often invade human tissues to gain access to a supply of amino acids, sugars, and other substances.

Pathogenic Effects of Bacteria

Bacterial infections can be harmful to host organisms in several ways.[23,34] Bacteria can multiply so they compete with host (human) cells for essential nutrients. Bacteria may directly harm human cells by releasing toxic substances. Bacteria may also cause an immune response that ultimately damages human tissues as well as the invading bacteria. Of course, not all bacteria in the human body are harmful. For instance, certain bacteria in the gastrointestinal system inhibit the growth of other microorganisms as well as assist in the digestion of food and synthesis of certain nutrients. Also, many bacteria that enter the body are adequately dealt with by normal immunologic responses. However, invasion of pathogenic bacteria can lead to severe infections and death, especially if the patient is debilitated or the body's endogenous defense mechanisms are unable to combat the infection. In some cases, bacteria may establish areas of growth or colonies that remain fairly innocuous for extended periods. This colonization may, however, begin to proliferate and become a health threat when the patient succumbs to some other disorder or illness. Consequently, the chance of severe, life-threatening infections is especially high in individuals who are debilitated or have some defect in their immune system.

Bacterial Nomenclature and Classification

Bacteria are usually named according to their genus and species with these names identified in italic typeset.[13] For instance, *Escherichia coli* refers to bacteria from the *Escherichia* genus, *coli* species. According to this nomenclature, the genus is capitalized and refers to bacteria with common genetic, morphologic, and biochemical characteristics. The species name is not capitalized and often refers to some physical, pathogenic, or other characteristic of the species. For example, *Streptococcus pyogenes* refers to bacteria from the *Streptococcus* genus that are commonly associated with pyogenic or pus-producing characteristics.

Because of the diverse bacterial genera, bacteria are often categorized according to common characteristics such as the shape and histologic staining of the bacterial cell. For example, *gram-positive cocci* refers to spherical bacteria (cocci) that retain the discoloration of a particular staining technique (Gram's method of staining). However, development of a comprehensive taxonomy that neatly categorizes all bacteria is difficult because of the diverse morphologic and biochemical characteristics of various bacterial families and genera.

For the purpose of this chapter, bacteria are categorized according to the criteria outlined in Table 33–1. This classification scheme does not fully identify all of the various characteristics of the many bacterial families. The classifications listed in Table 33–1 are only used here to categorize bacteria relative to the use of antibacterial agents, which are discussed later in this chapter under "Specific Antibacterial Agents."

TABLE 33–1 Types of Bacteria

Type	Principal Features	Common Examples
Gram-positive bacilli	Generally rod-shaped; retain color when treated by Gram's method of staining	*Bacillus anthracis, Clostridium tetani*
Gram-negative bacilli	Rod-shaped; do not retain color of Gram's method	*Escherichia coli, Klebsiella pneumoniae, Pseudomonas aeruginosa*
Gram-positive cocci	Generally spherical or ovoid in shape; retain color of Gram's method	*Staphylococcus aureus, Streptococcus pneumoniae*
Gram-negative cocci	Spherical or ovoid; do not retain color of Gram's method	*Neisseria gonorrhoeae* (gonococcus), *Neisseria meningitidis* (meningococcus)
Acid-fast bacilli	Rod-shaped; retain color of certain stains even when treated with acid	*Mycobacterium leprae, Mycobacterium tuberculosis*
Spirochetes	Slender, spiral shape; able to move about without flagella (intrinsic locomotor ability)	Lyme disease agent; *Treponema pallidum* (syphilis)
Actinomycetes	Thin filaments that stain positively by Gram's method	*Actinomyces israelii; Nocardia*
Others:		
Mycoplasmas	Spherical; lack the rigid, highly structured cell wall found in most bacteria	*Mycoplasma pneumoniae*
Rickettsiae	Small, gram-negative bacteria	*Rickettsia typhi, Rickettsia rickettsii*

TREATMENT OF BACTERIAL INFECTIONS: BASIC PRINCIPLES

Spectrum of Antibacterial Activity

Some drugs are effective against a variety of bacteria; these are usually referred to as *broad-spectrum agents*. For instance, a drug such as tetracycline is considered to have a broad spectrum of activity because this drug is effective against many gram-negative, gram-positive, and other types of bacteria. In contrast, a drug like isoniazid is fairly specific for the bacillus that causes tuberculosis (i.e., *Mycobacterium tuberculosis*), and its spectrum is relatively narrow. Hence, antibacterial spectrum is one property of an antibacterial drug that determines the clinical applications of that agent. Other factors, including patient tolerance, bacterial resistance, and physician preference, also influence the selection of a particular drug for a particular condition. The clinical use of antibacterial drugs relative to specific bacterial pathogens is discussed in "Clinical Use of Antibacterial Drugs: Relationship to Specific Bacterial Infections."

Bactericidal Versus Bacteriostatic Activity

The term **bactericidal** refers to drugs that typically kill or destroy bacteria. In contrast, drugs that do not actually kill bacteria but limit the growth and proliferation of bacterial invaders are referred to as **bacteriostatic**. Antibacterial drugs are usually classified as either bactericidal or bacteriostatic, depending on their mechanism of action. Also, the classification of whether or not a drug is bactericidal or bacteriostatic may depend on the dosage of the drug. For instance, drugs like erythromycin exhibit bacteriostatic activity at lower doses but are bactericidal at higher doses.

BASIC MECHANISMS OF ANTIBACTERIAL DRUGS

As mentioned previously, antibacterial and other antimicrobial drugs must be selectively toxic to the infectious microorganism, without causing excessive damage to human cells. Drugs that exert selective toxicity against bacteria generally employ one of the mechanisms shown in Figure 33–1. These mechanisms include (1) inhibition of bacterial cell wall synthesis and function, (2) inhibition of bacterial protein synthesis, and (3) inhibition of bacterial DNA/RNA function. The details of these mechanisms along with the reasons why each mechanism is specific for bacterial (versus human) cells are discussed subsequently.

Inhibition of Bacterial Cell Wall Synthesis and Function

Penicillin, cephalosporins, and several other commonly used drugs exert their antibacterial effects by inhibiting the synthesis of bacterial cell walls.[27] The selective toxicity of these drugs is accounted for by the fact that bacterial cell walls differ considerably from those of their mammalian counterparts. The membrane surrounding most bacterial cells (with the exception of the *Mycoplasma* genus) is a relatively rigid, firm structure. This rigidity appears to be essential in constraining the high osmotic pres-

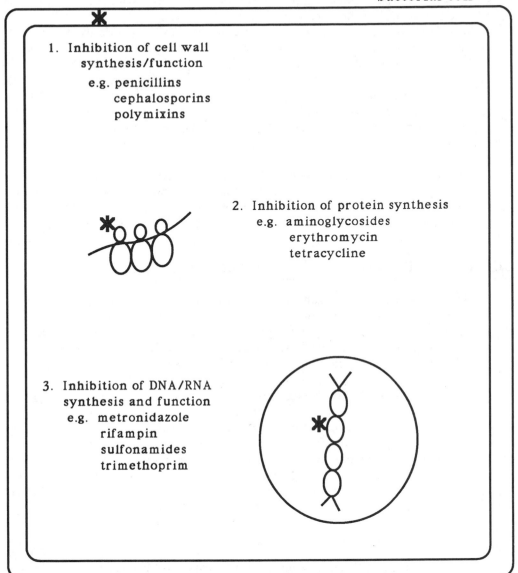

FIGURE 33-1. Primary sites of antibacterial drug action on bacterial cells. See text for discussion.

sure within the bacterial cell. This behavior contrasts with the relatively supple, flexible membrane encompassing the mammalian cell.

The increased rigidity of bacterial cells is caused by the presence of protein-polysaccharide structures known as *peptidoglycans*.[21,25] Peptidoglycan units within the cell wall are cross-linked to one another in such a way as to provide a remarkable amount of rigidity and firmness to the cell. If these peptidoglycans are not present, the bacterial cell may essentially burst apart and be destroyed. Also, the lack of adequate membrane cytoarchitecture appears to initiate a suicidal autolysis, whereby bacterial hydrolases released from lysosomes begin to break down the cell wall, thus further contributing to destruction of the microorganism.[33]

Consequently, drugs that cause inadequate production of peptidoglycans or other structural components within the cell membrane may produce a selective bactericidal effect. Also, a limited number of antibacterial agents directly punch holes in the bacterial cell membrane, destroying the selective permeability and separation of internal from external environment, which is crucial for the life of the microorganism.[15] These agents include the polymyxin antibiotics (polymyxin B, colistin). These drugs are cationic compounds that are attracted to negatively charged phospholipids in the bacterial cell membrane. The selectivity of these agents for bacterial cell membranes may be because of a greater attraction to certain bacterial phospholipids versus human cell membrane phospholipids. In any event, these drugs penetrate and disrupt the architecture and integrity of the surface membrane. In essence, these drugs act as detergents that break apart the phospholipid bilayer, creating gaps and leaks in the bacterial cell wall.[15,25] The loss of cell membrane integrity leads to rapid death of the bacteria.

Inhibition of Bacterial Protein Synthesis

Bacteria, like most living organisms, must continually synthesize specific proteins to carry out various cellular functions, including enzymatic reactions and membrane transport. A fairly large and well-known group of antibacterial agents work by inhibiting or impairing the synthesis of these bacterial proteins. Drugs that exert their antibacterial effects in this manner include the aminoglycosides (e.g., gentamicin, streptomycin), erythromycin, tetracyclines, and several other agents.[3,10,22,31]

Basically, drugs that inhibit bacterial protein synthesis enter the bacterial cell and bind to specific ribosomal subunits.[3,31] Antibacterial drugs that work by this mechanism have a much greater affinity for bacterial ribosomes than for human ribosomes, hence their relative specificity in treating bacterial infections. Binding the drug to the ribosome either blocks protein synthesis or causes the ribosome to misread the messenger RNA (mRNA) code, resulting in the production of meaningless or nonsense proteins.[11,18,22,31] The lack of appropriate protein production impairs bacterial cell membrane transport and metabolic function, resulting in retarded growth or death of the bacteria.

Inhibition of Bacterial DNA/RNA Synthesis and Function

As in any cell, bacteria must be able to replicate their genetic material to reproduce and function normally. An inability to produce normal DNA and RNA will prohibit the bacteria from mediating continued growth and reproduction. Drugs that exert their antibacterial activity by interfering with the structure, synthesis, and function of DNA and RNA in susceptible bacteria include rifampin, metronidazole, and several other agents.[14,32] These drugs are apparently able to selectively impair bacterial DNA/RNA function because they have a greater affinity for bacterial genetic material and enzymes related to bacterial DNA/RNA synthesis.

Several antibacterial drugs inhibit bacterial nucleic acid synthesis by inhibiting the production of folic acid.[35] Folic acid serves as an enzymatic cofactor in a number of reactions including synthesis of bacterial nucleic acids and certain essential amino acids. The pathway for synthesis of these folic acid cofactors is illustrated in Figure 33–2.

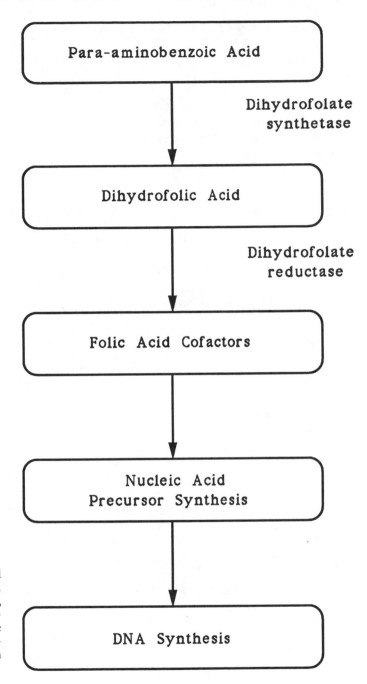

FIGURE 33–2. Folic acid metabolism in bacterial cells. Certain antibacterial drugs (e.g., sulfonamides and trimethoprim) inhibit the dihydrofolate synthetase and reductase enzymes, thus interfering with DNA biosynthesis.

Certain antibacterial drugs block specific steps in the folate pathway, thus impairing the production of this enzymatic cofactor and ultimately impairing the production of nucleic acids and other essential metabolites. Examples of drugs that exert antibacterial effects by this mechanism include trimethoprim and the sulfonamide drugs (sulfadiazine, sulfamethoxazole, etc.).[16]

SPECIFIC ANTIBACTERIAL AGENTS

Considering the vast number of antibacterial drugs, we cannot explore the pharmacokinetic and pharmacologic details of each individual agent. For the purposes of this chapter, the major groups of antibacterial drugs are categorized according to the basic modes of antibacterial action that were just discussed (inhibition of cell wall synthesis, etc.). Pertinent aspects of each group's actions, uses, and potential side effects are briefly discussed. For a more detailed description of any specific agent, the reader is referred to one of the current drug indices such as the *Physician's Desk Reference* (*PDR*).

ANTIBACTERIAL DRUGS THAT INHIBIT BACTERIAL CELL WALL SYNTHESIS AND FUNCTION

Table 33–2 lists drugs that exert their primary antibacterial effects by impairing bacterial cell membrane synthesis and function. Clinical use and specific aspects of these drugs are presented here.

Penicillins

Penicillin, the first antibiotic, was originally derived from mold colonies of the *Penicillium* fungus during the early 1940s. Currently, there are several forms of natural and semisynthetic penicillins (Table 33–2). These agents have a chemical structure and mode of action similar to the cephalosporin drugs and several other agents. Collectively, the penicillins and these other drugs are known as *beta-lactam antibiotics* because they share a common structure known as a *beta-lactam ring*.

Penicillin and other beta-lactam agents exert their effects by binding to specific enzymatic proteins within the bacterial cell membrane.[24,27,33] These enzymatic proteins are known as penicillin binding proteins (PBPs). PBPs are responsible for the normal synthesis and organization of the bacterial cell wall. In particular, PBPs help manufacture the peptidoglycans, which are essential for normal membrane structure and function. Penicillins and other beta-lactam drugs attach to the PBPs and inhibit their function. Thus, construction of the bacterial cell wall is impaired, and the cell dies from an inability of the membrane to serve as a selective barrier and contain the high internal osmotic pressure of the bacterial cell.

CLASSIFICATION AND USE OF PENICILLINS

As indicated in Table 33–2, penicillins can be classified according to their spectrum of antibacterial activity and pharmacokinetic features. The naturally occurring penicillins (penicillin G and V) can be administered orally but have a relatively narrow antibacterial spectrum. Some semisynthetic penicillins (amoxicillin, ampicillin) have been developed that have a broader antibacterial spectrum and may be administered either orally or parenterally, depending on the specific agent. Penicillinase-resistant forms of penicillin were developed to overcome strains of bacteria that contain an enzyme known as a penicillinase or beta-lactamase. This enzyme destroys natural and some semisynthetic penicillins, rendering these drugs ineffective in bacteria containing

TABLE 33–2 Drugs That Inhibit Bacterial Cell Membrane Synthesis

Penicillins	Cephalosporins	Other Agents
Natural penicillins Penicillin G (Bicillin, Wycillin, many others) Penicillin V (Beepen-VK, V-Cillin K, others) Penicillinase-resistant penicillins Cloxacillin (Cloxapen, Tegopen) Dicloxacillin (Cynapen, Pathocil) Methicillin (Staphcillin) Nafcillin (Unipen) Oxacillin (Bactocill, Prostaphlin) Aminopenicillins Amoxicillin (Amoxil, Polymox, others) Ampicillin (Omnipen, Polycillin, others) Bacampicillin (Spectrobid) Cyclacillin (Cyclapen-W) Extended-spectrum penicillins Azlocillin (Azlin) Carbenicillin (Geocillin, Geopen, Pyopen) Mezlocillin (Mezlin) Piperacillin (Pipracil) Ticarcillin (Ticar)	First-generation cephalosporins Cefadroxil (Duricef, Ultracef) Cefazolin (Ancef, Kefzol) Cephalexin (Keflex, Keftab) Cephalothin (Keflin) Cephapirin (Cefadyl) Cephradine (Anspor, Velosef) Second-generation cephalosporins Cefaclor (Ceclor) Cefamandole (Mandol) Cefmetazole (Zefazone) Cefonicid (Monocid) Ceforanide (Precef) Cefotetan (Cefotan) Cefoxitin (Mefoxin) Cefprozil (Cefzil) Cefuroxime (Kefurox, Zinacef) Third-generation cephalosporins Cefixime (Suprax) Cefoperazone (Cefobid) Cefotaxime (Claforan) Ceftazidime (Fortaz, Tazicef) Ceftizoxime (Cefizox) Ceftriaxone (Rocephin) Moxalactam (Moxam)	Aztreonam (Azactam) Bacitracin (Bacitracin ointment) Colistin (Coly-Mycin S) Cycloserine (Seromycin) Imipenem/cilastatin (Primaxin) Polymyxin B (generic) Vancomycin (Vancocin I.V., Vancoled)

509

this enzyme. In penicillinase-containing bacteria, semisynthetic forms of penicillin that are resistant to destruction by the penicillinase must be used (see Table 33–2).

Discussing all the clinical applications of the penicillins goes well beyond the scope of this chapter. These agents are a mainstay in the treatment of infection and remain the drugs of choice in a diverse array of clinical disorders. Tables 33–3a to 33–3d give some indication of the clinical uses of the penicillins. Clearly, these agents continue to be one of the most important and effective antibacterial regimens currently available.

ADVERSE EFFECTS

One of the primary problems with penicillin drugs is the potential for allergic reactions. **Hypersensitivity** to penicillin is exhibited by skin rashes, hives, itching, and difficulty breathing. In some individuals, these reactions may be fairly minor and can often be resolved by changing the type of penicillin or the method of administration. In some individuals, however, penicillin hypersensitivity may be quite severe and can lead to an *anaphylactic reaction* (severe bronchoconstriction and cardiovascular collapse).

During prolonged administration, penicillin drugs may also cause CNS problems (e.g., confusion, hallucinations), as well as certain blood disorders, such as hemolytic anemia and thrombocytopenia. Other relatively minor side effects of penicillin drugs include gastrointestinal problems such as nausea, vomiting, and diarrhea.

Cephalosporins

The cephalosporin drugs, which are also classified as beta-lactam antibiotics, exert their bactericidal effects in a manner similar to that of the penicillins (inhibition of PBPs resulting in inadequate peptidoglycan production). Generally, the cephalosporins serve as alternative agents to penicillins if penicillin drugs are ineffective or poorly tolerated by the patient. Cephalosporins may also be the drugs of choice in certain types of urinary tract infections (see Tables 33–3a to 33–3d).

Cephalosporins can be subdivided into first-, second-, and third-generation groups according to their spectrum of antibacterial activity (see Table 33–2). First-generation cephalosporins are generally effective against gram-positive cocci and may also be used against some gram-negative bacteria. Second-generation cephalosporins are also effective against gram-positive cocci, but they are somewhat more effective than first-generation agents against gram-negative bacteria. Third-generation cephalosporins have the broadest spectrum against gram-negative bacteria, but they have limited effectiveness against gram-positive cocci. Specific indications for cephalosporins are listed in Tables 33–3a to 33–3d.

ADVERSE EFFECTS

In some patients, cephalosporins may cause an allergic reaction similar to the penicillin hypersensitivity just described. Often a cross-sensitivity exists: a patient who is allergic to penicillin drugs will also display hypersensitivity to cephalosporin agents. Other principal adverse effects of cephalosporins consist of gastrointestinal problems including stomach cramps, diarrhea, nausea, and vomiting.

TABLE 33–3a Treatment of Common Infections Caused by Gram-Positive Bacilli*

Bacillus	Disease	Primary Agent(s)	Alternative Agent(s)
Bacillus anthracis	Anthrax; pneumonia	Penicillin G	Erythromycin; a tetracycline; a cephalosporin; chloramphenicol
Clostridium	Gas gangrene	Penicillin G	A cephalosporin; clindamycin; imipenem; chloramphenicol; a tetracycline
Clostridium tetani	Tetanus	Penicillin G	A tetracycline; erythromycin
Corynebacterium diphtheriae	Pharyngitis; laryngotracheitis; pneumonia; other local lesions	Penicillin G	Erythromycin, a cephalosporin; clindamycin; rifampin
Corynebacterium species	Endocarditis; infections in various other tissues	Penicillin G ± an aminoglycoside; vancomycin	Rifampin + penicillin G; ampicillin-sulbactam
Listeria monocytogenes	Bacteremia; meningitis	Ampicillin or penicillin G ± gentamicin	Trimethoprim-sulfamethoxazole; chloramphenicol; erythromycin; a tetracycline

*Adapted from Sande, MA, Kapusnik-Uner, JE, and Mandell, GL: Chemotherapy of microbial diseases. In Gilman, AG, et al (eds): The Pharmacological Basis of Therapeutics, ed 8. Pergamon Press, New York, 1990, with permission of McGraw-Hill, Inc.

Other Agents That Inhibit Bacterial Cell Wall Synthesis

Aztreonam. Aztreonam (Azactam) is considered to be a beta-lactam antibiotic with pharmacologic properties similar to penicillin and cephalosporin drugs. Aztreonam has a fairly limited spectrum, but it may be useful against serious infections caused by certain gram-negative bacilli (*Enterobacter aerogenes* and *Pseudomonas aeruginosa*). The principal problems associated with aztreonam include skin rashes, redness, and itching because of hypersensitivity in susceptible individuals.

Bacitracin. Bacitracin refers to a group of polypeptide antibiotics that have similar chemical and pharmacologic properties. These compounds inhibit bacterial cell wall synthesis by inhibiting the incorporation of amino acids and nucleic acid precursors into the bacterial cell wall. Bacitracin compounds, which have a fairly broad range of antibacterial activity, are effective against many gram-positive bacilli and gram-positive cocci, as well as several other microorganisms. Bacitracin is usually applied topically to prevent and treat infection in superficial skin wounds and certain ophthalmic infections. Commercial preparations containing bacitracin may also contain other antibiotics such as neomycin and polymyxin B. The primary problem associated with bacitracin is local hypersensitivity, as indicated by skin rashes and itching.

Colistin. Colistin (also known as *colistimethate* or *polymyxin E*) is similar to polymyxin B in terms of pharmacologic mechanism and antibacterial effects. Colistin is used primarily in combination with other agents (neomycin and hydrocortisone) to treat local infections of the external auditory canal. Adverse effects are relatively rare during local, topical use of this drug.

Cycloserine. Cycloserine inhibits bacterial wall synthesis by interfering with the final stage of peptidoglycan synthesis. Synthesis of peptidoglycans is completed by

TABLE 33–3b Treatment of Common Infections Caused by Gram-Negative Bacilli*

Bacillus	Disease	Primary Agent(s)	Alternative Agent(s)
Acinetobacter	Infections in various tissues; hospital-acquired infections	An aminoglycoside; imipenem	A cephalosporin
Bacteroides fragilis	Abscesses (brain, lung, intra-abdominal); bacteremia; empyema; endocarditis	Clindamycin; metronidazole	Cefoxitin or cefotetan; chloramphenicol; imipenem; other combinations
Bacteroides species	Abscesses (brain, lung); oral disease; sinusitis	Clindamycin; penicillin G	Cefoxitin; cefotetan or ceftizoxime; metronidazole; chloramphenicol; erythromycin; a tetracycline
Escherichia coli	Bacteremia; urinary tract infections; infections in other tissues	Ampicillin ± an aminoglycoside; trimethoprim-sulfamethoxazole; other combinations	An aminoglycoside; a cephalosporin; aztreonam; nitrofurantoin; a tetracycline
Flavobacterium meningosepticum	Meningitis	Vancomycin	Trimethoprim-sulfamethoxazole; rifampin
Fusobacterium nucleatum	Genital infections; gingivitis; lung abscesses; ulcerative pharyngitis	Penicillin G; clindamycin	A cephalosporin; metronidazole; chloramphenicol; erythromycin; a tetracycline
Klebsiella pneumoniae	Pneumonia; urinary tract infection	A cephalosporin ± an aminoglycoside	Mezlocillin or piperacillin; aztreonam; imipenem; trimethoprim-sulfamethoxazole
Legionella pneumophila	Legionnaires' disease	Erythromycin ± rifampin	Ciprofloxacin; trimethoprim-sulfamethoxazole
Pasteurella multocida	Abscesses; bacteremia; meningitis; wound infections (animal bites)	Penicillin G	A cephalosporin; a tetracycline; amoxicillin
Proteus mirabilis	Urinary tract and other infections	Ampicillin or amoxicillin	An aminoglycoside; a cephalosporin
Proteus, other species	Urinary tract and other infections	An aminoglycoside; a cephalosporin	A broad-spectrum penicillin; aztreonam; imipenem
Pseudomonas aeruginosa	Bacteremia; pneumonia; urinary tract infection	A broad-spectrum penicillin ± an aminoglycoside	An aminoglycoside; a cephalosporin; ticarcillin; aztreonam; imipenem
Streptobacillus moniliformis	Abscesses; bacteremia; endocarditis	Penicillin G	Streptomycin; a tetracycline; chloramphenicol; erythromycin

*Adapted from Sande, MA, Kapusnik-Uner, JE, and Mandell, GL: Chemotherapy of microbial diseases. In Gilman, AG, et al (eds): The Pharmacological Basis of Therapeutics, ed 8. Pergamon Press, New York, 1990, with permission of McGraw-Hill, Inc.

TABLE 33–3c Treatment of Common Infections Caused by Gram-Positive and Gram-Negative Cocci*

Gram-Positive Coccus	Disease	Primary Agent(s)	Alternative Agent(s)
Staphylococcus aureus	Abscesses; bacteremia; endocarditis; meningitis; osteomyelitis; pneumonia	Penicillin G (or a penicillinase-resistant penicillin); vancomycin	A cephalosporin; clindamycin; erythromycin; other combinations
Streptococcus agalactiae (group B)	Meningitis; septicemia	Ampicillin or penicillin G ± an aminoglycoside	A cephalosporin; chloramphenicol; erythromycin
Streptococcus bovis	Bacteremia; endocarditis	Penicillin G ± streptomycin or gentamicin	A cephalosporin; vanomycin
Streptococcus faecalis	Bacteremia; endocarditis; urinary tract infection	Ampicillin; penicillin G	Gentamicin; streptomycin; vancomycin
Streptococcus pneumoniae	Arthritis; otitis; pneumonia; sinusitis	Penicillin G or V	A cephalosporin; erythromycin; chloramphenicol; clindamycin; trimethoprim-sulfamethoxazole
Streptococcus pyogenes	Bacteremia; cellulitis; pharyngitis; pneumonia; scarlet fever; other local and systemic infections	Penicillin G or V	A cephalosporin; erythromycin; vancomycin
Streptococcus (anaerobic species)	Bacteremia; brain and other abscesses; endocarditis; sinusitis	Penicillin G	A cephalosporin; clindamycin; chloramphenicol; erythromycin
Streptococcus (*viridans* group)	Bacteremia; endocarditis	Penicillin G ± streptomycin or gentamicin	A cephalosporin; vancomycin
Neisseria gonorrhoeae (gonococcus)	Arthritis-dermatitis syndrome; genital infections	Ampicillin or amoxicillin + probenecid; penicillin G	Cefoxitin or cefotaxime; a tetracycline; trimethoprim-sulfamethoxazole; ciprofloxacin; erythromycin; spectinomycin
Neisseria meningitidis (meningococcus)	Bacteremia; meningitis	Penicillin G	A cephalosporin; chloramphenicol

*Adapted from Sande, MA, Kapusnik-Uner, JE, and Mandell, GL: Chemotherapy of microbial diseases. In Gilman, AG, et al (eds): The Pharmacological Basis of Therapeutics, ed 8. Pergamon Press, New York, 1990, with permission of McGraw-Hill, Inc.

TABLE 33–3d Treatment of Infections Caused by Acid-Fast Bacilli,
Spirochetes, Actinomycetes, and Other Microorganisms*

Microorganism	Disease	Primary Agent(s)	Alternative Agent(s)
Acid-fast bacillus			
Mycobacterium leprae	Leprosy	Dapsone + rifampin	Clofazimine
Mycobacterium tuberculosis	Pulmonary, renal, meningeal, and other tuberculosis infections	Isoniazid + rifampin + pyrazinamide	Ethambutol (added to the primary drugs); streptomycin (added to the primary drugs)
Spirochetes			
Treponema pallidum	Syphilis	Penicillin G	Ceftriaxone; a tetracycline
Leptospira Borrelia	Meningitis	Penicillin G	A tetracycline
burgdorferi	Lyme disease	A tetracycline	Penicillin G; ceftriaxone
Actinomycetes			
Actinomyces israelii	Cervicofacial, abdominal, thoracic, and other lesions	Penicillin G or ampicillin	A tetracycline; erythromycin
Nocardia	Brain abscesses; pulmonary and other lesions	A sulfonamide; trimethoprim-sulfamethoxazole	Minocycline ± a sulfonamide
Other microorganisms			
Chlamydia trachomatis	Blennorrhea; lymphogranuloma venereum; nonspecific urethritis; trachoma	A tetracycline; doxycycline	Erythromycin; a sulfonamide
Mycoplasma pneumoniae	"Atypical" pneumonia	Erythromycin; a tetracycline	—
Rickettsia	Q fever; rickettsialpox; Rocky Mountain spotted fever; typhus fever, other diseases	Chloramphenicol; a tetracycline	—

*Adapted from Sande, MA, Kapusnik-Uner, JE, and Mandell, GL: Chemotherapy of microbial diseases. In Gilman, AG, et al (eds): The Pharmacological Basis of Therapeutics, ed 8. Pergamon Press, New York, 1990, with permission of McGraw-Hill Inc.

adding two units of the amino acid D-alanine. Cycloserine, which is similar in structure to D-alanine, competitively inhibits the enzyme that adds the final D-alanine units onto the peptidoglycan structures. Cycloserine is considered to be a broad-spectrum antibiotic but is used primarily as an adjunct in the treatment of tuberculosis. The primary adverse effect of this drug is CNS toxicity, which may occur during prolonged use at relatively high dosage.

Imipenem and Cilastatin. Imipenem is a relatively new beta-lactam drug that is used in combination with cilastatin. Imipenem exerts bactericidal effects similar to those of penicillin and cephalosporins, that is, inhibition of PBP function and peptidoglycan synthesis. Cilastatin itself does not have any antibacterial activity, but it serves to enhance the bactericidal effects of imipenem by inhibiting metabolic inactivation of imipenem within the kidneys.[2] Imipenem, which has the broadest antibacterial spectrum of the beta-lactam drugs, may be useful against a variety of aerobic gram-positive and gram-negative bacteria, as well as some anaerobic bacterial strains.[1,8] Adverse side effects associated with imipenem include nausea, hypotension, and hypersensitivity (skin rashes, redness, itching). CNS abnormalities such as confusion, tremors, and even seizures have also been reported in certain patients.

Polymyxin B. Polymyxin antibiotics are cationic compounds that are attracted to negatively charged phospholipids in the bacterial cell membrane. These drugs penetrate and disrupt the architecture and integrity of the surface membrane. In essence, polymyxins act as detergents that break apart the phospholipid bilayer, creating gaps in the bacterial cell wall, which leads to the subsequent destruction of the bacteria.[15,25]

Polymyxin B is effective against many gram-negative bacteria including *E coli*, *Klebsiella*, and *Salmonella*. Systemic administration of this drug, however, is often associated with extreme nephrotoxicity. Hence, this agent is used primarily for the treatment of local, superficial infections of the skin, eyes, and mucous membranes. When applied topically for these conditions, adverse reactions are relatively rare. Polymyxin B is often combined with other antibiotics such as bacitracin and neomycin in commercial topical preparations.

Vancomycin. Vancomycin appears to bind directly to bacterial cell wall precursors such as D-alanine and to impair the incorporation of these precursors into the cell wall. Vancomycin is effective against gram-positive bacilli and cocci and serves primarily as an alternative to the penicillins in a variety of infections (see Tables 33–3a to 33–3d).[7] The primary adverse effects associated with this drug are hypersensitivity (e.g., skin rashes), a bitter or unpleasant taste in the mouth, and gastrointestinal disturbances (nausea and vomiting). Vancomycin also has the potential to cause nephrotoxicity and **ototoxicity.**

DRUGS THAT INHIBIT BACTERIAL PROTEIN SYNTHESIS

Drugs that exert their primary antibacterial effects by inhibiting protein synthesis are listed in Table 33–4 and are discussed here.

Aminoglycosides

The aminoglycosides are a group of antibacterial agents that include streptomycin, gentamicin, neomycin, and similar agents (see Table 33–4). These agents bind irreversibly to certain parts of bacterial ribosomes and cause several changes in protein synthesis including alterations in the ability of the ribosome to read the mRNA genetic code.[10,11] This misreading results in improper synthesis of proteins that control specific aspects of cell function such as membrane structure and permeability.[31] The lack of normal cell proteins leads to the death of the bacterial cell.

ANTIBACTERIAL SPECTRUM AND GENERAL INDICATIONS

Aminoglycosides have a very broad spectrum of antibacterial activity and are effective against many aerobic gram-negative bacteria including *E coli*, *Pseudomonas*, and *Salmonella*.[31] Aminoglycosides are also active against some aerobic gram-positive bac-

TABLE 33-4 Drugs That Inhibit Bacterial Protein Synthesis

Aminoglycosides	Erythromycins	Tetracyclines	Other Agents
Amikacin (Amikin)	Erythromycin (ERYC, E-Mycin, others)	Demeclocycline (Declomycin)	Chloramphenicol (Chloromycetin)
Gentamicin (Garamycin)	Erythromycin estolate (Ilosone)	Doxycycline (Doxy, Vibramycin, others)	Clindamycin (Cleocin)
Kanamycin (Kantrex)	Erythromycin ethylsuccinate (E.E.S., EryPed)	Minocycline (Minocin)	Ethionamide (Trecator-SC)
Neomycin (generic)	Erythromycin gluceptate (Ilotycin)	Oxytetracycline (Terramycin)	Lincomycin (Lincocin)
Netilmicin (Netromycin)	Erythromycin lactobionate (Erythrocin)	Tetracycline (Achromycin V, Sumycin, many others)	
Streptomycin (generic)	Erythromycin stearate (Erythrocin, Wyamycin-S)		
Tobramycin (Nebcin)			

teria, such as certain species of *Staphylococcus,* and many anaerobic bacteria. Consequently, aminoglycosides are used to treat a variety of tissue and wound infections (see Tables 33–3a to 33–3d).

ADVERSE EFFECTS

Aminoglycoside use is limited somewhat by problems with toxicity.[20] Nephrotoxicity, as indicated by bloody urine, increased urination, and so on, as well as ototoxicity, as indicated by dizziness and ringing or fullness in the ears, may occur. Toxicity may occur more frequently in certain individuals, such as patients with liver or kidney failure, or elderly patients. To reduce the risk of toxicity, drug levels in the bloodstream must be periodically monitored so dosages can be adjusted for individual patients. Other adverse effects include hypersensitivity (e.g., skin rashes, itching) in susceptible individuals.

Erythromycins

Erythromycin and its chemical derivatives inhibit bacterial protein synthesis by binding to specific parts of the ribosomes in susceptible bacteria. This binding impairs protein synthesis primarily by inhibiting the formation of peptide bonds between adjacent amino acids. In particular, erythromycin seems to encourage the dissociation of transfer RNA (tRNA) units from their binding site on the ribosome.[3,22] Normally the tRNAs bring amino acids to the ribosome, where the amino acids are linked together to form proteins. By stimulating the detachment of tRNA, peptide bond formation is averted.

ANTIBACTERIAL SPECTRUM AND GENERAL INDICATIONS

Erythromycin exhibits a very broad spectrum of antibacterial activity and is active against many gram-positive bacteria as well as some gram-negative bacteria. This agent is often used as the primary or alternative drug in a variety of clinical conditions (see Tables 33–3a to 33–3d). Erythromycin is especially useful in patients who are allergic to penicillin.

ADVERSE EFFECTS

When given in high (bactericidal) doses, gastrointestinal distress is a common problem during erythromycin administration. Stomach cramps, nausea, vomiting, and diarrhea may occur. Hence, erythromycins are usually only given in doses that impair the growth of bacteria (bacteriostatic doses). Various degrees of allergic reactions, ranging from mild skin rashes to acute anaphylaxis, may also occur with erythromycin use in susceptible individuals.

Tetracyclines

Tetracycline and tetracycline derivatives are listed in Table 33–4. These agents inhibit protein synthesis by binding to several components of the ribosomal apparatus in susceptible bacteria. Hence, these drugs may cause misreading of the mRNA code, as well as impair the formation of peptide bonds at the bacterial ribosome. Thus, tetracyclines are very effective in preventing bacterial protein synthesis.

ANTIBACTERIAL SPECTRUM AND GENERAL INDICATIONS

Tetracyclines are active against a variety of bacteria including many gram-positive and gram-negative bacteria, as well as other bacterial microorganisms (*Rickettsia*, spirochetes). Their use as a broad-spectrum antibiotic has diminished somewhat, however, because of the development of tetracycline-resistant bacterial strains. (The problem of drug-resistant bacteria is discussed in more detail in "Resistance to Antibacterial Drugs.") Currently, tetracyclines are used to treat specific infections relating to such bacilli as *Chlamydia, Rickettsia,* and certain spirochetes (see Tables 33–3a to 33–3d). Tetracyclines may also be used as alternative agents in bacterial strains that are resistant to other drugs such as chloramphenicol, streptomycin, and various penicillins.

ADVERSE EFFECTS

Gastrointestinal distress (nausea, vomiting, diarrhea) may be a problem with tetracycline use. Hypersensitivity reactions (such as rashes) may also occur, as well as increased sensitivity of the skin to ultraviolet light (photosensitivity). Tetracyclines form chemical complexes with calcium that may impair the growth and development of calcified tissues such as bone and teeth, especially in children. Tetracyclines also cause discoloration of teeth in children and pregnant women, apparently because of this tetracycline-calcium interaction. As mentioned previously, development of tetracycline-resistant strains and resulting superinfections may be a serious problem during tetracycline therapy.

Other Agents That Inhibit Bacterial Protein Synthesis

Chloramphenicol. Chloramphenicol (Chloromycetin) is a synthetically produced agent that exerts antibacterial effects similar to those of erythromycin; that is, it binds to the 50S subunit of bacterial ribosomes and inhibits peptide bond formation. Chloramphenicol is a broad-spectrum antibiotic that is active against many gram-negative and gram-positive bacteria. This drug is administered systemically to treat serious infections such as typhoid fever, *Hemophilus* infections such as osteomyelitis, rickettsial infections such as Rocky Mountain spotted fever, and certain forms of meningitis. Chloramphenicol may also be administered topically to treat various skin, eye, and ear infections.

The most serious problem associated with chloramphenicol is the potential for bone marrow aplasia, which can lead to aplastic anemia and possibly death. There is some suggestion that chloramphenicol may lead to chromosomal changes in certain tissues and that the possibility for genotoxicity with prolonged chloramphenicol use should be considered.[28]

Clindamycin. Clindamycin (Cleocin) is derived from lincomycin. Both drugs are similar in structure and function to erythromycin and inhibit protein synthesis by binding to the 50S ribosomal subunit of susceptible bacteria. These agents are effective against most gram-positive bacteria and some gram-negative microorganisms. Typically, clindamycin and lincomycin are reserved as alternative drugs (rather than primary agents) in the treatment of local and systemic infections and may be especially useful if patients are unable to tolerate either penicillin or erythromycin. The principal adverse effects associated with these drugs are gastrointestinal distress (nausea, diarrhea, colitis) and various allergic reactions ranging from mild skin rashes to anaphylactic shock.

Ethionamide. Ethionamide (Trecator-SC) appears to inhibit bacterial protein synthesis, but the exact mechanism of action is unknown. This drug may act in a manner similar to that of some of the other drugs discussed previously in this section (binding to bacterial ribosomes), or it may mediate its effect by some other means. Ethionamide is effective against *M tuberculosis* and is used primarily in the treatment of tuberculosis. This drug is usually used as a secondary agent when the primary antituberculosis drugs are ineffective. Gastrointestinal distress (nausea, vomiting) is the most frequent problem encountered with ethionamide use. CNS disorders (drowsiness, mental depression, etc.), as well as severe postural hypotension, may also occur.

Lincomycin. Lincomycin (Lincocin) is similar in mechanism of action, clinical indications, and adverse side effects to clindamycin (see previously in this section).

DRUGS THAT INHIBIT BACTERIAL DNA/RNA SYNTHESIS AND FUNCTION

Table 33–5 lists drugs that exert their primary antibacterial effects by impairing the synthesis and replication of bacterial DNA and RNA. These agents are presented here.

Aminosalicylic Acid

Aminosalicylic acid (PAS, Teebacin) exerts its effects in a manner similar to the sulfonamide drugs; that is, aminosalicylic acid is structurally similar to para-aminobenzoic acid (PABA) and inhibits folic acid synthesis by competing with PABA in tuberculosis bacteria. This drug is used as an adjunct to the primary antitubercular agents isoniazid and rifampin. Adverse effects are fairly common with aminosalicylic acid use and include gastrointestinal problems, hypersensitivity reactions, and **blood dyscrasias** (e.g., agranulocytosis, thrombocytopenia).

TABLE 33–5 Drugs That Inhibit Bacterial DNA/RNA Synthesis and Function

Fluoroquinolones	Sulfonamides	Others
Ciprofloxacin (Cipro)	Sulfacytine (Renoquid)	Aminosalicylic acid (Tubasal)
Enoxacin (Penetrex)	Sulfadiazine (Silvadene)	Clofazimine (Lamprene)
Lomefloxacin (Maxaquin)	Sulfamethizole (Thiosulfil Forte)	Dapsone (Avlosulfon)
Norfloxacin (Noroxin)	Sulfamethoxazole (Gantanol)	Ethambutol (Myambutol)
Ofloxacin (Floxin)	Sulfisoxazole (Gantrisin)	Metronidazole (Flagyl, Protostat, others)
		Rifampin (Rifadin, Rimactane)
		Trimethoprim (Proloprim, Trimpex)

Clofazimine

Although the exact mechanism of clofazimine (Lamprene) is unclear, this drug appears to bind directly to bacterial DNA in susceptible microorganisms. Binding of the drug may prevent the double-stranded DNA helix from unraveling to allow replication of the DNA genetic code. An inability to replicate its genetic material will prevent the bacteria from undergoing mitosis.

Clofazimine, which is effective against *Mycobacterium leprae*, is used primarily as an adjunct in the treatment of leprosy. During clofazimine therapy, many patients experience problems with red to brownish-black discoloration of the skin. Although this discoloration is reversible, it may take several months to years before skin color returns to normal after the drug is discontinued. Other adverse effects include abdominal pain, nausea, vomiting, and rough, scaly skin.

Dapsone

Dapsone (Avlosulfon) is a member of a class of chemical agents known as the sulfones. Dapsone is especially effective against *M leprae* and is used with rifampin as the primary method of treating leprosy. Dapsone appears to exert its antibacterial effects in a manner similar to that of the sulfonamide drugs; that is, dapsone impairs folic acid synthesis by competing with PABA in bacterial cells. Primary adverse effects associated with dapsone include peripheral motor weakness, hypersensitivity reactions (skin rashes, itching), fever, and blood dyscrasias such as hemolytic anemia.

Ethambutol

The mechanism of ethambutol (Myambutol) is not fully understood. This drug apparently suppresses RNA synthesis in susceptible bacteria, but the exact manner by which this occurs is unknown. Ethambutol is primarily effective against *M tuberculosis* infections and is a secondary agent in the treatment of tuberculosis. Adverse effects associated with this drug include joint pain, nausea, skin rashes/itching, and CNS abnormalities (dizziness, confusion, hallucinations).

Fluoroquinolones

The fluoroquinolone antibiotics include ciprofloxacin (Cipro), enoxacin (Penetrex), lomefloxacin (Maxaquin), norfloxacin (Noroxin), and ofloxacin (Floxin). These drugs inhibit the twisting or supercoiling of DNA that appears to be necessary for bacterial nucleic acid replication. Evidently, a specific enzyme known as DNA-gyrase is responsible for promoting the DNA supercoiling in bacterial cells. Fluoroquinolone antibiotics inhibit this DNA-gyrase enzyme, thus impairing normal DNA structure and function.[17,32]

Fluoroquinolones are effective against a wide range of gram-positive and gram-negative aerobic bacteria and are especially useful in urinary tract infections caused by *E coli*, *Klebsiella*, *Proteus*, and *Enterobacter aerogenes*.[29] Primary adverse effects include CNS toxicity, which is manifested as visual disturbances, headache, and dizziness.

Gastrointestinal distress (nausea, vomiting, diarrhea) and allergic reactions (skin rashes, itching) may also occur. These drugs produce photosensitivity and increase the skin's sensitivity to ultraviolet light.

Metronidazole

The exact mechanism of metronidazole (Flagyl, Protostat, others) is not fully understood. This drug appears to be incorporated into bacterial cells, where it undergoes chemical reduction. Apparently, the reduced metabolite of metronidazole interacts with bacterial DNA and causes the DNA to lose its characteristic double-helix structure. This leads to the disintegration of DNA molecules and a loss of ability to replicate and carry out normal genetic functions. Further details of this bactericidal effect remain to be determined, however.

Metronidazole is effective against most anaerobic bacteria and is useful in treating serious infections caused by *Bacteroides*, *Fusobacterium*, and other anaerobic bacteria. Metronidazole, which is also effective against certain protozoa, is discussed in Chapter 35 with regard to its antiprotozoal effects. Common side effects associated with metronidazole include gastrointestinal distress (nausea, diarrhea), allergic reactions (such as rashes), and CNS symptoms (confusion, dizziness, mood changes). This drug may also cause peripheral neuropathies as indicated by numbness and tingling in the hands and feet.

Rifampin

Rifampin (Rifadin, Rimactane) directly impairs DNA replication by binding to and inhibiting the DNA-dependent RNA polymerase enzyme in susceptible bacteria. This enzyme initiates the replication of genetic material by generating the formation of RNA strands from the DNA template. By inhibiting this enzyme, rifampin blocks RNA chain synthesis and subsequent replication of the nucleic acid code in bacterial cells.

Rifampin is effective against many gram-negative and gram-positive bacteria and is also one of the principal agents used in the treatment of tuberculosis and leprosy. Typically, this drug is combined with another agent, such as rifampin plus dapsone for leprosy, or rifampin plus isoniazid for tuberculosis, to increase effectiveness and prevent the development of resistance to rifampin. Rifampin is also used in combination with erythromycin to treat legionnaires' disease and certain forms of meningitis (see Tables 33–3a to 33–3d).

Common adverse effects with rifampin include gastrointestinal distress (nausea, vomiting, stomach cramps) and various hypersensitivity reactions (rashes and fever). Disturbances in liver function have also been noted, and serious hepatic abnormalities may occur in patients with pre-existing liver disease.

Sulfonamides

The sulfonamides include a number of agents such as sulfadiazine, sulfamethizole, and similar agents (see Table 33–5). Sulfonamides interfere with bacterial nucleic acid production by disrupting folic acid synthesis in susceptible bacteria. Sulfonamide drugs are structurally similar to PABA, which is the substance used in the first step of folic acid synthesis in certain types of bacteria (see Fig. 33–2). Sulfonamides either directly inhibit the enzyme responsible for PABA utilization or become a substitute for PABA and result in the abnormal synthesis of folic acid. In either case, folic acid synthesis is reduced and bacterial nucleic acid synthesis is impaired.

Sulfonamides have the potential to be used against a wide variety of bacteria including gram-negative and gram-positive bacilli and cocci. The development of resistance in various bacteria, however, has limited the use of these drugs somewhat. Currently, sulfonamides are used systemically to treat certain urinary tract infections and infections caused by *Nocardia* bacteria (see Tables 33–3a to 33–3d). Sulfonamides may also be applied topically to treat vaginal infections, burns, ophthalmic conditions, and other local infections.

The problems encountered most frequently with sulfonamide drugs include gastrointestinal distress, increased sensitivity of the skin to ultraviolet light, and allergic reactions. Fairly serious disturbances in the formed blood elements, including blood dyscrasias such as agranulocytosis and hemolytic anemia, may also occur during systemic sulfonamide therapy.

Trimethoprim

Trimethoprim (Proloprim, Trimpex) interferes with the bacterial folic acid pathway by inhibiting the dihydrofolate reductase enzyme in susceptible bacteria (see Fig. 33–2). This enzyme converts dihydrofolic acid to tetrahydrofolic acid during the biosynthesis of folic acid cofactors. By inhibiting this enzyme, trimethoprim directly interferes with the production of folic acid cofactors, and subsequent production of vital bacterial nucleic acids is impaired.

Trimethoprim is effective against several gram-negative bacilli including *E coli, Enterobacter, Proteus mirabilis,* and *Klebsiella.* Trimethoprim is used primarily in the treatment of urinary tract infections caused by these and other susceptible bacteria (see Tables 33–3a to 33–3d). Trimethoprim is frequently used in combination with the sulfonamide drug sulfamethoxazole.[26] Primary adverse effects associated with trimethoprim include headache, skin rashes/itching, decreased appetite, an unusual taste in the mouth, and gastrointestinal problems (nausea, vomiting, diarrhea).

OTHER ANTIBACTERIAL DRUGS

Several other antibacterial drugs work by mechanisms that are either unknown or are different from the classical antibacterial mechanisms described previously. These drugs are discussed individually here.

Capreomycin

Capreomycin (Capastat) is used as an adjunct or alternative drug in the treatment of tuberculosis. The mechanism of action of this drug is unknown. The primary problems associated with this drug include ototoxicity and nephrotoxicity.

Isoniazid

Isoniazid (INH, Nydrazid, other names) is one of the primary drugs used to treat tuberculosis. Although the exact mechanism of action is unknown, this drug appears to interfere with several enzymatic pathways involving protein, lipid, carbohydrate, and nucleic acid metabolism in susceptible bacteria. Adverse reactions to isoniazid are fairly common, and patients may develop disorders such as hepatitis and peripheral neuropathies.

Methenamine

Methenamine (Hiprex, Mandelamine, Urex) exerts antibacterial properties in a rather unique fashion. In an acidic environment, this drug decomposes into formaldehyde and ammonia. Formaldehyde is bactericidal to almost all bacteria, and bacteria do not develop resistance to this toxin. This mechanism enables methenamine to be especially useful in treating urinary tract infections, because the presence of this drug in acidic urine facilitates the release of formaldehyde at the site of infection (i.e., within the urinary tract). Use of methenamine is fairly safe, although high doses are associated with gastrointestinal upset and problems with urination (bloody urine, pain while urinating).

Pyrazinamide

Pyrazinamide (PZA) is used primarily as an adjunct to other drugs in treating tuberculosis. The mechanism of action of this drug against *M tuberculosis* is unknown. Problems associated with pyrazinamide include hepatotoxicity and lower-extremity joint pain.

Nitrofurantoin

Nitrofurantoin (Furalan, Macrodantin, others) is reduced by bacterial enzymes to a metabolite that is toxic to the bacterial cell. This toxic metabolite inhibits bacterial metabolic function by interfering with ribosomal function and other molecules involved in energy production and utilization in the bacterial cell. Nitrofurantoin is primarily used to treat urinary tract infections caused by a number of gram-negative and some gram-positive bacteria. Adverse effects associated with this drug include gastrointestinal distress (nausea, vomiting, diarrhea) and neurotoxicity (as indicated by headache, numbness, and excessive fatigue). Acute pneumonitis (as indicated by coughing, chills, fever, and difficulty breathing) may also occur soon after nitrofurantoin is initiated. This pneumonitis appears to be a direct chemical effect of the drug and usually disappears within hours after the drug is withdrawn.

CLINICAL USE OF ANTIBACTERIAL DRUGS: RELATIONSHIP TO SPECIFIC BACTERIAL INFECTIONS

There is an incredible array of antibacterial agents currently in clinical use. As mentioned previously, selection of a particular agent is based on the effectiveness of the drug against a range or spectrum of different bacteria. The clinical application of antibacterial drugs according to their effectiveness against specific bacteria is summarized in Tables 33–3a to 33–3d. As these tables indicate, various antibacterial drugs can serve as either the primary or alternative agents against specific bacterial infections. The actual selection of an antibacterial agent is often highly variable, depending on the particular patient, the type and location of the infection, the experience of the physician, and many other factors.

RESISTANCE TO ANTIBACTERIAL DRUGS

One of the most serious problems of antibacterial therapy is the potential for development of strains of bacteria that are resistant to one or more antibacterial agents.[19] Certain bacterial strains have a natural or acquired defense mechanism against specific antibacterial drugs. This enables the strain to survive the effects of the drug and continue to grow and reproduce similar resistant strains, thus representing a genetic selection process, where only the resistant strains survive the drug. As a result, bacteria that are invulnerable to the drug can breed. If other drugs are not effective against the resistant strain, or if cross-resistance to several antibacterial drugs occurs, the resistant bacteria become especially dangerous because of immunity from antibacterial chemotherapy.[30]

Bacterial resistance can occur as a result of several mechanisms.[4,19] Certain bacterial strains may be able to enzymatically destroy the antibacterial drug. The best example is the penicillinase enzyme that is found in penicillin-resistant bacteria. As previously discussed, this enzyme destroys certain penicillins such as the naturally occurring drugs (penicillin G and V). Resistance may also occur because of a defect in the intracellular binding of the antibacterial drug. For instance, penicillins, aminoglycosides, and other drugs must bind to intracellular proteins, ribosomes, and the like to exert their effect. Differences in the affinity of these binding sites may be acquired by bacterial mutation, thus decreasing the effectiveness of the drug. Bacteria may also develop resistance by decreasing the drug's ability to penetrate the bacterial cell. Most drugs must first penetrate the cell membrane and enter the bacterial cell to exert their bactericidal effects. Specific bacteria that have a natural or acquired opposition to drug penetration will render the drug useless, thus leading to the development of resistant strains. A combination of these and other factors may also be responsible for mediating the formation of bacterial resistance.

Consequently, bacterial resistance to penicillins, aminoglycosides, tetracyclines, and other antibacterial agents is a very serious problem in contemporary drug therapy.[5,6,12,36] In addition, the number of resistant bacterial strains continues to progressively increase in certain institutions.[9] To limit the development of resistant strains, antibacterial drugs should be used judiciously and not overused. For instance, the effort to perform culture and sensitivity tests on sputum, blood, and so on is worthwhile because the pathogenic bacteria can be identified and fairly selective agents can be used. Administering selective agents as opposed to broad-spectrum antibiotics may help attenuate and kill resistant strains more effectively. The selective use of current antibacterial drugs and the development of new bactericidal agents are needed to help control the problem of bacterial resistance.

SPECIAL CONCERNS IN REHABILITATION PATIENTS

Patients undergoing physical therapy and occupational therapy will be taking antibacterial drugs for any number of reasons. Antibacterial drugs may be administered to prevent or treat infection in conditions relating directly to the rehabilitation program. For instance, therapists are often involved with administering topical antibacterial agents (e.g., sulfadiazine) to patients with burns. Infection in other conditions that relate to rehabilitation, such as bone infections (osteomyelitis), infections sustained from trauma and various wounds, and infections following joint replacement and other types of surgery, will also require antibacterial therapy. Other types of infection not directly related to rehabilitation (e.g., urinary tract infection, pneumonia) are also very common, frequently occurring in hospitalized patients as well as in outpatients receiving physical therapy and occupational therapy. Consequently, therapists will routinely be working with patients who are undergoing antibacterial treatment.

Therapists should generally be aware of the possible adverse effects of antibacterial drugs. Many of these agents have the potential to cause hypersensitivity reactions including skin rashes, itching, and respiratory difficulty (such as wheezing). Therapists may help recognize the onset of such reactions when working with these patients. Other common side effects including gastrointestinal problems (nausea, vomiting, diarrhea) are usually not serious but may be bothersome if they continually interrupt physical therapy and occupational therapy. Therapists may have to alter the time of the rehabilitation session to work around these effects, especially if gastrointestinal and similar annoying side effects tend to occur at a specific time of the day (e.g., early morning, late afternoon).

Certain agents may have adverse effects that will directly interact with specific rehabilitation treatments. In particular, tetracyclines, sulfonamides, and fluoroquinolones (ciprofloxacin, norfloxacin, etc.) cause increased sensitivity of the skin to ultraviolet light. This problem is obvious if ultraviolet treatments are being administered by the therapist. Therapists must be especially careful to establish an accurate minimal erythemal dosage to ultraviolet light. Therapists should also be prepared to adjust the ultraviolet light treatments in accordance with changes in dosage of the antibacterial drug.

Finally, therapists play a vital role in helping prevent the spread of bacterial and other infections. Therapists must maintain appropriate sterile technique when dealing with open wounds. Adequate sterilization of whirlpools using strong disinfectants is also critical in preventing the spread of infection from patient to patient in a rehabilitation setting. Therapists must also recognize the importance of hand washing in preventing the spread of infection and must not neglect to wash their own hands between patients.

CASE STUDY

ANTIBACTERIAL DRUGS

Brief History. J.B. is a 40-year-old former truck driver who was injured in a traffic accident 5 years ago, sustaining a spinal cord transection that resulted in complete paraplegia at the L1-2 level. He underwent extensive physical rehabilitation, including vocational retraining, and had recently been working as a computer programmer when he began to develop a pressure sore in the region of the right ischial tuberosity. Despite conservative management, the pressure sore developed into a decubitus ulcer. Because the patient was in relatively good health otherwise, the decubitus was treated surgically by local debridement and reconstructive surgery using skin flaps. The patient was admitted to the hospital, and a routine preoperative culture of the ulcer revealed the presence of *E coli*. The patient had a history of sensitivity to penicillin drugs and was therefore given a tetracycline antibiotic (Tetracyn, 250 mg orally every 6 hours) to resolve the infection prior to surgery. Physical therapy and occupational therapy were also requested to help maintain the patient's upper body strength and functional activity while awaiting surgery. The physical therapist also suggested that ultraviolet radiation might be helpful in resolving the infection.

Problem/Influence of Medication. Tetracyclines and several other antibacterial agents increase the sensitivity of the skin to ultraviolet light.

Decision/Solution. The therapist carefully determined the minimal erythemal dosage in the patient prior to initiating ultraviolet treatments. Also, using careful draping techniques, the therapist confined the treatment to the ulcer site, so that a minimum of the surrounding skin was exposed to the ultraviolet light. This approach ensured that the surrounding tissues would not be endangered if the patient's response to the ultraviolet treatment changed during the course of tetracycline treatment. The combination of drug therapy and ultraviolet radiation quickly resolved the infection, allowing the surgery to proceed as planned.

SUMMARY

Antibacterial drugs are used to prevent and treat infection in a variety of clinical situations. Some drugs are effective against a fairly limited number of bacteria (narrow-spectrum), whereas other agents may be used against a relatively wide variety of bacterial pathogens (broad-spectrum). Specific agents may exert their antibacterial effects by inhibiting bacterial cell wall synthesis and function, inhibiting either bacterial protein synthesis or bacterial DNA/RNA synthesis and function. Although most bacterial infections can be effectively treated with one or more agents, the development of bacterial strains that are resistant to drug therapy continues to be a serious problem. Rehabilitation specialists will routinely treat patients receiving antibacterial drugs for conditions that are directly or indirectly related to the need for physical therapy and occupational therapy. Therapists should be cognizant of the potential side effects of these drugs and how these drugs may interfere with specific physical therapy and occupational therapy procedures.

REFERENCES

1. Barza, M: Imipenem: First of a new class of beta-lactam antibiotics. Ann Intern Med 103:552, 1985.
2. Birnbaum, J, et al: Carbapenems, a new class of beta-lactam antibiotics. Am J Med 78 (suppl 6A):3, 1985.
3. Brisson-Noel, A, Trieu-Cuot, P, and Courvalin, P: Mechanism of action of spiramycin and other macrolides. J Antimicrob Chemother 22(suppl B):13, 1988.
4. Bryan, LE: General mechanisms of resistance to antibiotics. J Antimicrob Chemother 22(suppl A):1, 1988.
5. Buu-Hoi, AY, Goldstein, FW, and Acar, JF: A seventeen year epidemiological survey of antimicrobial resistance in pneumococci in 2 hospitals. J Antimicrob Chemother 22(suppl B):41, 1988.
6. Carpenter, JL, et al: Antituberculosis drug resistance in south Texas. Annu Rev Respir Dis 128:1055, 1983.
7. Cheung, RPF and DiPiro, JT: Vancomycin: An update. Pharmacotherapy 6:153, 1986.
8. Clissold, SP, Todd, PA, and Campoli-Richards, DM: Imipenem/cilastatin: A review of its antibacterial activity, pharmacokinetic properties, and therapeutic efficacy. Drugs 33:183, 1987.
9. Cross, AS, Opal, S, and Kopecko, DJ: Progressive increase in antibiotic resistance of gram-negative bacterial isolates: Walter Reed Hospital, 1976–1980. Specific analysis of gentamicin, tobramycin, and amikacin resistances. Arch Intern Med 143:2075, 1983.
10. Davies, BD: The lethal action of aminoglycosides. J Antimicrob Chemother 22:1, 1988.
11. Davies, BD: Mechanism of bactericidal action of aminoglycosides. Microbiol Rev 51:341, 1987.
12. Duval, J: Evolution and epidemiology of MLS resistance. J Antimicrob Chemother 16(suppl A):137, 1985.
13. Freeman, BA: Textbook of Microbiology, ed 26. WB Saunders, Philadelphia, 1985.
14. Gale, EF, et al: The Molecular Basis of Antibiotic Action, ed 2. Wiley and Sons, New York, 1982.
15. Hancock, REW: Alterations in outer membrane permeability. Annu Rev Microbiol 38:327, 1984.
16. Harvey, RJ: Synergism in the folate pathway. Rev Infect Dis 4:255, 1982.
17. Hooper, DC and Wolfson, JS: Drug therapy: Fluoroquinolone antimicrobial agents. N Engl J Med 324:384, 1991.
18. Humbert, G, et al: Aminoglycosides. Semin Hop 62:1985, 1986.
19. Jacoby, GA and Archer, GL: Mechanisms of disease: New mechanisms of bacterial resistance to antimicrobial agents. N Engl J Med 324:601, 1991.
20. John, JF: What price success? The continuing saga of the toxic:therapeutic ratio in the use of aminoglycoside antibiotics. J Infect Dis 158:1, 1988.
21. Koch, AL: Biophysics of bacterial walls viewed as stress-bearing fabric. Microbiol Rev 52:337, 1988.
22. Menninger, JR: Functional consequences of binding macrolides to ribosomes. J Antimicrob Chemother 16(suppl A):23, 1985.
23. Merlin, TL, Gibson, DW, and Connor, DH: Infectious and parasitic diseases. In Rubin, E and Farber, JL (eds): Pathology, ed 2. JB Lippincott, Philadelphia, 1994.
24. Neu, HC: Relation of structural properties of beta-lactam antibiotics to antibacterial activity. Am J Med 79(suppl 2A):2, 1985.
25. Nikaido, H and Vaara, M: Molecular basis of bacterial outer membrane permeability. Microbiol Rev 49:1, 1985.
26. Quintilani, R, Levitz, RE, and Nightingale, CH: Potential role of trimethoprim-sulfamethoxazole in the treatment of serious hospital-acquired bacterial infections. Rev Infect Dis 9(suppl 2):S160, 1987.
27. Reynolds, PE: Inhibitors of bacterial cell wall synthesis. Symp Soc Gen Microbiol 38:13, 1985.
28. Rosenkrantz, HS: Chloramphenicol: Magic bullet or double-edge sword. Mutat Res 196:1, 1988.
29. Scully, BE: Pharmacology of the fluoroquinolones. Urology 35(suppl 1):8, 1990.
30. Seppala, H, et al: Resistance to erythromycin in group A streptococci. N Engl J Med 326:292, 1992.
31. Siegenthaler, WE, Bonetti, A, and Luthy, R: Aminoglycoside antibiotics in infectious diseases: An overview. Am J Med 80(suppl 6B):2, 1986.
32. Smith, JT: The mode of action of quinolone antibacterials. Infection 14(suppl 1):S3, 1986.
33. Tomasz, A: Penicillin-binding proteins and the antibacterial effectiveness of beta-lactam antibiotics. Rev Infect Dis 8(suppl):S260, 1986.
34. von Lichtenberg, F: Infectious diseases. In Robbins, SL, Cotran, RS, and Kumar, V (eds): Pathological Basis of Disease, ed 3. WB Saunders, Philadelphia, 1984.
35. Wolin, MJ and Miller, TL: Bacterial metabolism. In Freeman, BA: Textbook of Microbiology, ed 26. WB Saunders, Philadelphia, 1985.
36. Young, LS and Hindler, J: Aminoglycoside resistance: A worldwide perspective. Am J Med 80(suppl 6B):15, 1986.

CHAPTER 34

Treatment of Infections II: Antiviral Drugs

A virus is one of the smallest microorganisms, consisting only of a nucleic acid core surrounded by a protein shell. Several types of viruses commonly infect human cells and are responsible for a diverse range of pathologies. Viral infections extend from relatively mild disorders such as the common cold to serious, life-threatening conditions such as AIDS. Viruses are somewhat unique in that they must rely totally on the metabolic processes of the host (human) cell to function. Hence, the pharmacologic treatment of viral infections is complex, because selective destruction of the virus without destroying human cells is often difficult.

This chapter describes the basic characteristics of viruses and the relatively limited number of drugs that can act selectively as antiviral agents. Methods of preventing viral infections (antiviral vaccines) are also briefly discussed. Finally, the current methods of treating a specific viral-induced disease, AIDS, are presented. Rehabilitation specialists will often be treating patients who are in the active stages of viral infection as well as those suffering from the sequelae of viral disorders such as gastroenteritis, encephalitis, and influenza. Hence, the pharmacotherapeutic treatment and prophylaxis of viral infections should concern physical therapists and occupational therapists.

VIRAL STRUCTURE AND FUNCTION

Classification of Viruses

Viruses are classified according to several criteria including physical, biochemical, and pathogenic characteristics.[1,15,16] The classification of some of the more common viruses affecting humans and their associated diseases are listed in Table 34–1. This table shows that viruses can basically be divided into two categories, depending on the type of genetic material contained in the virus (DNA or RNA viruses). Families within each major subdivision are classified according to physical characteristics (con-

TABLE 34-1 Common Viruses Affecting Humans

Family	Virus	Related Infections
DNA viruses		
Adenoviridae	Adenovirus, types 1-33	Respiratory tract and eye infections
Hepatitis B	Hepatitis B virus	Hepatitis B
Herpesviridae	Cytomegalovirus	Cytomegalic inclusion disease (i.e., widespread involvement of virtually any organ, especially the brain, liver, lung, kidney, and intestine)
	Epstein-Barr virus	Infectious mononucleosis
	Herpes simplex, types 1 and 2	Local infections of oral, genital, and other mucocutaneous areas; systemic infections
	Varicella-zoster virus	Chickenpox; herpes zoster (shingles); other systemic infections
Poxviridae	Smallpox virus	Smallpox
RNA viruses		
Arenaviridae	Human respiratory virus	Respiratory tract infection
Hepatitis A	Hepatitis A virus	Hepatitis A
Orthomyxoviridae	*Influenzavirus*, types A, B, and C	Influenza
Paramyxoviridae	Measles virus	Measles
	Mumps virus	Mumps
	Respiratory syncytial virus	Respiratory tract infection in children
Picornaviridae	Polioviruses	Poliomyelitis
	Rhinovirus, types 1-89	Common cold
Retroviridae	Human immunodeficiency virus	(HIV) AIDS
Rhabdoviridae	Rabies virus	Rabies
Togaviridae	*Alphavirus*	Encephalitis
	Rubella virus	Rubella

figuration of the genetic material, shape of the virus capsule) and other functional criteria.

Characteristics of Viruses

Viruses are somewhat unique in structure and function when compared with other microorganisms. The basic components of viral microorganisms are illustrated in Figure 34-1. A virus essentially consists of a core of viral DNA or RNA.[16] The genetic core is surrounded by a protein shell, or *capsid*. This structure consisting of the capsid enclosing the nucleic acid core is referred to as the *nucleocapsid*. In some viruses, the nucleocapsid is also surrounded by a viral membrane, or envelope, which is composed of glycoproteins extending outward from a lipid bilayer.

The virus, however, does not contain any of the cellular components necessary to replicate itself or synthesize proteins and other macromolecules; that is, the virus lacks ribosomes, endoplasmic reticulum, and so on.[16] The virus only contains the genetic code (viral genome) that will produce additional viruses. To replicate itself, the virus must rely on the biochemical machinery of the host cell.[15] In essence, the virus invades the host cell, takes control of the cell's metabolic function, and uses the macromolecular-synthesizing apparatus of the host cell to crank out new viruses. Specific steps in the viral replication process are described in the next section.

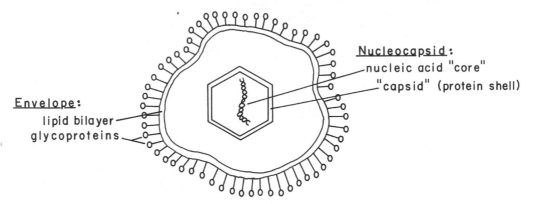

FIGURE 34–1. Basic components of a virus. Note the relative lack of most cellular organelles (ribosomes, endoplasmic reticulum, etc.).

Viral Replication

Self-replication of a virus occurs in several distinct steps.[16] These steps include (1) adsorption, (2) penetration and uncoating, (3) biosynthesis, and (4) maturation and release. These four basic steps are illustrated in Figure 34–2. Each step is also briefly discussed here.

Adsorption. Initially, the virus attaches or adsorbs to the surface of the host cell. Most viruses are attracted to the host cell because of the interaction between proteins on the outer surface of the virus and receptor-like proteins on the host-cell membrane. The interaction of the virus with these surface proteins causes the virus to adhere to the outer surface of the host-cell membrane.

Penetration and Uncoating. The virus enters the host cell either by passing directly through the cell membrane or by fusing with the host-cell membrane and releasing the viral genetic material into the host cell. Once inside the host cell, any coating that remains on the virus is removed, usually by proteolytic enzymes of the host cell.

Biosynthesis. When the viral genetic material is released within the host cell, the virus takes control of the cell's molecular synthesizing machinery to initiate the biosynthesis of new viral enzymes and proteins. Different viruses exert their effects on the host cell in different ways, but many viruses control the host cell through a direct effect on the cell's nucleus. Some viruses, including the virus that causes AIDS, actually insert their genetic material directly into the host cell's DNA, thereby becoming integrated within the genetic control of the infected cell.

Regardless of the exact mechanism of infection, the virus essentially commands the cell to synthesize enzymes that produce more copies of the viral DNA or RNA and to synthesize structural proteins that will ultimately be used to form new viral shells or capsids. Thus, the virus uses the biosynthetic machinery as well as the structural components and nutrients of the cell (amino acids, nucleic acids, etc.) to replicate itself. Likewise, the virus often incapacitates the cell so that the infected cell cannot carry out its normal physiologic activities.

Maturation and Release. The component parts of the virus (the genetic core and surrounding shell) are assembled into mature viruses and released from the host cell. In some cases the virus may be released by a process of exocytosis, leaving the host cell relatively intact (although still infected with the original virus). Alternatively, the host

FIGURE 34-2. Basic sequence of viral replication. See text for details.

cell may simply be destroyed (undergo lysis), thus releasing the viral offspring. Lysis of the host cell not only results in release of the virus and death of the cell but may also stimulate the production of inflammatory mediators (prostaglandins, kinins, etc.), which create a hypersensitivity response.

The steps involved in viral replication are important pharmacologically because antiviral drugs may help interrupt this process at one or more of the steps. Specific agents that are currently used as antiviral drugs and their pharmacodynamic aspects are discussed next.

SPECIFIC ANTIVIRAL DRUGS

The primary agents that are approved for use as antiviral drugs are listed in Table 34-2. Each agent is also briefly discussed below.

Acyclovir

Antiviral Efficacy and Clinical Use. Acyclovir (Zovirax) is effective against herpesvirus infections, especially those involving herpes simplex types I and II.[3,29,46,48,66] Acyclovir is the principal drug used to treat genital herpes and herpes simplex–

TABLE 34–2 Antiviral Drugs

Generic Name	Trade Name(s)	Principal Indication(s)
Acyclovir	Zovirax	Treatment of initial and recurrent herpesvirus infections (especially herpes simplex–related infections)
Amantadine	Symadine, Symmetrel	Prevention and treatment of influenza A infections (also used as an antiparkinsonism drug; see Chapter 10)
Didanosine	Videx	Treatment of human immunodeficiency (HIV) infection
Foscarnet	Foscavir	Treatment of cytomegalovirus (CMV) retinitis and other CMV and herpes virus infections in immuno-compromised patients
Ganciclovir	Cytovene	Treatment of CMV infections in immunocompromised patients
Ribavirin	Virazole	Treatment of severe viral pneumonia caused by respiratory syncytial virus in infants and young children
Vidarabine	Vira-A	Treatment of herpesvirus infections including systemic infections caused by herpes simplex, cytomegalovirus, and varicella zoster
Zalcitabine	HIVID	Treatment of HIV infection
Zidovudine	Retrovir	Treatment of HIV infection

related infections in other mucosal and cutaneous areas (lips and face).[13,29] Acyclovir is also effective against other members of the herpesvirus family including varicella-zoster and Epstein-Barr virus.[5,66] This agent may be used to treat varicella-zoster–related infections such as herpes zoster and chickenpox. Epstein-Barr virus infections including infectious mononucleosis may also respond to acyclovir.

Acyclovir can be applied topically as a cream to treat cutaneous and mucosal infections. This drug can also be administered systemically by the oral route or by intravenous administration in severe, acute infections.

Mechanism of Action. Acyclovir inhibits viral DNA replication by inhibiting the function of the DNA polymerase enzyme.[13–15] This drug is taken into virus-infected cells and converted to acyclovir triphosphate by an enzyme known as viral thymidine kinase.[30] The phosphorylated drug directly inhibits the function of the viral DNA polymerase, thus impairing the replication of viral genetic material. The virus also incorporates the drug into viral DNA strands, thus halting further production of DNA because of the presence of a false nucleic acid.[14]

The antiviral specificity of acyclovir is due to the much higher affinity of this drug for viral DNA polymerase rather than the analogous enzyme in human cells.[15] Also, the first step in the phosphorylation of acyclovir is greatly accelerated in virus-infected cells versus healthy cells. Hence, the amount of the activated (phosphorylated) form of acyclovir is much greater in the cells that really need it, that is, cells infected with the virus.

Adverse Effects. Topical application of acyclovir may produce local irritation of cutaneous and mucosal tissues. Prolonged systemic administration may cause headaches, dizziness, skin rashes, and gastrointestinal problems (nausea, vomiting, and diarrhea).

Amantadine

Antiviral Efficacy and Clinical Use. Amantadine (Symadine, Symmetrel) is used in the prevention and treatment of infections caused by the influenza A virus. This drug appears to be approximately 50 percent effective in preventing influenza A infections.[46] Also, amantadine is 70 to 100 percent effective in decreasing the severity of illness caused by influenza A virus.[5,46] As discussed in Chapter 10, amantadine is also effective in alleviating some of the motor abnormalities of Parkinson's disease. It is not exactly clear, however, why this antiviral agent is effective in treating parkinsonism.

Amantadine is administered to individuals already infected with influenza A to lessen the extent of the illness associated with this virus. Amantadine is also given prophylactically to individuals who may have been exposed to influenza A and to high-risk patients such as the elderly or patients with cardiopulmonary and other diseases. This drug is typically administered orally, either in capsule form or in a syrup preparation.

Mechanism of Action. The exact mechanism of amantadine's antiviral action is not fully understood. This drug appears to block the penetration of the influenza A virus into host cells.[16,30] Amantadine may also interfere with the uncoating of the virus and release of viral nucleic acid within the host cell.

Adverse Effects. Amantadine may produce CNS symptoms such as confusion, loss of concentration, mood changes, nervousness, dizziness, and light-headedness. These symptoms may be especially problematic in elderly patients. Excessive doses of amantadine may increase the severity of these CNS symptoms, and overdose may cause seizures.

Didanosine

Antiviral Efficacy and Clinical Use. Didanosine (Videx), also known as dideoxyinosine or ddI, is one of the three primary drugs currently used to slow the progression of HIV infection.[27,35] Didanosine, which was developed as an alternative to zidovudine, is typically used in patients who do not tolerate zidovudine or in cases where zidovudine is ineffective in controlling HIV infection.[27,33] Alternatively, didanosine and zidovudine can be given simultaneously, and the combination of these two anti-HIV drugs may provide the best treatment of some patients who are infected with HIV.[10]

Mechanism of Action. Didanosine is a reverse transcriptase inhibitor, meaning that this drug inhibits the enzyme that converts viral RNA to viral DNA (*reverse transcription*) (Fig. 34–3). Reverse transcription is one of the first steps needed for replication of HIV within host cells, and drugs that block this step help prevent HIV replication and proliferation. Through this action, didanosine and similar anti-HIV drugs may help delay the progression of HIV infection to full-blown AIDS.

Adverse Effects. Peripheral neuropathies and pancreatitis are fairly common side effects, especially when higher doses of didanosine are given.[11] Blood dyscrasias such as anemia, leukopenia, and thrombocytopenia can occur, especially if hematologic function has already been impaired by HIV infection. Other side effects associated with didanosine include CNS toxicity (headache, irritability, insomnia) and gastrointestinal disturbances (nausea, diarrhea).

FIGURE 34–3. Schematic illustration of HIV replication and the site of action of the anti-HIV drugs zidovudine, didanosine, and zalcitabine. These drugs interfere with the process of reverse transcription by inhibiting the enzyme that converts viral RNA (vRNA) to viral DNA (vDNA). See text for further discussion.

Foscarnet

Antiviral Efficacy and Clinical Use. Foscarnet (Foscavir) is primarily given to treat cytomegalovirus (CMV) retinitis in patients with AIDS. This agent may also help control other infections in patients with a compromised immune system, including serious cytomegaloviral infections (pneumonia, gastrointestinal infections) and some herpesvirus infections (herpes simplex, varicella-zoster).

Mechanism of Action. Foscarnet works somewhat like acyclovir and ganciclovir; that is, foscarnet inhibits the DNA polymerase enzyme necessary for viral DNA replication. Foscarnet differs from these other antiviral drugs, however, in that it does not require phosphorylation (activation) by enzymes such as viral thymidine kinase. Certain strains of viruses are thymidine-kinase deficient, meaning that these viruses lack the enzyme needed to activate antiviral agents such as acyclovir and ganciclovir. Hence, foscarnet is often used in patients who exhibit these thymidine-kinase–resistant viruses and do not respond to acyclovir or ganciclovir.

Adverse Effects. The primary problem associated with foscarnet is impaired renal function including acute tubular necrosis. Hematologic disorders (anemia, granulocytopenia, leukopenia), gastrointestinal disturbances (cramps, nausea, vomiting), and CNS toxicity (confusion, dizziness) may also occur during foscarnet treatment.

Ganciclovir

Antiviral Efficacy and Clinical Use. Ganciclovir (Cytovene) is given primarily to patients with AIDS to help treat problems related to CMV infection, including CMV retinitis, polyradiculopathy, and other systemic CMV infections.

Mechanism of Action. Ganciclovir works like acyclovir; these drugs both inhibit viral DNA replication by inhibiting DNA polymerase activity and by halting elongation of viral DNA chains.

Adverse Effects. The most serious problems associated with ganciclovir are anemia, granulocytopenia, thrombocytopenia, and related hematologic disorders. Ganciclovir may also cause gastrointestinal disturbances (anorexia, nausea) and CNS disturbances (mood changes, nervousness, tremor).

Ribavirin

Antiviral Efficacy and Clinical Use. Ribavirin (Virazole) is active against several RNA and DNA viruses, including respiratory syncytial virus (RSV).[5,46] Clinically, this drug is used to treat severe RSV pneumonia in infants and young children. Ribavirin may also be useful as a secondary agent in the treatment of influenza A and B in young adults.

Ribavirin is administered through oral inhalation. This drug is suspended in an aerosol form and administered to the patient by a mechanical aerosol generator and some sort of ventilation mask, mouthpiece, or hood.

Mechanism of Action. The mechanism of action of this drug is not fully understood. Ribavirin appears to impair viral messenger RNA synthesis, probably by selectively inhibiting enzymes responsible for RNA replication.[5,15] Inadequate viral mRNA production leads to impaired viral protein synthesis, which ultimately curtails viral replication.

Adverse Effects. Ribavirin produces relatively few adverse effects when administered by inhalation. Most of the drug's action is confined to local pulmonary tissues, and severe systemic effects are rare. One side effect that may occur is local irritation of the eyes (conjunctivitis) because of direct contact of the aerosol with the eyes. This occurrence may be a problem if the drug is administered via some sort of hood or tent that encloses the patient's entire head.

Vidarabine

Antiviral Efficacy and Clinical Use. Vidarabine (Vira-A) is effective against several members of the herpesvirus family, including CMV, herpes simplex virus, and varicella-zoster virus.[15] Clinically, this drug is used to treat systemic infections caused by these viruses including herpes simplex encephalitis, neonatal herpes simplex, and herpes zoster.[5] For treatment of systemic infections, vidarabine is usually administered by continuous intravenous infusion. This drug may also be applied by ophthalmic ointment to treat susceptible viral infections of the eye (e.g., herpes simplex keratoconjunctivitis).

Mechanism of Action. Vidarabine appears to exert its antiviral effects in a manner similar to acyclovir (see "Acyclovir"). Both drugs selectively inhibit viral enzymes that are responsible for viral DNA replication.[15]

Adverse Effects. The primary problems associated with systemic administration of vidarabine include gastrointestinal distress (nausea, vomiting, diarrhea) and CNS disturbances (dizziness, hallucinations, mood changes). Ophthalmic application may produce local irritation (itching, redness, swelling) in some individuals.

Zalcitabine

Antiviral Efficacy and Clinical Use. Zalcitabine (HIVID) is indicated for treatment of HIV infection. This agent is similar to other anti-HIV drugs (didanosine, zidovudine), but zalcitabine is typically reserved for patients with advanced cases of AIDS who begin to deteriorate despite treatment with zidovudine.[27] Zalcitabine is often combined with zidovudine,[27] or possibly alternated with zidovudine to provide the best anti-HIV effects with a lower incidence of toxicity and resistance.[58]

Mechanism of Action. Like other anti-HIV drugs, zalcitabine inhibits the reverse transcriptase enzyme that converts viral RNA to viral DNA (see Fig. 34–3). This action helps attenuate replication and proliferation of HIV and, it is hoped, will delay the progression of AIDS.

Adverse Effects. Side effects associated with zalcitabine are similar to those seen with didanosine. Peripheral neuropathies and pancreatitis are the primary adverse effects; other side effects include CNS toxicity, gastrointestinal disturbances, and hematologic disorders.

Zidovudine

Antiviral Efficacy and Clinical Use. Zidovudine (Retrovir), also known generically as azidothymidine or AZT, was the first drug approved for treating people who are infected with HIV.[27,60] Although this drug does not kill HIV, zidovudine appears to inhibit HIV replication and prolong the time before patients with HIV infection succumb to full-blown AIDS.[12] Likewise, the survival rate of patients with AIDS seems to be increased when zidovudine is given.[20,28,38,44] Treatment of AIDS using zidovudine and similar drugs (didanosine, zalcitabine) is discussed in more detail in "HIV and the Treatment of AIDS."

Mechanism of Action. Zidovudine inhibits HIV replication by inhibiting the reverse transcriptase enzyme that is needed to convert viral RNA to viral DNA (see Fig. 34–3). Specifically, zidovudine enters viral-infected cells, where it is progressively phosphorylated (activated) by various intracellular enzymes.[22] The phosphorylated version of this drug then acts as a false nucleic acid that competes with the real nucleic acid (thymidine) for incorporation into growing viral DNA strands. This competition slows down the reverse transcriptase enzyme because the enzyme cannot handle the false nucleic acid (zidovudine) as easily as the real nucleic acid (thymidine). Even if the reverse transcriptase is successful in incorporating zidovudine into viral DNA strands, this action prematurely terminates DNA strand synthesis because a false nucleic acid has been added to the viral DNA instead of the real nucleic acid. Thus, zidovudine impairs the ability of the virus to replicate and infect additional cells by slowing down the reverse transcriptase enzyme and halting the synthesis of viral DNA strands produced by this enzyme.

Adverse Effects. The most common problems associated with zidovudine are blood dyscrasias such as anemia and granulocytopenia. Other symptoms that may occur during zidovudine administration include fever, chills, nausea, diarrhea, dizziness, headache, and excessive fatigue. This drug may also cause myopathy as indicated by skeletal muscle tenderness, weakness, and atrophy. Considering, however, that this drug is often used in severely immunocompromised patients (such as patients with AIDS), some side effects may be caused by other sequelae of AIDS rather than directly by the effects of this drug.

CONTROLLING VIRAL INFECTION WITH VACCINES

Vaccines prevent viral infection by stimulating the endogenous production of immune factors that will selectively destroy the invading virus. Hence, the vaccine can be administered to healthy individuals to provide them with immunity from certain viral infections. Basically, a vaccine acts as an antigen that induces the immune system to generate virus-specific antibodies. The vaccine, however, does not cause any appreciable viral infection because the vaccine contains a virus that has been modified in some way so that it retains its antigenic properties, but lacks the ability to produce infection.[49] Thus, most antiviral vaccinations are accomplished by administering small amounts of the modified virus.

In general, it is somewhat easier to develop vaccines that prevent viral infection rather than develop drugs that destroy the virus once it has infected human cells. This notion is reasonable when one considers that the virus is essentially coexisting with the host cell. As indicated previously, there are currently only a limited number of drugs that are able to selectively inhibit the virus without harming the host cell. A more practical strategy is to use vaccines to enable the body to destroy the virus before an infection is established.

At present, vaccines are available for several serious viral infections including polio, smallpox, rabies, measles, mumps, rubella, hepatitis B, and influenza. In some situations, vaccination against certain viral infections is routine. For instance, schoolchildren must periodically show evidence of polio, measles, and other vaccinations according to state and local laws. In other cases, vaccines are administered prior to potential exposure to the virus, or in high-risk groups. For example, influenza vaccinations are usually not administered on a general basis but are reserved for elderly and debilitated patients during seasonal influenza outbreaks.[24,54]

Although vaccines exist for many serious viral infections, some drawbacks still exist. Some vaccines are only partially effective, and viral infection still occurs in a significant percentage of vaccinated individuals. Other vaccines require periodic readministration (boosters) to help maintain antiviral immunity. Also, certain types of viruses still lack an effective vaccination. For example, no vaccine currently exists for the HIV that causes AIDS. Hence, the improvement of existing vaccines and the development of new vaccines remain two of the more important aspects of antiviral chemotherapy.[68]

INTERFERONS

Interferons are a group of proteins that produce a number of beneficial pharmacologic and physiologic effects.[4,6,25] These agents were first recognized as endogenous substances that exert nonspecific antiviral activity; that is, interferons enable healthy cells to resist infection from a variety of viruses. Interferons produce other beneficial effects including controlling cell differentiation, limiting excessive cell proliferation, and activating certain immune processes.[25]

Human interferons are classified into three primary types: alpha, beta, and gamma (Table 34–3). Each primary type of interferon is produced by certain cells and tissues. Of these three types, alpha and beta interferons are more important in terms of

TABLE 34–3 Types of Interferons

Type	Endogenous Sources	Number of Subtypes	Physiologic/Pharmacologic Effects
Alpha	B and null lymphocytes; macrophages	15–20	Currently approved for use in certain leukemias (hairy cell, chronic myelocytic); certain neoplastic diseases (Kaposi's sarcoma, other cancers), and certain types of hepatitis
Beta	Fibroblasts; various epithelial cells	2	No current pharmacologic applications
Gamma	NK cells; T lymphocytes	1	Regulates lymphocyte proliferation/replication; used to treat infections associated with chronic granulomatous disease

antiviral activity. Gamma interferons appear to be more important in regulating certain aspects of the immune response and are responsible for promoting the growth of T lymphocytes.[36]

The possibility that interferons can be used as pharmacologic agents has aroused a great deal of interest. Recombinant DNA techniques and cell tissue cultures have been used to produce sufficient quantities of interferons for clinical drug trials. The rationale is that exogenously administered interferons will produce antiviral and other beneficial effects in healthy cells in a manner similar to their endogenously produced counterparts. Some of the pertinent aspects of interferon action and clinical applications are presented here.

Synthesis and Cellular Effects of Interferons

The basic sequence of events in the cellular production and antiviral action of interferons is illustrated in Figure 34–4. Cells that have been infected by a virus produce interferons that are subsequently released from the infected cell. These interferons then travel to noninfected cells, where they bind to specific receptors located on the surface of the healthy cells. Binding of the interferon induces the healthy cell to synthesize its own antiviral proteins. Interferons apparently direct the healthy cell to synthesize enzymes that inhibit viral messenger RNA and protein synthesis.[25] Thus, even if the virus does penetrate into the healthy cell, the virus cannot replicate because of an inability to synthesize viral proteins.

The manner in which interferons control cell growth and proliferation is not fully understood. Interferons appear to limit excessive cell division by controlling specific gene segments in normal and cancerous cells.[8,26] In particular, interferons may inhibit specific gene regulatory segments of tumor cells known as *oncogenes*. Inhibition of the oncogenes would attenuate the excessive proliferation and lack of cell differentiation that typify neoplastic disease.[25] Hence, interferons have proved effective in controlling several forms of cancer (see Table 34–3).

| 1. Virus infected cell produces interferons | 2. Interferons released, bind to non-infected cells. | 3. Interferons induce synthesis of new antiviral proteins in non-infected cell. |

FIGURE 34–4. Antiviral effects of interferons.

Pharmacologic Applications of Interferons

When interferons were first discovered, there was a great deal of optimism about their use as antiviral agents. To date, clinical trials with interferons have been somewhat disappointing. Exogenously administered interferons have been shown to be effective against several types of viruses including members of the herpesvirus family, hepatitis B virus, and the rhinovirus associated with the common cold (see Table 34–1).[4,31,42,61] The actual clinical effectiveness of interferons in treating viral infections, however, has not been overwhelming. These drugs are currently used as antiviral agents on only a limited basis such as systemic administration of interferons to treat certain forms of hepatitis. Yet, there is still a great deal of information to be gained about optimal methods of administration, dosage, and specificity of interferon subtypes for various viral infections. The clinical use of interferons as antiviral drugs should improve as more is learned about pharmacokinetic variables and other factors influencing their effectiveness.[31,40,59,61,67]

In contrast to the somewhat limited use of interferons in treating viral infections, these drugs have been approved for use in several forms of neoplastic disease. Interferons help control cell proliferation in certain leukemias, lymphomas, and several other forms of cancer (see Table 34–3). Interferon use in cancer chemotherapy is discussed in more detail in Chapter 36.

HIV AND THE TREATMENT OF AIDS

HIV is a member of the retrovirus family (see Table 34–1).[62,63] HIV selectively attacks certain cells in the immune system such as CD4+ (T-helper) lymphocytes.[17,32,55,64] Destruction of immune system components often leads to the severe immunocompromised state known as AIDS. Hence, HIV is also referred to informally as the "AIDS virus." Because there is currently no effective way to kill the AIDS virus in humans, there is no cure for AIDS.

AIDS is a life-threatening disorder because of the susceptibility of the immuno-compromised patient to severe infections and certain forms of cancer.[41,43,50,65] In partic-ular, patients with AIDS often suffer from severe viral infections (CMV, various her-pesvirus infections), bacterial infections (*Mycobacterium tuberculosis*), protozoal infections (*Pneumocystis carinii* pneumonia), and infections caused by various other mi-crobes and parasites. Patients with AIDS also develop relatively unusual neoplastic diseases, such as Kaposi's sarcoma.

There is also considerable neuromuscular involvement in patients with AIDS. Pe-ripheral neuropathies, myopathies, and various CNS manifestations (dementia, other psychologic manifestations) can occur directly from HIV infection or secondary to some other opportunistic infection. Likewise, peripheral neuropathies are a common side effect of certain anti-HIV drugs (didanosine, zalcitabine), and myopathies are a side effect of zidovudine therapy. Patients with HIV disease often have painful symp-toms including joint pain, back pain, and pain related to neuropathies and my-opathies.[47,56] Hence, HIV disease can often be regarded as a degenerative neuromuscu-lar disorder from the standpoint of a rehabilitation professional, and therapists can help improve function and decrease pain in patients with HIV infection and AIDS.[18,23,34,45,57]

Individuals who are infected with HIV may remain totally asymptomatic for sev-eral years before developing the full-blown clinical picture of AIDS. Even people ex-posed to HIV who do not initially develop AIDS carry the virus for the rest of their lives and are thus capable of transmitting the virus to others. Transmission of HIV from one individual to another occurs primarily through intimate sexual contact and through sharing intravenous needles. Transfusions using blood from HIV-infected donors are also a potential source of HIV transmission. Hence, practices such as safe sex, not sharing needles, and improved blood-screening techniques are crucial in pre-venting the transmission of HIV and the subsequent risk of developing AIDS.

The treatment of patients with AIDS and individuals infected by HIV is continu-ally being modified as new drugs become available and more information is gained about the nature of the AIDS virus. Currently, the pharmacologic management of HIV-infected patients consists of two principal strategies: (1) controlling the proliferation and effects of HIV in individuals infected with this virus and (2) treatment and pre-vention of various opportunistic infections that attempt to take advantage of the com-promised immune system in patients with AIDS. The pharmacologic methods used to accomplish these principal strategies are presented here.

Inhibiting HIV Proliferation in Infected Individuals

There are no drugs currently available that selectively kill HIV in humans, hence the lack of a cure for this viral infection. Nonetheless, several antiviral drugs are given to inhibit the replication of this virus, thus decreasing the morbidity and mortality of HIV infection. Zidovudine (Retrovir, AZT) was the first drug approved as an anti-HIV agent,[20,60] and didanosine (Videx, ddI) and zalcitabine (HIVID, ddC) were subse-quently approved to prevent HIV replication.[27] As discussed in "Specific Antiviral Drugs," these drugs share a common mechanism of action that is illustrated in Figure 34–3; that is, these drugs inhibit the reverse transcriptase enzyme that HIV uses to synthesize viral DNA from viral RNA. This action can impair one of the early steps in viral replication, thus slowing the progression of HIV infection and the development of AIDS.

Optimal strategies for the use of the anti-HIV medications continue to be explored. In general, zidovudine is the first drug used to control HIV proliferation.[43] It was originally held that rather high doses of zidovudine (upward of 1500 mg/day) were needed to control HIV infection, and these high doses often caused a number of side effects including flulike symptoms.[19] Various clinical trials were conducted to determine that much lower doses (500 to 600 mg/day) are often successful in limiting HIV growth, especially in the early (asymptomatic) stages of HIV infection.[9,52]

Hence, zidovudine therapy is often initiated fairly early to control HIV replication and delay the progression toward full-blown AIDS. Prolonged administration of zidovudine often results in development of resistance to this drug, however.[21,27,53] Hence, the other two antiviral agents, didanosine and zalcitabine, are typically reserved for use in patients who have become resistant to zidovudine or who are unable to tolerate zidovudine for some other reason.[27,33,43] Strategies continue to be explored to determine the best way to use these alternative drugs either alone or in combination with zidovudine to achieve optimal clinical effects.[2,10,58]

Regardless of which anti-HIV drugs are used, the preponderance of evidence indicates that zidovudine and similar drugs are successful in delaying the progression of AIDS. Most trials have seen favorable effects on immune system function (increased CD4 cell counts) and clinical outcome (fewer infections, prolonged survival) if zidovudine is given throughout the course of this disease.[12,38,44,52] There is some evidence, however, that outcome is the same regardless of whether zidovudine therapy is started early or late in the course of HIV infection.[1] Likewise, it has been suggested that benefits associated with a delay in the progression of HIV disease may be offset by a decrease in the quality of life caused by the side effects associated with zidovudine.[37,39] Clearly, a number of issues remain to be resolved about how zidovudine and other anti-HIV drugs can be used to provide optimal benefits for people with HIV infection and AIDS.

A number of other drugs are currently being investigated for their ability to attenuate the replication of the AIDS virus.[27,51,55] The basic strategy is to use any agent that has the potential to impair a key step in the HIV replication cycle.[55] For instance, some experimental drugs have been synthesized that block the attachment of HIV to host cells. Other drugs that impair the assembly of viral proteins in the HIV-infected cell may prove valuable. A group of agents that act in a manner similar to zidovudine and inhibit DNA strand synthesis are also currently being investigated. If clinical trials using these other drugs are favorable, they may also be approved for use in individuals infected with HIV. Likewise, as more drugs are added to the anti-HIV arsenal, we can begin to explore various combinations of different drugs to achieve the best clinical results.[27]

Nonetheless, we must remember that zidovudine and other drugs are not curative and may be helpful only in delaying or reducing AIDS-related deaths. A cure for AIDS, if at all possible, will take several years or even several decades before becoming a reality. As with many viruses, developing a vaccine against the AIDS virus is somewhat easier than making a drug that selectively destroys HIV. The development of an HIV vaccine, however, is still probably years away. Until a vaccine is developed, preventing transmission of HIV remains the best method of controlling the spread of AIDS.

Management of Opportunistic Infections

Because of a virtual lack of immunologic defenses, AIDS patients usually succumb to a variety of opportunistic infections.[32,43,65] Essentially, these patients simply do not have the ability to fight off various viral, bacterial, and other microbial invaders.[41] Consequently, much of the pharmacologic approach to the treatment of AIDS is associated with trying to curtail various infections using the respective antimicrobial drugs that are currently available.

It is beyond the scope of this chapter to give a detailed description of the pharmacologic treatment of all the possible opportunistic infections that occur in patients with AIDS. Nonetheless, some of the more common types of opportunistic infections and the drugs commonly used to treat them are listed in Table 34–4. Because the patient essentially lacks an endogenous defense system, drug therapy must often be continued indefinitely or the infection will recur. Also, early recognition of infectious symptoms is crucial in helping initiate drug therapy before the infection becomes uncontrol-

TABLE 34–4 Treatment of Opportunistic Infections in Patients with AIDS

Organism	Type of Infection	Drug Treatment*
Viral infections		
Cytomegalovirus	Pneumonia; hepatitis; chorio-retinitis; involvement of many other organs	Foscarnet, ganciclovir
Herpes simplex	Unusually severe vesicular and necrotizing lesions of muco-cutaneous areas and GI tract	Acyclovir
HIV	Infections of CNS and peripheral nerves; immune thrombocy-topenic purpura; lymph-adenopathy; other infections	Zidovudine, zalcitabine, didanosine
Varicella-zoster	Painful, vesicular eruption of skin according to dermatomal boundaries (shingles)	Acyclovir, vidarabine
Bacterial infections *Mycobacterium avium* complex	Involvement of bone marrow, reticuloendothelial tissues	Combination therapy using isoniazid, ethambutol, clofazimine, clar-ithromycin, and other antibacteri-als
Mycobacterium tuberculosis	Tuberculosis	Combination therapy using isoniazid, rifampin, and other drugs
Fungal infections *Candida*	Oral candidiasis; esophagitis; sys-temic infections	Clotrimazole, fluconazole, ketocona-zole, nystatin
Cryptococcus	Meningoencephalitis	Amphotericin B, fluconazole
Protozoal infections *Pneumocystis carinii*	Pneumonia	Trimethoprim-sulfamethoxazole, pentamidine
Toxoplasma	CNS infections (cerebral degen-eration meningoencephalitis)	Pyrimethamine and sulfadiazine

*Choice of specific drugs varies according to disease status, presence of other infections, and so forth. Pharmacotherapeutic rationale is also changing constantly as new agents are developed and tested.

lable.[43] Strategies for dealing with various infections are constantly changing, however, and drug therapy for these opportunistic infections will surely be modified as new antimicrobial agents are developed and new evidence is provided about how these agents can be used in various infections.

RELEVANCE OF ANTIVIRAL CHEMOTHERAPY IN REHABILITATION PATIENTS

The major significance of antiviral drugs to rehabilitation specialists and other health-care professionals is the potential for controlling or eliminating infectious disease at present and in the future. As indicated in this chapter, there are really only a few drugs that can effectively resolve viral infections in humans at the present time. Nonetheless, the development of new antiviral agents and the improved use of existing compounds such as the interferons are exciting and important areas of pharmacology. Also, viral prophylaxis through vaccinations has virtually eliminated some types of serious infections, and the possibility of new and improved antiviral vaccines may enhance the health and welfare of patients throughout the world.

Consequently, physical therapists and occupational therapists should keep abreast of advances in treating and preventing viral infections. This notion is especially true for the AIDS crisis, which promises to be a major health issue for some time. By keeping informed of current developments in antiviral pharmacology, health-care professionals will enrich their own knowledge while serving as a reliable source of information for their patients.

CASE STUDY

ANTIVIRAL DRUGS

Brief History. R.K. is a 28-year-old man who was infected with HIV through sexual contact and subsequently developed AIDS. He began a pharmacologic regimen of zidovudine (Retrovir) to help control HIV replication. Zidovudine was taken orally, 200 mg every 4 hours around the clock, for a total daily dosage of 1200 mg. Recently, the patient developed a fever and respiratory infection due to *Pneumocystis carinii* pneumonia. He was admitted to the hospital and treated with a combination of pentamidine and trimethoprim-sulfamethoxazole. The patient also exhibited muscular weakness and began to develop burning pain in both lower extremities. The weakness and pain were attributed to radiculopathy caused by infection of peripheral nerves by HIV or by some other opportunistic infection. Daily dosage of zidovudine was increased to 2400 mg. The physical therapy department was consulted to determine what could be done to alleviate the neuropathic pain and dysfunction.

Decision/Solution. The therapist initiated a program of transcutaneous electrical nerve stimulation (TENS) along the affected nerve pathways. The patient was instructed in the use of the TENS unit, and intensity and other stimulation parameters were adjusted to tolerance by the patient. The therapist also found that cold neon laser treatment helped decrease pain and increase function along the more severely affected nerves, and daily laser treatments were instituted. The combined use of TENS and laser helped decrease pain in this viral-related disorder, thus improving the patient's well-being without the use of additional pharmacologic agents (pain medications). Progressive involvement of other peripheral neurons occurred over the course of the next few weeks, however, and the patient eventually died of respiratory failure.

SUMMARY

Viruses present a unique problem in terms of the pharmacologic treatment of infectious disease. These microorganisms rely totally on the metabolic function of host (human) cells to function and replicate more viruses. Hence, there are currently only a limited number of effective antiviral agents that selectively kill or attenuate the virus without seriously harming the human cells. Developing and administering antiviral vaccines that stimulate immunity of the host to specific viral infections is often more practical. In the future, the development of new antiviral agents and vaccines may help treat and eliminate viral infections that currently pose a serious health threat.

REFERENCES

1. Aboulker, J-P and Swart, AM: Preminary analysis of the Concorde trial. Lancet 341:889, 1993.
2. Abrams DI, et al: A comparative trial of didanosine or zalcitabine after treatment with zidovudine in patients with human immunodeficiency virus infection. N Engl J Med 330:657, 1994.
3. Balfour, HH: Acyclovir and other chemotherapy for herpes group viral infections. Annu Rev Med 35:279, 1984.
4. Baron, S, et al: The Interferon System: A Current Review to 1987. University of Texas Press, Austin, 1987.
5. Bean, B: Antiviral therapy: New drugs and their uses. Postgrad Med 80:109, 1986.
6. Billiau, A: The interferon system as a basis for antiviral therapy or prophylaxis. Antiviral Res 1(suppl):131, 1985.
7. Brock, TD and Madigan, MT: Biology of Microorganisms, ed 6. Prentice-Hall, Englewood Cliffs, NJ, 1991.
8. Chang, C: Interferons, growth factors, and sarcolectins as regulators of coordinated growth. Reversion of cancer cells to non-malignancy. Med Mal Infect 17:664, 1987.
9. Collier, AC, et al: A pilot study of low dose zidovudine in human immunodeficiency virus infection. N Engl J Med 323:1015, 1990.
10. Collier, AC, et al: Combination therapy with zidovudine and didanosine compared with zidovudine alone in HIV-1 infection. Ann Intern Med 119:786, 1993.
11. Cooley, TP, et al: Once daily administration of 2',3'-dideoxyinosine (ddI) in patients with the acquired immunodeficiency syndrome or AIDS-related complex. N Engl J Med 322:1340, 1990.
12. Cooper, DA, et al: Zidovudine in persons with asymptomatic HIV infection and CD4+ cell counts greater than 400 per cubic millimeter. N Engl J Med 329:297, 1993.
13. Corey, L and Holmes, KK: Genital herpes simplex virus infections: Current concepts in diagnosis, therapy, and prevention. Ann Intern Med 98:973, 1983.
14. Darby, G: The acyclovir legacy: Its contribution to antiviral drug discovery. J Med Virol 1(suppl):134, 1993.
15. Deeter, RC and Khanderia, U: Recent advances in antiviral therapy. Clin Pharm 5:961, 1986.
16. Dorsett, PH: Fundamentals of animal virology. In Freeman, BA (ed): Textbook of Microbiology, ed 26. WB Saunders, Philadelphia, 1985.
17. Eales, L-J and Parkin, JM: Current concepts in the immunopathogenesis of AIDS and HIV infection. Br Med Bull 44:38, 1988.
18. Eidelberg, D, et al: Progressive polyradiculoneuropathy in acquired immune deficiency syndrome. Neurology 36:912, 1986.
19. Fischl, MA, et al: A randomized controlled trial of a reduced daily dose of zidovudine in patients with the acquired immunodeficiency syndrome. N Engl J Med 323:1009, 1990.

20. Fischl, MA, et al: The efficacy of azidothymidine (AZT) in the treatment of patients with AIDS and AIDS-related complex. N Engl J Med 317:185, 192, 1987.
21. Freifeld, AG and Ostrove, JM: Resistance of viruses to antiviral drugs. Annu Rev Med 42:247, 1991.
22. Furman, PA, et al: Phosphorylation of 3'-azido-3'-deoxythimidine and selective interaction of the 5'-triphosphate with human immunodeficiency virus reverse transcriptase. Proc Nat Acad Sci (USA) 83:8333, 1986.
23. Galantino, ML and Levy, JK: HIV infection: Neurological implications for rehabilitation. Clin Management Phys Ther 8:6, 1988.
24. Galbraith, AW: Influenza: Recent developments in prophylaxis and treatment. Br Med Bull 41:381, 1985.
25. Gastl, G and Huber, C: The biology of interferon actions. Blut 56:193, 1988.
26. Hersey, P: The evolving role of alpha interferon in the treatment of malignancies. Aust NZ J Med 16:425, 1986.
27. Hirsch, MS and D'Aquila, RT: Drug therapy: Therapy for human immunodeficiency virus infection. N Engl J Med 328:1686, 1993.
28. Hirsch, MS and Kaplan, JC: Treatment of human immunodeficiency virus infections. Antimicrob Agents Chemother 31:839, 1987.
29. Hirsch, MS and Schooley, RT: Treatment of herpes virus infections. N Engl J Med 309:963, 1034, 1983.
30. Hirsch, MS and Swartz, MN: Antiviral agents. N Engl J Med 302:903,949, 1980.
31. Ho, M: Interferon for the treatment of infections. Annu Rev Med 38:51, 1987.
32. Johnson, KJ, et al: Immunopathology. In Rubin, E and Farber, JL (eds): Pathology, ed 2. JB Lippincott, New York, 1994.
33. Kahn, JO, et al: A controlled trial comparing continued zidovudine and didanosine in HIV infection. N Engl J Med 327:581, 1992.
34. Koppel, BS, et al: Central nervous system involvement in patients with acquired immune deficiency syndrome (AIDS). Acta Neurol Scand 71:337, 1985.
35. Lambert, JS, et al: 2', 3'-dideoxyinosine (ddI) in patients with the acquired immunodeficiency syndrome or AIDS-related complex. N Engl J Med 322:1333, 1990.
36. Landolfo, S, et al: Interferon-gamma is not an antiviral, but a growth-promoting factor for T lymphocytes. Eur J Immunol 18:503, 1988.
37. Landor, M: Drug therapy for human immunodeficiency virus infection. Ann Allergy 71:341, 1993.
38. Lemp, GF, et al: Survival trends for patients with AIDS. JAMA 263:402, 1990.
39. Lenderking, WR, et al: Evaluation of the quality of life associated with zidovudine treatment in asymptomatic human immunodeficiency virus infection. N Engl J Med 330:738, 1994.
40. Mannering, GJ and Deloria, LB: The pharmacology and toxicology of the interferons: An overview. Ann Rev Pharmacol Toxicol 26:455, 1986.
41. Masur, H: The compromised host: AIDS and other diseases. In Walzer, PD and Genta, RM (ed): Parasitic Infections in the Compromised Host. Dekker, New York, 1989.
42. Mendelson, J, Clecner, B, and Eiley, S: Effect of recombinant interferon alpha-2 on clinical course of first episode genital herpes infection and subsequent recurrences. Genitourin Med 62:97, 1986.
43. Montauk, SL and Mandell, K: Clinical pharmacology: Update on drug therapy for HIV and related infections in adults. Am Family Phys 46:1772, 1992.
44. Moore, RD, et al: Zidovudine and the natural history of acquired immunodeficiency syndrome. N Engl J Med 324:1412, 1991.
45. Nath, A, Jankovic, J, and Pettigrew, LC: Movement disorders and AIDS. Neurology 37:37, 1987.
46. Nicholson, KG: Antiviral therapy: Respiratory infections, genital herpes, and herpetic keratitis. Lancet 2:617, 1984.
47. O'Neill, WM and Sherrard, JS: Pain in human immunodeficiency disease: A review. Pain 54:3, 1993.
48. Pallasch, TJ, Joseph, CE, and Gill, CJ: Acyclovir and herpesvirus infection: A review of the literature. Oral Surg 57:41, 1984.
49. Pearson, GR: Immunity, autoimmunity, and immunopathology. In Freeman, BA (ed): Textbook of Microbiology, ed 26. WB Saunders, Philadelphia, 1985.
50. Penn, I: Tumors of the immunocompromised patient. Annu Rev Med 39:63, 1988.
51. Pinching, AJ and Jeffries, DJ: Therapy for HIV infections and AIDS. Br Med Bull. 44:115, 1988.
52. Richman, DD: Antiviral therapy of HIV infections. Annu Rev Med 42:69, 1991.
53. Richman, DD, et al: Resistance to AZT and ddC during long-term combination therapy in patients with advanced infection with human immunodeficiency virus. J Acquired Immune Deficiency Syndrome 7:135, 1994.
54. Ruben FL: Prevention and control of influenza: Role of vaccine. Am J Med 82(suppl 6A):31, 1987.
55. Sarin, PS: Molecular pharmacologic approaches to the treatment of AIDS. Annu Rev Pharmacol Toxicol 28:411, 1988.
56. Singer, EJ, et al: Painful symptoms reported by ambulatory HIV-infected men in a longitudinal study. Pain 54:15, 1993.
57. Singh, BM, et al: Spinal cord syndromes in the acquired immune deficiency syndrome. Acta Neurol Scand 73:590, 1986.
58. Skowron, G, Bozzette, SA, and Lim, L: Alternating and intermittent regimens of zidovudine and dideoxycitidine in patients with AIDS or AIDS-related complex. Ann Intern Med 118:321, 1993.

59. Stuart-Harris, RC, Lauchlan, R, and Day, R: The clinical application of the interferons: A review. Med J Australia 156:869, 1992.
60. Symposium (various authors): Zidovudine and human immunodeficiency virus infections. Am J Med 85(suppl 2A):165, 1988.
61. Tyrrell, DAJ and Oxford, JS (eds): Symposium: Antiviral chemotherapy and interferon. Br Med J 41:307, 1985.
62. Vaishnav, YN and Wong-Staal, F: The biochemistry of AIDS. Annu Rev Biochem 60:577, 1991.
63. Weber, JN and Weiss, RA: The virology of human immunodeficiency viruses. Br Med Bull 44:20, 1988.
64. Weiss, A, Hollander, H, and Stobo, J: Acquired immunodeficiency syndrome: Epidemiology, virology, and immunology. Annu Rev Med 36:545, 1985.
65. White, DA and Gold, JWM (eds): Symposium: Medical management of AIDS patients. Med Clin 76:1, 1992.
66. Whitley, RJ and Gnann, JW: Drug therapy: Acyclovir—a decade later. N Engl J Med 327:782, 1992.
67. World Health Organization: Progress in the Development and Use of Antiviral Drugs and Interferon. Technical Report No. 754, WHO, Geneva, 1987.
68. World Health Organization: Viral Vaccines and Antiviral Drugs. Technical Report No. 693, WHO, Geneva, 1983.

CHAPTER 35

Treatment of Infections III: Antifungal and Antiparasitic Drugs

In additional to bacteria and viruses, several parasitic microorganisms may produce infections in humans. In particular, certain species of fungi, protozoa, and helminths (worms) frequently cause infections in humans. Although some types of parasitic infections are limited or unknown in developed nations such as the United States, parasitic infections generally represent the most common form of disease worldwide. These infections are especially prevalent in tropical and subtropical environments and in impoverished areas of the world where sanitation and hygiene are inadequate. Also, the incidence of serious fungal and other parasitic infections has been increasing even in industrialized nations because of the susceptibility of immunocompromised patients, such as patients with AIDS, to these infections.[18,20,29] Hence, effective pharmacologic treatment of these infections remains one of the most important topics in the global management of disease.

The pharmacologic treatment of parasitic infections is a fairly complex and extensive topic. In a limited space, it is difficult to describe the many species of each parasite, all the diseases caused by these parasites, and the chemical methods currently available to selectively destroy various fungi, protozoa, and helminths in humans. Consequently, the general aspects of each type of parasitic infection are reviewed briefly, followed by the primary drugs used to treat specific fungal, protozoal, and helminthic infections. This discussion will acquaint physical therapists and occupational therapists with the nature of these types of infections and the basic chemotherapeutic techniques and agents that are used to treat these problems.

ANTIFUNGAL AGENTS

Fungi are plantlike microorganisms that exist ubiquitously throughout the soil and air and in plants and animals. Although abundant in nature (about 100,000 species exist), only a few species produce infections in humans.[16,21] A disease that is caused by fungal infection is also referred to as a *mycosis*. Some fungal infections are relatively local or superficial, affecting cutaneous and mucocutaneous tissue. Examples of common superficial fungal infections include the tinea (ringworm) infections that cause problems such as athlete's foot. Common mucocutaneous fungal infections include candidiasis and yeast infections of vaginal tissues. Other fungal infections are deeper or more systemic. For instance, fungal infections may affect the lungs, CNS, or other tissues and organs throughout the body.[16]

Often, fungal infections are relatively innocuous because they can be destroyed by the body's normal immune defense mechanisms. Some infections require pharmacologic treatment, especially if the patient's endogenous defense mechanisms are compromised in some way. For instance, individuals undergoing immunosuppressive drug treatment with corticosteroids or certain antibiotics may develop systemic fungal infections. Also, diseases that attack the immune system, such as AIDS, leave the patient vulnerable to severe fungal infections (see Chapter 34). Hence, there is currently a significant need for effective systemic antifungal agents in certain high-risk patients.

The pharmacologic treatment of common fungal infections is summarized in Table 35–1. The clinical use, mechanism of action, and possible adverse effects of individual antifungal agents follow.

Amphotericin B

Clinical Use. Amphotericin B is the drug used most frequently to treat severe systemic fungal infections.[4,13,15,25] This drug is often chosen to treat systemic infections and meningitis caused by *Candida*, *Cryptococcus*, and several species of other pathogenic fungi (see Table 35–1). Typically, this drug is administered by slow intravenous infusion to treat systemic infections. Local and topical administration may also be used to treat more limited infections caused by susceptible fungi.

Mechanism of Action. Amphotericin appears to work by binding to specific

TABLE 35–1 Treatment of Common Fungal Infections

Type of Infection	Principal Sites of Infection	Principal Agent(s)	Secondary/Alternative Agent(s)
Aspergillosis	Lungs, body orifices	Amphotericin B	Itraconazole
Blastomycosis	Lungs, skin; may disseminate to other tissues	Ketoconazole	Amphotericin B, itraconazole
Candidiasis	Intestinal tract, skin, mucous membranes (especially vagina)	Amphotericin B, clotrimazole, miconazole	Fluconazole, flucytosine, ketoconazole
Coccidioidomycosis	Lungs, skin, subcutaneous tissues; may form disseminated lesion throughout the body	Amphotericin B	Ketoconazole, itraconazole, miconazole
Cryptococcosis	Lungs, meninges, other tissues	Amphotericin B	Flucytosine, fluconazole
Histoplasmosis	Lungs, spleen	Amphotericin B	Ketoconazole, itraconazole

steroidlike lipids (sterols) located in the cell membrane of susceptible fungi.[9,15] This binding causes increased permeability in the cell membrane, leading to a leaky membrane and loss of cellular components.

Adverse Effects. The effectiveness of amphotericin against serious systemic fungal infections is tempered somewhat by a high incidence of side effects.[4] Most patients experience problems such as headache, fever, muscle and joint pain, muscle weakness, and gastrointestinal distress (nausea, vomiting, and stomach pain or cramping). Some degree of nephrotoxicity may also occur in many patients. Considering, however, the life-threatening nature of some fungal infections such as meningitis, these adverse effects must often be tolerated while the drug exerts its antifungal actions.

Clotrimazole

Clinical Use. Clotrimazole (Canesten, Lotrimin, Mycelex Troches, many other names) is a broad-spectrum antifungal agent that cannot be given systemically because of toxicity, but is often applied topically or locally to treat various types of fungal infections. Clotrimazole is often applied vaginally to treat local *Candida* infections, and this agent is applied via creams and lotions to treat tinea infections that cause athlete's foot, jock rash, and the like. Clotrimazole can also be applied locally via lozenges to treat oral candidiasis that occurs in patients with a compromised immune system.

Mechanism of Action. Clotrimazole and other antifungal azoles (ketoconazole, fluconazole) work by inhibiting the synthesis of key components of the fungal cell membrane; that is, this drug impairs production of membrane sterols, triglycerides, and phospholipids. Loss of these components results in an inability of the membrane to maintain intracellular homeostasis.

Adverse Side Effects. Side effects are relatively few when these drugs are applied locally, but gastrointestinal distress (cramps, diarrhea, vomiting) can occur if clotrimazole lozenges are swallowed.

Fluconazole

Clinical Use. Fluconazole (Diflucan) is used to treat urinary tract infections, pneumonia, and infections of the mouth and esophagus caused by the *Candida* species of fungus. This agent may also be used to treat cryptococcal meningitis, and fluconazole may be used to help prevent recurrence of cryptococcal infections in patients with AIDS.

Mechanism of Action. Fluconazole and similar drugs (ketoconazole) inhibit certain enzymes in fungal cells that are responsible for the synthesis of important steroidlike compounds (sterols).[8,23] A deficiency of these sterols results in impaired membrane function and other metabolic abnormalities within the fungal cell. Fluconazole also causes direct damage to the fungal membrane by destroying certain membrane components such as triglycerides and phospholipids. Loss of normal membrane structure and function results in the destruction of the fungus.

Adverse Effects. Hepatotoxicity is the most serious side effect of fluconazole, and this drug should be used cautiously in patients with impaired liver function. Other common side effects include headache and gastrointestinal disturbances (abdominal pain, nausea, vomiting).

Flucytosine

Clinical Use. The antifungal spectrum of flucytosine (Ancobon) is limited primarily to the *Candida* and *Cryptococcus* species.[4,25] This drug is used systemically to treat endocarditis, urinary tract infections, and presence of fungi in the bloodstream (*fungemia*) during candidiasis. Flucytosine is also used to treat meningitis and severe pulmonary infections caused by cryptococcosis.

Mechanism of Action. Flucytosine is incorporated into susceptible fungi, where it then undergoes enzymatic conversion to fluorouracil.[4,13] Fluorouracil then acts as an antimetabolite during RNA synthesis in the fungus. Fluorouracil is incorporated into RNA chains but acts as a false nucleic acid. This event ultimately impairs protein synthesis, thus disrupting the normal function of the fungus.

Adverse Effects. Flucytosine may impair bone marrow function, resulting in anemia, leukopenia, and several other blood dyscrasias. This drug may also produce severe gastrointestinal disturbances including nausea, vomiting, diarrhea, and loss of appetite.

Griseofulvin

Clinical Use. Griseofulvin (Fulvicin, Grisactin, other names) is used primarily in the treatment of common fungal infections of the skin known as tinea or ringworm infections.[4,23] For example, this drug is administered to treat fungal infections of the feet (tinea pedis, or "athlete's foot"); infections in the groin area (tinea cruris, or "jock rash"); and similar infections of the skin, nails, and scalp. Griseofulvin is administered orally to treat these infections.

Mechanism of Action. Griseofulvin enters susceptible fungal cells and binds to the mitotic spindle during cell division. This binding impairs the mitotic process, thus directly inhibiting the ability of the cell to replicate itself.

Adverse Effects. Common side effects of griseofulvin administration include headache, which may be severe, and gastrointestinal disturbances (nausea, vomiting, and diarrhea). Some individuals may exhibit hypersensitivity to this drug as evidenced by skin rashes. Skin photosensitivity (increased reaction to ultraviolet light) may also occur.

Itraconazole

Clinical Use. Itraconazole (Sporanox) is one of the newer imidazole antifungals that is administered systemically to treat blastomycosis and histoplasmosis infections in the lungs and other tissues, especially in patients with a compromised immune system.

Mechanism of Action. Itraconazole works like ketoconazole and similar imidazoles; these drugs disrupt membrane function of the fungal cell by inhibiting the synthesis of key membrane components such as sterols and by directly damaging other membrane components such as phospholipids. Impaired membrane function leads to metabolic abnormalities and subsequent death of the fungal cell.

Adverse Effects. Side effects associated with itraconazole include headache, gastrointestinal disturbances (nausea, vomiting), and skin rash.

Ketoconazole

Clinical Use. Ketoconazole (Nizoral) is used to treat a variety of superficial and deep fungal infections.[4,13] This drug can be administered orally to treat pulmonary and systemic infections in candidiasis, coccidioidomycosis, and several other types of deep fungal infections. Oral administration is also used to treat tinea infections of the skin, scalp, and so on. Ketoconazole is also available in topical preparations for the treatment of tinea infections and other relatively localized infections including certain vaginal infections.

Mechanism of Action. Ketoconazole selectively inhibits certain enzymes in fungal cells that are responsible for the synthesis of important steroidlike compounds (sterols).[8,23] A deficiency of these sterols results in impaired membrane function and other metabolic abnormalities within the fungal cell. At higher concentrations, ketoconazole may also directly disrupt the cell membrane, resulting in the destruction of the fungus.

Adverse Effects. Systemic use of ketoconazole is associated with several common side effects. Gastrointestinal disturbances (e.g., nausea, vomiting, stomach pain) are the most common adverse effects of ketoconazole. Some degree of hepatotoxicity may occur, and severe or even fatal hepatitis has been reported on rare occasions. In large, prolonged doses, this drug may also impair testosterone and adrenocorticosteroid synthesis, resulting in breast tenderness and enlargement (gynecomastia) and decreased sex drive in some men.

Miconazole

Clinical Use. Miconazole (Monistat) is similar to ketoconazole in chemistry and the ability to treat a variety of fungal infections.[9] This drug is often applied topically for the treatment of skin infections (tinea) and other localized fungal disorders (certain vaginal infections). Miconazole may also be administered intravenously to treat severe systemic infections and meningitis caused by pathogenic fungi.

Mechanism of Action. Miconazole causes a thickening and subsequent decrease in the permeability of the cell membrane in susceptible fungi,[15] thus inhibiting the transport of important nutrients into the cell. At higher concentrations, this drug may also inhibit certain intracellular enzymes, resulting in the accumulation of cellular metabolites and subsequent damage and necrosis to the cell.

Adverse Effects. Intravenous administration of this drug may cause phlebitis and irritation/itching of the skin (pruritus). Other relatively common side effects of systemic administration include drowsiness, dizziness, blurred vision, and gastrointestinal distress (nausea, vomiting, and diarrhea).

Nystatin

Clinical Use. Nystatin (Mycostatin, Nilstat) has a wide spectrum of activity against various fungi and is used primarily to treat gastrointestinal infections caused by various fungi. Nystatin is administered topically to treat *Candida* infections of the skin and mucous membranes.[4]

Mechanism of Action. Nystatin exerts its antifungal effects in a manner similar to that of amphotericin B; that is, these drugs bind to sterols in the cell membrane, causing an increase in membrane permeability and loss of cellular homeostasis.

Adverse Effects. Systemic administration of nystatin may cause some gastrointestinal disturbances (nausea, vomiting, diarrhea), but these side effects are generally mild and transient.

Other Topical Antifungals

Several other agents are available for treating local fungal infections. These drugs are generally too toxic for systemic use, but they can be applied topically to treat vaginal and other local fungal infections. Examples include butoconazole (Femstat), terconazole (Terazol), and tioconazole (Vagistat). These agents, which are similar to other antifungal azoles such as clotrimazole and miconazole, are commonly used to treat vaginal candidiasis. Other topical antifungals include tolnaftate (Aftate, Tinactin, many other names), naftifine (Naftin), and natamycin (Natacyn), and these drugs are used to treat various topical fungal infections caused by tinea and certain other susceptible fungi.

ANTIPROTOZOAL AGENTS

Protozoa are single-celled organisms that represent the lowest division of the animal kingdom. Of the several thousand species of protozoa, there are approximately 35 that represent a threat of parasitic infection in humans.[5] One relatively common disease caused by protozoal infection is malaria. Malaria is caused by several species of a protozoan parasite known as plasmodia. Although this disease has been virtually eliminated in North America and Europe, malaria continues to be the primary health problem throughout many other parts of the world.[16] Individuals who live in these areas, as well as those traveling to parts of the world where malaria is prevalent, must often undergo antimalarial chemotherapy. Hence, drugs that prevent and treat malaria are extremely important.

In addition to malaria, several other serious infections may occur in humans because of parasitic invasion by protozoa.[16] Severe intestinal infections (dysentery) produced by various protozoa occur quite frequently, especially in areas where contaminated food and drinking water are prevalent. Infections in tissues such as the liver, heart, lungs, brain, and other organs may also occur because of protozoal infestation. As mentioned in the introduction to this chapter, individuals with a compromised immune system may be especially susceptible to these intestinal and extraintestinal infections.[29]

The primary agents used to treat protozoal infections are listed in Table 35–2, and each agent is described subsequently. Drugs that are used primarily to treat and prevent malaria are grouped together, followed by drugs that are used to treat other types of protozoal infections (intestinal and extraintestinal infections).

TABLE 35–2 Treatment of Protozoal Infections

Treatment of Malaria

Type of Malaria	Primary Agent(s)	Alternative/Secondary Agent(s)
Chloroquine-sensitive	Chloroquine	Primaquine
Chloroquine-resistant	Quinine, mefloquine, pyrimethamine-sulfadoxine	Antibiotics (e.g., tetracycline) may be added to the primary agent(s)

Treatment of Other Protozoal Infections

Type of Infection	Principal Site(s) of Infection	Primary Agent(s)	Alternative/ Secondary Agent(s)
Amebiasis	Intestinal tract; liver; lungs	Metronidazole	Diloxanide furoate,* Emetine
Balantidiasis	Lower gastrointestinal tract	Iodoquinol (tetracycline antibiotics are also effective)	Metronidazole
Giardiasis	Small intestine	Metronidazole; antimalarial drugs (e.g., quinacrine)	—
Leishmaniasis	Skin; mucocutaneous tissues, viscera	Sodium stibogluconate*	Amphotericin B, pentamidine
Pneumocystis carinii	Lungs (pneumonia)	Trimethoprim-sulfamethoxazole (see Chapter 33)	Pentamidine
Trichomoniasis	Vagina, genitourinary tract	Metronidazole	—
Toxoplasmosis	Lymph nodes, many organs and tissues	Pyrimethamine-sulfadiazine (see antimalarial drugs)	—
Trypanosomiasis (Chagas' disease; African sleeping sickness)	Heart, brain, many other organs	Nifurtimox,* melarsoprol,* suramin*	Pentamidine

*Only available in the United States from the Centers for Disease Control.

ANTIMALARIAL AGENTS

Chloroquine

Clinical Use. Chloroquine (Aralen) is currently the drug of choice in preventing and treating most forms of malaria.[8,33] This agent is routinely administered to individuals who are traveling to areas of the world where they may be exposed to malaria infection. Certain strains of the parasite that causes malaria (the *Plasmodium* ameba) are resistant to chloroquine, however.[30] If these chloroquine-resistant strains are encountered, other antimalarial drugs must be used (see Table 35–2).

Chloroquine is also used for the treatment of conditions other than malaria. This drug is effective against other types of protozoal infections such as amebiasis and may be used with iodoquinol or emetine to treat infections in liver and pericardium. As discussed in Chapter 16, chloroquine is effective in rheumatoid disease and is used in the treatment of conditions such as rheumatoid arthritis and systemic lupus erythematosus. However, the reasons why this antiprotozoal agent is also effective against rheumatoid disease are unclear. Chloroquine is administered orally.

Mechanism of Action. Although the exact mechanism is unknown, chloroquine binds directly to DNA within susceptible parasites, and inhibits DNA/RNA function and subsequent protein synthesis. Chloroquine may also impair metabolic and digestive function in the protozoa by becoming concentrated within subcellular vacuoles and raising the pH of these vacuoles.[22]

Adverse Effects. The most serious problem associated with chloroquine is the possibility of toxicity to the retina and subsequent visual disturbances. This issue is usually insignificant, however, when this drug is used for short periods of time in relatively low doses (see Chapter 16). Other relatively mild side effects may occur, including gastrointestinal distress (nausea, vomiting, stomach cramps, diarrhea), behavior and mood changes (irritability, confusion, nervousness, depression), and skin disorders (rashes, itching, discoloration).

Hydroxychloroquine

Hydroxychloroquine (Plaquenil) is derived chemically from chloroquine and is similar to it in clinical use, mechanism of action, and adverse effects. Hydroxychloroquine does not have any distinct therapeutic advantages over chloroquine, but it may be substituted in certain individuals who do not respond well to chloroquine.

Mefloquine

Clinical Use. Mefloquine (Lariam), a relatively new antimalarial agent, has been used in certain parts of the world.[10] This drug was developed to treat certain strains of malaria that are resistant to the primary antimalarial drugs such as chloroquine and quinine.[1] Mefloquine has shown activity against some but not all of these resistant strains, and this agent is used for both prophylaxis and treatment of certain types of malaria.

Mechanism of Action. The exact mechanism of action of this drug is unknown. Mefloquine may exert antimalarial effects by several mechanisms, including interaction with phospholipids in the host-cell membrane and interaction with heme components in host-cell erythrocytes.[1]

Adverse Effects. Although the information on this drug is somewhat limited, mefloquine is fairly safe and well tolerated. Some problems including gastrointestinal disturbances may occur, but these are usually minor.

Primaquine

Clinical Use. Primaquine is used in rather extreme circumstances to cure certain forms of malaria[1,32] and is generally administered in acute, severe exacerbations or when chloroquine is ineffective in suppressing malarial attacks. Primaquine may also be used to prevent the onset of malaria in individuals who are especially at risk because of prolonged exposure to this disease. This drug is administered orally.

Mechanism of Action. Primaquine appears to impair DNA function in susceptible parasites. The exact manner in which this occurs is unknown, however.

Adverse Effects. Gastrointestinal disturbances (nausea, vomiting, abdominal
pain), headache, and visual disturbances may occur during primaquine therapy. A
more serious side effect, acute hemolytic anemia, may occur in patients who have a deficiency in the enzyme glucose-6-phosphate dehydrogenase. This enzymatic deficiency
is more common in certain black, Mediterranean, and Asian individuals; hence there is
an increased risk of hemolytic anemia in these groups.[32]

Pyrimethamine

Clinical Use. When used alone, pyrimethamine (Daraprim) is only of minor use
relative to chloroquine in treating and preventing malaria. However, the antimalarial
effectiveness of pyrimethamine is increased dramatically by combining it with the antibacterial drug sulfadoxine.[32] The combination of these two drugs (known commercially as Fansidar) is the primary method of treating and preventing certain forms of
chloroquine-resistant malaria (see Table 35–2).[1,33] Pyrimethamine may also be combined with a sulfonamide drug like dapsone, sulfadiazine, or sulfamethoxazole to treat
protozoal infections that cause toxoplasmosis or *Pneumocystis carinii* pneumonia. These
agents are administered orally.

Mechanism of Action. Pyrimethamine blocks the production of folic acid in susceptible protozoa by inhibiting the function of the dihydrofolate reductase enzyme.
Folic acid helps catalyze the production of nucleic and amino acids in these parasites.
Therefore, this drug ultimately impairs nucleic acid and protein synthesis by interfering with folic acid production. The action of sulfadoxine and other sulfonamide antibacterial agents was discussed in Chapter 33. These agents also inhibit folic acid synthesis in certain bacterial and protozoal cells.

Adverse Effects. The incidence and severity of side effects from pyrimethamine-
sulfadoxine are related to the dosage and duration of therapy. Toxicity is fairly common when these drugs are given in high doses for prolonged periods, and adverse
effects include gastrointestinal disturbances (vomiting, stomach cramps, loss of appetite), blood dyscrasias (agranulocytosis, leukopenia, thrombocytopenia), CNS abnormalities (tremors, ataxia, seizures), and hypersensitivity reactions (skin rashes,
anaphylaxis, liver dysfunction). Hence, pyrimethamine-sulfadoxine is usually administered on a very limited basis such as giving a single dose at the onset of malarial symptoms.

Quinine

Clinical Use. Quinine (Quinamm, Quindan, and others) is one of the oldest forms
of antimalarial chemotherapy, having been obtained from the bark of certain South
American trees as early as the 1600s.[32] Although quinine was the principal method of
preventing and treating malaria for many years, the use of this drug has diminished
somewhat because of expense and relatively toxicity.[33] Hence, the routine use of this
drug has been replaced somewhat by newer, safer agents such as chloroquine and
pyrimethamine-sulfadoxine. Quinine, however, remains one of the most effective antimalarial drugs and is currently used to prevent and treat malaria that is resistant to

other drugs. Quinine sulfate is administered orally, and quinine dihydrochloride is administered by slow intravenous infusion.

Mechanism of Action. The exact mechanism of quinine is not known, although this drug probably exerts antimalarial effects similar to those of primaquine, that is, inhibition of DNA function in susceptible protozoa.

Adverse Effects. Quinine is associated with many adverse effects involving several primary organ systems. This drug may produce disturbances in the CNS (headache, visual disturbances, ringing in the ears), gastrointestinal system (nausea, vomiting, abdominal pain), and cardiovascular system (cardiac arrhythmias). Problems with hypersensitivity, blood disorders, liver dysfunction, and hypoglycemia may also occur in some individuals.

DRUGS USED TO TREAT PROTOZOAL INFECTIONS IN THE INTESTINES AND OTHER TISSUES

Emetine

Clinical Use. Emetine is used primarily to treat protozoal infections in the intestinal tract and extraintestinal sites such as the lungs and liver. This drug is a powerful amebicide and is generally reserved for severe, acute cases of intestinal amebiasis (dysentery).[1] Because of potential adverse effects, emetine is no longer marketed in the United States, and safer agents like metronidazole are often used in place of emetine. Emetine is typically administered by deep subcutaneous injection or intramuscular injection.

Mechanism of Action. Emetine exerts a direct effect on susceptible protozoa by causing degeneration of subcellular components such as the nucleus and reticular system within the parasite.

Adverse Effects. As indicated earlier, the effectiveness of emetine is limited by a number of potentially serious side effects. In particular, problems with cardiotoxicity may occur, as reflected by arrhythmias, palpitations, and other changes in cardiac conduction and excitability. Gastrointestinal disturbances such as diarrhea, nausea, and vomiting are also quite common. Generalized muscular aches and weakness may occur, as well as localized myositis near the site of administration. Hence, emetine is administered under close medical supervision and is withdrawn as soon as the amebicidal effects are apparent.

Iodoquinol

Clinical Use. Iodoquinol (Diquinol, Yodoxin) is primarily used to treat protozoal infections within the intestinal tract[1] and is often combined with a second tissue amebicide, which kills protozoa at extraintestinal sites. For instance, iodoquinol is routinely combined with metronidazole or emetine to ensure destruction of parasites throughout the body. Iodoquinol is usually administered orally.

Mechanism of Action. The mechanism of action of iodoquinol as an amebicide is unknown.

Adverse Effects. Iodoquinol is neurotoxic and may produce optic and peripheral neuropathies when administered in large doses for prolonged periods. Problems with muscle weakness and ataxia may also occur because of the neurotoxic effects of this drug. Other adverse effects include gastrointestinal distress (e.g., nausea, vomiting, cramps) and various skin reactions (rashes, itching, discoloration), but these effects are relatively mild and transient.

Paromomycin

Clinical Use. Paromomycin (Humatin) is used primarily to treat mild to moderate intestinal infections (amebiasis). This drug may also be used as an adjunct to other amebicides during the treatment of more severe protozoal infections. Paromomycin is also effective against some bacteria and tapeworms and may be used as a secondary agent in certain bacterial or helminthic infections. This drug is administered orally.

Mechanism of Action. Paromomycin acts selectively on protozoa within the intestinal lumen and destroys these parasites by a direct toxic effect.

Adverse Effects. Paromomycin is not absorbed from the intestine to any great extent, so adverse effects are fairly limited. Nonetheless, problems with gastrointestinal distress (nausea, vomiting, abdominal pain) may occur as this drug exerts amebicidal effects within the intestine.

Metronidazole

Clinical Use. Metronidazole (Flagyl, Protostat, other names) is effective against a broad spectrum of protozoa and is often the primary agent used against protozoal infections in intestinal as well as extraintestinal tissues.[1,7,17] Metronidazole is frequently combined with another amebicide, such as iodoquinol or diloxanide furoate, to ensure that the protozoal infection is destroyed throughout the body. Metronidazole is also the primary drug used to treat trichomoniasis, which is a sexually transmitted protozoal disease affecting the vagina and male genitourinary tract. As indicated in Chapter 33, metronidazole has bactericidal effects and is used in certain gram-negative bacterial infections. This drug may be administered orally or intravenously.

Mechanism of Action. The exact mechanism of action of this drug is not known. Metronidazole is believed to be reduced chemically within the parasitic cell to a metabolite that impairs nucleic acid and DNA synthesis.[7,17] The exact nature of this metabolite, however, and other features of the cytotoxic effects of this drug remain to be determined.

Adverse Effects. Gastrointestinal disturbances including nausea, vomiting, diarrhea, stomach pain, and an unpleasant taste in the mouth are relatively common with metronidazole. Other adverse effects such as hypersensitivity reactions, peripheral neuropathy, hematologic abnormalities, and genitourinary problems have been reported, but their incidence is relatively low.

Pentamidine

Clinical Use. Pentamidine (Pentam) is effective against several types of extraintestinal protozoal infections, including *P carinii* pneumonia, certain forms of trypanosomiasis (African sleeping sickness), and visceral infections caused by *Leishmania* protozoa. Typically, pentamidine is reserved as a secondary agent in treating these infections and is used when the principal drug in each case is not available or is poorly tolerated (see Table 35–2). Use of this drug as a primary agent has increased, however, in the treatment of *P carinii* infections in patients with AIDS.[6,14,28] This drug is usually administered by parenteral routes such as deep intramuscular injection or slow intravenous infusion. Pentamidine may also be administered by oral inhalation to treat lung infections, and this strategy is now commonly used as prophylaxis and treatment of *P carinii* pneumonia (PCP) in patients with AIDS.[12]

Mechanism of Action. The exact mechanism of this drug is not clear, and pentamidine may affect different parasites in different ways. Some possible antiprotozoal actions of this drug include inhibition of protein and nucleic acid synthesis, cellular metabolism, and oxidative phosphorylation in susceptible parasites.

Adverse Effects. The primary adverse effect of systemic pentamidine administration is renal toxicity. Renal function may be markedly impaired in some patients, but kidney function usually returns to normal when the drug is withdrawn. Other adverse effects include hypotension, hypoglycemia, gastrointestinal distress, blood dyscrasias (leukopenia, thrombocytopenia), and local pain and tenderness at the site of injection. Adverse effects are reduced substantially when this drug is given by inhalation, and this method of administration is desirable when pentamidine is used to prevent PCP in patients with HIV disease.

Other Antiprotozoal Drugs

Several additional agents have been developed to treat intestinal and extraintestinal infections caused by various protozoa. These agents include dehydroemetine, diloxanide furoate, melarsoprol, nifurtimox, sodium stibogluconate, and suramin. The use and distribution of these drugs, however, is quite different from the agents described above. In the United States, these additional drugs are available only from the Centers for Disease Control (CDC), in Atlanta, Georgia. At the request of the physician, the CDC dispenses the drug to the physician, who then provides the agent to the patient.

Clinical applications of individual drugs in this category are indicated in Table 35–2. In general, these drugs are reserved for some of the more serious or rare types of protozoal infections. As might be expected, adverse side effects of these drugs are quite common. Yet these drugs may be lifesaving in some of the more severe infections, which is why the CDC controls their distribution. For more information about specific agents in this group, the reader is referred to other sources.[31]

ANTHELMINTICS

Infection from helminths, or parasitic worms, is the most common form of disease in the world.[2,24,34] There are several types of worms that may invade and subsist from human tissues.[5,16] Common examples include tapeworms (cestodes), roundworms (nematodes), and flukes (trematodes). Worms can enter the body by various routes but often are ingested as eggs in contaminated food and water. Once in the body, the eggs hatch and adult worms ultimately lodge in various tissues, especially the digestive tract. Some types (flukes) may also lodge in blood vessels such as the hepatic portal vein. Depending on the species, adult worms may range anywhere from a few millimeters to several meters in length. The adult worms begin to steal nutrients from their human host and may begin to obstruct the intestinal lumen or other ducts if they reproduce in sufficient numbers.

Some of the common **anthelmintics** used to kill the basic types of worms in humans are listed in Table 35–3. These agents are often very effective, a single oral dose being sufficient to selectively destroy the parasite. Brief descriptions of the basic pharmacologic effects and possible adverse effects of the primary anthelmintic agents are presented here. The pharmacologic treatment of helminthic infections has also been reviewed extensively by several authors.[1–3,11,27]

Diethylcarbamazine

Diethylcarbamazine (Hetrazan) is used to treat certain roundworm infections of the lymphatics and connective tissues including loiasis, onchocerciasis, and Bancroft's filariasis. This agent immobilizes immature roundworms (microfilariae) and facilitates the destruction of these microfilariae by the body's immune system. Diethylcarbamazine is also effective against the adult forms of certain roundworms, but the mechanism of this anthelmintic action against mature nematodes is not known. Side effects associated with diethylcarbamazine include headache, malaise, weakness, and loss of appetite. More severe reactions (fever, acute inflammatory response) may also occur following diethylcarbamazine use, but these reactions may be caused by release of antigenic substances from the dying roundworms rather than from the drug itself.

Mebendazole

Mebendazole (Vermox) is effective against many types of roundworms and a few tapeworms that parasitize humans.[26] This drug appears to selectively damage intestinal cells in these worms, thus inhibiting the uptake and intracellular transport of glucose and other nutrients into these parasites. This occurrence leads to destruction of

TABLE 35–3 Treatment of Common Helminthic Infections

Parasite	Primary Agent(s)	Secondary Agent(s)
Roundworms (nematodes)		
Ascariasis (roundworm)	Mebendazole, pyrantel pamoate	Piperazine citrate
Pinworm	Mebendazole, pyrantel pamoate	Piperazine citrate
Hookworm	Mebendazole, pyrantel pamoate, thiabendazole	—
Trichinosis	Thiabendazole	Mebendazole
Tapeworms (cestodes)		
Beef tapeworm	Niclosamide, praziquantel	—
Pork tapeworm	Niclosamide, praziquantel	—
Fish tapeworm	Niclosamide, praziquantel	—
Flukes (trematodes)		
Blood flukes	Praziquantel	Oxamniquine
Fluke infections in other organs	Praziquantel	—

the epithelial lining and subsequent death of the parasite. Mebendazole is a relatively safe drug, although some mild, transient gastrointestinal problems may occur.

Niclosamide

Niclosamide (Niclocide) is effective against several types of tapeworm (see Table 35–3). This drug inhibits certain mitochondrial enzymes in these parasites. This inhibition ultimately results in the breakdown of the protective integument of the worm, thus allowing the digestive enzymes in the host (human) intestine to attack the parasite. Ultimately, the worm is digested and expelled from the gastrointestinal tract. There are relatively few adverse effects of niclosamide treatment, probably because the drug is not absorbed to any great extent from the human intestine. Thus, the drug remains in the intestinal lumen, where it can act directly on the tapeworm.

Oxamniquine

Oxamniquine (Vansil) is effective against a genus of parasitic worms known as blood flukes (schistosomes). These parasites typically adhere to the wall of blood vessels such as the hepatic portal vein. Oxamniquine inhibits muscular contraction of the sucker that holds the fluke to the vessel wall, thus allowing the worm to dislodge and travel to the liver. In the liver, the parasite is engulfed and destroyed by hepatic phagocytes. Common side effects associated with this drug include headache, dizziness, and drowsiness. These adverse effects are generally mild and transient, however.

Piperazine Citrate

Piperazine citrate is typically used as a secondary agent in ascariasis (roundworm) and enterobiasis (pinworm) infections (see Table 35–3). This drug appears to paralyze the worm by blocking the effect of acetylcholine at the parasite's neuromuscular junction. The paralyzed worm can then be dislodged and expelled from the host (human) intestine during normal bowel movements. Side effects such as headache, dizziness, and gastrointestinal disturbance may occur during piperazine citrate administration, but these effects are generally mild and transient.

Praziquantel

Praziquantel (Biltricide) is one of the most versatile and important anthelmintic agents[19] and is the drug of choice in treating all major trematode (fluke) infections and several common types of tapeworm infections (see Table 35–3). The exact mechanism of action of this drug is not known. Praziquantel may stimulate muscular contraction of the parasite, resulting in a type of spastic paralysis, which causes the worm to lose its hold on intestinal or vascular tissue. At higher concentrations, this drug may initiate destructive changes in the integument of the worm, allowing the host defense mechanisms (e.g., enzymes, phagocytes) to destroy the parasite. Praziquantel is associated with a number of frequent side effects including gastrointestinal problems (such as abdominal pain, nausea, vomiting), CNS effects (headache, dizziness), and mild hepatotoxicity. These adverse effects can usually be tolerated, however, for the relatively short period of time that the drug is in effect.

Pyrantel Pamoate

Pyrantel pamoate (Antiminth, several other names) is one of the primary agents used in several types of roundworm and pinworm infections (see Table 35–3). This drug stimulates acetylcholine release and inhibits acetylcholine breakdown at the neuromuscular junction, thus producing a prolonged state of excitation and muscular contraction that causes spastic paralysis of the worm. The worm is unable to retain its hold on the intestinal tissue and can be expelled from the digestive tract by normal bowel movements. This drug is generally well tolerated, with only occasional problems of mild gastrointestinal disturbances.

Thiabendazole

Thiabendazole (Mintezol) is the primary drug used in trichinosis and several other types of roundworm infections (see Table 35–3). The anthelmintic mechanism of this drug is not fully understood, but selective inhibition of certain key metabolic enzymes in susceptible parasites is probable. The most common side effects associated with this drug involve gastrointestinal distress (nausea, vomiting, and loss of appetite). Allergic reactions (e.g., skin rash, itching, chills) may also occur in some individuals.

SIGNIFICANCE OF ANTIFUNGAL AND ANTIPARASITIC DRUGS IN REHABILITATION

The drugs discussed in this chapter are relevant in that they relate largely to specific groups of patients seen in a rehabilitation setting. Therapists working in sports physical therapy may deal frequently with topical antifungal agents in the treatment of cutaneous ringworm infections. For instance, physical therapists and athletic trainers may be responsible for recognizing and helping treat tinea pedis, tinea cruris, and similar infections. Therapists and trainers can make sure the drugs are being applied in the proper fashion and as directed by the physician. Therapists may also play a crucial role in preventing the spread of these infections by educating athletes about how to prevent transmission among team members (e.g., not sharing towels and combs).

Physical therapists and occupational therapists working with patients who have AIDS will frequently encounter patients taking systemic antifungal and antiprotozoal drugs. The use of these agents is critical in controlling parasitic infections in patients with AIDS and other individuals with a compromised or deficient immune system.

Finally, the drugs discussed in this chapter will have particular importance to therapists working in or traveling to parts of the world where parasitic infections remain a primary health problem and source of human suffering. Therapists involved in the Peace Corps or similar organizations will routinely treat patients taking these drugs. Also, therapists working in these areas may be taking some of these drugs themselves, such as prophylactic antimalarial agents, like chloroquine. Hence, therapists should be aware of the pharmacology and potential side effects of these agents, both in their patients and in themselves. Of course, therapists working in North America should know that individuals who have returned from or immigrated from certain geographic areas may carry various fungal and parasitic infections and that these patients will also require chemotherapy using the drugs discussed in this chapter.

CASE STUDY

ANTIFUNGAL DRUGS

Brief History. A physical therapist working with a college football team was taping a team member's ankle when he noticed redness and inflammation between the athlete's toes. The athlete reported that the redness and itching had developed within the last few days and was becoming progressively worse. The therapist suspected a cutaneous fungal infection (probably tinea pedis) and reported this information to the team physician.

Decision/Solution. The physician prescribed a topical antifungal preparation containing miconazole (Monistat-Derm). The athlete was instructed to apply this preparation twice daily. The physical therapist also instructed the athlete in proper skin hygiene (such as thoroughly washing and drying the feet, wearing clean socks). In addition, the physical therapist had the locker room floors and shower areas thoroughly disinfected to prevent transmission of the fungus to other team members. This isolated case of tinea pedis was resolved without further incident.

SUMMARY

This chapter presented three general groups of drugs that are used to treat infection caused by specific microorganisms in humans. Antifungal drugs are used against local or systemic infections caused by pathogenic fungi. Antiprotozoal agents are used to prevent and treat protozoal infections such as malaria, severe intestinal infection (dysentery), and infections in other tissues and organs. Anthelmintic drugs are used against parasitic worms (tapeworm, roundworm, etc.) that may infect the human intestinal tract and other tissues. Although the use of some of these agents is relatively limited in the United States, these drugs tend to be some of the most important agents in controlling infection and improving health on a worldwide basis. Also, the use of some of these agents has increased lately in treating opportunistic fungal and protozoal infections in patients who have AIDS and other individuals with compromised immune systems. Physical therapists and occupational therapists may be involved with treating specific groups of patients taking these drugs, including patients with AIDS and patients located in geographic areas where these types of infections are prevalent.

REFERENCES

1. Campbell, WC: The chemotherapy of parasitic infections. J Parasitol 72:45, 1986.
2. Campbell, WC and Rew, RS (eds): Chemotherapy of Parasitic Diseases. Plenum Press, New York, 1986.
3. Cline, BL: Current drug regimens for the treatment of intestinal helminth infections. Med Clin North Am 66:721, 1982.
4. Drouhet, E and Dupont, B: Evolution of antifungal agents: Past, present, and future. Rev Infect Dis 9(suppl 1):S4, 1987.
5. Dusanic, DG: Medical parasitology. In Freeman, BA (ed): Textbook of Microbiology, ed 26. WB Saunders, Philadelphia, 1985.
6. Goa, KL and Campoli-Richards, DM: Pentamidine isethionate: A review of its antiprotozoal activity, pharmacokinetic properties, and therapeutic use in *Pneumocystis carinii* pneumonia. Drugs 33:242, 1987.
7. Goldman, P: Metronidazole. N Engl J Med 303:1212, 1980.
8. Harris, LF, Shasteen, WJ, and Lampert, R: Malaria: Recent experience in a community. South Med J 77:1121, 1984.
9. Hay, RJ: Antifungal chemotherapy. Med J Aust 143:287, 1985.
10. Howells, RE: Symposium on malaria: Advances in chemotherapy. Br Med Bull 38:193, 1982.
11. Janssen, PAJ and Van Den Bossche, H: Treatment of helminthiasis. Scand J Infect Dis 36(suppl):52, 1982.
12. Leoung, GS, et al: Aerosolized pentamidine for prophylaxis against *Pneumocystis carinii* pneumonia: The San Francisco prophylaxis trial. N Engl J Med 323:769, 1990.
13. Lyman, CA and Walsh, TJ: Systemically administered antifungal agents: A review of their clinical pharmacology and therapeutic applications. Drugs 44:9, 1992.
14. Masur, H: Drug therapy: Prevention and treatment of *Pneumocystis* pneumonia. N Engl J Med 327:1853, 1992.
15. Medoff, G, et al: Antifungal agents useful in the therapy of systemic fungal infection. Annu Rev Pharmacol Toxicol 23:303, 1983.
16. Merlin, TL, Gibson, DW, and Connor, DH: Infections and parasitic diseases. In Rubin, E and Farber, JL (eds): Pathology, ed 2. JB Lippincott, Philadelphia, 1994.
17. Molavi, A, LeFrock, JL, and Prince, RA: Metronidazole. Med Clin North Am 66:121, 1982.
18. Montauk, SL and Mandell, K: Clinical pharmacology: Update on drug therapy for HIV and related infections in adults. Am Fam Physician 46:1772, 1992.
19. Pearson, RD and Guerrnat, RL: Praziquantel: A major advance in anthelminthic therapy. Ann Intern Med 99:195, 1983.
20. Pinching, AJ: Clinical aspects of AIDS and HIV infection in the developed world. Br Med Bull 44:89, 1988.
21. Rippon, JW: Medical Mycology: The Pathogenic Fungi and the Pathogenic Actinomycetes. WB Saunders, Philadelphia, 1988.
22. Schlesinger, PH, Krogstad, DJ, and Herwaldt, BL: Antimalarial agents: Mechanisms of action. Antimicrob Agents Chemother 32:793, 1988.
23. Smith, EB and Henry, JC: Ketoconazole: An orally effective antifungal agent: Mechanism of action, pharmacology, clinical efficacy, and adverse effects. Pharmacotherapy 4:199, 1984.
24. Stephenson, LS and Holland, C: The Impact of Helminth Infections on Human Nutrition. Taylor & Francis, New York, 1987.
25. Utz, JP: Chemotherapy of the systemic mycoses. Med Clin North Am 66:221, 1982.
26. Van den Bossche, H, Rochette, F, and Horig, C: Mebendazole and related anthelminthics. Adv Pharmacol Chemother 19:67, 1982.
27. Van den Bossche, H, Thienpoint, D, and Janssens, PG (eds): Chemotherapy of Gastrointestinal Helminths. Springer-Verlag, Berlin, 1985.
28. Vohringer, HF and Arasteh, K: Pharmacokinetic opimisation in the treatment of *Pneumocystis carinii* pneumonia. Clin Pharmacokin 24:388, 1993.
29. Walzer, PD and Genta, RM (eds): Parasitic Infections in the Compromised Host. Dekker, New York, 1989.
30. Warhurst, DC: Antimalarial drugs: An update. Drugs 33:50, 1987.
31. Webster, LT: Drugs used in the chemotherapy of protozoal infections: Leishmaniasis, trypanosomiasis, and other protozoal infections. In Gilman, AG, et al (eds): The Pharmacological Basis of Therapeutics, ed 8. Pergamon Press, New York, 1990.
32. Webster, LT: Drugs used in the chemotherapy of protozoal infections: Malaria. In Gilman, AG, et al (eds): The Pharmacological Basis of Therapeutics, ed 8. Pergamon Press, New York, 1990.
33. World Health Organization: WHO Expert Committee on Malaria, Eighteenth Report. Technical Report No. 735, WHO, Geneva, 1986.
34. World Health Organization: Control of Schistosomiasis. Technical Report No. 728, WHO, Geneva, 1985.

CHAPTER 36

Cancer Chemotherapy

Cancer encompasses a group of diseases that are marked by rapid, uncontrolled cell proliferation and a conversion of normal cells to a more primitive and undifferentiated state.[17,31,51] Excessive cell proliferation may form large tumors, or *neoplasms*. Although some types of tumors are well contained, or benign, **malignant tumors** continue to proliferate within local tissues, as well as spreading (**metastasizing**) to other tissues in the body. *Cancer* specifically refers to the malignant forms of neoplastic disease that are often fatal as tumors invade and destroy tissues throughout the body. This notion does not mean that benign tumors cannot also be life-threatening; that is, a large benign tumor may produce morbidity and mortality by obstructing the intestinal tract, pressing on crucial CNS structures, and so on. Cancer cells, however, are unique in their progressive invasion of local tissues and ability to metastasize to other tissues.[51]

Cancer ranks second to cardiovascular disease as the leading cause of death in the United States.[31] There are many different types of cancer, and various malignancies are classified depending on the location and type of tissue from which the cancer originated.[31,51] For instance, cancers arising from epithelial tissues (e.g., skin, gastrointestinal lining) are labeled as *carcinomas*, and cancers arising from mesenchymal tissues (e.g., bone, striated muscle) are labeled as *sarcomas*. Also, cancers associated with the formed blood elements are connoted by the "-emia" suffix (e.g., "leukemia," cancerous proliferation of leukocytes). Many other descriptive terms are used to describe various malignancies, and certain forms of cancer are often named after a specific person (e.g., Hodgkin's disease, Wilms' tumor). We cannot, however, describe all the various types of malignancies. The reader may want to consult a pathology text[31,51] or similar reference for more information about the location and morphology of particular forms of cancer.

The exact cause of many cases of neoplastic disease is unknown. However, a great deal has been learned about possible environmental, viral, genetic, and other possible elements, or **carcinogens**, that may cause or increase the susceptibility to various types of cancer. Conversely, certain positive lifestyles that include adequate exercise, high-fiber diet, and not smoking cigarettes may be crucial in preventing certain forms of cancer. Of course, routine checkups and early detection play a crucial role in reducing cancer mortality.

When cancer is diagnosed, three primary treatment modalities are available: surgery, radiation treatment, and cancer chemotherapy. The purpose of this chapter is to describe the basic rationale of cancer **chemotherapy** and to provide an overview of the drugs that are currently available to treat specific forms of cancer. Rehabilitation specialists will routinely be working with patients undergoing cancer chemotherapy. For reasons that will become apparent in this chapter, these drugs tend to produce toxic effects that will directly influence physical therapy and occupational therapy procedures. Therefore, this chapter should provide therapists with a better understanding of the pharmacodynamic principles and beneficial effects as well as the reason for the potential adverse effects of these important drugs.

GENERAL PRINCIPLES

Cytotoxic Strategy

The basic strategy of anticancer drugs is to limit cell proliferation by killing or attenuating the growth of the cancerous cells. However, the pharmacologic treatment of cancer represents a unique and perplexing problem. Although cancer cells have become more primitive and have lost much of their normal appearance, these are still human cells that have simply gone wild and they cannot be easily destroyed without also causing some harm to the healthy human tissues. The concept of selective toxicity becomes much more difficult to achieve when using anticancer drugs versus drugs that attack foreign invaders and parasites such as antibacterial drugs or antiprotozoal drugs (see Chapters 33 through 35).

Hence, most anticancer drugs rely on the basic strategy of inhibiting DNA/RNA synthesis and function. The idea is that cells that undergo extremely rapid cell division (mitosis) must replicate their genetic material at a much greater rate than other cells. Since cancer cells undergo mitosis at a rate that is much higher than that of healthy cells, drugs that impair DNA synthesis and function will preferentially affect cancer cells.

Cell-Cycle–Specific Versus Cell-Cycle–Nonspecific Drugs

Antineoplastic drugs are sometimes classified according to whether they act at a specific phase of cell division.[59] Cancer cells and most normal cells typically undergo a life cycle that can be divided into several distinct phases: resting phase (G_0), pre-DNA synthesis phase (also the phase of normal cell metabolism—G_1), period of DNA synthesis (S), post-DNA synthesis phase (G_2), and the period of actual cell division or mitosis (M).[3,9,59] Certain antineoplastic drugs are referred to as cell-cycle–specific because they exert their effects only when the cancer cell is in a certain phase. For instance, most antimetabolites (cytarabine, methotrexate, others) act when the cell is in the S phase. Other drugs are classified as cell-cycle–nonspecific because they exert antineoplastic effects on the cell regardless of the phase of the cell cycle. Examples of cell-cycle–nonspecific agents include most alkylating agents and antineoplastic antibiotics.

The significance of cell-cycle specificity or nonspecificity is fairly obvious. Cell-cycle–specific drugs will be effective only in cells that are progressing through the cell cycle, that is, cells that are not remaining in the resting (G_0) phase. Cell-cycle–nonspecific agents will have a more general effect and should inhibit replication in all the cells reached by the drug.

Concepts of Growth Fraction and Total Cell Kill

Cancer cells are not all uniform in their rate of replication and proliferation. In any given tumor or type of disseminated cancer, certain cells do not proliferate, while other cells reproduce at variable rates. The term *growth fraction* refers to the percentage of proliferating cells relative to total neoplastic cell population.[32] The cells included in the growth fraction are more susceptible to antineoplastic drugs because these are the cells that must synthesize and replicate their genetic material. Fortunately, these are also the cells that must be killed in order to prevent the cancer from spreading.

The concept of *total cell kill* refers to the fact that virtually every tumor cell capable of replicating must be killed to eliminate the cancer totally.[3] Even one single surviving malignant cell could eventually replicate in sufficient numbers to cause death. The difficulty of achieving total cell kill is illustrated by the following example.[3] The number of malignant cells in a patient with acute lymphocytic leukemia could be as high as 10^{12} cells. If an anticancer drug kills 99.99 percent of these cells, one might think that the drug would be successful in resolving the cancer. However, 10^8, or approximately 1 billion, cells would still remain alive and capable of advancing the leukemia. Obviously, total cell kill is always a chemotherapeutic goal but may sometimes be difficult to achieve.

Incidence of Adverse Effects

Since antineoplastic agents also impair replication of normal tissues, these drugs are generally associated with a number of common and relatively severe adverse effects. Normal human cells must often undergo controlled mitosis to sustain normal function. This fact is especially true for certain tissues such as hair follicles, bone marrow, immune system cells, and epithelial cells in the skin and gastrointestinal tract. Obviously, these tissues will also be affected to some extent by most cancer chemotherapy agents. In fact, the primary reason for most of the common adverse effects (e.g., hair loss, anemia, anorexia) is that normal cells are also undergoing the same toxic changes as the tumor cells. The cancer cells, however, tend to suffer these toxic effects to a greater extent because they must synthesize and replicate their genetic material even more than the healthy cells. Still, healthy cells often exhibit some toxic effects even at the minimum effective doses of the chemotherapeutic agents.

Consequently, antineoplastic drugs typically have a very low therapeutic index compared to drugs that are used to treat less serious disorders (see Chapter 1). Considering that cancer is usually life-threatening, these toxic effects must be expected and tolerated during chemotherapeutic treatments. Occasionally, some side effects can be treated using other drugs. In particular, gastrointestinal disturbances (e.g., nausea, vomiting, loss of appetite) may be relieved to some extent by administering anticholinergic drugs like metoclopramide, corticosteroid drugs like dexamethasone, or a combination of these and other agents.[6,30,34,47] Also, support from medical, nursing, and other health-care providers (including physical therapists and occupational therapists) can help immeasurably in reassuring the patient that these side effects are normal—and even necessary—for the cancer chemotherapy drugs to exert their antineoplastic effects.

SPECIFIC DRUGS

Drugs used against cancer can be classified by their chemical structure, source, or mechanism of action.[8] The primary groups of antineoplastic drugs are the alkylating agents, antimetabolites, antineoplastic antibiotics, antineoplastic hormones, and several other miscellaneous drug groups and individual agents. These principal antineoplastic medications are presented here.

Alkylating Agents

Alkylating agents exert cytotoxic effects by inducing binding within DNA strands and by preventing DNA function and replication.[8,14,48] Essentially, the drug causes cross-links to be formed between the strands of the DNA double helix or within a single DNA strand (Fig. 36–1). In either case, these cross-links effectively tie up the DNA

FIGURE 36–1. Mechanism of action of anticancer alkylating agents. The alkylating agent (R) causes alkylation of guanine nucleotides located in the DNA strand. Cross-links are then formed between two alkylated guanines, thus creating strong bonds between or within the DNA strands that inhibit DNA function and replication.

molecule, eliminating the ability of the DNA double helix to untwist and allow replication of the genetic code. If the DNA double helix cannot unravel, the genetic code of the cell cannot be reproduced and cell reproduction is arrested. Also, cross-linking within the double helix impairs cellular protein synthesis since the DNA double helix cannot unwind to allow formation of messenger RNA strands. The cell soon dies because vital cellular proteins (enzymes, transport proteins, etc.) are no longer being produced.

Alkylating agents are so named because they typically generate a chemical alkyl group on one of the bases such as guanine in the DNA chain. This alkyl group acts as the bridge that ultimately links together two bases in the DNA molecule (see Fig. 36–1). The bonds formed by this cross-linking are strong and resistant to breakage. Thus the DNA double helix remains tied up for the life of the cell.

Anticancer drugs that work primarily as alkylating agents are listed in Table 36–1. As indicated, these agents represent the largest category of anticancer drugs and are used to treat a variety of leukemias, carcinomas, and other neoplasms. Common adverse side effects of alkylating agents are also listed in Table 36–1. As previously discussed, most of these adverse effects are caused by the effect of the alkylating agent on DNA replication in normal, healthy tissues.

Antimetabolites

Cells are able to synthesize genetic material (DNA, RNA) from endogenous metabolites known as purine and pyrimidine nucleotides (Fig. 36–2). Certain anticancer drugs are structurally similar to these endogenous metabolites and compete with these compounds during DNA/RNA biosynthesis. These drugs are therefore called **antimetabolites** because they interfere with the normal metabolites during cellular biosynthesis.[8,32]

Antimetabolites can impair the biosynthesis of genetic material in two primary ways.[56] First, the drug may be incorporated directly into the genetic material, thus forming a bogus and nonfunctional genetic product. This effect would be like baking a cake but substituting an inappropriate ingredient (salt) for a normal ingredient (flour). Obviously, the end product would not work (or taste) very well. A second manner in which antimetabolites may impair DNA/RNA biosynthesis is by occupying the enzymes that synthesize various components of the genetic material. These enzymes do not recognize the difference between the antimetabolite drug and the normal metabolite, and waste their time trying to convert the antimetabolite into a normal metabolic product. The enzyme, however, cannot effectively act on the drug, so the normal metabolic products are not formed. In either case, the cell's ability to synthesize normal DNA and RNA is impaired, and the cell cannot replicate its genetic material or carry out normal protein synthesis because of a lack of functional DNA and RNA.

Cancer chemotherapeutic agents that act as antimetabolites and the principal neoplastic diseases in which they are indicated are listed in Table 36–2. As indicated previously, these drugs interrupt cellular pathways that synthesize DNA and RNA, and the primary sites where specific antimetabolites interrupt these pathways are indicated in Figure 36–2. As with most anticancer drugs, these agents are especially toxic to cells that have a large growth fraction and undergo extensive replication. These cells have an especially great need to synthesize nucleic acids—hence the preferential effect of antimetabolites on these cells.

TABLE 36–1 Alkylating Agents

Generic Name	Trade Name	Primary Antineoplastic Indication(s)*	Common Adverse Effects
Busulfan	Myleran	Chronic myelocytic leukemia	Blood disorders (anemia, leukopenia, thrombocytopenia); metabolic disorders (hyperuricemia, fatigue, weight loss, other symptoms)
Carmustine	BCNU, BiCNU	Primary brain tumors; Hodgkin's disease; non-Hodgkin's lymphomas; multiple myeloma	Blood disorders (thrombocytopenia, leukopenia); GI distress (nausea, vomiting); hepatotoxicity; pulmonary toxicity
Chlorambucil	Leukeran	Chronic lymphocytic leukemia; Hodgkin's disease; non-Hodgkin's lymphomas	Blood disorders (leukopenia, thrombocytopenia, anemia); skin rashes/itching; pulmonary toxicity; seizures
Cisplatin†	Platinol	Carcinoma of bladder, ovaries, testicles, and other tissues	Nephrotoxicity; GI distress (nausea, vomiting); neurotoxicity (cranial and peripheral nerves); hypersensitive reactions (e.g., flushing, respiratory problems, tachycardia)
Cyclophosphamide	Cytoxan, Neosar	Acute and chronic lymphocytic leukemia; acute and chronic myelocytic leukemia; carcinoma of ovary, breast; Hodgkin's disease; non-Hodgkin's lymphomas; multiple myeloma	Blood disorders (anemia, leukopenia, thrombocytopenia); GI distress (nausea, vomiting, anorexia); bladder irritation; hair loss; cardiotoxicity; pulmonary toxicity
Dacarbazine	DTIC-Dome	Malignant melanoma; refractory Hodgkin's lymphomas	GI distress (nausea, vomiting, anorexia); blood disorders (leukopenia, thrombocytopenia)
Lomustine	CeeNU	Brain tumors; Hodgkin's disease	Blood disorders (anemia, leukopenia); GI disorders (nausea, vomiting)
Mechlorethamine	Mustargen, Nitrogen mustard	Bronchogenic carcinoma; chronic leukemia; Hodgkin's disease; non-Hodgkin's lymphomas	Blood disorders (anemia, leukopenia, thrombocytopenia); GI distress (nausea, vomiting); CNS effects (headache, dizziness, convulsions); local irritation at injection site

(Continued)

569

TABLE 36-1 Alkylating Agents—*Continued*

Generic Name	Trade Name	Primary Antineoplastic Indication(s)*	Common Adverse Effects
Melphalan	Alkeran	Ovarian carcinoma; multiple myeloma	Blood disorders (leukopenia, thrombocytopenia); skin rashes/itching
Procarbazine[†]	Matulane	Hodgkin's disease	Blood disorders (leukopenia, thrombocytopenia); GI distress (nausea, vomiting); CNS toxicity (mood changes, incoordination, motor problems)
Streptozocin	Zanosar	Pancreatic carcinoma	Nephrotoxicity; GI distress (nausea, vomiting); blood disorders (anemia, leukopenia, thrombocytopenia); local irritation at injection site
Thiotepa	—	Carcinoma of breast, ovary, and bladder; Hodgkin's disease	Blood disorders (anemia, leukopenia, thrombocytopenia, pancytopenia)
Uracil mustard	—	Chronic lymphocytic leukemia; chronic myelocytic leukemia; non-Hodgkin's lymphomas	Blood disorders (anemia, leukopenia, thrombocytopenia); GI distress (nausea, vomiting, diarrhea, anorexia)

*Only the indications listed in the U.S. product labeling are included here. Many anticancer drugs are used for additional types of neoplastic disease.
[†]These drugs are not classified chemically as alkylating agents (i.e., they do not produce an "alkyl" group). However, they appear to form cross-links within DNA similar to alkylating drugs; hence their inclusion here.

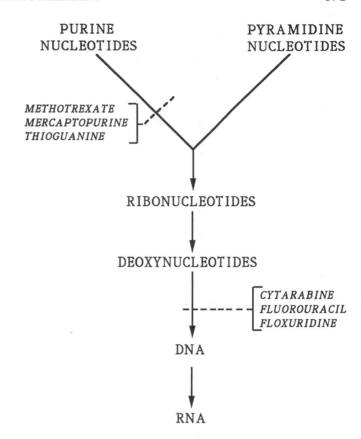

FIGURE 36-2. Sites of action of anticancer antimetabolites. Various drugs interfere with DNA/RNA production by inhibiting nucleic acid biosynthesis at specific sites indicated by the dashed lines.

Antibiotics

Several anticancer drugs are chemically classified as antibiotics but are usually reserved for neoplastic diseases because of the relatively high toxicity of these agents. In general, these drugs act directly on DNA by becoming intercalated (inserted) between base pairs in the DNA strand. This insertion causes a general disruption or even lysis of the DNA strand, thus preventing DNA replication and RNA synthesis.[8,32,56] Antibiotic agents used primarily for cancer chemotherapy are listed in Table 36-3.

Hormones

Several forms of cancer are referred to as hormone sensitive, because they tend to be exacerbated by certain hormones and attenuated by others. In particular, adrenocorticosteroids (see Chapter 29) and the sex hormones (androgens, estrogens, and progesterone; see Chapter 30) may influence the proliferation of certain tumors. Hence, drugs that either mimic or block (antagonize) the effects of these hormones may be useful in treating certain hormone-sensitive forms of cancer.[4,32,44,52,56] The primary drugs that inhibit neoplasms via hormonal mechanisms are listed in Table 36-4. In some cases, these drugs may work by negative feedback mechanisms

TABLE 36–2 Antimetabolites

Generic Name	Trade Name	Primary Antineoplastic Indication(s)*	Common Adverse Effects
Cytarabine	Cytosar-U	Several forms of acute and chronic leukemia; non-Hodgkin's lymphomas	Blood disorders (anemia, megaloblastosis, reticulocytopenia, others); GI distress (nausea, vomiting); skin rashes; hair loss
Floxuridine	FUDR	Carcinoma of the GI tract and liver	GI disorders (nausea, vomiting, anorexia); skin disorders (discoloration, rashes, hair loss)
Fluorouracil	Adrucil	Carcinoma of colon, rectum, stomach, and pancreas	GI distress (anorexia, nausea); blood disorders (anemia, leukopenia, thrombocytopenia); skin disorders (rashes, hair loss)
Mercaptopurine	Purinethol	Acute lymphocytic and myelocytic leukemia; chronic myelocytic leukemia	Blood disorders (anemia, leukopenia, thrombocytopenia); GI distress (nausea, anorexia); hepatotoxicity
Methotrexate	Folex, Mexate	Acute lymphocytic leukemia; meningeal leukemia; carcinoma of head and neck region, lung; non-Hodgkin's lymphomas	Blood disorders (anemia, leukopenia, thrombocytopenia); GI distress (including ulceration of GI tract); skin disorders (rashes, photosensitivity, hair loss); hepatotoxicity; CNS effects (headaches, drowsiness, fatigue)
Thioguanine	Lanvis	Acute lymphocytic leukemia; acute and chronic myelocytic leukemia	Blood disorders (anemia, leukopenia, thrombocytopenia); GI distress (nausea, vomiting); hepatotoxicity

*Only the indications listed in the U.S. product labeling are included here. Many anticancer drugs are used for additional types of neoplastic disease.

TABLE 36–3 Antineoplastic Antibiotics

Generic Name	Trade Name	Primary Antineoplastic Indication(s)*	Common Adverse Effects
Bleomycin	Blenoxane	Carcinoma of head, neck, cervical region, skin, penis, vulva, and testicle; Hodgkin's disease; non-Hodgkin's lymphomas	Pulmonary toxicity (interstitial pneumonitis); skin disorders (rashes, discoloration); mucosal lesions; fever; GI distress; general weakness and malaise
Dactinomycin	Cosmegen	Carcinoma of testicle and endometrium; carcinosarcoma of kidney (Wilms' tumor); Ewing's sarcoma; rhabdomyosarcoma	Blood disorders (leukopenia, thrombocytopenia, others); GI distress (nausea, vomiting, anorexia); mucocutaneous lesions; skin disorders (rashes, hair loss); local irritation at injection site
Daunorubicin	Cerubidine	Several forms of acute leukemia	Blood disorders (anemia, leukopenia, thrombocytopenia); cardiotoxicity (arrhythmias, congestive heart failure); GI distress (nausea, vomiting, GI tract ulceration); hair loss
Doxorubicin	Adriamycin RDF	Acute leukemias; carcinoma of bladder, breast, ovary, thyroid, and other tissues; Hodgkin's disease; non-Hodgkin's lymphomas; several sarcomas	Similar to daunorubicin
Idarubicin	Idamycin	Acute myelocytic leukemia	Similar to daunorubicin
Mitomycin	Mutamycin	Carcinoma of stomach and pancreas; chronic myelocytic leukemia	Blood disorders (leukopenia, thrombocytopenia); GI distress (nausea, vomiting, GI irritation and ulceration); nephrotoxicity; pulmonary toxicity
Plicamycin	Mithracin	Testicular carcinoma	Blood disorders (leukopenia, thrombocytopenia); GI distress (nausea, vomiting, diarrhea, GI tract irritation); general weakness and malaise

*Only the indications listed in the U.S. product labeling are included here. Many anticancer drugs are used for additional types of neoplastic disease.

TABLE 36-4 Antineoplastic Hormones

Types of Hormones	Primary Antineoplastic Indication(s)*	Common Adverse Effects
Adrenocorticosteroids Prednisone Prednisolone	Acute lymphoblastic leukemia; chronic lymphocytic leukemia; Hodgkin's disease	Adrenocortical suppression; general catabolic effect on supporting tissues (see Chapter 29)
Androgens Fluoxymesterone Methyltestosterone Testolactone Testosterone	Advanced, inoperable breast cancer in postmenopausal women	Masculinization in women (see Chapter 30)
Antiandrogens Flutamide	Inhibits the cellular uptake and effects of androgens in advanced, metastatic prostate cancer	Nausea, vomiting, diarrhea; decreased sex drive
Estrogens Chlorotrianisene Diethylstilbestrol Estradiol Others	Advanced, inoperable breast cancer in selected men and postmenopausal women; advanced, inoperable prostate cancer in men	Cardiovascular complications (including stroke and heart attack—especially in men); many other adverse effects (see Chapter 30)
Antiestrogens Tamoxifen	Acts as an estrogen antagonist to decrease the recurrence of cancer following mastectomy or to reduce tumor growth in advanced stages of breast cancer	Nausea, vomiting, hot flashes (generally well tolerated relative to other antineoplastic hormones)
Gonadotropin-releasing hormone drugs Leuprolide Goserelin	Work by negative feedback mechanisms to inhibit testosterone production; used primarily in advanced prostate cancer	Hot flashes; bone pain; CNS effects (e.g., headache, dizziness); GI disturbances (nausea, vomiting)

*Administration of hormonal agents in neoplastic disease is frequently palliative; that is, these drugs may offer some relief of symptoms but are not curative. Also, hormones are usually combined with other antineoplastic drugs or are used as an adjunct to surgery and radiation treatment.

to decrease endogenous hormonal stimulation of the tumor. In the majority of cases, however, the exact way that hormonal drugs inhibit tumor growth is unknown.[32] Hormonal anticancer drugs are typically used as adjuvant therapy; that is, they are used in conjunction with surgery, radiation treatments, and other anticancer drugs.

Interferons

The chemistry and pharmacology of the interferons was discussed in Chapter 34. Basically, these peptide compounds exert a number of beneficial effects including antiviral and antineoplastic activity. Interferons may be produced endogenously to help regulate cell growth. Pharmacologic administration of biosynthetically produced interferons may produce a similar antiproliferative effect. These agents are currently used to treat certain types of leukemias, lymphomas, Kaposi's sarcoma, and cancer in other organs and tissues (Table 36–5).[1,55,65] Interferons are also being tested in other forms of neoplastic disease, and these drugs will probably be approved for treating other cancers in the future.[2,40,42,46]

Plant Alkaloids

Alkaloids are nitrogen-based compounds frequently found in plants. The primary plant alkaloids used in treating cancer in humans are vincristine and vinblastine (see Table 36–5). These agents bind to cellular microtubules and initiate destruction and dissolution of these microtubules.[4,8] In particular, these drugs cause destruction of microtubules that are involved in the mitotic apparatus of the cell (the mitotic spindle). By disrupting the mitotic apparatus, the cell is unable to undergo normal cell division. In fact, when the cell attempts to divide, the nuclear material becomes disrupted and dispersed throughout the cytosol. This effect causes damage directly to the chromosomes, leading to subsequent cell dysfunction and death.

Aspirin and Other NSAIDs

There is considerable evidence that aspirin and similar nonsteroidal anti-inflammatory drugs (NSAIDs) may help prevent cancer in the colon and rectum.[37,63,64] This effect seems to be dose-related, with increased protection occurring in people who use aspirin on a regular basis.[57,62] The exact reason for this anticancer effect is not known. As indicated in Chapter 15, aspirin and similar drugs inhibit the cyclooxygenase enzyme that synthesizes prostaglandins in various cells in the body. It is not clear, however, if these drugs reduce the risk of colorectal cancer by inhibiting prostaglandin synthesis or through some other mechanism that remains to be determined. More information will surely be forthcoming about how aspirin and other NSAIDs can help prevent specific types of cancer.

TABLE 36–5 Other Antineoplastic Drugs

Drug(s)	Primary Antineoplastic Indication(s)*	Common Adverse Effects
Interferons Interferon alfa-2a (Roferon-A) Interferon alfa-2b (Intron-A)	Hairy-cell leukemia, Kaposi's sarcoma, chronic myelocytic leukemia, renal and bladder cancers	Flulike syndrome (mild fever, chills, malaise)
Plant alkaloids Vinblastine (Velban, Velsar	Carcinoma of breast, testes, other tissues; Hodgkin's disease; non-Hodgkin's lymphomas; Kaposi's sarcoma	Blood disorders (primarily leukopenia); GI distress (nausea, vomiting); hair loss; central and peripheral neuropathies; local irritation at injection site
Vincristine (Oncovin, Vincasar)	Acute lymphocytic leukemia; neuroblastoma; Wilms' tumor; Hodgkin's disease; non-Hodgkin's lymphomas; Ewing's sarcoma	Neurotoxicity (peripheral neuropathies, CNS disorders); hair loss; local irritation at injection site
Miscellaneous agents Asparaginase (Elspar)	Acute lymphocytic leukemia	Allergic reactions; renal toxicity; hepatic toxicity; delayed hemostasis; CNS toxicity (fatigue, mood changes); GI distress (nausea, vomiting); pancreatitis
Etoposide (VePesid)	Carcinoma of lung, testes	Blood disorders (anemia, leukopenia, thrombocytopenia); GI distress (nausea, vomiting); hypotension, allergic reactions; hair loss; neurotoxicity (peripheral neuropathies, CNS effects)
Hydroxyurea (Hydrea)	Carcinoma of the ovaries, head/neck region, other tissues; chronic myelocytic leukemia; melanomas	Blood disorders (primarily leukopenia); GI distress (nausea, vomiting, anorexia, GI tract irritation and ulceration); skin rashes
Mitotane (Lysodren)	Suppresses adrenal gland; used primarily to treat adrenocortical carcinoma	GI distress (nausea, vomiting, diarrhea, anorexia); CNS toxicity (lethargy, fatigue, mood changes); skin rashes

*Only the indications listed in the U.S. product labeling are included here. Many anticancer drugs are used for additional types of neoplastic disease.

Miscellaneous Agents

Asparaginase. Asparaginase (Elspar) is an enzyme that converts the amino acid asparagine into aspartic acid and ammonia. Most normal cells are able to synthesize sufficient amounts of asparagine in order to function properly. Some tumor cells (especially certain leukemic cells) must rely on extracellular sources for a supply of asparagine, however. By breaking down asparagine in the bloodstream and extracellular fluid, asparaginase deprives tumor cells of their source of asparagine, thus selectively impairing cell metabolism in these cells.[8,32] Asparaginase is used primarily in the treatment of acute lymphocytic leukemia (see Table 36–5).

Etoposide. The exact antineoplastic action of etoposide (VePesid) is not known.[41] This drug does appear to cause damage to DNA structure, possibly by stimulating endogenous enzymes that cleave the DNA strands.[4] Clinical applications of etoposide are listed in Table 36–5.

Hydroxyurea. Hydroxyurea (Hydrea) is believed to impair DNA synthesis by inhibiting a specific enzyme (ribonucleoside reductase) that is involved in synthesizing nucleic acid precursors.[4] Uses of hydroxyurea are listed in Table 36–5.

Mitotane. Although the exact mechanism of this drug is unknown, mitotane (Lysodren) selectively inhibits adrenocortical function. This agent is used exclusively to treat carcinoma of the adrenal cortex.

Mitoxantrone. This agent binds to DNA and becomes intercalated (inserted) between base pairs, thus producing breaks in the DNA strand and inhibition of DNA and RNA synthesis. Mitoxantrone (Novantrone) is used primarily in the treatment of various forms of acute leukemia.

COMBINATION CHEMOTHERAPY

Frequently, several different anticancer drugs are administered simultaneously. This process of combination chemotherapy increases the chance of successfully treating the cancer because of an additive and synergistic effect of each agent. Often, different types of anticancer drugs are combined in the same regimen to provide optimal results.[15] For instance, a particular drug regimen may include an alkylating agent, an antineoplastic antibiotic, a hormonal agent, or some other combination of anticancer drugs.

Some common anticancer drug combinations and the types of cancer in which they are used are listed in Table 36–6. These drug combinations are often indicated by an acronym of the drug names. For instance, "FAC" indicates a regimen of fluorouracil, Adriamycin (doxorubicin), and cyclophosphamide. These abbreviations are used to summarize drug therapy in a patient's medical chart, so therapists should be aware of the more common chemotherapy combinations.

USE OF ANTICANCER DRUGS WITH OTHER TREATMENTS

Cancer chemotherapy is only one method of treating neoplastic disease. The other primary weapons in the anticancer arsenal are surgery and radiation treatment. The choice of one or more of these techniques depends primarily on the patient, type of cancer, and location of the tumor. In many situations chemotherapy may be the primary or sole form of treatment in neoplastic disease, especially for certain advanced or inoperable tumors, or in widely disseminated forms of cancer, such as leukemia or lymphoma.[32] In other situations, chemotherapy is used in combination with other techniques, as an adjuvant to surgery and radiation treatment.[29,36] Primary examples of adjuvant cancer chemotherapy include using anticancer drugs following a mastectomy or surgical removal of other carcinomas.[13,24,43,60]

Whether anticancer drugs are used as the primary treatment or as adjuvant ther-

TABLE 36–6 Frequently Used Combination Chemotherapy Regimens

Type of Cancer	Therapy	Components of Therapy Regimen
Breast	FAC	5-Fluorouracil, doxorubicin (Adriamycin), cyclophosphamide (Cytoxan)
	CMF	Cyclophosphamide (Cytoxan), methotrexate, 5-fluorouracil
	Cooper's regimen (CVFMP)	5-Fluorouracil, methotrexate, vincristine (Oncovin), cyclophosphamide (Cytoxan), prednisone
Hodgkin's disease	MOPP	Mustargen (mechlorethamine), Oncovin (Vincristine), procarbazine, prednisone
	ABVD	Doxorubicin (Adriamycin), bleomycin (Blenoxane), vinblastine (Velban), dacarbazine (DTIC)
Leukemia	OAP	Oncovin, Ara-C (cytarabine), prednisone
	COAP	Cyclophosphamide, Oncovin (vincristine), Ara-C (cytarabine), prednisone
	Ad-OAP	Adriamycin (doxorubicin), Oncovin (vincristine), Ara-C (cytarabine), prednisone
Multiple myeloma	VBAP	Vincristine, BCNU (carmustine), Adriamycin (doxorubicin), prednisone
	VCAP	Vincristine, Cytoxan (cyclophosphamide), Adriamycin (doxorubicin), prednisone
Non-Hodgkin's lymphomas (vincristine)	CHOP	Cytoxan (cyclophosphamide), doxorubicin, Oncovin*, prednisone
	COP	Cytoxan (cyclophosphamide), Oncovin (vincristine), prednisone
Testicular tumors	VB-3	Vinblastine (Velban), bleomycin (Blenoxane)

*The H in this regimen refers to hydroxyldaunorubicin, the chemical synonym for doxorubicin.
From Moraca-Sawicki, AM: Antineoplastic chemotherapy. In Kuhn, MA: Pharmacotherapeutics: A Nursing Process Approach, ed 3. FA Davis, Philadelphia, 1994, p 1225, with permission.

apy, a common general strategy is upheld. To achieve a total cell kill, all reasonable means of dealing with the cancer are employed as early as possible. Cancer is not the type of disease where a wait-and-see approach can be used. The general strategy is more aligned with the idea that a barrage of anticancer modalities (i.e., surgery, radiation, and a combination of several different antineoplastic drugs) may be necessary to achieve a successful outcome. In addition, a multimodality approach (combining chemotherapy with radiation or using several drugs simultaneously) may produce a synergistic effect between these modalities. For instance, certain drugs may sensitize cancer cells to radiation treatment.[22,54] Likewise, several drugs working together may increase the antineoplastic effects of one another through a synergistic cytotoxic effect.[11]

SUCCESS OF ANTICANCER DRUGS

Various forms of cancer exhibit a broad spectrum of response to antineoplastic medications (Table 36–7). Some forms of cancer (choriocarcinoma, Wilms' tumor) can be cured in more than 90 percent of the affected patients. In other neoplastic disorders, chemotherapy may not cure the disease but may succeed in mediating remission and prolonging survival in a large percentage of patients (see Table 36–7). Of course, other

TABLE 36–7 Spectrum of Effectiveness of Cancer Chemotherapy

Disease	Survival
Neoplasms cured by chemotherapy	Patients with normal survival (%)
Choriocarcinoma	>90
Wilms' tumor	90
Testicular tumors	90
Hodgkin's disease	60
Rhabdomyosarcoma (childhood)	60
Burkitt's lymphoma	60
Acute lymphocytic leukemia	50–60
Diffuse histiocytic lymphoma	30
Ewing's sarcoma	30
Acute myelogenous leukemia	20
Ovarian cancer	20
Metastatic neoplasms with chemotherapy induced prolongation in survival (some cures)	Showing benefit (%)
Small-cell lung cancer	75
Non-Hodgkin's lymphomas	60–80
Chronic granulocytic leukemia	90
Multiple myeloma	50
Breast cancer	75
Head and neck cancer	50

From Spiegel and Muggia,[56] 1983, p 338, with permission.

factors such as early detection of the cancer will greatly influence the success of chemotherapy drugs.

There are, however, several types of cancer that do not seem to respond very well to anticancer drugs. For instance, the majority of metastatic cancers cannot be cured by current chemotherapeutic methods or by any other type of treatment.[18] As indicated in Table 36–7, chemotherapy drugs cure ovarian cancer and acute myelogenous leukemia in only about 20 percent of the patients. In addition, some of the most common forms of adult neoplastic disease, including lung, colorectal, prostate, breast, bladder, and pancreatic cancer, are difficult to cure using anticancer drugs.[20,21,23,27,39] Exactly why some forms of cancer are more difficult to treat pharmacologically remains unclear. Differences in the biochemistry, genetics, and location of certain cancer cells may make them less sensitive to the toxic effects of anticancer drugs.[5,10] Resistance to anticancer drugs (see "Resistance to Cancer Chemotherapy Drugs") is also a primary reason why certain cancers respond poorly to chemotherapy. Consequently, investigations of how to improve the efficacy of existing agents and the development of new anticancer drugs remain major foci in pharmacologic research. Some of the primary strategies in improving cancer chemotherapy are discussed in "Future Perspectives."

RESISTANCE TO CANCER CHEMOTHERAPY DRUGS

As indicated previously, certain cancers do not respond well to cancer chemotherapy. A primary reason for this fact is that cancers may develop resistance to a broad range of chemotherapeutic agents (multiple drug resistance), thus rendering these drugs ineffective in treating the cancer.[18,53] Cancers can become resistant to drugs through several different mechanisms. One primary mechanism occurs when the cancer cell synthesizes a glycoprotein that acts as a drug efflux pump.[18,25,53] This glycoprotein pump is inserted into the cancer cell's membrane and effectively expels different types of anticancer drugs from the cancer cell. Thus, cancer chemotherapeutic agents are ineffective because they are removed from the cell before they have a chance to exert cytotoxic effects.

Cancer cells also use other mechanisms to induce drug resistance, including production of specific substances (glutathione, glutathione-S-transferases) that inactivate anticancer drugs within the cancer cell, or by developing mechanisms that repair DNA that is damaged by anticancer drugs.[25,53] Essentially, cancer cells are often capable of developing methods for self-preservation against a broad range of cytotoxic drugs. Hence, various strategies are being explored to prevent or overcome multiple drug resistance during cancer chemotherapy. These strategies include altering the dosage, timing, and sequence of administration of different medications and using different combinations of medications to combat resistance.[33,45,50] Use of these strategies along with the development of new anticancer agents that do not cause resistance should help increase the effectiveness of chemotherapy in certain types of cancer.

FUTURE PERSPECTIVES

A major focus of cancer research is to increase the selective toxicity of currently available anticancer drugs. As discussed previously, most of these drugs are not only toxic to tumor cells, but also to normal cells. Nonetheless, if the drug can be delivered or targeted specifically for tumor cells, the drug will produce a more selective effect. One way that this targeting can be accomplished is by attaching the drug to another substance that is attracted specifically to tumor cells. For instance, joining the drug with an antibody that recognizes receptors only on cancerous cells may prove to be an effective method of delivering the drug directly to the neoplastic tissues.[28,35] Drugs may also be delivered more effectively to cancerous cells by attaching the drug to other chemicals (e.g., activated carbon particles), or by encapsulating the drug in a microsphere that becomes lodged in the tumor.[19,26,38] For the most part, these delivery techniques have not been overwhelmingly successful in improving the delivery of anticancer drugs.[28] Variations on these techniques and other delivery methods continue to be explored and may someday be used on a widespread basis to increase the effectiveness while decreasing the toxicity of anticancer drugs.

Another new and exciting approach to treating cancer is the development of methods that stimulate endogenous defense mechanisms against cancerous cells.[7,16] If the body's immune system recognizes the cancer cell as an invader, then various endogenous immune responses can be initiated to combat the cancerous cells. Hence, various strategies are being explored to help stimulate this immunologic response, including genetic modification of the cancer cells to increase their antigenic properties and expose these cells to immune attack.[7,12,49,58] Increased knowledge about the nature of cancer combined with a better understanding of the endogenous control of cell replication may ultimately provide drugs that are safe and effective in curing all forms of cancer.

IMPLICATIONS OF CANCER CHEMOTHERAPY IN REHABILITATION PATIENTS

The major way in which antineoplastic drugs will affect physical therapy and occupational therapy is through the adverse side effects of these agents. These drugs are routinely associated with a number of severe toxic effects including gastrointestinal problems, blood disorders, and profound fatigue. Also, neurotoxic effects including CNS abnormalities (such as convulsions and ataxia) and peripheral neuropathies may be a problem, especially with the plant alkaloids (vinblastine, vincristine). In terms of physical rehabilitation, these side effects typically are a source of frustration to both the patient and therapist. On some days, the patient undergoing cancer chemotherapy will simply not be able to tolerate even a relatively mild rehabilitation session. This reality can be especially demoralizing to patients who want to try to overcome their disease and actively participate in therapy as much as possible. Physical therapists and occupational therapists must take into account the debilitating nature of these drugs and be sensitive to the needs of the patient on a day-to-day basis. At certain times, the therapist must simply back off in trying to encourage active participation from the patient. Therapists, however, can often be particularly helpful in providing psychologic support to patients undergoing antineoplastic drug treatment. Therapists can reassure the patient that the side effects of these drugs are usually transient and that there will be better days when rehabilitation can be resumed.

Therapists may also be helpful in treating other problems associated with neoplastic disease. In particular, therapists may be involved in reducing the severe pain typically associated with many forms of cancer. Therapists may use transcutaneous electric nerve stimulation (TENS) or other physical agents as a nonpharmacologic means to attenuate pain. This approach may reduce the need for pain medications, thus reducing the chances that these drugs will cause additional adverse side effects and drug interactions with the anticancer drugs. As previously mentioned, physical therapists and occupational therapists also play a vital role in providing encouragement and support to the patient with cancer. This support can often help immeasurably in improving the quality of life of the cancer patient.

CASE STUDY

CANCER CHEMOTHERAPY

Brief History. R.J. is a 57-year-old woman with metastatic breast cancer, diagnosed 1 year ago, at which time she underwent a modified radical mastectomy followed by antineoplastic drugs. The cancer, however, had evidently metastasized to other tissues, including bone. She recently developed pain in the lumbosacral region that was attributed to metastatic skeletal lesions in the lower lumbar vertebrae. She was admitted to the hospital to pursue a course of radiation treatment to control pain and minimize bony destruction at the site of the skeletal lesion. Her current pharmacologic regimen consists of an antineoplastic antimetabolite (doxorubicin) and an antiestrogen (tamoxifen). She was also given a combination of narcotic and nonnarcotic analgesics (codeine and aspirin) to help control pain. Physical therapy was consulted to help control pain and maintain function in this patient.

Problem/Influence of Medication. The patient began to experience an increase in gastrointestinal side effects including nausea, vomiting, anorexia, and epigastric pain. These problems may have been caused by the analgesic drugs or by the combination of the analgesics and the antimetabolite. The patient, however, was experiencing adequate pain relief from the aspirin/codeine combination and was reluctant to consider alternative medications. The persistent nausea and anorexia had a general debilitating effect on the patient, and the physical therapist was having difficulty engaging the patient in an active general conditioning program.

Decision/Solution. The therapist instituted a program of local heat (hot packs) and TENS to help control pain in the lumbosacral region. This approach provided a nonpharmacologic means of alleviating pain, thereby decreasing the patient's analgesic drug requirements and related gastrointestinal problems. The patient was able to actively participate in a rehabilitation program throughout the course of her hospitalization, thus maintaining her overall strength and physical condition.

SUMMARY

Most antineoplastic drugs limit excessive growth and proliferation of cancer cells by impairing DNA synthesis and function. To replicate at a rapid rate, cancer cells must synthesize rather large quantities of DNA and RNA. Hence, cancer cells tend to be affected by antineoplastic drugs to a somewhat greater extent than normal cells. Normal cells, however, are also frequently affected by these drugs, resulting in a high incidence of adverse side effects. Currently, cancer chemotherapy is effective in reducing and even curing many neoplastic diseases. Other forms of cancer are much more difficult to treat pharmacologically, however. In the future, the development of methods that target the antineoplastic drug directly for cancer cells may improve the efficacy and safety of these agents. Rehabilitation specialists should be aware of the general debilitating nature of these drugs, and therapists must be prepared to adjust their treatment based on the ability of the patient to tolerate the adverse effects of cancer chemotherapy.

REFERENCES

1. Agarwala, SS and Kirkwood, JM: Interferons in the therapy of solid tumors. Oncology 51:129, 1994.
2. Borden, EC: Effects of interferons in neoplastic diseases in man. Pharmacol Ther 37:213, 1988.
3. Calabresi, P and Chabner, BA: Chemotherapy of neoplastic diseases: Introduction. In Gilman, AG, et al (eds): The Pharmacological Basis of Therapeutics, ed 8. Pergamon Press, New York, 1990.
4. Calabresi, P and Chabner, BA: Antineoplastic agents. In Gilman, AG, et al (eds): The Pharmacological Basis of Therapeutics, ed 8. Pergamon Press, New York, 1990.
5. Calabresi, P, Dexter, DL, and Heppner, GH: Clinical and pharmacological implications of cancer cell differentiation and heterogeneity. Biochem Pharmacol 28:1933, 1979.
6. Cersosimo, RJ and Karp, DD: Adrenal corticosteroids as antiemetics during chemotherapy. Pharmacotherapy 6:118, 1986.
7. Chabner, BA: Biological basis for cancer treatment. Ann Intern Med 118:633, 1993.
8. Chabner, BA and Meyers, CE: Clinical pharmacology of cancer chemotherapy. In DeVita, VT, Hellman, S, and Rosenberg, SA (ed): Cancer: Principles and Practice of Oncology, ed 3. JB Lippincott, Philadelphia, 1989.

9. Cormack, DH: Ham's Histology, ed 9. JB Lippincott, New York, 1987.
10. Curt, GA, Clendeninn, NJ, and Chabner, BA: Drug resistance in cancer. Cancer Treat Rep 68:87, 1984.
11. Damon, LE and Cadman, EC: The metabolic basis for combination chemotherapy. Pharmacol Ther 38:73, 1988.
12. Deisseroth, AB: Current trends and future directions in the genetic therapy of human neoplastic disease. Cancer 72:2069, 1993.
13. Ervin, TJ, et al: An analysis of induction and adjuvant chemotherapy in the multidisciplinary treatment of squamous-cell carcinoma of the head and neck. J Clin Oncol 5:10, 1987.
14. Farmer, PB: Metabolism and reactions of alkylating agents. Pharmacol Ther 35:301, 1987.
15. Fisher, RI, et al: Comparison of a standard regimen (CHOP) with three intensive chemotherapy regimens for advanced non-Hodgkin's lymphoma. N Engl J Med 328:1002, 1993.
16. Goey, SH, Wagstaff, J, and Pinedo, HM: Biological approaches to the treatment of cancer. Neth J Med 33:41, 1988.
17. Goldfarb, S: Pathology of neoplasia. In Kahn, SB, et al (eds): Concepts in Cancer Medicine. Grune & Stratton, New York, 1983.
18. Gottesman, MM: How cancer cells evade chemotherapy. Cancer Res 53:747, 1993.
19. Hagiwara, A and Takahashi, T: A new drug-delivery system of anticancer agents: Activated carbon particles absorbing anticancer agents. In Vivo 1:241, 1987.
20. Hainsworth, JD and Greco, FA: Drug therapy: Treatment of patients with cancer of an unknown primary site. N Engl J Med 329:257, 1993.
21. Hill, GJ, Omura, GA, and Bartolucci, AA: Treatment of gastrointestinal cancer: The Southeastern Cancer Study Group experience. South Med J 79:1197, 1986.
22. Hofer, KG, et al: Radiosensitizing and cytocidal effects of midonidazole: Evidence for seperate mode of action. Radiat Res 111:130, 1987.
23. Ihde, DC: Drug therapy: Chemotherapy of lung cancer. N Engl J Med 327:1434, 1992.
24. James, AG: How effective is adjuvant cancer chemotherapy? Arch Surg 121:1233, 1986.
25. Johnson, SW, Ozols, RF, and Hamilton, TC: Mechanisms of drug resistance in ovarian cancer. Cancer 71(suppl 2):644, 1993.
26. Jones, C, Burton, MA, and Gray, BN: Albumin microspheres as vehicles for the sustained and controlled release of doxorubicin. J Pharm Pharmacol 41:813, 1989.
27. Kearsley, JH: Cytotoxic chemotherapy for common adult malignancies: "The Emperor's New Clothes" revisited? Br Med J 293:871, 1986.
28. Kemshead, JT and Hopkins, K: Uses and limitations of monoclonal antibodies (MoAbs) in the treatment of malignant disease: A review. J R Soc Med 86:219, 1993.
29. Koutcher, JA, et al: Potentiation of a three drug chemotherapy regimen by radiation. Cancer Res 53:3518, 1993.
30. Krebs, H-B, et al: Combination antiemetic therapy in cisplatin-induced nausea and vomiting. Cancer 55:2645, 1985.
31. Kumar, V, Cotran, RS, and Robbins, SL: Basic Pathology, ed 5. WB Saunders, Philadelphia, 1992.
32. Lane, M: Chemotherapy of cancer. In del Regato, JA, Spjut, HJ, and Cox, JD (eds): Cancer: Diagnosis, Treatment, and Prognosis, ed 6. CV Mosby, St. Louis, 1985.
33. Lauer, SJ, et al: Intensive alternating drug pairs for treatment of high-risk childhood acute lymphoblastic leukemia: A pediatric oncology group pilot study. Cancer 71:2854, 1993.
34. Lazlo, J (ed): Symposium: Chemotherapy-induced emesis: Focus on metoclopramide. Drugs 25(suppl 1):1, 1983.
35. Levy, R: Biologicals for cancer treatment: Monoclonal antibodies. Hosp Pract 20:67, 1985.
36. Link, MP, et al: Results of treatment of childhood localized Hodgkin's lymphoma with combination chemotherapy with or without radiotherapy. N Engl J Med 322:1169, 1990.
37. Logan, RFA, et al: Effect of aspirin and nonsteroidal anti-inflammatory drugs in colorectal adenomas: Case-control study of subjects participating in the Nottingham faecal occult blood screening programme. Br Med J 307:285, 1993.
38. McArdle, CS, et al: Cytotoxic-loaded albumin microspheres: A novel approach to regional chemotherapy. Br J Surg 75:132, 1988.
39. Morton, RP and Stell, PM: Cytotoxic chemotherapy for patients with terminal squamous carcinoma: Does it influence survival? Clin Otolaryngol 9:175, 1984.
40. Oberg, K, et al: Treatment of malignant carcinoid tumors with human leukocyte interferon: Long-term results. Cancer Treat Rep 70:1297, 1986.
41. O'Dwyer, PJ, et al: Etoposide (VP-16-213). Current status of an active anticancer drug. N Engl J Med 312:692, 1985.
42. Oldham, RK: Biologicals for cancer treatment: Interferons. Hosp Pract 20:71, 1985.
43. Olivotto, IA, et al: Adjuvant systemic therapy and survival after breast cancer. N Engl J Med 330:805, 1994.
44. Parazzini, F, et al: Treatment with tamoxifen and progestins for metastatic breast cancer in postmenopausal women: A quantitative review of published randomized clinical trials. Oncology 50:483, 1993.

45. Perez, RP, et al: Mechanisms and modulation of resistance to chemotherapy in ovarian cancer. Cancer 71(suppl 4):1571, 1993.
46. Polli, E and Cortelezzi, A: Therapy with interferons in blood disease. Acta Haematol 78(suppl 1):64, 1987.
47. Richards, PD, et al: The antiemetic efficacy of secobarbital and chlorpromazine compared to metoclopramide, diphenhydramine, and dexamethasone: A randomized trial. Cancer 58:959, 1986.
48. Roberts, JJ and Friedlos, F: Quantitative estimation of cisplatin-induced DNA interstrand cross-links and their repair in mammalian cells: Relationship to toxicity. Pharmacol Ther 34:215, 1987.
49. Rosenberg, SA, et al: Gene transfer into humans: Immunotherapy with advanced melanoma using tumor-infiltrating lymphocytes modified by retroviral gene transduction. N Engl J Med 323:570, 1990.
50. Ross, DD, et al: Enhancement of daunorubicin accumulation, retention, and cytotoxicity by verapamil or cyclosporin-A in blast cells from patients with previously untreated acute myeloid leukemia. Blood 82:1288, 1993.
51. Rubin, E and Farber, JL: Neoplasia. In Rubin, E and Farber, JL (eds): Pathology, ed 2. JB Lippincott, Philadelphia, 1994.
52. Santen, RJ: Clinical review 37: Endocrine treatment of prostate cancer. J Clin Endocrinol Metab 75:685, 1992.
53. Schneider, E and Cowan, KH: Multiple drug resistance in cancer therapy. Med J Aust 160:371, 1994.
54. Severin, E and Hagenhoff, B: Synchronization of tumor cells with 5-fluorouracil plus uracil and with vinblastine and irradiation of synchronized cultures: A contribution concerning combined radiochemotherapy. Strahlenther Onkol 164:165, 1988.
55. Solal-Celigny, P, et al: Recombinant interferon alfa-2b combined with a regimen containing doxorubicin in patients with advanced folliclar lymphoma. N Engl J Med 329:1608, 1993.
56. Spiegel, RJ and Muggia, FM: Cancer chemotherapy. In Kahn, SB, et al (eds): Concepts in Cancer Medicine. Grune & Stratton, New York, 1983.
57. Suh, O, Mettlin, C, and Petrelli, NJ: Aspirin use, cancer, and polyps of the large bowel. Cancer 72:1171, 1993.
58. Symposium (various authors): Gene therapy for neoplastic diseases. Ann NY Acad Sciences 716:1, 1994.
59. Tannock, IF: Principles of cell proliferation: Cell kinetics. In DeVita, VT, Hellman, S, and Rosenberg, SA (eds): Cancer: Principles and Practice of Oncology, ed 3. JB Lippincott, Philadelphia, 1989.
60. The Department of Veteran's Affairs Laryngeal Cancer Study Group: Induction chemotherapy plus radiation compared with surgery and radiation in patients with advanced laryngeal cancer. N Engl J Med 324:1685, 1991.
61. The Italian Cooperative Study Group on Chronic Myeloid Leukemia: Interferon alfa-2a as compared with conventional chemotherapy for the treatment of chronic myeloid leukemia. N Engl J Med 330:820, 1994.
62. Thun, MJ, et al: Aspirin use and risk of fatal cancer. Cancer Res 53:1322, 1993.
63. Thun, MJ, Namboodiri, M, and Heath, C: Aspirin use and reduced risk of fatal colon cancer. N Engl J Med 325:1593, 1991.
64. Turner, D and Berkel, HJ: Nonsteroidal anti-inflammatory drugs for the prevention of colon cancer. Can Med Assoc J 149:595, 1993.
65. Worman, CP, et al: Interferon is effective in hairy-cell leukemia. Br J Haematol 60:759, 1985.

CHAPTER 37

Immunosuppressive Agents

The immune system is responsible for controlling the body's response to various types of injury and for defending the body from invading pathogens including bacteria, viruses, and other parasites.[15] The importance of this system in maintaining health is illustrated by the devastating effects that can occur in people who lack adequate immune function, such as patients with AIDS. It is sometimes necessary, however, to suppress immune function pharmacologically to prevent immune-mediated injury to certain tissues or organs. This need is especially true following organ transplants and tissue grafts, where the immune system may cause rejection of tissues transplanted from other donors (*allografts*) or from other sites in the patient's body (*autografts*). Likewise, immunosuppression may be helpful in treating certain conditions where, for some reason, the immune system causes damage to the body's own tissues. Such conditions are often referred to as *autoimmune diseases*, and many clinical disorders including rheumatoid arthritis, myasthenia gravis, and systemic lupus erythematosus are now recognized as having an autoimmune basis.[15]

Hence, a limited number of immunosuppressive drugs, or **immunosuppressants**, are currently available to prevent rejection of transplants or to treat specific diseases caused by an autoimmune response. Clearly, these drugs must be used very cautiously because too much suppression of the immune system will increase the susceptibility of the patient to infection from foreign pathogens. Likewise, these drugs are rather toxic and often cause a number of adverse side effects to the kidneys, lungs, musculoskeletal system, and other tissues. Nonetheless, immunosuppressive agents are often lifesaving because of their ability to prevent and treat organ rejection and to decrease immune-mediated tissue damage in other diseases.

This chapter provides a brief overview of the immune response and the drugs that are currently available to control and suppress this response. Physical therapists and occupational therapists may be involved in the rehabilitation of patients who have received organ transplants, skin grafts, or similar procedures that necessitate the use of immunosuppressant drugs. Likewise, rehabilitation specialists often treat patients with autoimmune disorders that affect the musculoskeletal system, and these patients will also likely be undergoing immunosuppressive treatment. Hence, this chapter will provide therapists with knowledge about the pharmacology of these drugs and how drug effects and side effects can impact on physical rehabilitation.

OVERVIEW OF THE IMMUNE RESPONSE

As indicated, one of the primary responsibilities of the immune system is to protect the body from bacteria, viruses, and other foreign pathogens. This responsibility is often referred to as *acquired immunity* because the immune system must recognize invading microorganisms and initiate specific steps to attack and destroy the invading cell.[15] The immune system's ability to recognize and deal with foreign pathogens involves an incredibly complex interaction between various cellular and chemical components.[38,41] I cannot give a detailed description of the intricacies of how these components work together because such a description is beyond the scope of this chapter and because many aspects of the immune response are still being investigated. An overview of key elements that mediate acquired immunity is illustrated in Figure 37–1, and these elements are described briefly here.

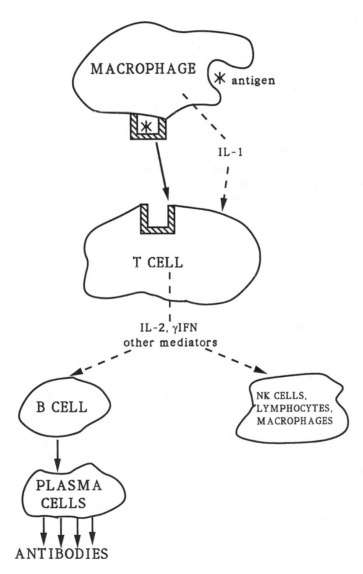

FIGURE 37–1. Schematic diagram of some of the key cellular and humoral elements involved in the immune response. Macrophages engulf and process antigens and present these antigens to T lymphocytes (T cells). Macrophages also stimulate T-cell function by releasing interleukin-1 (IL-1). T cells synthesize and release a number of humoral factors including interleukin-2 (IL-2), gamma interferon (γIFN), and other mediators. These mediators activate other lymphocytes (B cells) and cause B cells to differentiate into plasma cells, which produce various antibodies. T-cell–derived mediators also stimulate the activity of other immune system cells such as natural killer (NK) cells, other cytotoxic lymphocytes, and other macrophages. See text for further explanation.

1. *Antigen ingestion, processing, and presentation:* An invading substance (*antigen*) is engulfed by phagocytes such as macrophages.[16] The macrophage then processes the antigen by forming a complex between the antigen and specific membrane proteins known as major histocompatibility complex (MHC) proteins. The antigen-MHC complex is placed on the surface of the macrophage, where this complex can be presented to other lymphocytes such as the T cells. The macrophage also synthesizes and releases chemical mediators such as interleukin-1 (IL-1), which acts on other immune cells (T cells) to amplify the response of these cells to immune mediators.

2. *Antigen recognition and T-cell activation:* Lymphocytes derived from thymic tissues (hence the term *T cell*) recognize the antigen-MHC complex that is presented to the T cell on the surface of the macrophage. This recognition activates certain T cells (T helper cells), which begin to synthesize and release a number of chemical mediators known as **lymphokines**.[24,27] The lymphokines include mediators such as interleukin-2 (IL-2), other interleukins, gamma interferon, B-cell growth and differentiation factors, and other chemicals that stimulate the immune system. Certain T cells (T killer cells) are also activated by the macrophage presentation, and these T killer cells directly destroy targeted antigens.

3. *Proliferation, amplification, and recruitment:* The T cells continue to replicate and proliferate, thus producing more lymphokines, which further amplify T-cell effects. These lymphokines also recruit lymphocytes derived from bone marrow, that is, B cells.[6] Under the direction of IL-2 and other lymphokines, B cells proliferate and differentiate into plasma cells. Plasma cells ultimately release specific antibodies known as *immunoglobulins* (IgG, IgA, IgM, and the like). Likewise, T-cell and macrophage-derived lymphokines recruit additional cellular components, including other macrophages, other cytotoxic lymphocytes (natural killer, or NK, cells), and various other cells that can participate in the destruction of the foreign antigen.

Clearly, the immune response is an intricate sequence of events that involves a complex interaction between a number of cellular and humoral components. The overview provided here is just a brief summary of how some of the primary components participate in mediating acquired immunity, so readers are referred to additional sources for more information on this topic.[15,41]

PHARMACOLOGIC MODIFICATION OF THE IMMUNE RESPONSE

Drugs are used to suppress the immune system for two basic reasons (Table 37–1). First, the immune response is often attenuated pharmacologically following transplantation of organs or tissues to prevent rejection of these tissues.[9,30,32] Organs and other tissues can sometimes be attacked by the recipient's immune system even if these tissues appear to be cross-matched between donor and recipient. This rejection is often because of membrane proteins on the donor tissue that are recognized as antigens by the host's immune system.[15] Hence, drugs that suppress the cellular and chemical response to these membrane proteins can help prevent these responses from destroying the transplanted tissues and causing additional injury to the host's tissues.

Often, several different types of immunosuppressants are used together in fairly high doses to prevent or treat transplant rejection.[1,5,18,28] For instance, a glucocorticoid such as prednisolone is often administered with nonsteroidal drugs such as azathio-

TABLE 37–1 Common Immunosuppressive Agents

Generic Name	Trade Name(s)	Primary Indications*	
		Prevention or Treatment of Transplant Rejection	Diseases That Have an Autoimmune Response
Antibodies	Names vary according to specific lymphocyte targets	Bone marrow, other organ transplants	Idiopathic thrombocytic purpura, other hemolytic disorders
Azathioprine	Imuran	Kidney, heart	Rheumatoid arthritis, inflammatory bowel disease, myasthenia gravis, systemic lupus erythematosus (SLE), others
Cyclophosphamide	Cytoxan	Bone marrow	Rheumatoid arthritis, multiple sclerosis, SLE, dematomyositis, glomerulonephritis, hematologic disorders
Cyclosporine	Sandimmune	Kidney, liver, heart, lung, pancreas, bone marrow	Psoriasis, rheumatoid arthritis, inflammatory bowel disease, glomerulonephritis, others
Glucocorticoids	See Table 37–2	Heart, kidney, liver, bone marrow	Multiple sclerosis, rheumatoid arthritis, SLE, inflammatory bowel disease, hemolytic disorders, others.
Methotrexate	Folex, Mexate, Rheumatrex	—	Rheumatoid arthritis, psoriasis
Sulfasalazine	Azulfidine, others	—	Rheumatoid arthritis, inflammatory bowel disease
Tacrolimus	Prograf	Liver	—

*Indications vary considerably and many indications listed here are not in the U.S. product labeling for each drug; optimal use of these drugs alone or in combination with each other continues to be investigated.

prine and cyclosporine to provide optimal success and viability of the transplant. Of course, giving several powerful drugs at high doses often causes unpleasant or even toxic side effects. These effects must often be tolerated, however, considering the limited number of organs that are available for transplantation and the need to ensure survival of the transplant as much as possible.

A second major indication for these drugs is to limit immune-mediated damage to the body's tissues, that is, suppression of an autoimmune response.[25,32,42] Autoimmune responses occur when the immune system loses the ability to differentiate the body's own tissues from foreign or pathogenic tissues.[15] Exactly what causes this defect in immune recognition is often unclear, but prior exposure to some pathogen such as a virus may activate the immune response in a way that causes the immune system to mistakenly attack normal tissues while trying to destroy the virus. This autoimmune activation may remain in effect even after the original pathogen has been destroyed, thus leading to chronic immune-mediated injury to the body's tissues.

Autoimmune responses seem to be the underlying basis for a number of diseases including rheumatoid arthritis, diabetes mellitus, myasthenia gravis, systemic lupus erythematosus, scleroderma, polymyositis/dermatomyositis, and several other disorders.[15] As indicated previously, it is not exactly clear what factors cause autoimmune responses, and the reasons why certain individuals are more prone to autoimmune-related diseases remain to be elucidated. Nonetheless, drugs that suppress the immune system can limit damage to various other tissues, and these drugs may produce dramatic improvements in patients with diseases that are caused by an autoimmune response.

SPECIFIC IMMUNOSUPPRESSIVE AGENTS

Drugs commonly used to suppress the immune system are listed in Table 37–1, and the pharmacology of specific agents is described subsequently.

Azathioprine

Clinical Use. Azathioprine (Imuran) is a cytotoxic agent that is structurally and functionally similar to certain anticancer drugs like mercaptopurine.[10] Azathioprine is used primarily to prevent rejection of transplanted organs, especially in patients with kidney transplants. Azathioprine may also be used to suppress the immune response in a wide range of other conditions such as systemic lupus erythematosus, dermatomyositis, inflammatory myopathy, hepatic disease, myasthenia gravis, and ulcerative colitis. As indicated in Chapter 16, azathioprine is also used as an antiarthritic disease modifying agent.

Mechanism of Action. Although the exact mechanism of azathioprine is unknown, this drug probably interferes with DNA synthesis in cells that mediate the immune response. Azathioprine appears to act like the antimetabolite drugs used in cancer chemotherapy (see Chapter 36). The cell normally uses various endogenous substances such as purines as ingredients during DNA synthesis. Azathioprine is structurally similar to these purines, and this drug acts as a false ingredient that competes with the naturally occurring substances to slow down and disrupt DNA synthesis. Impaired nucleic acid synthesis slows down the replication of lymphocytes and other key cellular components that direct the immune response. Thus, azathioprine directly limits cellular proliferation through this inhibitory effect on DNA synthesis and ultimately limits the production of humoral components (antibodies) produced by these cells.

Adverse Effects. The primary side effects of azathioprine are related to suppression of bone marrow function, and these side effects include leukopenia, megaloblastic anemia, and similar blood dyscrasias. Other side effects include skin rash and gastrointestinal distress (appetite loss, nausea, vomiting), and hepatic dysfunction can also occur when higher doses are used.

Cyclophosphamide

Clinical Use. Cyclophosphamide (Cytoxan) is an anticancer alkylating agent that is commonly used in a variety of neoplastic disorders (see Chapter 36). This drug may also be helpful in suppressing the immune response during certain autoimmune diseases such as multiple sclerosis, systemic lupus erythematosus, and rheumatoid arthritis.[32] High doses of cyclophosphamide are also used to prevent tissue rejection in patients receiving bone marrow transplants and other organ transplants.

Mechanism of Action. The mechanism of cyclophosphamide as an anticancer alkylating agent was described in Chapter 36. This drug causes strong cross-links to be formed between strands of DNA and RNA, thus inhibiting DNA/RNA replication and function. Cyclophosphamide probably exerts immunosuppressant effects in a similar manner; that is, this drug inhibits DNA and RNA function in lymphocytes and other key cells, thus limiting the rapid proliferation of these cells during the immune response.

Adverse Effects. Cyclophosphamide is used very cautiously as an immunosuppressant because of the possibility of severe side effects including carcinogenic effects during long-term use. Other serious side effects include hematologic disorders (leukopenia, thrombocytopenia), cardiotoxicity, nephrotoxicity, and pulmonary toxicity.

Cyclosporine

Clinical Use. Cyclosporine (Sandimmune) is one of the primary medications used to suppress immune function following organ transplantation.[1,19,32,37] This medication can be used alone or combined with glucocorticoids, azathioprine, and other immunosuppressants to prevent rejection of kidney, lung, liver, heart, pancreas, and other organ transplants. Cyclosporine is used to a somewhat lesser extent in treating autoimmune diseases, but it may be helpful in conditions such as psoriasis, rheumatoid arthritis, inflammatory bowel disease, and glomerulonephritis.[4,19,23,32] As indicated in Chapter 32, cyclosporine has been used in the early stages of type I diabetes mellitus to help control immune-mediated destruction of pancreatic B cells, thus decreasing the severity of this disease in some patients.[3,7]

Mechanism of Action. Cyclosporine binds to specific proteins in lymphoid tissues and blocks the production of IL-2.[8,14] IL-2 plays a critical role in the immune response because this substance promotes the growth and proliferation of activated T lymphocytes and other immune cells such as natural killer (NK) cells (see Fig. 37–1). Thus, cyclosporine is one of the premier immunosuppressants because this drug is relatively selective for T cells and inhibits production of a key mediator of the immune response (IL-2).[8,19] This relatively specific inhibition is often advantageous compared to other nonselective drugs such as azathioprine, cyclophosphamide, and glucocorticoids that inhibit virtually all the cells and chemical mediators involved in the immune response.

Adverse Effects. The primary problem associated with cyclosporine is nephrotoxicity, which can range from mild, asymptomatic cases to severe kidney dysfunction that necessitates discontinuing this drug.[29] Hypertension is also a common adverse effect, especially when cyclosporine is used for prolonged periods.[29,33] Other problems include neurotoxicity, gingival hyperplasia, hair growth (hirsutism), and increased infections. These problems, however, tend to be less severe with cyclosporine than with other less selective immunosuppressants.

Glucocorticoids

Clinical Use. As described in Chapter 29, glucocorticoids are powerful anti-inflammatory and immunosuppressive drugs. Glucocorticoids exert a rather nonspecific inhibition of virtually all aspects of cell-mediated and chemical-mediated immunity, thus enabling these drugs to be used in a variety of situations where it is necessary to suppress immune function. Hence, these drugs are a mainstay in preventing transplant rejection and in the treatment of various diseases associated with an autoimmune response. Glucocorticoids commonly used as immunosuppressants are listed in Table 37–2.

Mechanism of Action. Although the exact mechanism of immunosuppression is unclear, glucocorticoids probably interrupt the immune response in several ways. These drugs inhibit the migration of leukocytes and macrophages to the location of a foreign tissue or antigen, and glucocorticoids inhibit the ability of macrophages to ingest and process antigens.[11] Glucocorticoids also inhibit T-cell activation and suppress the ability of these cells to synthesize and respond to chemical mediators such as interleukins and interferons.[2,13,21,22] The ability of T cells to proliferate and activate other immune components (B cells, other lymphocytes) is therefore inhibited. Hence, these drugs disrupt the initial steps in antigen recognition, and they also interfere with the complex interaction that normally occurs between various cellular components of the immune response. Please refer to Chapter 29 for more details about how glucocorticoids exert their effects on various cells and tissues.

Adverse Effects. The immunosuppressive effects of these drugs are balanced by several serious side effects. As indicated in Chapter 29, glucocorticoids typically produce a catabolic effect on collagenous tissues, and breakdown of muscle, bone, skin, and various other tissues is a common adverse effect. Glucocorticoids also produce other side effects including hypertension, adrenocortical suppression, increased chance of infection, glaucoma, decreased glucose tolerance, and gastric ulcer. These side effects can be especially problematic when glucocorticoids are used to prevent transplant rejection because these drugs are often given in fairly high doses for extended periods of time. Hence, efforts are often made to progressively decrease glucocorticoid dosage so that immunosuppression is achieved using the lowest possible dose. Likewise, glucocorticoids are often combined with other nonsteroidal immunosuppressants such as cyclosporine and azathioprine so that synergistic effects can be obtained and immunosuppression can be achieved using relatively lower doses of each drug.

Methotrexate

Clinical Use. Methotrexate (Folex, Mexate, Rheumatrex) was developed originally as an anticancer agent (see Chapter 36), but this drug is also used in certain noncancerous conditions that have an autoimmune component.[10] As indicated in Chapter 16, methotrexate is commonly used as a disease-modifying drug in rheumatoid arthritis, and methotrexate is also approved for use in psoriasis. Methotrexate is not typically

TABLE 37–2 Glucocorticoids Used as Immunosuppressive Agents*

Betamethasone (Celestone)	Methylprednisolone (Medrol)
Corticotropin (Acthar)	Paramethasone (Haldrone)
Cortisone (Cortone)	Prednisolone (Hydeltrasol, Predate)
Dexamethasone (Decadron)	Prednisone (Deltasone)
Hydrocortisone (Cortef)	Triamcinolone (Aristocort)

*Common trade names are shown in parentheses.

used to prevent transplant rejection, but this drug may be used to help prevent the recurrence of leukemia (anticancer effects) following bone marrow transplants.

Mechanism of Action. The pharmacology of methotrexate is described in Chapter 36. This drug acts as an antimetabolite that interferes with the production of DNA and RNA precursors in rapidly proliferating cells. This interference produces a general inhibition of the replication of lymphocytes inherent to the immune response.

Adverse Effects. The major problems associated with methotrexate include hepatic and pulmonary toxicity. These problems are dose-related, however, and serious adverse effects tend to occur less frequently at doses used for immunosuppression as compared to anticancer doses.

Sulfasalazine

Clinical Use. Sulfasalazine (Azulfidine, other names) has unique properties in that it has some antibacterial characteristics similar to sulfonamide drugs (see Chapter 33) and some anti-inflammatory characteristics similar to the salicylates (see Chapter 15). This drug is used primarily to suppress the immune response that underlies rheumatoid arthritis and inflammatory bowel disease.

Mechanism of Action. The exact mechanism of this drug in immune-related disorders is not fully understood. Sulfasalazine may affect key components in the immune system, including suppression of NK cells. Other effects may be related to the breakdown of this drug into active metabolites, including sulfapyridine and mesalamine, which exert antibiotic and anti-inflammatory effects, respectively.

Adverse Effects. Primary side effects include headache, blood dyscrasias (agranulocytosis, anemia, thrombocytopenia), increased sensitivity to ultraviolet light, and hypersensitivity reactions (fever, skin rashes/itching). Hypersensitivity can be severe or even fatal in susceptible individuals.

Tacrolimus

Clinical Use. Tacrolimus (Prograf) is a fairly new immunosuppressant that was developed under the investigational name FK-506.[12] This drug is similar to cyclosporine in structure and immunosuppressive effects, but tacrolimus is approximately 10 to 100 times more potent than cyclosporine.[35,39] Tacrolimus may be somewhat less toxic than cyclosporine and other immunosuppressants, although serious side effects may still occur at higher doses (see "Adverse Effects" in this section). Tacrolimus is used primarily to prevent rejection of liver transplants, but this drug may also be useful in rescuing other organ transplants that do not respond to other immunosuppressive drugs.[17,36]

Mechanism of Action. Tacrolimus acts like cyclosporine by binding to specific proteins in lymphoid tissues and inhibiting the production of key immune mediators such as IL-2.[39] This binding provides a somewhat more selective inhibition of immune function compared to other drugs that exert a general or nonselective inhibition of the immune response.

Adverse Effects. Common side effects of tacrolimus include gastrointestinal disturbances (cramps, nausea, diarrhea or constipation), muscle and joint pain, and skin rashes/itching. More serious problems include fever, CNS toxicity (headache, anxiety, nervousness, seizures), and pulmonary toxicity. These effects, however, are generally less severe than those of similar immunosuppressants such as cyclosporine.

Other Methods of Immunosuppression

Immune function can also be suppressed using antibodies that interact with specific immune system cells and interfere with the function of these cells.[20,32,34] These antibodies can be obtained from animal sources and cell culture techniques (monoclonal antibodies) to provide a rather selective method of suppressing immune function. For example, antibodies such as Rh(D) immunoglobulin are routinely used to suppress the immune response in mothers who have been exposed to an incompatible blood type from their fetus. This immunosuppression prevents the mother from developing antibodies that will be passed on to the fetus or to a fetus in a subsequent pregnancy, thus blocking the production of maternal antibodies that can attack the fetus's blood and cause a potentially fatal condition known as hemolytic anemia of the newborn.[32] Antibodies have also been developed that are very selective for antigens located on the surface of specific T cells and other lymphocytes, and these antibodies inhibit cell function or cause destruction of the cell.[26,34,40] These anti–T-cell antibodies are primarily used to help prevent rejection of organ and bone marrow transplants.[31,40] For more information on the use of specific antibodies in specific disorders, please refer to other sources on this topic.[10,32]

A variety of other agents have cytotoxic effects that can also be used to suppress the immune system. These drugs include chlorambucil (Leukeran), dactinomycin (Cosmegen), mercaptopurine (Purinethol), and vincristine (Oncovin, Vincasar). These agents are similar to methotrexate; they exert cytotoxic effects that interfere with the proliferation of immune system cellular components. Hence, these drugs are used primarily as anticancer agents, but they may be helpful in certain autoimmune disorders or to prevent rejection of tissue/organ transplants. The pharmacology of antineoplastic drugs that also have immunosuppressive effects is described in more detail in Chapter 36.

SIGNIFICANCE OF IMMUNOSUPPRESSIVE AGENTS IN REHABILITATION

Physical therapists and occupational therapists are often involved in the physical rehabilitation of patients who have received heart, liver, kidney, and other organ transplants. Therapists also frequently deal with patients who have received autologous grafts such as skin grafts for treating burns and bone marrow transplants during treatment of certain cancers. Hence, therapists frequently deal with patients taking drugs to prevent tissue rejection.

Therapists also deal with the rehabilitation of musculoskeletal disorders that are caused by an autoimmune response. Many such diseases attack connective tissues, and various autoimmune diseases such as rheumatoid arthritis, dermatomyositis, and systemic lupus erythematosus are often the primary reason that patients are undergoing rehabilitation. Hence, these drugs are frequently used in a large population of patients receiving physical therapy and occupational therapy.

The most significant impact of these drugs on rehabilitation is related to the side effects of these agents. Immunosuppressants are typically used in high doses to produce immunosuppressive effects, and these effects are often achieved at the expense of a number of serious and toxic side effects. Many immunosuppressants exert catabolic effects on bone, muscle, and other tissues, and this fact is especially true for the glucocorticoids. Other immunosuppressants such as cyclosporine and tacrolimus are neurotoxic and may cause peripheral neuropathies and CNS-related problems in balance and posture.

Hence, rehabilitation specialists can play a critical role in helping offset some of these adverse effects. Therapists can institute strengthening and general conditioning exercises to prevent breakdown of muscle, bone, and other tissues as well as to help maintain cardiovascular function. Problems associated with peripheral neuropathies such as pain and weakness may respond to TENS and other electrotherapeutic treatments. Balance and gait training may also help patients overcome problems caused by CNS toxicity and vestibular problems. Thus, therapists can implement specific strategies as required to help patients cope with adverse drug effects associated with immunosuppressive agents.

CASE STUDY

IMMUNOSUPPRESSIVE AGENTS

Brief History. A.S. is a 47-year-old concert musician who experienced a progressive decline in renal function that ultimately led to renal failure. Kidney function was maintained artificially through renal dialysis until a suitable kidney transplant became available from a donor who died in an automobile accident. The kidney was transplanted successfully and A.S. was placed on a prophylactic regimen of three different immunosuppressive drugs to prevent rejection of the transplanted kidney. At the time of the transplant, cyclosporine was initiated at a dose of 10 mg per kilogram of body weight each day. After 15 days, cyclosporine dosage was decreased to 8 mg/kg per day, and dosage was progressively decreased over the next 2 months until a maintenance dosage of 2 mg/kg per day was achieved. On the day of surgery, he also received an intravenous dose of 0.5 g of methylprednisolone. Oral doses of methylprednisolone were then administered in dosages of 16 mg/day for the first 3 months, 12 mg/day for the next 3 months, and 8 mg/day thereafter. Azathioprine was administered at a dosage of 1 mg/kg per day throughout the posttransplant period. Physical therapy was initiated in the intensive care unit (ICU) 1 day after the transplant to help increase strength and facilitate recovery from the surgery.

Problem/Influence of Medication. The therapist noted that several drugs were being used to prevent rejection including rather high doses of methylprednisolone, a glucocorticoid agent. Glucocorticoids are notorious for their catabolic effects, and the therapist was aware that a program of strengthening and weight-bearing exercise would help offset the breakdown of muscle and bone that can often occur with prolonged glucocorticoid administration.

Decision/Solution. Gentle resistance exercises were initiated in the ICU as soon as the patient was alert and could follow basic instructions. Strengthening exercises were progressively increased using manual resistance, and various weights and exercise machines were incorporated into the strengthening regimen as tolerated by the patient. The therapist also initiated weight-bearing activities as soon as the patient was able to tolerate standing in the ICU. Weight-bearing activities were progressively increased, and the patient was able to walk independently for distances up to 1000 feet and climb two flights of stairs at the time of discharge. The therapist also worked closely with the patient and the patient's family to make sure that strengthening exercises and a progressive ambulation program were continued in the patient's home. The patient did not experience any problems related to tissue rejection, and he was able to resume his musical career and maintain an active lifestyle that included daily walks and regular visits to a health club, where he participated in a supervised program of strength training.

SUMMARY

Our knowledge of how the immune system functions in normal and disease states has increased dramatically over the last several decades, and we now have drugs that can moderate the effects of the immune response in certain clinical situations. Immunosuppressants are a mainstay in preventing tissue rejection, and much of the current success of organ transplants is because of the judicious use of immunosuppressive drugs. These drugs are also beneficial in a number of diseases that have an autoimmune basis, and immunosuppressants can help alleviate symptoms or possibly even reverse the sequelae of certain diseases such as rheumatoid arthritis. These drugs are not without problems, however, because many immunosuppressants cause a rather nonspecific inhibition of immune function, which leads to a number of rather serious side effects. As more is learned about the details of immune function, it is hoped that new drugs will be developed that are more selective in their ability to prevent immune-mediated injury without causing a generalized suppression of the immune system.

REFERENCES

1. Barry, JM: Immunosuppressive drugs in renal transplantation: A review of the regimens. Drugs 44:554, 1992.
2. Besedovsky, H, et al: Immunoregulatory feedback between interleukin-1 and glucocorticoid hormones. Science 233:652, 1986.
3. Bougneres, PF, et al: Factors associated with early remission of type I diabetes in children treated with cyclosporine. N Engl J Med 318:663, 1988.
4. Brynskov, J, et al: A placebo-controlled, double-blind, randomized trial of cyclosporine therapy in active chronic Crohn's disease. N Engl J Med 321:845, 1989.
5. Chao, NJ, et al: Cyclosporine, methotrexate, and prednisone compared with cyclosporine and prednisone for prophylaxis of acute graft-versus-host disease. N Engl J Med 329:1225, 1993.
6. Cooper, MD: B lymphocytes: Normal development and function. N Engl J Med 317:1452, 1987.
7. Feutren, G, et al: Cyclosporine increases the rate of remissions in insulin-dependent diabetes of recent onset: Results of a multicentre double-blind trial. Lancet 2:119, 1986.
8. Gelfand, EW, Cheung, R, and Mills, GB: The cyclosporines inhibit lymphocyte activation at more than one site. J Immunol 138:1115, 1987.
9. Hall, BM, et al: Comparison of three immunosuppressive regimens in cadaver renal transplantation: Long-term cyclosporine, short-term cyclosporine followed by azathioprine and prednisolone, and azathioprine and prednisolone without cyclosporine. N Engl J Med 318:1499, 1988.
10. Handschumacher, RE: Immunosuppressive agents. In Gilman, AG, et al (eds): The Pharmacologic Basis of Therapeutics, ed 8. Pergamon Press, New York, 1990.

11. Haynes, RC: Adrenocorticotropic hormone; adrenocortical steroids and their synthetic analogs; inhibitors of the synthesis and actions of adrenocortical hormones. In Gilman, AG, et al (eds): The Pharmacologic Basis of Therapeutics, ed 8. Pergamon Press, New York, 1990.
12. Hooks, MA: Tacrolimus, a new immunosuppressant: A review of the literature. Ann Pharmacother 28:501, 1994.
13. Horst, H-J and Flad, HD: Corticosteroid-interleukin 2 interactions: Inhibition of binding of interleukin 2 to interleukin 2 receptors. Clin Exp Immunol 68:156, 1987.
14. Jenkins, MK, Schwartz, RH, and Pardoll, DM: Effects of cyclosporine A on T cell development and clonal deletion. Science 241:1655, 1988.
15. Johnson, KJ, et al: Immunopathology. In Rubin, E and Farber, JL (eds): Pathology, ed 2. JB Lippincott, Philadelphia, 1994.
16. Johnston, RB: Current concepts in immunology: Monocytes and macrophages. N Engl J Med 318:747, 1988.
17. Jordan, ML, Shapiro, R, and Vivas, CA: FK 506 "rescue" for resistant rejection of renal allografts under primary cyclosporine immunosuppression. Transplantation 57:860, 1994.
18. Kahan, BD: Development of synergistic immunosuppressive drug regimens based upon cyclosporine. Kidney Int 44(suppl 43):S12, 1993.
19. Kahan, BD: Cyclosporine. N Engl J Med 321:1725, 1989.
20. Larick, JW: Potential of monoclonal antibodies as pharmacological agents. Pharmacol Rev 41:539, 1989.
21. Lee, SW, et al: Glucocorticoids selectively inhibit the transcription of the interleukin 1-beta gene and decrease stability of interleukin 1-beta messenger RNA. Proc Natl Acad Sci 85:1204, 1988.
22. Lew, W, Oppenheim, JJ, and Matsushima, K: Analysis of the suppression of IL-1 alpha and IL-1 beta products in human peripheral blood mononuclear adherent cells by a glucocorticoid hormone. J Immunol 140:1895, 1988.
23. Lichtiger, S and Present, DH: Preliminary report: Cyclosporine in treatment of severe active ulcerative colitis. Lancet 336:16, 1990.
24. Lipsky, PE: The control of antibody production by immunomodulatory molecules. Arthritis Rheum 32:1345, 1989.
25. Luqmani, R, Gordon, C, and Bacon, P: Clinical pharmacology and modification of autoimmunity and inflammation in rheumatoid disease. Drugs 47:259, 1994.
26. Mathieson, PW, et al: Monoclonal antibody therapy in systemic vasculitis. N Engl J Med 323:250, 1990.
27. Miyajima, A, et al: Coordinate regulation of immune and inflammatory responses by T cell-derived lymphokines. FASEB J 2:2462, 1988.
28. Montagnino, G, et al: A randomized trial comparing triple-drug and double-drug therapy in renal transplantation. Transplantation 58:149, 1994.
29. O'Grady, JG, et al: An analysis of cyclosporine efficacy and toxicity after liver transplantation. Transplantation 45:575, 1988.
30. Opelz, G: Effect of the maintenance immunosuppressive drug regimen on kidney transplant outcome. Transplantation 58:443, 1994.
31. Ortho Multicenter Transplant Study Group: A randomized clinical trial of OKT3 monoclonal antibody for acute rejection of cadaveric renal transplants. N Engl J Med 313:337, 1985.
32. Salmon, SE: Immunopharmacology. In Katzung, BG (ed): Basic and Clinical Pharmacology, ed 5. Appleton & Lange, Norwalk, CT, 1992.
33. Scherrer, U, et al: Cyclosporine-induced sympathetic activation and hypertension after heart transplantation. N Engl J Med 323:693, 1990.
34. Seaman, WE, and Wofsy, D: Selective manipulation of the immune response in vivo by monoclonal antibodies. Annu Rev Med 39:231, 1988.
35. Singh, N, et al: Infectious complications in liver transplant recipients on tacrolimus. Transplantation 58:774, 1994.
36. Starzl, TE: FK 506 for liver, kidney, and pancreas transplantation. Lancet 2:1000, 1989.
37. Symposium (various authors): Second International Congress on Cyclosporine. Transplant Proc 20:3, 1988.
38. Thomson, AW, Woo, J, and Cooper, M: Mode of action of immunosuppressive drugs with particular reference to the molecular basis of macrolide-induced immunosuppression. In Thomson, HW (ed): The Molecular Biology of Immunosuppression. John Wiley & Sons, New York, 1992.
39. Tocci, MJ, et al: The immunosuppressant FK 506 selectively inhibits expression of early T cell activation genes. J Immunol 143:718, 1989.
40. Waldman, TA: Immune receptors: Targets for therapy of leukemia/lymphoma, autoimmune diseases, and for the prevention of allograft rejection. Annu Rev Immunol 10:675, 1992.
41. Warrens, AN and Lechler, RI: Key molecular events in the induction and expression of the immune response. In Thomson, HW (ed): The Molecular Biology of Immunosuppression. John Wiley & Sons, New York, 1992.
42. Wraith, D and Cooke, A: Molecular intervention in the therapy of autoimmune disease. In Thomson, HW (ed): The Molecular Biology of Immunosuppression. John Wiley & Sons, New York, 1992.

Drugs Administered by Iontophoresis and Phonophoresis

Listed here are some drugs that may be administered by iontophoresis and phonophoresis. Administration of these agents by these techniques is largely empirical. Use of these substances in the conditions listed is based primarily on clinical observation and anecdotal reports in the literature. Likewise, the preparation strengths given here are merely suggestions based on currently available information.

Drug	Principal Indication(s)	Treatment Rationale	Iontophoresis	Phonophoresis
Acetic acid	Calcific tendinitis	Acetate is believed to increase solubility of calcium deposits in tendons and other soft tissues	2–5% aqueous solution from negative pole	—
Calcium chloride	Skeletal muscle spasms	Calcium stabilizes excitable membranes; appears to decrease excitability threshold in peripheral nerves and skeletal muscle	2% aqueous solution from positive pole	—
Dexamethasone	Inflammation	Synthetic steroidal anti-inflammatory agent (see Chapter 29)	4 mg/mL in aqueous solution from negative pole	0.4% ointment
Hydrocortisone	Inflammation	Anti-inflammatory steroid (see Chapter 29)	0.5% ointment from positive pole	0.5–1.0% ointment
Iodine	Adhesive capsulitis and other soft-tissue adhesions; microbial infections	Iodine is a broad-spectrum antibiotic, hence its use in infections, etc.; the sclerolytic actions of iodine are not fully understood	5–10% solution or ointment from negative pole	10% ointment
Lidocaine	Soft-tissue pain and inflammation (e.g., bursitis, tenosynovitis)	Local anesthetic effects (see Chapter 12)	4–5% solution or ointment from positive pole	5% ointment

Magnesium sulfate	Skeletal muscle spasms; myositis	Muscle relaxant effect may be caused by decreased excitability of the skeletal muscle membrane and decreased transmission at the neuromuscular junction	2% aqueous solution or ointment from positive pole	2% ointment
Hyaluronidase	Local edema (subacute and chronic stage)	Appears to increase permeability in connective tissue by hydrolyzing hyaluronic acid, thus decreasing encapsulation and allowing dispersement of local edema	Reconstitute with 0.9% sodium chloride to provide a 150 μg/mL solution from positive pole	—
Salicylates	Muscle and joint pain in acute and chronic conditions (e.g., overuse injuries, rheumatoid arthritis)	Aspirin-like drugs with analgesic and anti-inflammatory effects (see Chapter 15)	10% trolamine salicylate ointment or 2–3% sodium salicylate solution from negative pole	10% trolamine salicylate ointment or 3% sodium salicylate ointment
Tolazoline hydrochloride	Indolent cutaneous ulcers	Increases local blood flow and tissue healing by inhibiting vascular smooth muscle contraction	2% aqueous solution from positive pole	—
Zinc oxide	Skin ulcers, other dermatologic disorders	Zinc acts as a general antiseptic; may increase tissue healing	20% ointment from positive pole	20% ointment

APPENDIX B

Potential Interactions Between Physical Agents and Therapeutic Drugs

Listed here are some potential interactions between physical agents used in rehabilitation and various pharmacologic agents. Considering the vast array of therapeutic drugs, it is impossible to list all the possible relationships between these drugs and the procedures used in physical and occupational therapy. However, some of the more common interactions are indicated here.

Modality	Desired Therapeutic Effect	Drugs with Complementary/ Synergistic Effects	Drugs with Antagonistic Effects	Other Drug-Modality Interactions
Cryotherapy Cold/ice packs Ice massage Cold baths Vapocoolant sprays	Decreased pain, edema, and inflammation	Anti-inflammatory steroids (glucocorticoids); nonsteroidal anti-inflammatory analgesics (aspirin and similar NSAIDs)	Peripheral vasodilators may exacerbate acute local edema	Some forms of cryotherapy may produce local vasoconstriction that temporarily impedes diffusion of drugs to the site of inflammation
	Muscle relaxation and decreased spasticity	Skeletal muscle relaxants	Nonselective cholinergic agonists may stimulate the neuromuscular junction	—
Superficial and deep heat Local application Hot packs Paraffin Infrared	Decreased muscle/joint pain and stiffness Decreased muscle spasms	NSAIDs; opioid analgesics; local anesthetics Skeletal muscle relaxants	— Nonselective cholinergic agonists may stimulate the neuromuscular junction	—
Fluidotherapy Diathermy Ultrasound	Increased blood flow to improve tissue healing	Peripheral vasodilators	Systemic vasoconstrictors (e.g., alpha-1 agonists) may decrease perfusion of peripheral tissues	—
Systemic heat Large whirlpool Hubbard tank	Decreased muscle/joint stiffness in large areas of the body	Opioid and nonopioid analgesics; skeletal muscle relaxants	—	Severe hypotension may occur if systemic hot whirlpool is administered to patients taking peripheral vasodilators and some antihypertensive drugs (e.g., alpha-1 antagonists, nitrates, direct-acting vasodilators, calcium channel blockers (*Continued*)

Modality	Desired Therapeutic Effect	Drugs with Complimentary/ Synergistic Effects	Drugs with Antagonistic Effects	Other Drug-Modality Interactions
Ultraviolet radiation	Increased wound healing	Various systemic and topical antibiotics	—	Antibacterial drugs generally increase cutaneous sensitivity to ultraviolet light (i.e., photosensitivity)
	Management of skin disorders (acne, rashes)	Systemic and topical antibiotics and anti-inflammatory steroids (glucocorticoids)	Many drugs may cause hypersensitivity reactions that result in skin rashes, itching	Photosensitivity with antibacterial drugs
Transcutaneous electrical nerve stimulation (TENS)	Decreased pain	Opioid and nonopioid analgesics	Opioid antagonists (naloxone)	—
Functional neuromuscular electrical stimulation	Increased skeletal muscle strength and endurance	—	Skeletal muscle relaxants	—
	Decreased spasticity and muscle spasms	Skeletal muscle relaxants	Nonselective cholinergic agonists may stimulate the neuromuscular junction	—

APPENDIX **C**

Use of the *Physicians' Desk Reference*

Several drug indices are available that can supplement this text by serving as a detailed source of information about individual drugs. One of the most readily available and frequently used indices is the *Physicians' Desk Reference*, or *PDR*. The *PDR* is published annually by Medical Economics Data Production Company, Inc., Montvale, NJ, 07645.

Basically, drug manufacturers submit information about the indications, dosage, adverse effects, and so on, of individual agents for inclusion into the *PDR*. The *PDR* is then published annually, providing a relatively current source of information. The *PDR* is also updated within a given year through periodic supplements.

The *PDR* begins by listing all the manufacturers who submitted information to the *PDR* in the Manufacturers' Index. Immediately following the Manufacturers' Index, drugs are listed according to the Product Name Index and the Product Category Index. These listings are followed by detailed descriptions of the drugs in the Product Information Section. The Product Information section constitutes the bulk of the *PDR*.

Using the *PDR* for the first time can be somewhat confusing because drugs are listed in several different ways. The brief outline provided here may help individuals use the *PDR* more effectively to obtain information about specific agents.

1. If the Trade Name or Brand Name of the Drug Is Known. Begin by looking in the Product Name Index in the front of the *PDR*, easily found by locating the PINK pages. Drugs are listed alphabetically according to the name given by the drug manufacturer (trade or brand name) as well as by the generic name (see section 2). Each trade name is followed by the name of the manufacturer (in parentheses) and by a page number, which indicates where the drug is described in the Product Information section. Some trade names are preceded by a small diamond and will usually have two page numbers following the name. This diamond indicates that a color photograph of the actual medication is also provided in the special section of the *PDR* known as the Product Identification section. The first page number following the drug name is the page that illustrates a picture of the drug, and the second page number is where the written information can be found.

Many drugs listed in the Product Name Index have several variations on the trade name, depending on different forms of the drug and routes of administration. For example, a drug that is available in tablets, capsules, and injectable forms may have slight variations on the trade name that reflect these different preparations.

2. If the Generic or Chemical Name Is Known. If you are using an edition of the *PDR* published in 1994 or later, begin by looking in the Product Name Index (PINK pages). This section integrates generic names into the alphabetical listing of trade names. The generic name of each drug is followed by the trade name, manufacturer (in parentheses), and pages where the drug is illustrated and described. Often the generic heading in this section is followed by several different trade names, indicating that the drug is marketed by several different manufacturers.

Older editions of the *PDR* (1993 and earlier) listed generic and chemical names in a separate section called the Generic and Chemical Name Index, which was marked by YELLOW pages. If you are using an older edition, consult this section if you only know the generic name.

3. To Find Out What Drugs Are Available to Treat a Given Disorder. The best place to begin is the Product Category Index located in the BLUE pages. Here, drugs are listed according to the principal pharmacologic classifications, such as anesthetics, laxatives, sedatives, and so on. Major categories in this section are often subdivided into more specific subcategories. For example, cardiovascular preparations are subdivided into antianginals, antihypertensives, antiarrhythmics, and so on. Drugs in each category (or subcategory) are listed according to their trade name followed by the manufacturer (in parentheses) and pages on which the drug is illustrated and described.

4. If You Want to Contact the Manufacturer for More Information about the Drug. Look in the Manufacturers' Index located in the WHITE pages at the very beginning of the *PDR*. Manufacturers who have contributed to the *PDR* are listed alphabetically, giving an address and phone number that serve as a source for inquiries. Also, a partial listing of the products available from each manufacturer is included following the manufacturer's name and address.

5. If You Want to Identify the Name of a Specific Pill, Capsule, or Tablet. Locate the Product Identification section, which is composed of glossy, color photographs of many of the drugs. Drugs are categorized alphabetically according to their manufacturer. Often, individual pills, tablets, and the like have the name of the manufacturer scored or printed directly on the medication. An unknown medication can be identified by matching the drug to the pictures listed under that manufacturer.

APPENDIX D

Drugs of Abuse

Some of the more frequently abused drugs are listed here. Agents such as cocaine, the cannabinoids, and the psychedelics are illicit drugs with no major pharmacotherapeutic value. Other drugs such as the barbiturates, benzodiazepines, and opioids are routinely used for therapeutic reasons but have a strong potential for abuse when taken indiscriminately. Finally, drugs such as alcohol, caffeine, and nicotine are readily available in various commercial products but may also be considered drugs of abuse when consumed in large quantities for prolonged periods.

Drug(s)	Classification/Action	Route/Method of Administration	Effect Desired by User	Principal Adverse Effects	Additional Information
Alcohol	Sedative-hypnotic	Oral, from various beverages (wine, beer, other alcoholic drinks)	Euphoria; relaxed inhibitions; decreased anxiety; sense of escape	Physical dependence; impaired motor skills; chronic degenerative changes in brain, liver, and other organs	See Chapter 6
Barbiturates Nembutal Seconal Others	Sedative-hypnotic	Oral or injected (IM, IV)	Relaxation and a sense of calmness; drowsiness	Physical dependence; possible death from overdose; behavior changes (irritability, psychosis) following prolonged use	See Chapter 6
Benzodiazepines Valium Librium Others	Similar to barbiturates	Similar to barbiturates	Similar to barbiturates	Similar to barbiturates	Similar to barbiturates
Caffeine	CNS stimulant	Oral, from coffee, tea, other beverages	Increased alertness; decreased fatigue; improved work capacity	Sleep disturbances; irritability; nervousness; cardiac arrhythmias	See Chapter 26
Cocaine	CNS stimulant (when taken systemically)	"Snorted" (absorbed via nasal mucosa); smoked (in crystalline form)	Euphoria; excitement; feelings of intense pleasure and well-being	Physical dependence; acute CNS and cardiac toxicity; profound mood swings	See Chapter 12

Drug	Description	Route	Effects	Adverse effects	Reference
Cannabinoids Hashish Marijuana	Psychoactive drugs with mixed (stimulant and depressant) activity	Smoked; may also be eaten	Initial response: euphoria, excitement, increased perception; later response: relaxation, stupor, dreamlike state	Heavy use may lead to endocrine changes (decreased testosterone in males) and changes in respiratory function similar to chronic cigarette smoking	—
Narcotics Demerol Morphine Heroin Others	Natural and synthetic opioids; analgesics	Oral or injected (IM, IV)	Relaxation; euphoria; feelings of tranquility; prevent onset of opiate withdrawal	Physical dependence; respiratory depression; high potential for death due to overdose	See Chapter 14
Nicotine	CNS toxin: produces variable effects via somatic and autonomic nervous system interaction	Smoked or absorbed from tobacco products (cigarettes, cigars, chewing tobacco)	Relaxation; calming effect; decreased irritability	Physical dependence; possible carcinogen; associated with pathologic changes in respiratory function during long-term tobacco use	—
Psychedelics LSD Mescaline Phencyclidine (PCP) Psilocybin	Hallucinogens	Oral; may also be smoked or inhaled	Altered perception and insight; distorted senses; disinhibition	Severe hallucinations; panic reaction; acute psychotic reactions	—

APPENDIX E

Common Drug Suffixes

Medications that are chemically and functionally similar often have generic names that share a common ending or suffix. Listed here are some drug classes that contain groups of drugs that share a common suffix. Please note that some members of a drug class may have a suffix that is different from the one indicated; for instance, not all benzodiazepines end with "-epam" or "-olam" and so on.

Drug Class	Suffix	Common Examples	Primary Indication or Desired Effect (Chapter in Parentheses)
Angiotensin-converting enzyme (ACE) inhibitors	-pril	Captopril, enalapril	Antihypertensive (21), congestive heart failure (24)
Barbiturates	-barbital	Phenobarbital, secobarbital	Sedative-hypnotic (6), antiseizure (9)
Benzodiazepines	-epam or -olam	Diazepam, temazepam, alprazolam, triazolam	Sedative-hypnotic (6), antianxiety (6), antiseizure (9)
Beta blockers	-olol	Metoprolol, propranolol	Antihypertensive (21), antianginal (22), antiarrhythmic (23)
Bronchodilators (adrenergic)	-erol	Albuterol, pirbuterol	Bronchodilation (26)
Bronchodilators (xanthine derivatives)	-phylline	Theophylline, aminophylline	Bronchodilation (26)
Calcium channel blockers (dihydropyridine group)	-ipine	Nifedipine, nicardipine	Antihypertensive (21), antianginal (22)
Glucocorticoids	-sone or -olone*	Cortisone, dexamethasone, prednisone, prednisolone, triamcinolone	Anti-inflammatory (16, 29), immunosuppressants (37)
Histamine H_2-receptor blockers	-idine	Cimetidine, ranitidine	Gastric ulcers (27)
Local anesthetics	-caine	Lidocaine, bupivicaine	Local anesthetic (12), antiarrhythmics (23)
Oral hypoglycemics	-amide	Chlorpropamide, tolbutamide	Antidiabetic (type II diabetes mellitus) (32)
Penicillin antibiotics	-cillin	Penicillin, ampicillin, amoxicillin	Bacterial infections (33)
Tetracycline antibiotics	-cycline	Tetracycline, doxycycline	Bacterial infections (33)
Various other antibacterials	-micin or -mycin[†]	Streptomycin, gentamicin, erythromycin	Bacterial infections (33)

*Some anabolic steroids also end with -olone, e.g., nandrolone, oxymetholone (Chapter 30).
[†]Some antibiotics ending with "-mycin" or "rubicin" are used as antineoplastics (Chapter 36).

Glossary

Listed here are some common terms related to pharmacology and a brief definition of each term. Synonyms (SYN), antonyms (ANT), and common abbreviations (ABBR) are also included, whenever applicable.

Acetylcholine: A neurotransmitter in the somatic and autonomic nervous systems; principal synapses using acetylcholine include the skeletal neuromuscular junction, autonomic ganglia, and certain pathways in the brain.

Adenylate cyclase: An enzyme located on the inner surface of many cell membranes; it is important in mediating biochemical changes in the cell in response to drug and hormone stimulation (SYN: adenyl cyclase).

Adrenergic: Refers to synapses or physiologic responses involving epinephrine and norepinephrine.

Adrenocorticosteroids: The group of steroid hormones produced by the adrenal cortex. These drugs include the glucocorticoids (cortisol, cortisone), mineralocorticoids (aldosterone), and the sex hormones (androgens, estrogens, and progestins).

Affinity: The mutual attraction between a drug and a specific cellular receptor.

Agonist: A drug that binds to a receptor and causes some change in cell function (ANT: antagonist).

Akathisia: A feeling of extreme motor restlessness and an inability to sit still; may occur as a result of antipsychotic drug therapy.

Allergy: A state of hypersensitivity to foreign substances (e.g., environmental antigens and certain drugs), manifested by an exaggerated response of the immune system.

Alpha receptors: A primary class of the receptors that are responsive to epinephrine and norepinephrine. Alpha receptors are subclassified into alpha-1 and alpha-2 receptors based on their sensitivity to various drugs.

Anabolic steroids: Natural and synthetic male hormones that may be misused in an attempt to increase muscle size and improve athletic performance (SYN: androgens).

Analgesia: To lessen or relieve pain. Drugs with this ability are known as *analgesics*.

Androgen: A male steroid such as testosterone.

Angina pectoris: Severe pain and constriction in the chest region, usually associated with myocardial ischemia.

Antagonist: A drug that binds to a receptor but does not cause a change in cell activity (SYN: blocker).

610

Anthelmintic: A drug that destroys parasitic worms (e.g., tapeworms, roundworms) in the gastrointestinal tract and elsewhere in the body.

Anticholinergic: Drugs that decrease activity at acetylcholine synapses. These agents are often used to diminish activity in the parasympathetic nervous system (SYN: parasympatholytic).

Anticoagulation: To decrease the capacity of the blood to coagulate (clot). Drugs with this ability are known as *anticoagulants*.

Antimetabolite: The general term for drugs that impair function in harmful cells and microorganisms by antagonizing or replacing normal metabolic substrates in those cells. Certain anti-infective and antineoplastic agents function as anti-metabolites.

Antineoplastic: A drug that prevents or attenuates the growth and proliferation of cancerous cells.

Antipyresis: To reduce fever. Drugs with this ability are known as *antipyretics*.

Antitussive: A drug that reduces coughing.

Asthma: A chronic disease of the respiratory system characterized by bronchoconstriction, airway inflammation, and formation of mucous plugs in the airway.

Bactericidal: An agent that kills or destroys bacteria.

Bacteriostatic: An agent that inhibits the growth and proliferation of bacteria.

Beta receptor: A primary class of the receptors that are responsive to epinephrine and (to a lesser extent) norepinephrine. Beta receptors are subclassified into beta-1 and beta-2 receptors based on their sensitivity to various drugs.

Bioavailability: The extent to which a drug reaches the systemic circulation following administration by various routes.

Biotransformation: Biochemical changes that occur to the drug within the body, usually resulting in breakdown and inactivation of the drug (SYN: drug metabolism).

Bipolar syndrome: A psychologic disorder characterized by mood swings from excitable (manic) periods to periods of depression (SYN: manic-depression).

Blood-brain barrier: The specialized anatomic arrangement of cerebral capillary walls which serves to restrict the passage of some drugs into the brain.

Blood dyscrasia: A pathologic condition of the blood, usually referring to a defect in one or more of the cellular elements of the blood.

Carcinogen: Any substance that produces cancer or increases the risk of developing cancer.

Catecholamine: A group of chemically similar compounds that are important in the modulation of cardiovascular activity and many other physiologic functions. Common catecholamines include epinephrine, norepinephrine, and dopamine.

Cathartic: An agent that causes a relatively rapid evacuation of the bowels.

Ceiling effect: The point at which no further increase in response occurs as drug dose is progressively increased; this effect is represented by a plateau on the drug's dose-response curve (SYN: maximal efficacy).

Chemical name: The drug name that is derived from the specific chemical structure of the compound. Chemical names are not used clinically but are shortened in some way to form the drug's generic name.

Chemotherapy: The use of chemical agents to treat infectious or neoplastic disease.

Cholinergic: Refers to synapses or physiologic responses involving acetylcholine.

Cholinesterase: The enzyme that breaks down acetylcholine (SYN: acetylcholinesterase).

Clearance: The process by which the active form of the drug is removed from the bloodstream by either metabolism or excretion.

Congestive heart failure: A clinical syndrome of cardiac disease that is marked by decreased myocardial contractility, peripheral edema, shortness of breath, and decreased tolerance for physical exertion.

Cretinism: A congenital syndrome of mental retardation, decreased metabolism, and impaired physical development secondary to insufficient production of thyroid hormones.

Cyclic adenosine monophosphate (ABBR: cAMP): The ring-shaped conformation of adenosine monophosphate, it is important in acting as a second messenger in mediating the intracellular response to drug stimulation.

Demand dose: Amount of drug administered when a patient activates certain drug delivery systems such as those used during patient-controlled analgesia.

Desensitization: A fairly brief and transient decrease in the responsiveness of cellular receptors to drug effects.

Diabetes insipidus: A disease marked by increased urination (polyuria) and excessive thirst (polydipsia) due to inadequate production of antidiuretic hormone (ADH) and/or a decrease in the renal response to ADH.

Diabetes mellitus: A disease marked by abnormal metabolism of glucose and other energy substrates caused by a defect in the production of insulin and/or a decrease in the peripheral response to insulin.

Diuretic: A drug that increases the formation and excretion of urine.

Dopa decarboxylase: The enzyme that converts dihydroxyphenylalanine (dopa) into dopamine.

Dopamine: A neurotransmitter located in the CNS that is important in motor control as well as certain aspects of behavior. The presence of endogenous or exogenous dopamine in the periphery also affects cardiovascular function.

Dosage: The amount of medication that is appropriate for treating a given condition or illness.

Dose: The amount of medication that is administered at one time.

Dose-response curve: The relationship between incremental doses of a drug and the magnitude of the reaction that those doses will cause.

Down-regulation: A prolonged decrease in the number and/or sensitivity of drug receptors, usually occurring as a compensatory response to overstimulation of the receptor.

Drug holiday: A period of several days to several weeks in which medications are withdrawn from the patient to allow recovery from drug tolerance or toxicity; sometimes used in patients with advanced cases of Parkinson's disease.

Drug microsomal metabolizing system (ABBR: DMMS): A series of enzymes located on the smooth endoplasmic reticulum that are important in catalyzing drug biotransformation.

Dysentery: The general term for severe gastrointestinal distress (diarrhea, cramps, bloody stools) usually associated with the presence of infectious microorganisms in the intestines.

Eicosanoids: The general term for the group of 20-carbon fatty acids that includes the prostaglandins, thromboxanes, and leukotrienes. These substances are involved in mediating inflammation and other pathologic responses.

Emetic: A drug that initiates or facilitates vomiting.

End-of-dose akinesia: A phenomenon in Parkinson's disease in which the effectiveness of the medication wears off toward the end of the dosing interval, resulting in a virtual lack of volitional movement from the patient.

Enteral administration: Administration of drugs by way of the alimentary canal.

Enzyme induction: The process wherein some drugs provoke cells to synthesize more drug metabolizing enzymes, thus leading to accelerated drug biotransformation.

Epidural nerve block: Administration of local anesthesia into the spinal canal between the bony vertebral column and the dura mater (i.e., the injection does not penetrate the spinal membranes but remains above the dura).

Epilepsy: A chronic neurologic disorder characterized by recurrent seizures that are manifested as brief periods of altered consciousness, involuntary motor activity, or vivid sensory phenomena.

Epinephrine: A hormone synthesized primarily in the adrenal medulla, mimicking the peripheral effects of norepinephrine. Epinephrine is involved in the sympathetic nervous system response to stress and is especially effective in stimulating cardiovascular function (SYN: adrenaline).

Estrogens: The general term for the natural and synthetic female hormones such as estradiol and estrone.

Expectorant: A drug that facilitates the production and discharge of mucous secretions from the respiratory tract.

First-pass effect: The phenomenon in which drugs absorbed from the stomach and small intestine must pass through the liver before reaching the systemic circulation. Certain drugs undergo extensive hepatic metabolism due to this first pass through the liver.

Food and Drug Administration (ABBR: FDA): The official government agency involved in regulating the pharmaceutical industry in the United States.

Gamma-aminobutyric acid (ABBR: GABA): An inhibitory neurotransmitter in the brain and spinal cord.

Generic name: The name applied to a drug, which is not protected by a trademark, usually being a shortened version of the drug's chemical name (SYN: nonproprietary name).

Glucocorticoid: The general class of steroid agents that affect glucose metabolism and are used pharmacologically to decrease inflammation and suppress the immune system. Principal examples include cortisol and corticosterone.

Glycosuria: The presence of glucose in the urine.

Gonadotropin: A hormone that produces a stimulatory effect on the gonads (ovaries and testes); primary gonadotropins include luteinizing hormone (LH) and follicle-stimulating hormone (FSH).

G proteins: Proteins that bind with guanine nucleotides and regulate cell activity. G proteins often serve as a link between surface receptors and intracellular enzymes such as adenylate cyclase.

Half-life: The time required to eliminate 50 percent of the drug existing in the body.

Histamine: A chemical produced by various cells in the body, it is involved in the modulation of certain physiologic responses (e.g., secretion of gastric acid) as well as in the mediation of hypersensitivity (allergic) responses.

Hypercalcemia: An excessive concentration of calcium in the bloodstream (ANT: hypocalcemia).

Hyperglycemia: An excessive concentration of glucose in the bloodstream (ANT: hypoglycemia).

Hypersensitivity: An exaggerated response of the immune system to a foreign substance (SYN: allergic response).

Hypertension: A pathologic condition characterized by a sustained, reproducible increase in blood pressure.

Hypnotic: A drug that initiates or maintains a relatively normal state of sleep.

Hypokalemia: An abnormally low concentration of potassium in the bloodstream (ANT: hyperkalemia).

Hyponatremia: An abnormally low concentration of sodium in the bloodstream (ANT: hypernatremia).

Immunosuppressant: A drug used to attenuate the body's immune response. These agents are often used to prevent rejection of organ transplants or to treat diseases caused by overactivity in the immune system.

Interferon: A member of the group of proteins that exert a number of physiologic and pharmacologic effects including antiviral and antineoplastic activity.

Intrathecal: Administration of substances within a sheath; typically refers to injection into the subarachnoid space surrounding the spinal cord.

Laxative: An agent that promotes peristalsis and evacuation of the bowel in a relatively slow manner (as opposed to a cathartic).

Loading dose: Amount of drug administered at the onset of treatment to rapidly bring the amount of drug in the body to therapeutic levels.

Lockout interval: The minimum amount of time that must expire between each dose of medication that is administered by patient-controlled analgesia (PCA). The PCA pump is inactivated during the lockout interval so that the patient cannot self-administer excessive amounts of drugs.

Lymphokines: Chemicals released from activated lymphocytes that help mediate various aspects of the immune response. Common lymphokines include the interleukins and gamma interferon.

Malignancy: A term usually applied to cancerous tumors, which tend to become progressively worse.

Maximal efficacy: The maximum response a drug can produce; the point at which the response does not increase even if dosage continues to increase (SYN: ceiling effect).

Median effective dose (ABBR: ED_{50}): The drug dosage that produces a specific therapeutic response in 50 percent of the patients in whom it is tested.

Median lethal dose (ABBR: LD_{50}): The drug dosage that causes death in 50 percent of the experimental animals in which it is tested.

Median toxic dose (ABBR: TD_{50}): The drug dosage that produces a specific adverse (toxic) response in 50 percent of the patients in whom it is tested.

Metabolite: The compound that is formed when the drug undergoes biotransformation and is chemically altered by some metabolic process.

Metastasize: The transfer or spread of diseased (i.e., cancerous) cells from a primary location to other sites in the body.

Mineralocorticoid: A steroid hormone (e.g., aldosterone) that is important in regulating fluid and electrolyte balance by increasing the reabsorption of sodium from the kidneys.

Monoamine oxidase (ABBR: MAO): An enzyme that breaks down monoamine neurotransmitters such as dopamine, norepinephrine, and serotonin.

Mucolytic: A drug that decreases the viscosity and increases the fluidity of mucous secretions in the respiratory tract, thus making it easier for the patient to cough up secretions.

Muscarinic receptor: A primary class of cholinergic receptors that are named according to their affinity for the muscarine toxin. Certain cholinergic agonists and antagonists also have a relatively selective affinity for muscarinic receptors.

Myxedema: The adult or acquired form of hypothyroidism characterized by decreased metabolic rate, lethargy, decreased mental alertness, weight gain, and other somatic changes.

Neuroleptic: A term frequently used to describe antipsychotic drugs, referring to the tendency of these drugs to produce a behavioral syndrome of apathy, sedation, decreased initiative, and decreased responsiveness (SYN: antipsychotic).

Nicotinic receptor: A primary class of cholinergic receptors, named according to their affinity for nicotine, as well as certain other cholinergic agonists and antagonists.

Norepinephrine: A neurotransmitter that is important in certain brain pathways and in the terminal synapses of the sympathetic nervous system (SYN: noradrenaline).

On-off phenomenon: The fluctuation in response seen in certain patients with Parkinson's disease, in which the effectiveness of the medications may suddenly diminish at some point between dosages.

Opioid: An analgesic drug with morphinelike effects; commonly refers to the synthetic forms of these analgesics (SYN: narcotic).

Orthostatic hypotension: A sudden fall in blood pressure that occurs when the patient stands erect; this is a frequent side effect of many medications.

Ototoxicity: The harmful side effect of some drugs and toxins influencing the hearing and balance functions of the ear.

Over-the-counter drugs (ABBR: OTC): Drugs that can be purchased directly by the consumer without a prescription (SYN: nonprescription drugs).

Parenteral administration: Administration of drugs by routes other than via the alimentary canal: by injection, transdermally, topically, and so on.

Parkinson's disease or **parkinsonism:** The clinical syndrome of bradykinesia, rigidity, resting tremor, and postural instability associated with neurotransmitter abnormalities within the basal ganglia.

Pharmacodynamics: The study of how drugs affect the body; that is, the physiologic and biochemical mechanisms of drug action.

Pharmacokinetics: The study of how the body handles drugs; that is, the manner in which drugs are absorbed, distributed, metabolized, and excreted.

Pharmacologic dose: An amount of drug given that is much greater than the amount of a similar substance produced within the body; this increased dosage is used to exaggerate the beneficial effects normally provided by the endogenous compound.

Pharmacotherapeutics: The study of how drugs are used in the prevention and treatment of disease.

Pharmacy: The professional discipline dealing with the preparation and dispensing of medications.

Physical dependence: A phenomenon that develops during prolonged use of addictive substances, signified by the onset of withdrawal symptoms when the drug is discontinued.

Physiologic dose: The amount of drug given that is roughly equivalent to the amount of a similar substance normally produced within the body; this dosage is typically used to replace the endogenous substance when the body is no longer able to produce the substance.

Placebo: A medication that contains inert or inactive ingredients but is used to pacify a patient or test the patient's psychophysiologic response to treatment.

Potency: The dosage of a drug that produces a given response in a specific amplitude. When two drugs are compared, the more potent drug will produce a given response at a lower dosage.

Progestins: The general term for the natural and synthetic female hormones such as progesterone.

Psychosis: A relatively severe form of mental illness characterized by marked thought disturbances and an impaired perception of reality.

Receptor: The component of the cell (usually a protein) to which the drug binds, thus initiating a change in cell function.

Salicylate: The chemical term commonly used to denote compounds such as aspirin that have anti-inflammatory, analgesic, antipyretic, and anticoagulant properties.

Second messenger: The term applied to compounds formed within the cell such as cyclic AMP. The second messenger initiates a series of biochemical changes within the cell following stimulation of a receptor on the cell's outer surface by drugs, hormones, and so on.

Sedative: A drug that produces a calming effect and serves to pacify the patient. These agents are sometimes referred to as minor tranquilizers.

Seizure: A sudden attack of symptoms usually associated with diseases such as epilepsy. Epileptic seizures are due to the random, uncontrolled firing of a group of cerebral neurons, which results in a variety of sensory and motor manifestations.

Selective toxicity: A desired effect of antineoplastic and anti-infectious agents, wherein the drug kills the pathogenic organism or cells without damaging healthy tissues.

Serotonin: A neurotransmitter located in the CNS that is important in many functions including mood, arousal, and inhibition of painful stimuli (SYN: 5-hydroxytryptamine).

Side effect: Any effect produced by a drug that occurs in addition to the principal therapeutic response.

Spinal nerve block: Administration of local anesthesia into the spinal canal between the arachnoid membrane and the pia mater (i.e., the subarachnoid space).

Status epilepticus: An emergency situation characterized by a rapid series of epileptic seizures that occur without any appreciable recovery between seizures.

Steroid: The general term used to describe a group of hormones and their analogs that have a common chemcial configuration but are divided into several categories depending on their primary physiologic effects. Common types of steroids include the glucocorticoids (cortisone, prednisone, many others), mineralocorticoids (aldosterone), androgens/anabolic steroids (testosterone), and steroids related to female physiologic function (estrogen, progesterone).

Supersensitivity: An increased response to drugs and endogenous compounds caused by an increase in the number and/or sensitivity of receptors for that drug.

Sympatholytics: Drugs that inhibit or antagonize function within the sympathetic nervous system.

Sympathomimetics: Drugs that facilitate or increase activity within the sympathetic nervous system.

Tardive dyskinesia: A movement disorder characterized by involuntary, fragmented movements of the mouth, face, and jaw (i.e., chewing, sucking, tongue protrusion, and the like). This disorder may occur during the prolonged administration of antipsychotic drugs.

Therapeutic index (ABBR: TI): A ratio used to represent the relative safety of a particular drug; the larger the therapeutic index, the safer the drug. It is calculated as the median toxic dose divided by the median effective dose. (In animal trials, the median lethal dose is often substituted for the median toxic dose.)

Therapeutic window: The range of drug concentrations in the body that will promote optimal beneficial effects. Drug concentrations less than the lower end of this range will be ineffective, and concentrations greater than the upper end of this range will create excessive side effects.

Thyrotoxicosis: Abnormally high production of thyroid hormones resulting in symptoms such as nervousness, weight loss, and tachycardia (SYN: hyperthyroidism).

Tolerance: The acquired phenomenon associated with some drugs, in which larger doses of the drug are needed to achieve a given effect when the drug is used for prolonged periods.

Toxicology: The study of the harmful effects of drugs and other chemicals.

Trade name: The name given to a drug by the pharmaceutical company which is protected by a trademark and used by the company for marketing the drug (SYN: proprietary name).

Vaccine: A substance typically consisting of a modified infectious microorganism that is administered to help prevent disease by stimulating the endogenous immune defense mechanisms against infection.

Viscosupplementation: Injection of a polysaccharide (hyaluronin) into osteoarthritic joints to help restore the viscosity of synovial fluid.

Volume of distribution (ABBR: V_d): A ratio used to estimate the distribution of a drug within the body relative to the total amount of fluid in the body. It is calculated as the amount of drug administered divided by the plasma concentration of the drug.

Withdrawal syndrome: The clinical syndrome of somatic and psychologic manifestations that occur when a drug is removed from a patient who has become physically dependent on the drug (SYN: abstinence syndrome).

INDEX

The Drug and Agent Index appears on p. xxxv. An "f" following a page number indicates a figure; a "t" following a page number indicates a table.

A

Abbokinase, 351 t
Abitrate, 359t, 360
Accupril, 299t
Absence seizures, 108t, 109
Access port, 235–236, 236f
Accupril, 299t
ACE inhibitors. *See* Angiotensin-converting enzyme (ACE) inhibitors
acebutolol, 282, 282t, 295t, 314t, 328t, 330
acetaminophen, 5t, 13, 33t, 166, 177, 194, 207–208, 209, 225
acetic acid, 598
acetohexamide, 490t
acetophenazine, 98t, 99t
Acetylcholine (ACh), 65t, 66, 252, 254f
acetylcysteine, 373
ACh. *See* Acetylcholine
Achromycin V, 516t
Acid-fast bacilli, 503t, 514t
Acitinomycetes, 503t, 514t
Aclovate, 427t
Acquired immunity, 586
ACTH. *See* Adrenocorticotropic-releasing hormone
Acthar, 591t
Actidil, 372t
Actifed, 371t
Action potentials, 68, 323–325, 324f, 326f
Active transport, 24
Acutrim, 278
acyclovir, 531–532, 532t, 542t
Adalat, 299t
Adapin, 86t
Addiction, 188, 190
Adenosine triphosphate (ATP), 47f, 48, 253, 482
Adenylate cyclase-cAMP system, 47f, 48
ADH. *See* Antidiuretic hormone
Adipose tissue, 26
Adrenal cortex, 407t, 409, 419, 422f
Adrenal gland, 409–410
Adrenal medulla, 250–251, 407t, 410
Adrenal steroids. *See* Adrenocorticosteroids
Adrenalin, 278
Adrenergic drugs, 271–285
    agonists, 271, 272t, 273–279
        alpha, 273–275, 277–279, 370, 371t
        beta, 275–279, 373–374, 374f, 375t, 376, 382
    antagonists, 272t, 279–284

alpha, 279–281, 295t, 296–297
    See also Beta antagonists
    receptors, 252f, 253, 254–256, 254f, 255t, 272–273, 272t
        alpha, 254f, 255–256, 255t, 272, 272t, 296–298
        beta, 254f, 255t, 256, 272–273, 272t, 313–314
Adrenocortical suppression, 430
Adrenocorticosteroids, 419
    biosynthesis of, 420–421, 420f
    for cancer, 574t
    case study of, 435–436
    drugs inhibiting production of, 431–432
    special concerns, 434–435
    See also Glucocorticoids; Mineralocorticoids
Adrenocorticotropic-releasing hormone (ACTH), 406t, 407, 409, 413, 421, 422f, 428, 432
Adriamycin, 577, 578t
Adriamycin RDF, 573t
Adrucil, 572t
Adsorbents, 394–395, 394t
Adsorbocarpine, 262t
Advil, 205t
AeroBid, 380t, 427t
Aerolate, 378t
Affective disorders, 83–95
Affinity, definition of, 49
African sleeping sickness. *See* Trypanosomiasis
Afrin, 273, 371t
Aftate, 552
Age, 41
Agonists, 180, 181t, 414
    adrenergic, 271, 272t, 273–279
    alpha, 273–275, 277–279, 370, 371t
    versus antagonists, 51–52, 51f
    beta, 275–277, 277–279, 373–374, 374f, 375t, 376, 382
    definition of, 51
    partial, 52–53
Agoral, 396t
AIDS (autoimmune deficiency syndrome), 357, 528, 529t, 536, 537, 548, 585
    opportunistic infections with, 542–543, 542t
    treatment of, 539–540, 549, 558, 561
    See also HIV
Airway obstruction, 373–383
Akathisia, 103
Akineton, 129t
albuterol, 276, 375t, 609

619